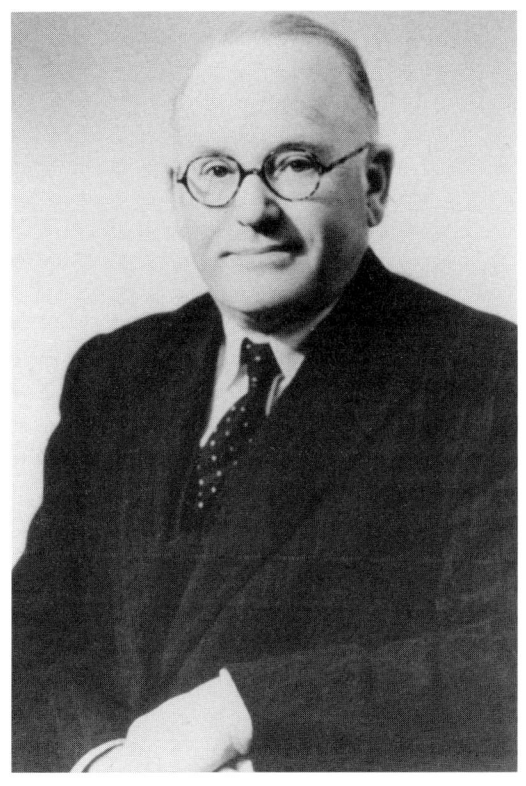

Henry Walter Featherstone, (1894 - 1967)
O.B.E., M.D., L.L.D.(Hon), F.F.A.R.C.S. (Hon),
D.A., J.P.

Founder of the Association of Anaesthetists of Great
Britain and Ireland, 1932

The Association of Anaesthetists of Great Britain and Ireland 1932-1992
and
The Development of the Specialty of Anaesthesia

Sixty years of progress and achievement in the context of scientific, political and social change

THOMAS B. BOULTON

*Past President
Association of Anaesthetists of Great Britain and Ireland*

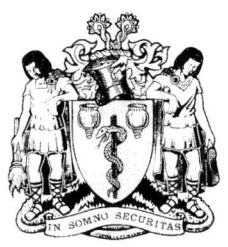

Chapter 10 "A postscript for the years 1993-1997"
compiled by
*Anna-Maria Rollin
Past Vice President
Association of Anaesthetists of Great Britain and Ireland*
and
Appendix A "Henry Walter Featherstone 1894-1967"
by
*E T Mathews
Consultant Anaesthetist Birmingham General Hospital*

Association of Anaesthetists of Great Britain and Ireland, London, WC1B 3RA, 1999

Published by:

*The Association of Anaesthetists of Great Britain and Ireland
9 Bedford Square
London, WC1B 3RA
England*

All rights reserved. no part of this publication may be reproduced, stored in a retrieval system, or transmitted, in any form or by any means, electronic, mechanical, photocopying, recording, or otherwise, without the prior permission of The Association of Anaethestists of Great Britain and Ireland

Produced by:

*Rotadex Print
3-5 Fortnum Close
Kitts Green
Birmingham, B33 0JL
England*

*First Published 1999
Copyright Thomas B. Boulton*

ISBN 0 9536639 0 6

Foreword
by
Professor T. Cecil Gray
C.B.E., OStJ., K.C.S.G., M.D., F.R.C.S., F.R.C.P., F.R.C.A.,
Hon. F.F.A.R.C.S.I., Hon. F.A.N.Z.C.A., D.A.

It seems a long time since Dr Boulton let me see a draft of the first 135 pages of this monumental work, with Appendix A by Dr Mathews reviewing the career of Dr Henry Featherstone, the founder of the Association. Those pages brought the record up to 1957, the year of the Silver Jubilee of the foundation of the Association. He still had forty eventful years to cover with the meticulous accuracy which was obvious in those early pages, which are of special and absorbing interest to all who have been fortunate enough to serve our specialty through those stirring times. There can be no doubt that their excellence has been continued throughout the book.

The Council of the Association is to be congratulated on its wisdom in choosing its archivist, Dr Boulton, to write this history. His work would obviously produce an invaluable record of the influence and achievements of the Association over the most productive and exciting years in the development of anaesthesia. He had already shown his literary ability and soundness of judgement during his periods as Editor of *Anaesthesia* and his work in the same field is also shown by his contributions to the Classical File as Associate Editor of *Survey of Anesthesiology* and his Editorship of two Symposia on the history of medicine.

Dr Boulton has contributed to the progress of anaesthesia not only in the United Kingdom but also through his worldwide travels, teaching and lecturing in many centres in Europe, North America, Asia and Africa - travels which have included work with Children's Medical Relief International in Saigon during the Vietnam War. That he is not lacking in commitment was recognised by his award of a Mention in Dispatches for his work with the RAMC in Malaysia and now further by his acceptance of the prodigious task finally brought to its conclusion.

This history will remain a necessary "Source Reference" for serious researchers and for any who are interested in the development of the specialty in the United Kingdom from 1932 to 1997. It is a tale of how a discipline,

Foreword

which, at the inception of the British National Health Service in 1948, was considered a Cinderella specialty, doubtfully of equal standing with others in Medicine and Surgery, was transformed into the scientific specialty now extended into the fields of intensive therapy and the treatment and study of pain. In these developments the Association, of course with the Faculty and now the Royal College of Anaesthetists, have played key parts. The evolution of our Faculty into a Royal College, despite the misgivings of some of its more conservative members, which have been proven to be unfounded, has owed a very great deal indeed to the Officers and Members of the Council of the Association.

Dr Boulton has all the assets necessary for an expert and trustworthy historian: he is modest, veracious and meticulous, despite the seven Presidencies of learned societies which he has enjoyed and his six Honorary Memberships of important medical and dental societies.

Like many who write as non-professional historians, his task will have been completed with some relief. However, there is no doubt that the result of his labours will be regarded as one of his outstanding contributions and one for which he will be rewarded by the gratitude of future generations of those who are interested in the domestic history of our specialty, whether professional or dilettante.

T CECIL GRAY
President 1956-1959
Association of Anaesthetists of Great Britain and Ireland
9 Bedford Square
London WC1 3RA
1998

Author's Preface

I was pleased and honoured to be asked in 1991 to undertake the preparation of a history of the Association of Anaesthetists of Great Britain and Ireland to mark its Diamond Jubilee in 1992. I was aware that this was a formidable task as a history of the Association had been attempted by at least two previous authors but, since I had retired from clinical practice in 1990, I accepted the challenge optimistically, in the belief that I might have a better chance of succeeding than my predecessors; in the event, the undertaking has proved to be laborious but fascinating, although, regretfully, it has taken far longer than even I, or the Officers of the Association, anticipated, and I am grateful to them for their forbearance.

The late Gwen Wilson's well written history of the first fifty years (1934-1984) in the life of the Australian Society of Anaesthetists had been published in 1987, well before I began my work. It was helpful to me in the planning of this volume and, latterly, I have taken heart from the fact that it was published three years after the Golden Jubilee which it celebrates! David Shepherd and Nargin Parbhoo produced their histories of the Canadian and South African societies of anaesthetists on time for their respective Golden Jubilees in 1993 and these also gave me assistance and encouragement. These three authors are, however, like myself, anaesthetists, and neither I nor they could hope to approach the detached objectivity which the professional historian Jennifer Beinart demonstrated in researching and writing her outstanding *History of the Nuffield Department of Anaesthetics, Oxford 1937-1987*, from which, as an amateur, I have been privileged to learn a great deal.

This volume is then, unashamedly an account of the foundation and progress of an organisation seen through the eyes of one who was aged seven when the Association was founded, who had his first experience of general anaesthesia as a patient some eight years later, who qualified in medicine and became an anaesthetist in 1949, coincident with the introduction of the British National Health Service, and was increasingly close to the events which are described during the forty odd years thereafter. Every effort has been made to research and reference the historical details accurately but, if the reader should feel that the author's proximity to events has unduly influenced his opinions (in particular in respect of his analysis of the attitudes of

Author's Preface

politicians, administrators and other medical disciplines), this is regretted; whenever possible reference has been made to the views of others but, when references are not supplied, the comments must be accepted as solely conveying the opinions of the writer; on no account must they be considered to be the views of the Officers and Council Members or others of the Association past or present.

I decided at the start, and perhaps rather ambitiously, to try to set the history of the Association of Anaesthetists and the conduct of its business in the context of the general and medicopolitical history of the period, and the development of medicine as a whole, and of anaesthesia in particular. The six chapters (four to nine) which cover the chronological history of the Association leading up to its Diamond Jubilee in 1992 are consequently deliberately not precisely coincident with the first six decades under consideration. Each culminates in accounts of events which had special important significance for the Association and the British specialty of anaesthesia - the outbreak of the Second World War in 1939, the inauguration of the British National Health Service in 1948, the introduction of the combination of external cardiac compression and external cardiac defibrillation in 1960, the Fourth World Congress of Anaesthesiologists hosted by the Association in 1968, the Golden Jubilee of the Association and the Sixth European Congress of Anaesthesia in London in 1982, and its Diamond Jubilee and the initiation of the major reorganisation of the National Health Service in 1992.

I am grateful to Anna-Maria Rollin of Epsom, a Past Vice President of the Association, for compiling Chapter 10 as a postscript to account for the years 1993 to 1997 which have elapsed since the Diamond Jubilee of the Association was celebrated in 1992.

Dr Edward T Mathews of Birmingham, a pupil and colleague of Henry Walter Featherstone, has provided an admirable biography of the Founder of the Association as Appendix A, but biographical material concerning other individuals has only been included when it relates directly to the development of the Association of Anaesthetists or the specialty of anaesthesia. References are provided to the obituaries of those who are no longer living, but I would particularly also like to mention the names of four individuals who have died

Author's Preface

in 1998 during the final stages of the preparation of this volume. Each of them, in his own particular way, made important contributions to the history and development of the Association of Anaesthetists. They are Vernon F Hall (1904-1998) who was President from 1962 to 1965, W Derek Wylie (1918-1998), President 1980-1982, who was closely concerned with the purchase of 9 Bedford Square as the Headquarters of the Association of Anaesthetists, George H Ellis (1909-1998) Chairman of the Organising Committee of the 4th World Congress in London in 1968 and Vice President 1969-71, and Michael P Coplans (1923-1998) who was Honorary Secretary from 1970 to 1972 at a particularly important time in the development of the Association. Current volumes of the *Medical Directory*, *Who's Who*, and other reference works must be consulted for details of the careers, some of them very distinguished, of living persons. The tedious, repetitious use of the title "Doctor" has been avoided, but other honorific titles are noted. If an individual did not actually have the title at the time of his or her particular action or pronouncement, the convention has been adopted of placing the title in parenthesis, for example (Sir).

"The Association of Anaesthetists of Great Britain and Ireland" is a very long title. There are other "associations" and other "Associations of Anaesthetists", but I have taken the liberty in this volume of using the title of "Association of Anaesthetists" to refer exclusively to the Association of Anaesthetists of Great Britain and Ireland, and I have employed the designation "Association" to a very limited degree only when the context makes the meaning absolutely obvious.

The constant use of acronyms in modern corporate speech and writing is sometimes useful (*Royal College of Anaesthetists Newsletter* No **41**: July 1998: pp 1-3), but they are quite often employed in an attempt to demonstrate the putative superior knowledge of a topic by the originator, and this can be extremely irritating. I have endeavoured to overcome this difficulty by being as careful as I can to define an acronym when it is first employed in a passage, and limiting its use to the immediate vicinity of the term or title to which it refers; in addition, a list of acronyms and other abbreviations is provided. There are also names and subject indices at the end of the volume.

Author's Preface

The development of the Association of Anaesthetists has taken place during a period of continual inflation, except during the period 1932 to 1939 immediately preceding the Second World War, The purchasing power of £1.00 sterling was, in fact, about thirty five items that of £1.00 in 1996 (the latest figure available in the table of "Cost of living and inflation rates" on page 604 of *Whitaker's Almanack 1997*). It is important to bear this in mind when comparing the relative values of benefactions, salaries, fees, and other costs as the years have passed; I have therefore included the 1996 purchasing power in parenthesis for each such item.

The Association of Anaesthetists of Great Britain and Ireland is an outstandingly successful organisation. It is moreover a tolerant, friendly and supportive body (a band of brothers and sisters rather than a hierarchy), of which it has been a privilege and pleasure to be a member. I have enjoyed researching and telling the story of the Association, from the inspiration of its founder Henry Featherstone to its present important position in British national as well as in international medicine. I hope that others will find the tale as interesting and inspiring as I have done in relating it.

THOMAS B BOULTON
President 1984-1986
Association of Anaesthetists of Great Britain and Ireland
9 Bedford Square,
London WC1 3RA
1998

Acknowledgments

I would like to thank the Officers of the Association of Anaesthetists of Great Britain and Ireland for the inspiration which led me to research and write this history, as well as for their considerable patience in waiting for the completion of the volume. I also acknowledge with gratitude the contributions of Anna-Maria Rollin and Eddie Mathews to the book which are mentioned in the Preface.

Thanks are also due to the many past and present Officers, Members of Council and Ordinary Members of the Association of Anaesthetists who have answered my innumerable questions both in writing and verbally. They have many times countered my erroneous impressions and told me "how it really was." I am particularly grateful to Maldwyn Morgan, Editor of *Anaesthesia* and now (1998) President of the Association of Anaesthetists, and Ed Charlton, Editor of *Anaesthesia News,* who have proof read the volume and caused me to blunt some of my wilder prejudices!

Mrs Una J Spanner, formerly the Librarian of the Royal Berkshire Hospital, was my Personal Assistant when I was Editor of the journal *Anaesthesia*, and subsequently during my Presidency of the Association and the latter part of my clinical career, right up to the time in 1990 when we thought that we had both retired; however, as she is the only person who can consistently interpret my handwriting, she courageously returned to the fray and has meticulously typed every word of this book with the exception of this acknowledgment. She has in the process corrected innumerable spelling and other errors in my manuscript. The extensive knowledge of the specialty of anaesthesia and its personnel and organisations, which she acquired in our editorial years, has been of invaluable assistance. I am deeply grateful for her patience and support.

I am indebted to the three Administration Managers, Miss Ann Muir, Mrs Sally Collins and Mrs Lesley Ogg, who have reigned serenely at the headquarters of the Association of Anaesthetists at 9 Bedford Square during the production of the book and have been responsible for smoothing the administrative and technical difficulties. I am also grateful to their staff, both permanent and temporary, who have converted the typescript into camera-ready copy; in the latter context I would particularly like to thank Mrs Karen

Acknowledgments

Rogers who has borne the burden of the final stages of preparation.

I would like to thank the photographers and organisations who have granted permission for the publication of various photographs; acknowledgments are made in the list of illustrations. The illustrations have been prepared for publication by Lionel Williams and his staff of the Medical Illustration Department of the Royal Berkshire Hospital. They have my thanks for their usual willingness and helpful skill.

My thanks are also due to the staff of Rotadex Print of Birmingham for their courteous professionalism.

Last, but not least, I am eternally grateful to my wife Helen, who has borne my repeated absences in libraries and elsewhere with the never failing equanimity which she has shown throughout my career, although she must have many times had cause to wonder whether I had actually retired!

The title "The Association of Anaesthetists of Great Britain and Ireland 1932-1992 and the development of the specialty of anaesthesia" has been approved by the MD Committee of the University of Cambridge for a proposed dissertation for the degree of Doctor of Medicine.

T.B.B.

Contents

	Foreword	v
	Author's Preface	vii
	Acknowledgements	xi
	Illustrations	xiv
	Acronyms and Abbreviations	xvii
1.	Introductory	1
2.	Whys and Wherefores	5
3.	The Foundation. January to July 1932	16
4.	The Prewar Years. 2 July 1932 to 2 September 1939	28
5.	War and Peace. 3 September 1939 to 31 December 1948	62
6.	Consolidation and Progress. 1 January 1949 to 31 December 1959	114
7.	Expansion. 1 January 1960 to 31 December 1969	177
8.	Turbulent Years. 1 January 1970 to 31 December 1982	279
9.	The Sixth Decade. 1 January 1983 to 31 December 1992	413
10.	Yesterday, Today and Tomorrow. 1 January 1993 to 30 June 1997 Compiled by Anna-Maria Rollin	601
	References	626
	Appendices:	
A.	Henry Walter Featherstone (1894-1967) By E T Mathews	704
B.	The Arms of the Association of Anaesthetists of Great Britain and Ireland	710
C.	Honours and Awards of the Association of Anaesthetists of Great Britain and Ireland	715
D.	Eponymous Lecturers of the Association of Anaesthetists of Great Britain and Ireland	746
E.	Members of the Council of the Association of Anaesthetists of Great Britain and Ireland	754
	Name Index	767
	Subject Index	780

Illustrations

Detailed information concerning individual illustrations will be found in the legends printed with the figures and in the text.

Copyright acknowledgement is made with gratitude in italics under relevant figures. Other figures are filed in the archives of the Association of Anaesthetists.

Frontispiece:	Henry Walter Featherstone, OBE (1894-1967)
Figure 1:	J Frederick Silk (1848-1943)
Figure 2:	Hyman Morris Cohen (1875-1929)
Figure 3:	Henry Walter Featherstone, OBE (1894-1967)
Figure 4:	W Howard Jones (1895-1935)
Figure 5:	Sir Ivan Whiteside Magill, KCVO (1888-1986)
Figure 6:	Professor Sir Robert Reynolds Macintosh (1897-1989)
Figure 7:	Air Commodore R R Macintosh, RAF (1941-1945)
Figure 8:	The Oxford Vaporiser (1942)
Figure 9:	SS Queen of the Channel (c. 1938) *National Maritime Museum*
Figure 10:	SS Amsterdam, Hospital Carrier 64 (c. 1938) *National Maritime Museum*
Figure 11:	RAMC Regional Advisors in India (c. 1943)
Figure 12:	Badge of the President of the Association of Anaesthetists of Great Britain and Ireland (presented 1946)
Figure 13:	Ronald Jarman, DSC (1898-1972) at the 26th Congress of Anesthetists of the Anesthesia Research Society in London in 1951
Figure 14:	Professor T Cecil Gray, CBE as President of the Association of Anaesthetists, 1956-1959
Figure 15:	(Sir) Geoffrey and (Lady) Organe welcoming Mr Martin Clover (grandson of the British pioneer anaesthetist Joseph T Clover) and his daughter at the celebrations to mark the 10th anniversary of the foundation of the Faculty of Anaesthetists, 1958

Illustrations

Figure 16: The Royal College of Surgeons of England. Headquarters of the Secretariat of the Association of Anaesthetists 1944 to 1971 *Phil McCarthy Photography, London*

Figure 17: The Organising Committee of the 4th World Congress of Anaesthesiology, London in 1968

Figure 18: British Medical Association House. Headquarters of the Council of the Association of Anaesthetists 1971-1985

Figure 19: Philip J Helliwell (1915-1994) as President of the Association, 1973-1976

Figure 20: Z Lett (Hong Kong) and Cyril F Scurr, CBE (President) at the Annual Meeting of the Association of Anaesthetists in 1978

Figure 21: HRH The Princess Margaret, Countess of Snowdon (Patron), W D Wylie (President of the Association of Anaesthetists) and a representative from the extensive Trade Exhibition at the 6th European Congress of Anaesthesiology in London in 1982

Figure 22: J S M Zorab (Secretary General of the WFSA and of the 6th European Congress of Anaesthesiologists) with Mrs Zorab and Filipino delegates during the Congress in London in 1982

Figure 23: Robert Hare (President of the Australian Society of Anaesthetists) and W D Wylie (President) at the Golden Jubilee Celebrations of the Association in 1982

Figure 24: 9 Bedford Square, London. Headquarters of the Association of Anaesthetists since 1985 *Drawing reproduced with the permission of Glaxo Wellcome PLC*

Figure 25: Officers of the Association of Anaesthetists at the time of the official opening of 9 Bedford Square, 1987 *Phil McCarthy Photography, London*

Figure 26: Presentation to the Association of Anaesthetists of the portrait of H W Featherstone (Founder President) by the Dean of the Faculty of Anaesthetists (Aileen K Adams, CBE), 1988 *Phil McCarthy Photography, London*

Illustrations

Figure 27:   The first and second recipients of the Sir Ivan Magill Gold Medal. J F Nunn (1988) and Michael Rosen, CBE (1993)
Figure 28:   Michael Rosen, CBE (President of the College of Anaesthetists) and Sir Ian Todd, KBE (President of the Royal College of Surgeons of England) at the inauguration of the College of Anaesthetists in 1988 *Jalmar Photographers, London*
Figure 29   The five members of the Association of Anaesthetists of Great Britain and Ireland who were concurrently Presidents of United Kingdom, European, and World Anaesthetic Organisations in 1991 *Phil McCarthy Photography, London*
Figure 30:   HRH The Princess Margaret, Countess of Snowdon (Patron), and Peter Baskett (President) during the Diamond Jubilee celebrations of the Association of Anaesthetists in 1992 *Phil McCarthy Photography, London*
Figure 31:   The reigning President with Past Presidents of the Association of Anaesthetists in 1997 *Phil McCarthy Photography, London*

Acronyms and Abbreviations

Acronyms and Abbreviations

The employment of acronyms and abbreviations in this volume is generally restricted to the immediate vicinity of the use of a term or title in a particular passage and repeated elsewhere as necessary. Acronyms or abbreviations used in the brief explanatory notes in parenthesis in this table are cross referenced.

AAGBI	Association of Anaesthetists of Great Britain and Ireland
A&E	Accident and Emergency (medical specialty or department: UK)
AHA	Area Health Authority (NHS 1974-1984)
AIDS	Acquired immune deficiency syndrome
ANZCA	Australian and New Zealand College of Anaesthetists (before 1992 FARACS)
AOTT	Association of Operating Theatre Technicians (UK)
AP	Academic Press (international publishers)
ASA	American Society of Anesthesiologists
ASA	Australian Society of Anaesthetists
ASCAB	Armed Services Consultant Advisory Board (UK)
ATLS	Advanced trauma life support (international courses)
BAODA	British Association of Operating Department Assistants
BAREMA	British Association of Anaesthetic and Respiratory Equipment Manufacturers
BCL	Bachelor of Civil Law
BDA	British Dental Association
BJA	British Journal Of Anaesthesia
BMA	British Medical Association
BMJ	British Medical Journal
BSE	Bovine Spongiform Encephalopathy
BSI	British Standards Institution
BSP/BS	Blackwell Scientific Publications (later Blackwell Scientific: Publishers: UK)
BST	Basic specialist training (UK)
BUPA	British United Provident Association (Health insurers: UK)
CABG	Coronary artery bypass graft
CBE	Commander of the Order of the British Empire (UK)
CCHMS	Central Council for Hospital Medical Services (later the Central Consultants and Specialists Committee: BMA)
CCICMS	Council for the Coordination of International Congresses of Medical Sciences (WHO)
CCSC	Central Consultants and Specialists Committee (BMA, formerly CCHMS)
CCST	Certificate of Completion of Specialist Training (EU & UK)
CCU	Coronary Care Unit
CEPOD	Confidential Enquiry into Perioperative Deaths (UK)
CFS	Chronic fatigue syndrome (synonym for ME)
CHC	Community Health Council (NHS)
CJD	Creutzfeldt-Jakob disease (a human disease linked to BSE)
CME	Continuing medical education (UK)
CNO	Chief Nursing Officer (UK)
COHSE	Confederation of Health Service Employees (UK)
CPSM	Council for Professions Supplementary to Medicine (UK)

Acronyms and Abbreviations

CSM	Committee on the Safety of Medicines (UK)
CVP	Central venous pressure
DA	Diploma in Anaesthetics (UK)
DDC	Doctor with domestic commitment (NHS)
DH	Department of Health
DHA	District Health Authority (NHS)
DHSS	Department of Health and Social Security (UK)
DM	Doctor of Medicine (MD of the University of Oxford: UK)
DMT	District Management Team (NHS)
DMU	Directly Managed Units (NHS)
DNA	Desoxyribonucleic acid (genetics)
DNR	"Do not resuscitate"
DRG	Diagnostically related groups
EBAR	European Board in Anaesthesiology, Reanimation and Intensive Care (EU)
EEA	European Economic Area
EEC	European Economic Community (later EU)
EFTA	European Free Trade Area
EMS	Emergency Medical Service (World War II: UK)
EMU	European Monetary Union
ENB	English Nursing Board
ERM	Exchange Rate Mechanism
EU	European Union (formerly EEC)
F....	Fellow of .... (see also ANZCA, FARACS, FARCS, RCA, RCOG, RCS, RCSE and RCSI)
FARACS	Faculty of Anaesthetists of the Royal Australasian College of Surgery (after 1992 ANZCA)
FARCS	Faculty of Anaesthetists of the Royal College of Surgeons of England (after 1992 RCA)
FARCSI	Faculty of Anaesthetists of the Royal College of Surgeons in Ireland
FDA	Food and Drugs Administration (USA)
FHSA	Family Health Service Authority (NHS)
FST	Field Surgical Team (Military: UK)
GAT	Group of Anaesthetists in Training (of the AAGBI: formerly JAG)
GDC	General Dental Council (UK)
GDR	German Democratic Republic (East Germany)
GMC	General Medical Council (UK)
GMSC	General Medical Services Committee (BMA)
GNP	Gross National Product (economics)
GP	General (primary care) Practitioner (UK)
GPT	General (specialist) Postgraduate Training (UK)
HCA	Health Care Assistant (nursing assistant: UK)
HDU	High Dependency Unit
HIV	Human immunodeficiency virus (infection)
HMC	Hospital Management Committee (NHS)
HMO	Health Maintenance Organisation (USA)
HPT	Higher (specialist) Professional Training (UK)
HST	Higher (Specialist) Training (UK)
IARS	International Anesthesia Research Society (Based in USA)
ICS	Intensive Care Society

Acronyms and Abbreviations

ICU	Intensive Care Unit (synonym for ITU)
IMF	International Monetary Fund
ISO	International Standards Organisation
IRA	Irish Republican Army (terrorist organisation)
ITU	Intensive Therapy Unit (synonym for ICU)
JAG	Junior Anaesthetists Group of the AAGBI (later GAT)
JBCNC	Joint Board of Clinical Nursing Studies (UK)
JCC	Joint Consultants' Committee (NHS)
JCHTA	Joint Committee for Higher Training in Anaesthesia
JDC	Junior Doctors Committee (BMA)
JP	Justice of the Peace (Magistrate: UK)
KCSG	Knight Commander of the Order of Saint Gregory (Papal)
KCVO	Knight Commander of the Victorian Order (UK)
LCC	London County Council (England)
LLB	Bachelor of Laws
LLD	Doctor of Laws
LMA	Laryngeal mask airway
MA	Master of Arts
MD	Doctor of Medicine (see also DM)
ME	Myalgic encephalitis (synonym for CFS)
MMC	Monopolies and Mergers Commission (UK)
MP	Member of Parliament (UK)
MRCA	Member of the Royal College of Anaesthetists (the postnominals denoting the achievement of a certain stage in PGME were proposed but not implemented)
MRCP	Member of the Royal College of Physicians of London, Edinburgh or physician member of the Royal College of Physicians and Surgeons of Glasgow
MRSA	Methicillin resistant staphylococcus aureus
MTO	Medical Technical Officer (see also ODA: UK)
MVO	Member of the Victorian Order (later LVO - Lieutenant of he Victorian Order: UK)
NATN	National Association of Theatre Nurses (UK)
NCEPOD	National Confidential Enquiry into Perioperative Deaths (UK)
NCVQ	National Council for Vocational Qualification
NHS	National Health Service (UK)
NHSTA	National Health Service Training Authority (UK)
NTBR	"Not to be resuscitated"
NVQ	National Vocational Qualification (see also NCVQ: UK)
OBE	Order of the British Empire
ODA	Operating Department Assistant (see also MTO, ODO, OTT, SODA, TODA: NHS)
ODA	Overseas Development Administration (UK)
ODO	Operating Department Orderly (see also ODA: NHS)
ODP	Operating Department Practitioner (see also ODA: NHS)
OECD	Organisation for Economic Cooperation and Development (UN)
OSB	Order of Saint Benedict (Roman Catholic)
OStJ	Officer of the Order of the Hospital of St John of Jerusalem
OTT	Operating Theatre Technician (NHS)
PCA	Patient controlled analgesia

Acronyms and Abbreviations

PGME	Postgraduate medical education (UK)
PME	Postgraduate medical Education (UK)
PPC	Progressive patient care
PPP	Private Patients Plan (health insurers: UK)
RA	Relative analgesia (with low concentrations of nitrous oxide)
RAF	Royal Air Force (UK)
RAMC	Royal Army Medical Corps (UK)
RAWP	Research Allocation Working Party (NHS)
RCA	Royal College of Anaesthetists (formerly FARCS: UK)
RCOG	Royal College of Obstetricians and Gynaecologists (UK)
RCS	Royal College of Surgeons (of England)
RCSE	Royal College of Surgeons of Edinburgh (Scotland)
RCSI	Royal College of Surgeons in Ireland
REA	Regional Education Adviser (to the Council of the RCA: UK)
RGN	Registered General Nurse (formerly SRN: UK)
RHA	Regional Health Authority (NHS)
RMI	Resource Management Initiative (NHS)
RN	Royal Navy (UK)
RNO	Regional Nursing Officer (NHS)
RSM	Royal Society of Medicine (UK)
SAAD	Society for the Advancement of Anaesthesia in Dentistry (UK)
SAMO	Senior Administrative Medical Officer (NHS)
SEN	State Enrolled Nurse (former title of assistant nurse: UK)
SHMO	Senior Hospital Medical Officer (NHS)
SHO	Senior Hospital Officer (NHS)
SI	Système International of unit measurement
SODA	Senior Operating Department Assistant (see also ODA: NHS)
SpR	Specialist Registrar (NHS)
SR	Senior Registrar (NHS)
SRN	State Registered Nurse (later RGN: UK)
STA	Specialist Training Authority of the Medical Royal Colleges (UK)
TIVA	Total intra-venous anaesthesia
TODA	Trainee Operating Department Assistant (see also ODA: NHS)
TPN	Theatre Personnel Nationwide (formerly National Association of Professional and Technical Theatre Personnel: UK)
UDI	Unilateral declaration of independence
UEMS	Union Européene des Médicins Spécialistes (EU)
UK	United Kingdom of Great Britain and Northern Ireland
UKCC	United Kingdom Committee of the Central Council for Nursing, Midwifery and Health Visiting
UMT	Unit of Medical Time (NHS)
UN	United Nations
UNESCO	United Nations Educational, Scientific and Cultural Organisation
USA	United States of America
USSR	Union of Soviet Socialist Republics
VAT	Value Added Tax (UK and EU)
VHI	Voluntary Health Insurance Board (Republic of Ireland)
WFSA	World Federation of Societies of Anaesthesiologists
WHO	World Health Organisation

1

Introductory

"...I have had to revise drastically the opinion I formed of anaesthetists forty years ago when I first began to practise. Then they were at the bottom of the professional hierarchy, with a high proportion of dimwits, no-hopers and drunks. Now they are near the top, with a range of professional skills that make the obstetrician a member of the lumpen proletariat."

Arnold K Klopper, Emeritus Professor of Reproductive Endocrinology, University of Aberdeen

"Taking it all to heart" *Anaesthesia News,* April 1991

The Association of Anaesthetists of Great Britain and Ireland was founded in 1932 by Dr Henry W Featherstone of Birmingham (1894-1967).[1-3] He was one of the relatively few medical practitioners of that era who devoted his professional life exclusively to the practice of anaesthesia (Appendix A).[4]

The Association of Anaesthetists cannot claim to be the oldest surviving national society of anaesthetists (that honour properly belongs to the Scottish Society of Anaesthetists founded in 1914). It is, however, probably the oldest international society to be founded outside North America as it serves the United Kingdom of England, Wales, Scotland and Northern Ireland as well as the independent Republic of Ireland; only the International Anesthesia Research Society, which was founded in the United States in 1925, predates it. The Association of Anaesthetists was certainly one of the first independent societies of anaesthetists to take a leading role in the medicopolitical development of the specialty and the training and conditions of service of its members.

British anaesthetists now collectively constitute the largest hospital specialty in the British National Health Service (NHS);[5] almost 13% (2,271) of the 17,662 consultants in the NHS were anaesthetists at the end of 1992 (the year in which the Association of Anaesthetists celebrated its Diamond Jubilee). Their professional responsibilities not only cover the pre-, intra-

and postoperative care of patients undergoing surgery, but extend into the field of intensive care, in which they are in clinical and administrative charge of over 85% of the units in the United Kingdom.[6] They also play a leading part in the rapidly developing areas of resuscitation, emergency and disaster medicine and acute and chronic pain control (about 90% of pain clinics are the responsibility of anaesthetists).[6] The specialty has led the medical profession in the conduct of clinical audit, quality control, and the care of the sick doctor and the protection of his or her patients, and its members are increasingly in demand as medical administrators in the re-organised NHS.[6]

Things were different in the early thirties![7] Featherstone and his colleagues could not have foreseen the developments which were to take place in medicine and surgery which would require to be paralleled or preceded by advances in anaesthesia, but they realised that the importance of anaesthetic technique in the operating theatre was undervalued even in the leading University hospitals, and that the standard training available for anaesthetists was woefully inadequate.

The Association achieved much in the first decade of its existence, including the establishment of the Diploma in Anaesthetics in 1935 - the first such qualification in the world - and improvements in conditions of service and training facilities;[6,8] even after a decade, however, the activities and influence of anaesthetists was confined largely to the administration of general anaesthesia in the operating theatre. This fact is emphasised by the adoption of the rather ambiguous motto "in somno securitas" ("secure in sleep") when the Association of Anaesthetists was granted the right to bear arms in 1945 (Appendix B).

The author of the quotation at the head of this chapter had undergone a cardiac operation in 1990. He contrasts the status of anaesthetists when he qualified in South Africa in 1946 with the present time. He also correctly describes the lack of recognition accorded to the specialty at that time, but he unfairly overemphasises the "proportion of dimwits, no-hopers and drunks" amongst anaesthetists in the nineteen thirties and forties. Lack of recognition there certainly was but, by 1946, British anaesthesia at any rate, prompted by the activities of the Association, had met the challenge of the Second World War very effectively indeed. The small number of specialist anaesthetists serving in the prewar university hospitals had used their expertise to train a large corps of competent physician anaesthetists for the field surgical teams of the armed services. These young specialists returned to civilian life ready to take their places as Consultants in the British NHS which was to be inaugurated in 1948. There was in fact no shortage of enthusiastic and well qualified anaesthetists; all that was needed was recognition of their value and equality as specialist consultants in the new service. It is fortunate that the necessary recognition was forthcoming after considerable pressure from the Association of Anaesthetists and the support of surgical colleagues. British anaesthesia has never looked back; it has facilitated the major postwar developments in surgical techniques (notably in cardiac, neurological, paediatric and geriatric surgery) and, through the participation of anaesthetists in intensive therapy, the care of the critically ill has been immeasurably improved.[6]

The Association of Anaesthetists has played an important part in this dramatic progress. It represents the medical and political aspirations of a very considerable majority of anaesthetists in the United Kingdom and the Republic of Ireland and, through its overseas membership, it has close contact with, and has exerted, and still exerts, a considerable influence on the practice of anaesthesia in many countries both inside and outside the British Commonwealth. The Association of Anaesthetists does not have, and has never sought to have, direct statutory powers, either academic, negotiating or coordinating. Its role has been to initiate change and, through its broad constitution and relatively informal procedures, to prompt and encourage other bodies to further the academic and clinical advance of anaesthesia and the political welfare of anaesthetists. It can be truly said that no major development has taken place in British or Irish anaesthesia since the foundation of the Association of Anaesthetists sixty years ago, which has not been either proposed or promoted under its auspices. These developments include, besides those already mentioned, the publication and development of the international journal *Anaesthesia*, the foundation of the Faculty of Anaesthetists of the Royal College of Surgeons of England in 1948 and its metamorphosis into the independent Royal College of Anaesthetists in 1992, the foundation of the Faculty (now College) of Anaesthetists of the Royal College of Surgeons in Ireland in 1960, the establishment of the Junior Anaesthetists' Group (now Group of Anaesthetists in Training) in 1967 and the Linkman organisation in

1976, both of which are the envy of other medical disciplines; in more recent times there has been the publication of a series of important and authoritative guideline booklets, armed with which many anaesthetists have been able to influence policy in their Hospitals, Districts and Regions.

The Association of Anaesthetists of Great Britain and Ireland has already served anaesthetists, and through them their patients, in a period of dramatic developments in medicine generally, but even more so, in the practice of the specialty itself, and against a background of major social and political change. It is an exciting story worth telling but, unlike an individual after sixty years of service, the Association remains ever young and vigorous as enthusiastic generation of members succeeds enthusiastic generation. Who knows what the next sixty years will bring? One thing is certain, the Association of Anaesthetists will not be found wanting!

2

Whys and Wherefores

"There is occasions and causes why and wherefore in all things"

William Shakespeare (1564-1616) *King Henry V,* V.i.

Early British Anaesthesia Societies

The first Society "for the study of anaesthetics and to promote and encourage friendly relations among members" was formed in London in 1893 on the initiative of J Frederick W Silk, MD (1848-1943), at that time anaesthetist to Guy's Hospital and later to King's College Hospital.[1,2] This Society included in its membership a number of practitioners from provincial cities who held hospital appointments in anaesthesia, and some from British dominions and colonies, Europe, and North America. The business of the Society was mainly concerned with the practical and academic aspects of anaesthesia, but it actively promoted the concept that instruction in the administration of anaesthesia should be a compulsory subject in the undergraduate medical curriculum. Regulations to this end were adopted in due course by the Royal Colleges and the University of London, and ultimately by the General Medical Council. This was a very necessary measure at a time when any medical practitioner was deemed to be capable of administering an anaesthetic immediately on qualification. All pretensions to engage in political activity ceased, however, when, in 1909, the Society of Anaesthetists joined twenty-two other specialist societies and the Royal Medical and Chirurgical Society to become a section of the Royal Society of Medicine confined by Charter to academic discussion.

Clinically orientated meetings of a Section of Anaesthetics were a feature of the Annual Meeting of the British Medical Association (BMA) from 1912 onwards; in which year, at the Liverpool meeting, the proceedings were under the Presidency of the veteran pioneer Dudley W Buxton of the University College Hospital, London, who was a founder member and former President of the Society of Anaesthetists.[3,4]

The British Journal of Anaesthesia

The next really significant event in the progress towards corporate organisation of anaesthesia in the United Kingdom was the foundation of the *British Journal of Anaesthesia* in 1923. This independent journal was first published by Sherratt and Hughes of Manchester.[5-7] The first Editor, and probable initiator, was Hyman Morris Cohen (1875-1929).[7,8] The Editorial Board included the acknowledged doyen of British anaesthesia Dudley Buxton (1835-1931)[4] and other prominent anaesthetists;[6,7] amongst them Henry Edmund Gaskin Boyle (1875-1941)[9] and Joseph Blomfield (1870-1948)[10] who were to play an important part in the inauguration of the Association of Anaesthetists in 1932.

Cohen was from New York and had both British and American qualifications. He had married an English lady and had settled down to practise anaesthesia in Manchester with an appointment at St Mary's Hospital in that city.[6,8] He retained close links with the United States and was probably impressed by the various disparate attempts of F H McMechan of New York and others to organise anaesthetists in North America in the early twenties.[11,12] Societies founded in that period included the formation of the National Anesthesia Research Society founded in 1919 which became the International Anesthesia Research Society in 1925. This Society first published *Current Researches in Anesthesia and Analgesia* in 1922. The *British Journal of Anaesthesia* was thus the second journal in the world solely devoted to anaesthesia.

Cohen's very first Editorial in 1923 includes a plea for the formation of a British Society of Anaesthetists.[5] He returned to this theme on several occasions, including setting his sights even higher for an Association of Anaesthetists of the British Empire in an address to the "Sixth Annual Congress of the Associated Anaesthetists of the United States and Canada and the International Anaesthesia Research Society" in Washington DC, USA.[13] Cohen's journal also concerned itself with other organisational considerations; these included the teaching of medical students, the aetiology and recording of deaths under anaesthesia and the conduct of coroners' inquests and other legal matters. Cohen suffered from hypertension and died suddenly, if not unexpectedly, in 1929.[6,8] He was succeeded by Joseph Blomfield[10] of St

George's Hospital, London. Blomfield, a deeply respected pioneer who had kept abreast of newer techniques and developments, was destined to become the second President of the Association of Anaesthetists of Great Britain and Ireland. His policies as an Editor were similar to Cohen's. He outlined the scientific, economic, and academic difficulties facing anaesthetists in an Editorial entitled "Anaesthetists' worries" on the eve of the inauguration of the Association of Anaesthetists in January 1932.[14] Later in the same volume he welcomed the forthcoming formation of the Association of Anaesthetists in an Editorial[15] and recorded the proceedings of the provisional meeting "held in the rooms of the London Medical Society in Chandos Street on 28 April 1932" (Chapter 3).[16]

It is difficult to overemphasise the importance of the *British Journal of Anaesthesia* as the mouthpiece of the emergent specialty from 1923 until the establishment of the Association of Anaesthetists in 1932, and thereafter in recording the proceedings of the Association after its inauguration until the publication of its own journal *Anaesthesia* in 1946. Blomfield continued as Editor of the *British Journal of Anaesthesia* until shortly before he died in 1948. The Association of Anaesthetists of Great Britain and Ireland owes him a considerable debt.[10]

What were the scientific, economic and academic difficulties facing anaesthetists, to which Joseph Blomfield referred in his 1932 Editorial just before the initial steps to form the Association of Anaesthetists were taken?[15] It is not difficult to find an answer!

Clinical medicine and surgery in 1932

Medical treatment was at the crossroads at the beginning of the nineteen thirties. There were very few specific remedies; salvarsan for syphilis and quinine for malaria were virtually the only chemotherapeutic agents, and insulin treatment had been developed for the management of diabetes. Vaccination against smallpox and immunisation against diphtheria were available, but poliomyelitis, pneumonia (including postoperative pneumonia) and tuberculosis were still potential killers, against which only rest and placebos were available. Body surface, orthopaedic, and abdominal surgery were well advanced; they were, however, not yet supported by chemotherapy. Sepsis, both primary and secondary to surgery, was common, and operations for incision and drainage of large and small abscesses formed a major part of the surgeon's work. Septicaemia after surgery was an ever present threat which could be counteracted only by asepsis and antisepsis, and the sterilisation of surgical instruments was still largely accomplished by boiling and the use of chemical solutions.

Phrenic nerve crush operations, artificial pneumothoraces and the mutilating operation of thoracoplasty were carried out to rest the tuberculous lung, but operations inside the pleural cavity were rarities even in major centres except for empyema drainage. Cardiac surgery was two decades into the future. Neurosurgery, apart from the use of the trephine for head injury, was practised only in major centres.

Hospital organisation and staffing and the anaesthetist in 1932

Lloyd George's National Health Insurance Act of 1911 had provided the majority of general practitioners with a basic income and, coupled with subsequent legislation and the development of municipal and voluntary hospital outpatient clinics, had done much to regularise outpatient care for the majority of the working population in the lower income groups. The income of general practitioners was supplemented to a greater or lesser degree, depending on the locality of practice, by private fees for attendance on middle and upper class patients.

Hospital care was a very different matter. In the early thirties the voluntary hospitals, and privately run nursing homes for the better off sector of the population, provided the beds available for the acutely ill. These institutions ranged from the prestigious teaching hospitals in London and the largest cities, through county hospitals, to minute cottage hospitals and small private concerns. Patients were expected to contribute something for treatment at the voluntary hospitals according to their means; many paid into voluntary contributory insurance schemes for public ward treatment and there were also private beds. The chronically ill were nursed at home, except in the case of special statutory provision made for tuberculosis and mental illness, in private or charitable institutions, or in the local authority workhouse infirmaries. An Act of Parliament which was to stimulate the provision of municipal general hospitals by local authorities (including the vast London County Council empire) had been passed in 1929, but was only just beginning to be operative in 1932.[17]

The number of fully qualified surgeons engaged in exclusive consultant practice was not large in proportion to the population of the British Isles, and they were mainly to be found in the teaching hospitals in London and the larger provincial cities. They contributed their services free, or received a very nominal honorarium, as members of the staffs to voluntary hospitals, and relied financially on developing a reputation and referral from the many former students who passed through their wards, most of whom went out into general practice. A medical education was expensive and a drain on the family purse of a middle class family in those days before grant aided university education. The quickest way to earn money was therefore buying into a general practice, often immediately after qualification. Specialisation in surgery, on the other hand, added many years of training at peppercorn salaries as assistants before a reputation could be built and hospital appointments secured. This often meant that those who were able to train as specialists came from more moneyed classes than those who entered general practice.[18]

The position outside major cities was different. Many of the hospitals were staffed by general practitioner surgeons. These were often partners in practices from middle class areas in which the element of National Health Insurance "panel" patients, in comparison to fee paying patients, was small; this therefore constituted a form of class distinction even amongst general practitioners.[18] Work in the provincial voluntary hospital for general ward patients was unpaid; the financial rewards came from fee paying private patients, both in the private wings of voluntary hospitals and in the independent nursing homes. Referral of fee paying patients to the local surgeon would be both from his own practice, if he was a partner, or from other general practitioners in the area; the consequence was that, since all medical men at that time were supposed, by reason of their undergraduate training, to be capable of administering anaesthesia, general practitioners often claimed the right to give the anaesthetic to their fee paying patients and, indeed, patients often asked them to do so. This practice continued for many years, even when a visiting anaesthetist or a general practitioner from a rival practice had actually been appointed to the entirely honorary post of Visiting Anaesthetist in the local hospital. Several now very senior specialist anaesthetists, who started as general practitioners with a special interest in anaesthesia, have recollections of waiting in the doctor's room to start a list of public patients, while an unskilled practitioner from another practice struggled to provide adequate conditions for the surgeon by inhalation anaesthesia administered to a resisting fee-paying patient. Those few anaesthetists in provincial towns who chose to limit their practice to the administration of anaesthetics were certainly brave men![19]

The circumstances in which the few specialist honorary anaesthetists worked in association with the prestigious voluntary teaching hospitals in great cities varied, but they often did not enjoy the same status as physicians and surgeons on the Honorary Staff and frequently did not have direct representation on the all-powerful medical committees. The work they did in the voluntary hospital was unpaid or for a nominal honorarium and they were expected to make a living from private cases initiated by the surgeons with whom they worked in public hospitals.[20-22] This was not a happy situation in the circumstances of a large city in which a surgeon had many competing anaesthetists to choose from! It was small wonder that it was said of a well-known London anaesthetist that he would run a mile at the rustle of a five pound note (J Alfred Lee, personal communication)! It is true that close relationships between surgeons and anaesthetists often grew up, but more than one anaesthetist who practised at that time, has recalled living in dread lest one day he should read in his morning newspaper that the surgeon, from whom he derived the bulk of his income, had had a coronary and died! Many prominent anaesthetists, like their provincial counterparts, were also general practitioners.

A particular bone of contention at the time that the Association of Anaesthetists was founded in 1932 was the position of anaesthetists who were attached to the newly established university academic units; in these all the medical personnel were salaried except for the visiting anaesthetists who had perforce to work for long hours without fee, and without even the prospect of attracting private practice. This issue invoked considerable correspondence in the columns of the *Lancet* in 1931.[21-25] It is a sad fact that Dr William Howard Jones,[26] who initiated this correspondence,[21] and who was to become the first Honorary Secretary of the Association of Anaesthetists, died by his own hand in 1935. A bitter Editorial lamenting his death,[27] in terms that would probably be unacceptable today, makes no secret of the fact that he died "in pauperdom" despite his brilliance as a clinician and innovator, and it attributes his death to the "unjust and inadequate rewards which are meted out to much of our work as anaesthetists". The writer of this Editorial continues:-

> "It may be that some such catastrophe was necessary before.... men, could be brought to realise that many anaesthetists do a vast amount of work in conditions which are unfair, and for remuneration which is inadequate or actually non existent.... It may be that.... this death was not in vain and that Howard Jones will have helped his fellows even as he was always ready to help them in life."[27]

The position regarding the administration of anaesthesia for emergency cases in relation to the prevailing practice conditions was also an important cause for concern in the years immediately before the foundation of the Association of Anaesthetists. George Edwards, anaesthetist to St George's Hospital, London, investigated the status of those who administered anaesthesia for emergency operations in four categories of hospitals over a six month period.[28] His findings can be summarised as follows (the term "House Officer" refers to general House Surgeons and Physicians and not to House Anaesthetists) and, despite the anonymity, it can be assumed that the category D (and possibly the category C) hospital was a teaching hospital:-

Category A. A provincial general hospital of 80 beds.
All anaesthetics routine and emergency given by the 2 resident House Officers.
(Number of emergency cases not stated).

Category B. A London suburban general hospital of 200 beds.
Medical staff included 4 "Visiting Anaesthetists" and 5 House Officers.
10 serious emergency cases in the 6 months.
All emergency cases administered by House Officers.

Category C. A London General Hospital of 200 beds.
Medical staff included 5 "Honorary Anaesthetists", 1 Resident Anaesthetist, and 11 House Officers.
36 serious emergency cases in the 6 months.
None anaesthetised by Honorary Anaesthetists.
15 anaesthetised by the Resident Anaesthetist.
21 anaesthetised by the House Officers.

Category D. London General Hospital of 650 beds.
Medical staff included 5 "Honorary Anaesthetists", 1 "Senior Resident Anaesthetist", 4 "Casualty Officers on anaesthetic duty" and 20 House Officers.
56 serious emergency cases in the 6 months.
5 anaesthetised by Honorary Anaesthetists.
31 anaesthetised by Resident "Anaesthetists".
20 anaesthetised by House Officers.

Edwards points out that in categories A and B, 100%; in category C, 58%; and in category D, 36%; of these serious cases "fell to the lot of the House Physicians and House Surgeons, whose anaesthetic experience at the beginning of their period of office was probably confined to the twenty administrations required during training". Edwards goes on to explain the reasons for this unfortunate state of affairs and, in particular, why it was that Honorary Surgeons were able to attend voluntary hospitals for both routine and emergency cases whilst Visiting Anaesthetists were usually only able to anaesthetise for scheduled cases on set operating lists. He tells us that "some [probably many] anaesthetists have private general [or anaesthetic] practices to attend to; some surgeons prefer not to work with certain [visiting] anaesthetists; the surgeon arranges the hour at which he will operate and fits it in with other engagements, whilst the anaesthetist has to work in the surgeon's time; often the decision is not made until the patient is seen by the surgeon and such decision may be against operation, in which case either the anaesthetist has been called unnecessarily, or else the theatre has to wait his arrival".[28] The Editorial covering this article is even more forthright.[29] It points out that the remuneration of Visiting Anaesthetists (both direct and indirect) from the institution and their position in it are considered to be inferior to those of the surgeons and, consequently, "it would be inequitable to demand emergency work from them unless some compensation for this was provided". Edwards' article[28] and the Editorial[29] gave rise to correspondence. A letter from Edward Moir of the City of Manchester,[30] where all the seven Honorary Anaesthetists lived "fairly near the Infirmary", tells us that they attended emergency cases on a daily rota basis, and that the "Board" (on which unusually an anaesthetist sat) had agreed to pay Visiting Anaesthetists £1.11s.6d. for administrating anaesthesia or supervising House Surgeons administering anaesthesia for urgencies (sic). This remuneration of "one and a half guineas" would amount to about £52 per case in terms of 1996 purchasing power, and Moir tells us that anaesthetists "have been known to administer or supervise as many as ten cases on one day" - money indeed in those days! Each House Surgeon had to administer anaesthesia to twelve urgencies (sic) under supervision.[30] Francis Waddy[19] writing from a provincial town, wrote to say that, though he did not receive payment or an honorarium of any kind for his services as the only Honorary Anaesthetist appointed to the Northampton General Hospital, he attended the hospital five mornings and four afternoons a week, taking off what time was needed for private work, and regarded himself as being on continuous call for "urgency cases" which were too "dangerous and difficult" for the House Surgeon to anaesthetise. He stated further that he had never failed to answer a hospital call during the previous eighteen months.[19]

The state of the art of anaesthesia in 1932 and the teaching of anaesthesia.

Perusal of the relevant volumes (7 to 9) of the *British Journal of Anaesthesia* (1929-1933), the third edition of the popular *Handbook of Anaesthetics* (1929)[31] "for the student and practitioner",[31] and of the first edition of Langton Hewer's *Recent Advances in Anaesthesia and Analgesia* (1932)[32] provide us with an insight into current British practice over the period of the inauguration of the Association of Anaesthetists.

All patients breathed spontaneously. Neuromuscular blocking agents, though used by physiologists in their experiments for many years, were not accepted into anaesthetic practice for another decade, and there was doubt over the advisability of routinely employing endotracheal inhalation for abdominal cases.[33,34] There was also considerable disagreement over the wisdom of using "machines" (continuous flow nitrous oxide and oxygen apparatus with chloroform and/or ether vaporization).[34-38]

Ether was generally accepted to be safer than chloroform but the advantages of the latter, particularly for hastening induction, were considered to be indispensable.[34,39,40] Cyclopropane had not yet come into the picture but ethylene was on trial in the major cities.[41,42] The introduction of halothane was, of course, twenty years into the future. Hypoxic nitrous oxide anaesthesia was the only technique that would secure a rapid recovery for the dental and minor surgical outpatient, but the physiological principles were well understood by the principal exponents.[43,44] Anaesthesia for neurosurgery[45] and thoracic surgery[46] was undertaken only at major centres; high flow insufflation techniques with narrow bore catheters were used in both instances. Spinal (subarachnoid) anaesthesia was frequently employed using a variety of techniques and agents including the newly introduced "Percaine", which, as cinchocaine (Nupercaine), was destined to be the principal agent used by British anaesthetists for this technique for many years.[47,48]

There was a great deal of interest in what was then termed "premedication", but what would now be referred to as basal narcosis (that is, methods of induction designed to avoid the patient being aware of subsequent inhalation of ether or chloroform if this was required at all). The aim was to render the patient "unconscious in his bed"! These techniques fell in two categories, rectal and intravenous,[32,41,49] Paraldehyde and bromethol (Avertin) were the principal rectal agents and they were used particularly for toxic thyroid surgery.[49] Reference to the first intravenous barbiturates at that time is of still greater interest as they represent the dawn of intravenous induction as we know it today. The agents available were sodium 2 bromallyl-barbiturate (Pernocton), amylobarbitone (Amytal), and pentobarbitone (Nembutal). Hexobarbitone (Evipan) and thiopentone (Pentothal) were not introduced into practice until a year or two later.[32]

Intravenous blood volume or electrolyte replacement in the operating theatre was almost unheard of, but rectal fluids were administered pre- and postoperatively.[32] The aetiology of traumatic, operative and postoperative shock was still imperfectly understood. The emphasis was on the administration of anaesthesia in the face of shock, rather than measures designed to resuscitate the patient before operation. The theoretical concepts and practical teaching of the American surgeon George W Crile with regard to the neurological origin of shock and its management by anoci-association (the combination of light general with local anaesthesia) were accepted dogma.[31,32,50]

Treatment of respiratory arrest in the operating theatre was by Sylvester's or Schafer's chest compression methods, although mouth to mouth respiration was occasionally used to resuscitate the neonate. The treatment of cardiac arrest was by the use of stimulants and direct compression of the heart, usually through the diaphragm, and the intracardiac injection of drugs.[31,32,51]

Training. The practice of anaesthesia was beginning to change in 1932. The introduction of new agents and techniques during the next decade was to culminate in the promotion of curare and, ultimately, in the use of controlled respiration; however in 1932 the leaders of the specialty were faced with a situation in which, outside the major centres, anaesthesia was administered chiefly by House Surgeons and General Practitioners whose only training was as part of an undergraduate syllabus, which, even in those days, was considered to be crowded.[40,52,53] Better training was needed to improve even this rudimentary provision. Ross MacKenzie of Aberdeen[54] considered the problem of what and how to teach medical students in an erudite article[40] and was supported by an Editorial.[52] It is fortunate that, given the stage in development of surgery and attitudes as to what was and was not an acceptable operative risk, particularly in respect of age, the more straightforward inhalational techniques were surprisingly successful in the hands of a trained administrator. The techniques which were being developed at the major centres were however the harbingers of those which would be required to meet the surgical challenges that lay ahead. Ross MacKenzie called for better training for medical students but, in order that this could be accomplished he saw a need for an enhanced academic status for anaesthetists themselves, including the establishment of a qualification in anaesthesia - a Diploma in Anaesthetics.[40]

There is no doubt that by 1932 the time was ripe academically, politically and economically for the formation of a corporate organisation of anaesthetists; fortunately men of vision were on hand who could achieve that objective.

3

The Foundation

January to July 1932

"Mighty things from small beginnings grow"

John Dryden (1631-1700) *Annus Mirabilis*

The Founding Fathers

There is no doubt that Henry (Harry) Walter Featherstone (1894-1967) was the founder of the Association of Anaesthetists; "he was the mainspring in its creation".[1] He became its first President (1932-1935) and also took on the role of Honorary Secretary after the sudden and untimely death of W Howard Jones in 1935, until he was mobilised with the reserve Territorial Army in 1939 at the outbreak of the Second World War.[2]

Featherstone (Appendix A) was the son of a Birmingham General Practitioner who was also an Alderman on the City Council and prominent in several commercial enterprises. Harry Featherstone qualified from the Universities of Cambridge and Birmingham in 1916 and saw service with the Royal Army Medical Corps in Salonika and Flanders in the Great War (1914-1918). He was well qualified academically and was awarded the Cambridge MD in 1927. He returned to Birmingham in 1919 and was appointed as Honorary Anaesthetist to the Birmingham General Hospital and other hospitals in the area.[1-4] He built up an extensive private anaesthetic practice, but it is probable that his financially sound family background enabled him to limit his professional activities to anaesthesia in his early years despite the draw-backs (Chapter 2), and to devote time to writing, travel, and to taking an active part in the transactions of the Anaesthetic Section of the Royal Society of Medicine in London. He was on the Council of the Section from 1924 to 1929 and became its President in November 1930. His Presidential address was on the extensive tour of hospitals in Canada and of the Mayo Clinic which he had undertaken the previous summer.[5,6]

Featherstone followed the rules of the Royal Society of Medicine in his Presidential address and confined his remarks to the clinical practice of anaesthesia, but there is no doubt that it was as a result of his active Presidency, and the contacts which this brought with most of the leading anaesthetists of the day, that the need for action in relation to the problems discussed in Chapter 2 was impressed upon him.[2,7,8]

Harry Featherstone, writing in the first issue of *Anaesthesia* in 1946[7] summarises the conditions in which anaesthesia was practised at that time as follows:-

> *"The position in 1930 was this : the science and art of anaesthetics, and also the bulk of anaesthetic practice, had extended enormously - the latter being in part a result of the new Poor Law Reform and the consequent growth of general hospitals under county council and municipal authorities - but the practitioners of this branch of medicine had no means of organising their department nor of representing the needs of the anaesthetic service. No standard of service had been laid down, and there was little means of distinguishing trained workers from unskilled but optimistic novices. This was unsatisfactory for patients, for surgeons, and for hospital authorities, while skilled anaesthetists were inclined to feel that the devotion to this branch of the Profession had exposed them to an unstable career where "goodwill" could not be established, the problems of routine work could not be voiced, and there was no official body representative of anaesthetists, to whom medical and lay authorities could look for guidance".[7]*

Featherstone was the man of the moment. He had the authority, will, and ability to improve the lot of the majority of anaesthetists who were less favourably placed financially than he was himself. Featherstone's concern for the welfare of others was fully consistent with his generous character, epitomised by his life of public service[3-5]

The seed that was to grow into the Association of Anaesthetists of Great Britain and Ireland was sown at the Annual Conference of the BMA at Eastbourne in July 1931, when Featherstone raised the subject with William Howard Jones and George Ramsay Phillips.[7,8]

Howard Jones was destined to become the first Honorary Secretary of the Association; he was Senior Surgeon Anaesthetist to Charing Cross Hospital, a prominent member of Council of the Section of Anaesthetics and a frequent speaker at its meetings, as well as a contributor to the literature.[9] Ramsay Phillips was Senior Anaesthetist to St Mary's Hospital. He was less politically or academically inclined than Howard Jones, but he had succeeded Featherstone as President of the Section of Anaesthetics. He became one of the first Council members of the Association.

Howard Jones and Ramsay Phillips responded favourably to Featherstone's approach and they determined to give further consideration to the matter.

An informal discussion

Featherstone, Howard Jones and Ramsay Phillips met again informally in London in January 1932 and invited three other prominent London anaesthetists to join them. These were Henry Edmund Gaskin Boyle of St Bartholomew's Hospital, Zebulon Mennell of St Thomas', and Claude Woodham Morris of the University College and Royal Free Hospitals.

Boyle's is undoubtedly the most well known name amongst the six who attended this meeting because of its eponymous connection with British apparatus for the delivery of continuous flow nitrous oxide, oxygen, and ether mixtures; whatever the ins and outs of the argument concerning priority,[10] it was Boyle who promoted this technique in the United Kingdom during and after the Great War and he had been appointed an Officer of the Order of the British Empire (OBE) for his services. Boyle was Honorary Anaesthetist to St Bartholomew's Hospital, London, he had been a member of the original Society of Anaesthetists (Chapter 2), and had been President of the Section of Anaesthetics in 1923. He had travelled in the United States and was probably internationally the best known British anaesthetist.[11,12] He subsequently became a Member of the first Council of the Association. He never held Office but he was elected to Honorary Membership in 1939.

Zebulon Mennell[13] was Honorary Anaesthetist to St Thomas's Hospital and the National Hospital for the Paralysed and Epileptic (later the Hospital for Nervous Diseases), Queens Square, London.[13] He was a distinguished senior figure and notable literary contributor and speaker. He had been

President of the Section of Anaesthetics for the 1926-27 session and travelled widely on lecture tours both in the United States and Australia.[14] He had an important link with the past in that he, too, had been a member of the original Society of Anaesthetists. He also combined the practice of anaesthesia with general practice throughout his career. He owned a 'charming home' overlooking Hyde Park.[13] One suspects that, in the thirties, this must have been evidence of the success of his fashionable general practice rather than of his earnings as an Honorary Anaesthetist! Zebulon Mennell became the first Honorary Treasurer and third President of the Association, and, as a member of the Central Medical War Committee, he played an important part in mobilising the specialty in the Second World War (Chapter 5).[13]

Claude W Morris had had a distinguished career as an anaesthetist in the Royal Navy during the Great War and had been appointed as an Officer of the Order of the British Empire (OBE) for his services. He was Honorary Anaesthetist to the Royal Free and University College Hospitals, London, and in 1932 he was a Member of the Council of the Section of Anaesthetics.[15] Morris was elected to a resignation vacancy on the first Council of the Association in 1933.

All those present at this informal meeting were intimately connected with the Section of Anaesthetics of the Royal Society of Medicine (the reigning President, two ex-Presidents and three current members of its Council), but they were unanimous in their opinion that the Section was not, indeed could not be, the correct forum for discussion of the medicopolitical interests of anaesthetists. They were "convinced that anaesthetists must possess an autonomous body of their own, free from integration with the BMA, the Royal College of Surgeons [of England], the Society of Apothecaries or other self-governing medical institutions". They were also determined that anaesthetists must be free to select the members of such a body to be entirely representative of their wishes.[2,8]

Featherstone was reassured by the support he had received and proceeded to take positive action. He wrote a personal letter to "a hundred anaesthetists on the staffs of the main teaching hospitals" in the United Kingdom and the Irish Free State (now the Republic of Ireland) inviting them "to attend a meeting for the purpose of forming an association which would meet their needs".[7,8]

Featherstone, writing in 1946, clearly remembered wondering what he had started when he dropped the bundle of letters into a post-box at Atherstone, Warwickshire while motoring through that town.[8]

The Preliminary Meeting 27 April 1932

The time was ripe! Featherstone's proposal was greeted with enthusiasm. The preliminary meeting was held at the house of the Medical Society of London, 11 Chandos Street, London W1 on Wednesday 27 April 1932.[16] The venue was chosen to emphasise that the proceedings were not related to those of the Section of Anaesthetics of the Royal Society of Medicine. The time (8.00 pm) surely emphasised the pressure under which anaesthetists worked in their public and private practices!

The minutes of the meeting records the names of sixteen leading anaesthetists who were present.[16] They were headed by Sir Francis Shipway KCVO (Knight Commander of the Victorian Order) of Guy's Hospital, London.[17] He was the same age as Boyle and had been responsible for introducing many parallel innovations. He owed his title to having anaesthetised King George V on two occasions in 1928, but he certainly deserved his position in the first rank of British anaesthesia. He, too, had been a President of the Section of Anaesthetics, in 1926.

Mennell, Boyle and Howard Jones also supported Featherstone and, in addition, there attended from London, Joseph Blomfield of St George's Hospital and Editor of the *British Journal of Anaesthesia*, John H Chaldecott (St Thomas's), Cecil H M Hughes (King's College), Ashley S Daly (The London) who was later President of the Association, Charles F Hadfield (St Bartholomew's), Ivan W Magill (Westminster), Raymond J Clausen (Charing Cross), C Langton Hewer (St Bartholomew's) - later Editor of the journal *Anaesthesia* - and Harold P Crampton (Middlesex).[16]

The only named representative from the provinces besides Featherstone himself was E Falkner Hill of Manchester, a future Editor of the *British Journal of Anaesthesia*, but there were apologies from anaesthetists in Leeds and Birmingham as well as from Edinburgh, Glasgow and Aberdeen in Scotland expressing strong support. The minute also mentions that "others" were present but their names are not recorded.

Harry Featherstone was voted into the Chair and made his by then familiar general statement on the need for a formation of an association to represent anaesthetists.

The following resolutions were then passed:-

"That an association of anaesthetists be formed which will deal with the problems of the organisation of this branch of medicine".

"That the title of the association shall be the Association of Anaesthetists of Great Britain and Ireland".

"That anaesthetists from the Colonies [sic] should be admitted as corresponding members".

"That the new body should in no way conflict with the objects of the Section of Anaesthetics of the Royal Society of Medicine".

"That in dealing with other bodies such as hospital committees, it would endeavour to act either through the British Medical Association or by advising and helping anaesthetists in their own negotiations with their several hospitals".[16]

It is obvious from these resolutions that the impetus for founding the Association was to improve the terms and conditions of service of anaesthetists. The resolve of the meeting to avoid conflicting with the objects of the Section of Anaesthetics also reflects this view. The role of the Association of Anaesthetists in promoting training and further education was in the future.

One can sympathise with Featherstone and others, who initially would have preferred the designation "Guild" or "Craft" rather than "Association", but, in the end, a title based on those used by other professional bodies, such as the Association of Surgeons and the Association of Clinical Pathologists, was accepted. The pathologists belonged to another clinical service group whose status and remuneration were poorly defined in public hospitals. It is also noteworthy that, in those days before the National Health Service, negotiation would often be with individual hospital boards.[16]

The desire of those present at the preliminary meeting to include both Northern Ireland and the *de facto* independent Irish Free State (Republic of Ireland), reflects how close the professional bonds were (and are) with that country, and the reference to the "colonies" (despite the already well established existence of the self-governing dominions) is a reminder of the intimate relationship that existed between the members of the British Empire in the years between the First and Second World Wars. Those were the days, before the establishment of the Royal Australasian Colleges and similar bodies, in which the dominions, as well as the colonies, looked to the Royal Colleges of the mother country for specialist medical education and qualification.

A Provisional Council was then elected with Featherstone as President and charged with drawing up a set of rules for submission to an Inaugural General Meeting[3] including, significantly, limiting qualifications for membership (see below).

This preliminary meeting was recorded in a notice in the *British Journal of Anaesthesia*[18] and welcomed in an Editorial.[19]

The Provisional Council

Those elected to the Provisional Council were:-

President: H W Featherstone (Birmingham)[1-4]

Honorary Treasurer: Z Mennell (St Thomas', London)[13]

Honorary Secretary : W Howard Jones (Charing Cross, London)[9]

Council Members: Sir Francis Shipway (Guy's, London)[17]
Joseph Blomfield (St George's, London)[20]
E Falkner Hill (Manchester)[21]
H E G Boyle (St Bartholomew's London)[11]
Ashley S Daly (The London Hospital)[22]
G Ramsay Phillips (St Mary's, London)
John H Chaldecott (St Thomas', London)[23]

A further five Members were proposed for cooption at the first meeting of the Provisional Council and subsequently all of them accepted election,

C F Hadfield (St Bartholomew's, London), R E Apperly (Middlesex Hospital, London), H P Fairlie (Glasgow), H Torrance Thompson (Edinburgh), and J Ross Mackenzie (Aberdeen).[16]

Apperly had been Featherstone's predecessor and Ramsey Phillips his successor as President of the Section of Anaesthetics for 1929-1930, and Hadfield was President Elect for the 1932-1933 session.

The Provisional Council held meetings on 4 May and 27 May 1932.[16] Both of these were on neutral ground at the London Clinic. Rules for submission to the Inaugural Meeting were prepared; these were based on those of the Association of Surgery. An entrance fee of £1 (1996 equivalent £36) was levied on all the Council Members to create a fund for immediate requirements, and invitations were sent out to "about 300" anaesthetists on the staffs of the Schools of Medicine to attend the Inaugural Meeting and to become Members of the Association.

The Inaugural Meeting 1 July 1932

The Inaugural Meeting was "a representative gathering of about 70 of those who had responded to the invitation to become Members". It was held at the London Clinic at 8.30 pm on Friday 1 July 1932 with Featherstone in the Chair. "Numerous letters" of support had also been received by the Provisional Honorary Secretary.[16]

The resolution passed by the Provisional Meeting to form the Association of Anaesthetists of Great Britain and Ireland was approved, and all those who had immediately accepted the invitation to become Members were deemed to be elected.

The rules of the Association of Anaesthetists prepared by the Provisional Council were then considered in detail, modified as necessary, and duly accepted.

The objects of the Association were stated to be:-[16]

(a) To promote the development of this branch of medicine (i.e. anaesthesia).

(b) To co-ordinate the activities of anaesthetists.

(c) To represent anaesthetists and promote their interests.

(d) To favour the establishment of a Diploma in Anaesthetics.

(e) To encourage friendship amongst anaesthetists.

These objectives are rather wider than those originally considered at the Preliminary Meeting. They allow for the possibility of holding scientific meetings and, most important of all, they introduce the idea of the inauguration of a Diploma in Anaesthetics.

Membership was to consist of four categories.

Ordinary Members were to be selected "from anaesthetists who are actively engaged in the teaching of anaesthetics at the Schools of Medicine and Hospitals recognised by the University of Cambridge" and, further, the number of Members was to be limited to 150.[16] It is interesting that five of the original members from the provinces did not meet the requirement of being on the staff of a School of Medicine, but reference to the *Medical Directory* reveals that all of them were rare individuals for the time who were engaged whole time in anaesthetic practice without being also either general practitioners or on the staff of a teaching hospital. One of these was Francis F Waddy of Northampton (Chapter 4). After the initial elections the teaching hospital rule was strictly enforced until 1943 (Chapter 5).

The reference to "hospitals recognised by the University of Cambridge" was considered necessary because, although Cambridge had a preclinical school, it sent its students to recognised hospitals for their clinical training before they proceeded to their qualifying medical degree. It is doubtful whether this provision was really necessary, however, as the University of Cambridge was unlikely to recognise a hospital which was not also associated with an undergraduate medical school. The University of Oxford did not have an undergraduate medical school in 1932.

The limitation of membership to 150, without provision for a less exalted category of associates with an interest in anaesthesia, appears to be very restrictive, but it is larger than the one hundred possible Members to whom Featherstone sent his original invitation. Founder membership was on a "first come first served" basis. The limitation to anaesthetists with teaching hospital appointments, other than the initial exceptions mentioned above, is understandable; in the absence of a qualifying diploma the founders were obviously anxious that Membership of the Association of Anaesthetists of Great Britain and Ireland should indicate a certain status as a reputable anaesthetist. It did, however, exclude from any form of membership the large numbers of General Practitioners and other medical men who were administering anaesthesia in voluntary and municipal hospitals. It must be said, in defence of this policy of exclusiveness, that the Association of Anaesthetists was prepared to give advice and support in its early years to other anaesthetists who were not eligible for membership, especially in matters related to their terms of service.

The restriction to 150 Ordinary Members remained in force until after the outbreak of the Second World War when the expansion of the specialty made a change imperative (Chapter 5).

Senior Members were to be elected from amongst those who had retired from active teaching or research (but not necessarily from the practice of anaesthesia).[16]

Both Ordinary and Senior Members were to be elected by a rather cumbersome process. They were to be proposed in writing by any member of the Association, seconded by a Member of Council, balloted upon by Council (two adverse votes resulting in rejection), and then voted upon by the membership by postal ballot[8] before their names were announced at a General Meeting. Both Ordinary and Senior Members were eligible for election to Council. The entrance fee was to be £1 and the annual subscription £1 (1996: £35).

Honorary Members were to be nominated by Council and elected at the Annual General Meeting.[16]

Corresponding Members were also to be nominated by Council from "anaesthetists in established position who practise in other parts of the British Empire or [significantly] in foreign countries".[16]

Council was to consist of a President, Vice President, Honorary Treasurer and Honorary Secretary, and twelve other members, to be elected annually. The President was to hold office for a maximum of three years and Council Members for three years, but no limitation was placed on the length of time that the Vice President, Honorary Treasurer or Honorary Secretary could serve (see Chapter 8).[16]

Election of Officers and Council for 1932-1933

Featherstone[1-4] was formally elected as President and Mennell[13] and Howard Jones[9] as Honorary Treasurer and Honorary Secretary respectively. Joseph Blomfield[20] was elected Vice President. Sir Francis Shipway[17], having played his part faithfully as a member of the Preliminary Council, asked to be allowed to resign from Council. Two Council vacancies were thus created.

The remaining Members of the Provisional Council were then elected *en bloc,* and the two vacancies were filled by the election of A L Flemming of Bristol and C H M Hughes of King's College Hospital, London. E W Gandy (Westminster Hospital, London) proposed a hearty vote of thanks to Featherstone for all his hard work. This was passed with acclamation.[16] Seldom has such acknowledgment been so richly deserved.

Summary

It was thus that the Association of Anaesthetists of Great Britain and Ireland came into being nearly a decade after Hyman Cohen had expressed the need for such an organisation in his first Editorial in the *British Journal of Anaesthesia* in 1923[24] (Chapter 2); and almost exactly a year after Harry Featherstone had made his initial proposal.

The body that emerged was an exclusive organisation based on the teaching hospitals. The selection process guaranteed that a practitioner elected to membership was a leading member of the specialty; however the Association of Anaesthetists was prepared to concern itself with the problems of all anaesthetists. It was inevitable that the first Council included a high proportion of members from the London teaching hospitals because of the distribution of specialist anaesthetists at that time, but efforts had been made to include the interests of the whole of the United Kingdom (England, Scotland, Wales and Northern Ireland) as well as the Irish Free State (later the Republic of Ireland).

Featherstone must have been well satisfied with his achievement, but even he could not have foreseen the extent of the part the Association of Anaesthetists of Great Britain and Ireland was to play in the development of the scientific, political and social organisation of the specialty of anaesthesia in particular, and of British and Irish medicine in general, in the ensuing sixty years.

4

The Prewar Years

2 July 1932 to 2 September 1939

"For the cause that lacks assistance,
For the wrong that needs resistance,
For the future in the distance,
And the good that I can do."

George Linnaeus Banks (1821-1881) *What I live for*

The Executive Officers

Presidents:- H W Featherstone (1932-1935)[1]
J Blomfield (1935-1938)[2]
Z Mennell (1938-1941)[3]

Honorary Treasurers:- Z Mennell (1932-1938) &
(1941-1947)[3]
H Sington (1938-1941)[4]

Honorary Secretaries:- W Howard Jones (1932-1935)[5]
H W Featherstone (1935-1939)[1]

Political hopes and fears in the nineteen thirties

Nineteen thirty two, the year that the Association of Anaesthetists was born, was a climacteric year. The great financial depression was beginning to recede but the next year was to see Adolph Hitler come to power in Germany. The decade was one of gradually increasing prosperity, but this was an illusion because it was partly based on the need for preparation for the inevitable war as the German, Italian and Japanese dictators made territorial annexation after annexation.

Medicopolitical developments in the nineteen thirties

A succession of Acts of Parliament led to local authorities taking up an increasing burden for health care for the lower income groups in such areas as maternity and child welfare. These responsibilities included vaccination and immunisation, district nursing, fever hospitals, tuberculosis sanatoria and provision for the physically handicapped.[6,7]

Municipal authorities, led by the London County Council were, moreover, developing their own hospitals financed by public funds as a result of the 1929 Act (Chapter 2). These employed paid sessional and wholetime salaried medical staff. Voluntary hospitals were increasingly catering for those patients who were able to contribute financially. It is estimated that, whereas in 1891 88% of the revenue of provincial voluntary hospitals was derived from voluntary gifts and investments, by 1938 the proportion was 33%. Visiting staff continued to be unpaid for the work they did for public patients, though the number of patients accommodated in private wards was increasing.[7]

A greater awareness of the need for specialist knowledge, and the growth of pay-beds, led to a gradual tendency for general practitioners without specialist qualifications and experience to be excluded from hospital practice in the bed-owning specialties.[8] This trend was, however, much less marked so far as anaesthesia was concerned for obvious reasons. The limitation of the privilege of the administration of anaesthetics in provincial hospitals to those general practitioners who had specific appointments was by no means generally accepted, even towards the end of the decade; this was especially true where private practice was concerned. There had probably been a small increase in the number of wholetime residential appointments however, although W S Sykes, writing in 1936, mentions a teaching hospital with an annual operating list of 12,000 cases where there was no Resident Anaesthetist, and emergencies were often anaesthetised by "unskilled and unsupervised students".[9,10]

Clinical medicine in the nineteen thirties

The development of chemotherapy in the mid-thirties marked the historical divide between practice largely dominated by preventative medicine and symptomatically orientated pharmacology, and modern curative therapeutic medicine.[11,12] The German Gerhard Dogmagh introduced prontosil in 1935 and, by the end of the decade, sulphonamides were available that were effective against a variety of dreaded diseases including streptococcal infections, pneumonia, meningitis, gonorrhoea, typhoid and dysentery.

Alexander Fleming made his first observations on bacterial inhibiting powers of the penicillin mould in 1929 and, by the late thirties, (Sir) Howard Florey and E B Chain were working on its therapeutic application. The effect of their work, culminating in the publication of their first results in human subjects in practice, was to be profound both in prophylaxis against, and in treatment of surgical sepsis, and greatly extended the work of the surgeon and his anaesthetist colleague.[11,12]

The use of artificial respiration in the treatment of poliomyelitis as an additional responsibility for the British anaesthetist two decades later was foreshadowed in the nineteen thirties. Drinker, McKhann, and Shaw of the United States described the first really practical negative pressure respirator (the "Iron Lung") in 1928.[13] This, and apparatus derived from it, was used extensively in the thirties in the United States where poliomyelitis was prevalent; but such machines were rarities in the United Kingdom before 1938 when an epidemic highlighted British deficiencies.[13] Professor (Sir) Robert Macintosh (1897-1989), the then recently appointed first Nuffield Professor of Anaesthetics at Oxford[14] was asked by his benefactor Lord Nuffield, who had seen a newspaper article on the subject, whether the provision of iron lungs on a large scale would save lives. Macintosh believed it would. Nuffield rose to the occasion and proceeded to manufacture Both negative pressure respirators at his Morris Motor Works at Cowley as a gift to any hospital in the United Kingdom or British Dominions which asked to have one. Over 1600 machines were manufactured and distributed;[13-15] however, though one of the first professors of anaesthetics to be appointed in the world was concerned with the treatment of poliomyelitis in 1938, anaesthetists did not become deeply involved in intensive care until intermittent positive pressure ventilation (IPPV) replaced the negative pressure technique during and after the Copenhagen epidemic in 1952[13] (Chapter 6).

The practice of clinical anaesthesia 1932-1939

It must be appreciated that there were wide differences in sophistication between the anaesthetic techniques practised in leading teaching hospitals and those employed in the average provincial town. The contrast which was apparent at the time of the foundation of the Association of Anaesthetists in 1932 (Chapter 2)[16], persisted throughout the nineteen thirties and throughout the Second World War until the establishment of the NHS in 1948. It is even likely that the gap increased. There was, however, probably an increase in the use of continuous flow oxygen, nitrous oxide and ether and/or chloroform anaesthesia in larger hospitals where Boyle's machines had been purchased. Open drop chloroform and ether (often preceded by ethyl chloride or divinyl ether to facilitate a rapid induction) were still widely used, as were Clover's and Hewitt's simple air-ether inhalers.[16-18] The dilemma of what to teach medical students was a serious problem. The specialist anaesthetist in the teaching hospital naturally wished to provide the safest and best possible conditions for surgery with the latest agents and apparatus, for patients who had probably been referred for more complicated surgical procedures than were likely to be undertaken in the small town hospital; on the other hand, if he was conscientious, he would aim to instruct his student in the less complicated techniques which he was likely to be asked to use as a general practitioner.[16,19,20] W Stanley Sykes[10] details the organisational and pecuniary difficulties faced by anaesthetists in the thirties and makes proposals (very modest by 1998 standards) for improving clinical practice and training. This is a brilliant paper as one would expect from the man who was to write the classic history text *Essays on the first hundred years of anaesthesia*.[21]

Really important innovations were, however, made in the nineteen thirties. Cyclopropane, a wonderful new agent, was introduced from the leading hospitals in the United States. It brought with it the closed absorption techniques. The use of the agent had been popularised by Ralph Milton Waters in Wisconsin and by Harold Randall Griffith in Montreal from the early 1930's onwards.[22,23] It was introduced into the United Kingdom by Stanley Rowbotham, Honorary Anaesthetist to the Royal Free and Cancer (later renamed the Royal Marsden) Hospitals in London in 1935.[24] Cyclopropane was first mentioned in the *British Journal of Anaesthesia* in the July 1934 issue.[25,26] Cyclopropane was explosive but there was certainly a more relaxed attitude to the possibility of an explosion in those days; to quote Griffith, "It would be just as difficult to cause an explosion by the use of cautery in the abdomen as it would be to light the gas in one's kitchen by striking a match at the other side of the room".[23] The other feature of cyclopropane was that, although it gave a smooth inhalation induction, produced excellent relaxation, and was followed by a hitherto unprecedented rapid recovery, it induced respiratory depression and respiratory arrest with a frequency unknown with nitrous oxide, ether, or chloroform. The anaesthetist learned to withdraw the anaesthetic and to gently "squeeze the bag"[18,22] rather than resort to the old manual methods of artificial respiration which were previously employed. This in turn led to deliberate controlled ventilation techniques with cyclopropane for thoracic anaesthesia in the early nineteen forties, long before paralysis with curare and controlled ventilation was popularised (Chapter 5).[27,28]

Hexobarbitone (Evipan) was introduced in Germany by Helmut Weese in 1932,[29] and thiopentone (Pentothal) in the USA by John S Lundy of the Mayo Clinic[30] and by Ralph M Waters of Wisconsin[31] in 1934. Both were first used in the United Kingdom by Ronald Jarman - a future President of the Association of Anaesthetists - hexobarbitone in 1933[32] and thiopentone in 1935.[33] The first mention of hexobarbitone in the *British Journal of Anaesthesia* alludes to a report of the "Anaesthetics Committee, Medical Research Council and Royal Society of Medicine" in the October 1933 issue.[34] A paper on thiopentone in the *British Journal of Anaesthesia* in October 1937 by Wesley Bourne of Montreal, Canada described its use as an oral preparation in the first stage of labour![35] A note on its intravenous use appears in the same volume of the *British Journal of Anaesthesia* in the January 1938 number.[36] The Research Committee report on hexobarbitone mentions its possible intravenous use before inhalational anaesthesics[34], but it is clear from the other reports that, initially, hexobarbitone and thiopentone were generally used as sole agents, either in single doses for short operations, or intermittently or by infusion for longer procedures.[32,33] They were also used to cover spinal anaesthesia.[37] Preoperative intravenous administration of hexobarbitone and thiopentone with the patient in bed was considered to be acceptable.[37]

Electrolyte infusions were rarely given during surgery, postoperative rectal or subcutaneous saline being preferred. Blood transfusion was only used in severe cases of hypovolaemic shock or anaemia; however, the principles of the modern drip infusion were established by Marriott and Kekwick in their classic article in the *Lancet* in 1935.[38] It is interesting that the Laurie glass drip chamber which they employed, had been described in 1909 for rectal and subcutaneous infusions.[39]

Much technical and clinical progress had been made by the specialty of anaesthesia in the United Kingdom by 1939 but, as the Second World War approached, the knowledge of the latest advances was confined to relatively few specialist anaesthetists, the majority of whom were members of the Association of Anaesthetists; outside the main teaching centres and larger hospitals anaesthesia was practised much as it had been in the days before the Great War. The story of the way in which this small group of experts acted as the leaven which produced the large number of anaesthetists required to meet the challenge of the war years belongs to the next chapter; for the moment, however, we must return to 1932 to consider the early events in the life of the nascent Association.

The business of the Association 1932-1939

The business of the Association in the first seven years of its existence was largely concerned with the medicopolitical matters which were the immediate reason for its formation, and it was regarded by others to be a political organisation rather than a scientific body.[40] It promoted the image of anaesthesia and established itself as the recognised national mouthpiece of the specialty on matters concerning what are now known as "terms and conditions of service".[41] The clinical matters which were discussed, such as the introduction of nitrous oxide and air analgesia for use by midwives, had political overtones. Scientific meetings were not held. This is not surprising as the majority of its leading members were also Fellows of the Section of Anaesthetics of the Royal Society of Medicine with whose objectives the Association had resolved from the start not to conflict. A proposal to hold provincial scientific meetings from Henry Brennan of Manchester was firmly rejected by Council on 2 February 1939.[42]

The transactions of the Association were very business like throughout this period. The suggestion that "a dinner or supper should be held in conjunction with the annual meeting" was not raised until the 7th Annual General Meeting on 28 October 1938.[43] "The proposal received general approbation" but, alas, before the next Annual General Meeting was due to be held in October 1939, war had been declared.

The pattern in the early years was to hold an Annual General Meeting in October and a General Meeting in the Spring of the following year. The purpose of the General Meeting was to present an update of the proceedings of Council and to elect new members by the rather cumbersome procedure which the rules ordained (Chapter 3). The practice of holding General Meetings between Annual General Meetings seems to have lapsed after 1937. Attendance at Annual General and General Meetings in the prewar period (1932-1939) rarely rose above fifty members.[42]

Public Relations

The first act of the Council of the Association at its first meeting on 5th August 1932 was to announce its existence. The minutes record that a deputation of anaesthetists had already been sympathetically received by Dr Bone, the Chairman of the Medicopolitical Committee of the BMA, and it was agreed that the President should write to Dr Bone and the Editors of the *British Medical Journal* and the *Lancet* announcing the formation of the Association.[42]

Dr Featherstone's Presidential letter was published in both the *British Medical Journal* and the *Lancet* on 3rd September 1932. This communication announced the formation of the Association of Anaesthetists with the defined objective "promoting the development of this branch of medicine". It also outlined the conditions of membership, listed the names of the Officers and Council Members, and invited those who were eligible to apply for membership.[44,45]

The formation of the Association of Anaesthetists was welcomed by a powerful annotation in the editorial columns of the *Lancet*.[46] This piece is anonymous, but one suspects that it might have come from the pen of the Vice President of the Association Joseph Blomfield, Editor of the *British Journal of Anaesthesia*.[2] It says it all! Surprise is expressed that "surgeons themselves have not played a more active part in promoting the interests of specialist anaesthetists" when it was considered how great a part the correct selection and administration of the anaesthetic played in the welfare of the patient, and in "the completely successful outcome of the operation".

The passage on teaching is worth quoting :-

"[Anaesthetists] are painfully conscious of the limitations imposed upon them, which may lead to a choice of not teaching at all or displeasing the surgeon for whom they are working. If they consider the interests of the student they are apt seriously to damage their own interests [of being asked to anaesthetise for paying patients]......."

"The surgeon naturally dislikes it if the anaesthetist talks; the student complains if he does not. Facilities should be provided for such remunerated anaesthetists' attendances as would give them opportunities for practical teaching during some of the less important operations, those for example carried out by resident medical officers".[46]

A notice in the October 1932 issue of the *British Journal of Anaesthesia* records the formation of the Association of Anaesthetists, expresses the debt which anaesthetists owe to Featherstone, and tells us that up to that date 100 of the maximum 150 members have been recruited.[47]

The reply to the letter which Featherstone sent to the BMA, read at the second meeting of Council on 6 October 1932, was unexpectedly unenthusiastic. It was signed by a Dr Forbes, the Assistant Medical Secretary. We do not have the text of this missive, but the minute book tells us that he hinted that the new Association should be dissolved and a "group council" formed within the BMA. Featherstone reported that he had replied that he believed that anaesthetists "required an independent body in which there could be free discussion of the many problems which appeared to be peculiar to their branch of work and above all a certain amount of exclusiveness". Council endorsed Featherstone's reply (as did the subsequent first Annual General Meeting of the Association held on 28th October 1932).[42] It is to the credit of both the BMA and the Association of Anaesthetists of Great Britain and Ireland that this initial difference of opinion was soon forgotten; as early as March 1933 the BMA invited the Association of Anaesthetists to send a representative to attend the Committee of Consultants to discuss the inadequate sessional remuneration offered by the London County Council Service.[42] The two associations have subsequently maintained very close cooperation over the years with regard to matters of mutual concern; in 1998 the Anaesthetics Subcommittee of the Central Consultants and Specialist Committee of the BMA is chaired by a member of the Council of the Association of Anaesthetists. This committee is the link with the Government through the BMA which is the official negotiating body over terms and conditions of service in the modern British NHS.

The Association of Anaesthetists quickly established itself as the representative organisation of anaesthesia; by the end of the decade they had been consulted by the Home Office, the London County Council, the British (now Royal) College of Obstetricians and Gynaecologists, the Central Midwives' Board, Universities and many other organisations and Hospital Boards.[43]

Membership

The policy of limiting membership to 150 anaesthetists from the recognised medical schools of the United Kingdom and Ireland was maintained throughout the prewar period, and by 1937 there were 140 "Members". This category presumably included Senior (retired) Members as well as active Ordinary Members since a distinction is not drawn. The question of possible revision of the rules governing membership was raised only once in the prewar period. This was when George Edwards of St George's Hospital London at the 5th Annual General Meeting on 30 October 1936 gave notice "that he wished to propose that the rule limiting membership be rescinded at the next General Meeting".[42] He was discouraged by both Joseph Blomfield (the President) and Zebulon Mennell (the Honorary Treasurer). The latter stated that the Associations of Surgeons, Physicians and Pathologists all had limited membership and it was suggested that a solution might be to introduce a category of Associate Member. The matter was considered again at the Council meeting on 22 January 1937; no mention was made of the possibility of Associates but the idea of extending membership beyond 150 was firmly rejected. Council received a letter from George Edwards on 9 April 1937 stating that he did not intend to proceed further with the matter. No further action was taken.[42]

Geographical representation

The question of geographical representation has been destined to be a matter for discussion many times in the history of the Association of Anaesthetists. The Council, which was confirmed in office at the Second Annual General Meeting on 20 October 1933, was composed of eleven members representing all the London teaching hospitals, and five of the English provincial medical schools (Birmingham, Manchester, Liverpool, Leeds and Bristol). The President reported at the 1936 Annual General Meeting (30 October 1936) that the decision to reimburse the "third class" rail fares of provincial Members of Council taken at the 1935 Annual General Meeting had resulted in the regular attendance of provincial members.[42]

Very early on consideration was given to the question of securing the involvement of all the teaching hospitals in Scotland, Wales and Ireland and the remaining English provinces. The agreed solution was to appoint "District Representatives" from Edinburgh, Glasgow and Aberdeen in Scotland, from Cardiff in Wales, and from Dublin in the Irish Free State (now the Republic of Ireland) as well as from Sheffield, Oxford and Cambridge. The District Representatives were charged with coordinating local opinion and communicating directly with Council.[42] The scheme was abandoned during the Second World War, but it can be considered to be a forerunner of the Linkman scheme, which today provides wide National Health Service District representation. This was introduced in 1976 (Chapter 8) and now forms a most important part of the organisation of the Association.

Honorary Membership

The Association elected five Honorary Members at its inaugural meeting on 25 October 1932.[42] Four of them were eminent retired senior London anaesthetists. J F Silk of King's College Hospital - the founder and sometime President of the original Society of Anaesthetists (Chapter 2), R J Probyn-Williams of the London Hospital, C Carter Braine of Charing Cross Hospital, and Richard Gill of St. Bartholomew's Hospital. The other Honorary Member was an interesting choice. This was Francis H McMechan of New York. He was the first Editor of *Current Researches in Anaesthesia and Analgesia* and an inveterate founder of societies of anaesthesia in North America (Chapter 5).[48] The young Association of Anaesthetists was sparing in the election of Honorary Members in its early years however. Viscount Nuffield became an Honorary Member in 1936. This was the year in which he made his munificent gift to Oxford University which led to the foundation of the Chair of Anaesthetics and the appointment of Professor (Sir) Robert Macintosh.[15] Ralph M Waters of Madison, Wisconsin was also elected in 1936. He was the first anaesthetist in the world to hold a Professorial Chair and was greatly respected by the British anaesthetists of the nineteen thirties. Many of them visited his Department and admired its organisation, research, teaching and clinical activities; it was their ideal of how a Department ought to be run.[49] Macintosh[15] and Stanley Sykes[10] were amongst those who made the pilgrimage to Madison, and Macintosh incorporated many of Waters' ideas into the structure of his Oxford Department. Waters visited London in 1936. He lectured on and demonstrated closed circuit anaesthesia with cyclopropane. He was also elected to Honorary Membership of the Section of Anaesthetics of the Royal Society of Medicine.[50] The only other Honorary Member of the Association of Anaesthetists to be elected before the Second World War was the beloved H E G ("Cocky") Boyle of St Bartholomew's Hospital. He was elected in 1939 when his health was already failing. He died in 1941.[42,51]

Corresponding Membership and international relations

Two Corresponding Members were elected on 25 October 1932 at the first Annual General Meeting.[42] J T Gwathmey of New York[52] had been closely associated with British Military Hospitals in the Great War. He is probably best remembered in the United Kingdom for his promotion of continuous flow nitrous oxide, oxygen and ether techniques, which Boyle later developed.[53] Wesley Bourne, an anaesthetist from Montreal with a classical and philosophical turn of mind, was also elected. He had been President of the International Anesthesia Research Society and was awarded the first Henry Hill Hickman Medal of the Royal Society of Medicine in 1935. In 1942 he became the only President of the American Society of Anesthesiologists who was not an American citizen. He was elected an Honorary Member of the Association of Anaesthetists of Great Britain and

Ireland in 1955.[54]

The further election of Corresponding Members in the period 1932 to 1939 was confined to anaesthetists from countries in the British Empire. Corresponding Members from New Zealand and Adelaide, South Australia, were elected at the 1934 Annual General Meeting (31 October 1934). Council initiated cordial relations with the newly formed Australian[55] and Italian Societies (which were founded in 1934 and 1935 respectively) at its meeting on 20 March 1935.[42] The Honorary Treasurer (Mennell) visited Australia and the Far East in 1935.[55,56] He delivered a paper at the First Annual General Meeting of the Australian Society and also the Second Embley Memorial Lecture at the University of Melbourne - a lecture dedicated to E H Embley a pioneer Australian anaesthetist. Mennel's lectures tended to be conservative and were apparently not particularly well received by an audience eager to learn of innovations from Europe, but a proposal for affiliation with the British Association was greatly appreciated; on his return corresponding members from Sydney (New South Wales), Melbourne (Victoria), Perth (Western Australia) and Singapore (Straits Settlements) were elected on 20 December 1935.[57] A further Australian Corresponding Member, Geoffrey Kaye of Melbourne,[57] was chosen at the 6th Annual General Meeting on 29 October 1937. The minute states that he was elected on a personal basis and not as the founding Honorary Secretary of the Australian Society.[42] It is of interest that, though Kaye was much younger than Featherstone (31 as compared to 58) when his inspiration led to the foundation of the Australian Society in 1934, he too had travelled widely in North America and had the benefit of a private income. This, as was the case with Featherstone, enabled him to pursue his purpose without serious financial implication in medicopolitical circumstances which closely resembled those in the United Kingdom.[55,57]

Status and remuneration

There is no doubt that some ambivalence attended the foundation of the Association of Anaesthetists. Anaesthetists found satisfaction in their calling and they certainly wished to improve their techniques and their opportunities for teaching, as well as to ensure that patients had the benefit of professionalism. The financial rewards were so meagre, however, and so dependant on the whim of another specialist - the surgeon - that they lacked the means to improve their situation.

The tradition of the specialist in British hospital medicine was to give professional service to patients in the lower income groups in the voluntary hospitals, but to charge fees to the middle and upper classes; at the time the Association was founded in 1932 it was therefore considered to be almost unethical for specialists to press for remuneration for services to public patients. If, however, payment or an honorarium was accepted by an anaesthetist the chances of achieving a place on the all powerful medical committee of a teaching or voluntary hospital receded.

Times were changing however. The new local authority hospitals introduced under the 1929 Act (Chapter 2) were being established with sessional payments or whole time employment of medical staff, the provision of private wards in voluntary hospitals was increasing as more of the poorer patients were treated in municipal hospitals, and voluntary "contributory" schemes for the lower income groups and "provident" schemes for the middle classes were becoming popular. These provided cash benefits during hospitalisation.[8,58] It was considered legitimate to press for reasonable fees in all these areas. The local authorities had limited funds however and often at first offered very small rewards to anaesthetists in comparison to those paid to surgeons. Throughout the period 1932-1939 the Association of Anaesthetists was active in pressing the claims of anaesthetists with individual hospital authorities, both directly and through the BMA, with some success.[42] It is only possible to outline a few examples however. It must be remembered that inflation was negligible in the decade leading up to the Second World War; the sum mentioned below must be multiplied more than thirtyfold to arrive at equivalent 1996 purchasing power (i.e. £1 in 1932 = about £35 in 1996). The fees are quoted in the traditional guinea (£1.1s.0d old currency = £1.05 decimal equivalent). The London County Council (LCC) had agreed with the BMA in 1932 that the minimum fee offered to sessional specialists should be $2\frac{1}{2}$ guineas (1996: £71) for sessions not exceeding 2 hours and one guinea (1996: £36) for every hour or part of an hour thereafter, yet anaesthetists were offered only $1\frac{1}{2}$ guineas (1996: £51) to begin with in 1932. The Honorary Secretary (Howard Jones) was invited to a meeting of the BMA Committee of Consultants composed of physicians and surgeons who backed the protest made by the Association of Anaesthetists. This was rather a surprising decision considering the small size of the anaesthetist's fee for anaesthesia in comparison with the surgeon's fee which was customary in private practice at the time; but, of course, this was "someone else's money"! Further negotiations took place and the President was able to report at the 3rd Annual General Meeting in 1934 (20 October 1934) that a "satisfactory" revision had been obtained.[42] The advice of the Association of Anaesthetists was also sought by the LCC with regard to wholetime resident anaesthetists. A recommendation was made that their salary should be the same as for other specialists with whom they were working, and that they should have six weeks holiday each year!

Plymouth City Council accepted the BMA recommendations (2nd Annual General Meeting 20 October 1933).[42] Manchester City Council, after negotiation, agreed to a payment of £250 (1996: £9,500) per annum for two sessions per week of not more than 3 hours with adequate holiday provision (Council Meeting 10 October 1935).[42]

The policy on remuneration of part-time consultants and specialists working on a sessional basis in Local Authority hospitals was reviewed by the BMA in 1936.[59] One session per week was to be rewarded by "not less than" £125 (1996: £4,750) per annum and 6 regular attendances by "not less than" £500 (1996: £19,000) per annum. Unspecified mileage payments for over 2 miles of travel from "residence or consulting room" and "seasonal" annual holidays with locum provision was to be arranged. "Anaesthetics, treatment of venereal disease and x-ray examination and treatment" are specifically included as being eligible for these payments. There was a less satisfactory provision for tonsil and adenoid operations involving a general anaesthetic (one wonders whether tonsils were still sometimes being removed without anaesthesia as in the writer's grandfather's time about 1890, or were some tonsillectomies done under local anaesthesia as was still popular for adults in the USA up to the nineteen fifties?) The "total fee for the two practitioners concerned" presumably the surgeon and the anaesthetist, was to be, £1.11s.6d (1996: £57) per case for less than four cases; or £5.5s.0d (1996: £200) per session at which the average number of cases per session to be dealt with is agreed locally, such agreed number to be not more than eight".

It is also strange that, as anaesthetists' fees in Local Authority hospitals were specifically equated with the surgeons' on an annual sessional basis, occasional per case payment for an isolated anaesthetic was to be much less. The anaesthetist, for anaesthetics other than for tonsils and adenoids and for minor out-patient dental procedures using nitrous oxide (see below), was to receive a minimum of £1.1s.0d (1996: £38) whatever the nature, or length, of the anaesthetic, while the surgeon's fee was to be a minimum of £5.5s.0d (1996: £200) for a minor operation and a minimum of £10.10s.0d (1996: £400) for a major operation![59]

The Association of Anaesthetists endorsed this policy (Council 22 May 1936), but pointed out, in answer to an enquiry from Liverpool, that these rates were a minimum, and that some hospitals were paying more.[42]

Fees for the administration of anaesthetics to dental out-patients under the National Insurance Schemes have been woefully inadequate in proportion to the skill required in sharing the airway with the surgeon, and a matter for dispute between the Association of Anaesthetists and the BMA, on one hand, and the Government authorities on the other, throughout almost the whole of the history of the Association of Anaesthetists. There are several references to dissatisfaction with the regulations and fees in the reports of meetings in the Association minute book in the nineteen thirties (e.g. 10 October 1935, 29 October 1937 and 18 February 1938)[42] and further reference is made in subsequent chapters. The Association of Anaesthetists endeavoured to influence the BMA in their negotiations in these early years, but frustration at the intransigence of officialdom is evident from the resolutions and debates at the Annual Representative Meetings of the BMA of 1937 and 1938. The rate for the job was half a guinea (1996: £20) for the first patient in a session irrespective of the number of teeth, and 7s.6d (1996: £14.50) for each subsequent patient for the administration of (at that time) the usual brief nitrous oxide anaesthetics. One guinea (1996: £40) could be earned for the other longer anaesthetics.[61,62] It is an amazing fact, however, that, in purchasing power, these rates were more than those paid in the period after the Second World War, and bear comparison with those offered in 1992 by the NHS

(Chapter 9).

The "sliding scale" related to the number of patients anaesthetised per session was particularly disliked, as was the rule which confined the right to earn National Insurance fees to specifically contracted practitioners - much was said about the freedom of choice of patients![61,62]

The payment of the anaesthetists to academic professorial surgical units was one of the issues which prompted Harry Featherstone to found the Association of Anaesthetists in 1932 (Chapter 2). It was a problem which particularly applied to certain London teaching hospitals (St Bartholomew's, St Mary's, University College, the Royal Free and St Thomas') and it pervades the pages of the minute book throughout the whole period 1932-1939.[42]

Investigation of the problem was delegated to a subcommittee of Council composed of Charles Hadfield (St Bartholomew's), Ramsay Phillips (St. Mary's) and Claude Morris (University College) at the Council meeting on 16 February 1934, and all anaesthetists from the hospitals having academic surgical units were invited to a meeting on 7 May 1934.[42]

Morris reported to Council on 11 May and Hadfield on 21 June 1934. Their reports are detailed in the minute book.[42] This was a University matter and it will not surprise those who have experience of the Machiavellian procedural contortions of academic boards and committees, that endless procrastination and buck-passing took place. Amongst those consulted officially or unofficially were the Academic Registrar of London University, the Board of the Faculty of Medicine and its Chairman and individual members, Directors of the Medical and Surgical units at St Bartholomew's, the Board of Studies of the University of London, (Sir) Girling Ball, Dean of St Bartholomew's Medical College, the University Grants Committee, St Bartholomew's Medical College Committee, and Dr Dudgeon, Dean of St Thomas' Medical School.[42]

Almost all the individuals and bodies expressed sympathy but declared themselves powerless to act. The only positive result that ever seems to have accrued over the years 1932-1939 was the appointment of a wholetime anaesthetist to the Surgical Professorial Unit at University College Hospital "largely through the influence of Dr Claude Morris" (Report of Council for the year 1934-1935 presented at the Annual General Meeting on 31 October 1935).[42] This anaesthetist was to be paid £250 per year (1996: £9,550) (Council 5 July 1935). This was considered inadequate and it was agreed that an effort should be made to secure an increase in salary to £400 per annum (1996: £15,300). The result of this modest representation is not subsequently reported in the minutes. The authorities at St Thomas' and St Bartholomew's were apparently still resisting payments to anaesthetists to their surgical units in 1939 (Council 11 May 1939).[42]

Private fees for anaesthesia were usually collected by the surgeon, the general practitioner or even the matron of a nursing home and passed on to the anaesthetist. It is unfortunate that payment through the surgeon persists even in 1998. In some quarters this practice tends to diminish the importance of anaesthesia in the eyes of the patient. This was even more the case in the thirties when the anaesthetist often did not see the patient before operation.[10,62] The policy of some modern provident societies of providing a global sum to cover both the anaesthetist's and the surgeon's fees is an archaic survival of this practice, which is still a matter of concern to the Association of Anaesthetists even in the nineteen nineties.[63]

It is interesting that as early as the Second Annual General Meeting (20 October 1933) a resolution proposing the separation of the fees of surgeons and anaesthetists was debated. This is not surprising. The anaesthetist's fee could be as low as 10% of the surgeon's as was made clear at a special General Meeting called to consider private practice on 18 June 1937. The Report of Council at the Sixth Annual General Meeting on 29 October 1937 records that an article favourable to anaesthetists and supporting their claim for better remuneration had been published in the lay press "without instigation from the Association".[42] One wonders, however, how much unofficial "instigation" had been brought to bear by Blomfield,[2] the reigning President! The following resolution was drawn up by Council of the Association of Anaesthetists at its meeting on 18 February 1938 and submitted first to the Consultants Group of the BMA and through them to the 1938 Annual Representative Meeting of the BMA.[42,62]

> *"The Association [i.e. the BMA)] appreciates the value of the specialist anaesthetist as an essential unit in medical practice both in hospital and in private practice and recognises the right of the anaesthetist to assess and collect his own fees".*

Professor A H Burgess of Manchester (a surgeon who was Chairman of the Consultants Group of the BMA) presented a reasonable assessment of the progress anaesthesia had made since the foundation of the Association of Anaesthetists of Great Britain and Ireland in 1932. He drew particular attention to the establishment of the Diploma in Anaesthetics in 1935 (see below) which could be used to distinguish the specialist anaesthetist. The motion was passed but not without protest from Dr A B Murray (a General Practitioner from Banff, Scotland) who, significantly, succeeded in having the word "important" substituted for "essential" in the above motion.[62]

The passing of this motion was reported with some satisfaction to the Annual General Meeting of the Association of Anaesthetists on 28 October 1938.[42] It was, however, pointed out by Francis Waddy of Northampton that this resolution was in contrast to the policy of the BMA concerning the provision made by provident society schemes agreed by the BMA. These schemes did not define the need for specialist status of the anaesthetist and authorised fees of one, one and a half and two guineas (1996: £36.50, £57 and £73) according to the minor, intermediate, or major severity of the operation. Further representations were made to the BMA. Zebulon Mennell, who was by now the President of the Association of Anaesthetists, attended two meetings of the BMA Provident Scheme Subcommittee. He described the attitude of its members as "very difficult". He was, however, able to report to the Association Council meeting of 11 May 1939 (the last held before the declaration of the Second World War on 3 September 1939) that "the following plan was settled by the Provident Scheme Subcommittee and provisionally accepted by the King's Fund Provident Committee"[42]:-

1. Fees strictly net (i.e. not including anaesthetics and other charges).
2. Anaesthetic fees are in respect of administration by anaesthetists of specialist rank only.
3. In so far as the scheme applies to nursing homes these are grant-in-aid payments to patients direct, the fees of the consultants and specialists remaining a matter of arrangement between the doctor and the patient.
4. The major and intermediate operations will be grouped together for anaesthetic purposes and a fee of three guineas[1996: £109] paid.
5. Dissection of tonsils will come under the major heading whatever the age of the patient.

Mennell commented that, in view of the fact that the global benefit available from the provident schemes, for surgeons' and anaesthetists' fees together, was likely to average "less than fourteen pounds [1996: £485], it was felt that the terms represented a very satisfactory advance" towards the objective of ensuring that the anaesthetist's fee should be 20% of the surgeon's fee.[42]

Representation on hospital medical boards and committees

The Report of Council at the Second Annual General Meeting on 20 October 1933 and subsequent Council minutes state that several Liverpool hospitals had coopted anaesthetists to their Medical Boards after representations made by the President and the Honorary Secretary of the Association of Anaesthetists.[42]

A circular letter was initiated at a General Meeting of the Association on 26 June 1936 and sent to hospitals and medical schools and lay management boards.[42] It is sad that the text of this communication has not survived, but it can be deduced from the Report of the Sixth Annual General Meeting on 30 October 1936, that it concerned both status (in particular representation on the Medical Boards of the hospitals or medical schools), and the need for reasonable recompense either in terms of likelihood of consequential private practice or adequate fees from private or provident patients within the hospital, or even payment for public sessions if there was little possibility of generating private practice. The Sixth Annual Report of Council (Annual General Meeting 30 October 1936) states that many anaesthetists had written to say that the letter had had a good effect.[42]

The Diploma in Anaesthetics

There is no doubt that the jewel in the crown of the Association in the first few years of its existence was the introduction of the Diploma in Anaesthetics. No other single measure was as important in establishing anaesthesia as a specialty in British medicine in the eyes of other disciplines.[40,63,64] The Diploma was also destined to become the key to the recognition of physician anaesthetists as specialists in the armed services in the Second World War, and ultimately, as Consultants of equal status on the establishment of the NHS in 1948.

The rapidity with which the Diploma was established once the initial steps had been taken, is not only evidence that the time was right and the need well recognised by the medical profession, but it also testifies to the good sense and administrative expertise of the Association of Anaesthetists itself and the Royal Colleges of Physicians and Surgeons which sponsored it.

The inauguration of a Diploma had been the ambition of enlightened anaesthetists since at least the early thirties, and was one of the five objectives when Featherstone founded the Association (Chapter 3). It is therefore rather surprising that the Report of Council presented at the Second General Meeting of the Association on 20 October 1933[42] states rather cryptically: -

"It is felt generally that the time is not yet ripe for the introduction of a Diploma in Anaesthetics. Some of us think, however, that the advantages of having a special qualification will soon be great enough to justify its introduction".

It may be that some members with established practices had lobbied the Officers because they feared that they might have to sit an examination! Whatever the reason for this cautious statement, less than two months later, on 15 December 1933, when Council discussed the matter, it was resolved that "Mr Magill [at that time a Council Member but who was not present at the meeting] be asked to produce the correspondence he had had with the Society of Apothecaries relating to this proposal".[42]

Ivan Whiteside Magill (1888-1986) - later Sir Ivan Magill, KCVO - of Westminster Hospital, London is rightly revered as one of the most influential figures in the development of anaesthesia in the twentieth century.[65] He was Honorary Secretary of the Section of Anaesthetics of the Royal Society of Medicine in 1931 when Featherstone, the founder of the Association, was President of the Section.1,[65,66] Magill proposed to Council of the Section that the possibility of establishing a diploma in anaesthetics should be explored but this was not possible under the provisions of the Charter of the Society.[65] Featherstone founded the Association in 1932 with the idea of a diploma very much in mind; meanwhile, it seems that Magill had had correspondence with the Society of Apothecaries (a chartered diploma granting body) on his own account.

At the Council Meeting of the Association of Anaesthetists on 16 February 1934, Magill proposed that steps should be taken to inaugurate a Diploma in Anaesthetics. This proposal was accepted and a subcommittee was appointed consisting of Magill,[65] Hadfield[67] and Blomfield[2] to make recommendations. The subcommittee presented draft proposals to Council on 20 April 1934 and these were considered at a General Meeting on 11 May 1934 at which about forty members were present. The subcommittee had prepared the ground very thoroughly indeed. The President of the Royal College of Surgeons of England (Sir Holburt Waring of St Bartholomew's Hospital) had been consulted unofficially. He had reacted favourably and had suggested that an official approach be made to his College by the Association. A letter had also been sent to the Association's American Honorary Member, Francis H McMechan, asking him to provide information about the position with regard to the specialist certification of physician anaesthetists in the United States. His reply was not helpful in the context of the United Kingdom and, indeed, the evidence is that there was considerable confusion over the issue in the USA at that time.[48]

The Subcommittee made the following suggestions "as a working basis":-

1. *Every candidate must be a Registered Medical Practitioner.*

2. *The Diploma should be intended for those practitioners the major part of whose professional work was concerned with anaesthesia.*

3. *Every candidate should be required to produce evidence that he had held a responsible anaesthetic post in a hospital or hospitals of not less than one hundred beds, for a period of not less than two years.*

4. *Each candidate must produce evidence that he has personally administered 2,000 anaesthetics since qualification, of which more than half shall be for major surgical procedures.*

5. *The examination should consist of:- (a) a written paper, (b) a viva voce and (c) a practical demonstration.*

6. *In the first instance the Diploma should be granted to any practising anaesthetist who applied for it who had held a post as a visiting anaesthetist to a teaching hospital for a period of ten years.*

A proposal was made at the General Meeting suggesting that application should be made to the Royal College of Surgeons of Edinburgh as well as the Royal College of Surgeons of England, but this was defeated, and it was agreed that only the Royal College of Surgeons of England should be approached. It can be seen with hindsight, that this was a very significant decision; unlike the specialist qualifications of the surgeons, the diplomas granted today by the Royal College of Anaesthetists cover the whole of the United Kingdom.

A joint meeting of the Association of Anaesthetists and the representatives of the Royal College of Surgeons of England was convened on Friday 2 November 1934. The Association was represented by Featherstone,[1] Magill,[65] Blomfield,[2] and Hadfield,[67] and the Royal College by the President (Sir Holburt

Waring), the two Vice Presidents (Professor G E Gask of St Bartholomew's and Mr Wilfred Trotter (of University College Hospital), Mr Victor Bonney (gynaecologist of the Middlesex Hospital), and Mr Hugh Lett (surgeon to the London Hospital). The proposals of the Association were favourably received, and the representatives of the Royal College suggested that the Diploma should be put under the wing of the Conjoint Examining Board in England of the Royal College of Physicians of London and the Royal College of Surgeons of England. This was agreed and Featherstone subsequently interviewed Mr Horace Rew, Secretary of the Examining Board. Consultations took place between the two Colleges with Professor Samson Wright (the eminent physiologist from the Middlesex Hospital) representing the physicians.[42] The regulations were agreed by May 1935 and published in the *British Journal of Anaesthesia* in the following July.[68] These regulations were based on those originally submitted by the Association Subcommittee but with certain refinements and modifications.

Candidates were required either to have a qualification in medicine, surgery and midwifery registerable in the United Kingdom, or be "graduates in medicine and surgery (MD or MB, BS) of an Indian, Colonial or Foreign University recognised by the Examining Board in England but whose degrees were not recognisable in the United Kingdom".

Candidates were required also to have "held resident appointments in recognised general hospitals for not less than twelve months of which six months shall have been as a Resident Anaesthetist". This is a much reduced qualification from "the two years in a responsible anaesthetic post" originally proposed, and especially so when one remembers that there was no compulsory preregistration year of house appointments at that time. The required number of recorded anaesthetics was also reduced from 2,000 to 1,000, but a detailed list of the operations and type of anaesthesia was required with a confirmatory certificate, signed by the Senior Anaesthetist of a general hospital associated with a medical school, or the Senior Surgeon of any other recognised general hospital.

There were to be examinations in May and November each year and the subjects to be examined both in a written paper and in an oral examination were:-

(a) Human anatomy and physiology considered in relation to anaesthesia.

(b) The history, theory and practice of anaesthesia including - inhalation anaesthesia, intravenous, rectal, and other methods of inducing anaesthesia; local regional and spinal anaesthesia in all varieties; anaesthesia in relationship to disease.

(c) Pre-operative investigation, preparation and medication; the recognition of post-operative complications and their treatment in so far as they are related to anaesthesia.

(d) The pharmacology and elementary chemistry of drugs used for, or in association with, anaesthesia.

A note followed to the effect that candidates would be required to demonstrate their knowledge of the use of various types of apparatus employed in anaesthesia.[68]

The first examination was held on 8 November 1935. There were two examiners, both anaesthetists. C W Morris (nominated by the Royal College of Physicians of London) and H E G Boyle[51] (nominated by the Royal College of Surgeons of England). The examination fee was £6.6s.0d (1996: £240). The last examination fee for Part 1 of the examination for the Diploma of Fellowship of the Royal College of Anaesthetists (the equivalent of the original Diploma in Anaesthetics), which was discontinued in 1996, was £265.

There were 46 successful candidates at the first examination, of whom seven were ladies and two were future Presidents of the Association (John Gillies and Ronald Jarman). Other subsequently famous names in the group were H J Brennan of Manchester, W S McConnell of Guy's Hospital and M D Nosworthy of St Thomas'.[69]

The *British Journal of Anaesthesia* published some of the questions from the paper set in the first examination "as a guide to future candidates".[69] These were:-

1. *Give the points for and against spinal anaesthesia. Describe the technique which you employ, with doses.*

2. *You are called to a case of intestinal obstruction with almost constant vomiting. It is decided to do an exploratory laparotomy. What will you do? Describe in detail.*

3. *Write a short essay on the history and present position of rectal anaesthesia and analgesia.*

4. *What premedication and anaesthetic would you employ in a case of bad toxic goitre?*

Questions one and two would not be out of place in a modern examination, but the technique defined in the third question is almost obsolete, and 4 would be phrased differently in the light of modern preoperative preparation.

Award of the Diploma in Anaesthetics without examination

The proposal of the Council of the Association of Anaesthetists that Visiting Anaesthetists to teaching hospitals who had been in post for at least ten years should be granted the Diploma in Anaesthetics without examination was accepted, but not without some opposition, particularly from the Royal College of Physicians. The Council minute for the meeting of 8 February 1935[42] records that it was only agreed to after Claude Morris, who represented the Association, had been strongly supported by Mr Victor Bonney representing the Royal College of Surgeons. A time-limit was put on the concession however (three years from the publication of the regulations on 1 May 1935). The award of the Diploma without examination was to be made by the two "Royal Colleges on the recommendation of the Examining Board".[42] The first list of 16 leading teaching hospital anaesthetists to be awarded the Diploma without examination appeared in the October 1935 *British Journal of Anaesthesia* but neither of the two examiners (Boyle and

Morris) were included![69] This surprising omission is remedied in the full list published the next year;[70] presumably by then they had come up with their six guineas! One hundred and thirty seven diplomas were awarded without examination. One hundred and five of these were to anaesthetists from the medical schools of the British Isles, 12 were from Australia, 8 from Canada, 7 from India, 2 each from New Zealand and South Africa and one each from Malta and Egypt.[70-72]

The minutes of the Council meeting of 18 February 1938[42] report correspondence with the Examining Board about the possibility of extending the deadline for applications for the award of the Diploma without examination. Council were of the opinion that the date should not be postponed but decided to ask the Examining Board to take permanent power to award the Diploma to "certain specialist anaesthetists of distinction". The President (Blomfield),[2] the Honorary Secretary (Featherstone)[1] and Ivan Magill[65] were asked to meet the Management Committee of the Examining Board to convey their views. It was reported to Council on 7 July 1938 that, in the event, the Examining Board had postponed the deadline temporarily, but declined to set up permanent machinery for the award of the Diploma without examination.[42]

An Editorial in the April 1939 issue of the *British Journal of Anaesthesia*,[73] presumably written by Blomfield,[2] records that the time had finally expired for applications for the award of the Diploma without examination. It goes on to regret the "hard cases"; for example those who have failed to reach the required ten years by "a few months or even, perhaps, a few weeks", or those whose hospital was not recognised as fulfilling the necessary requirements, or individuals who can not furnish evidence of having given the necessary number of major anaesthetics. It is of further interest that the Editorial also foreshadows the conduct of overseas examinations, but only, at that stage, to accommodate candidates from the far flung corners of the British Empire such as Canada, Australia and New Zealand.[73]

The hardest case of all with regard to the award of the Diploma without examination was that of Professor (Sir) Robert Macintosh. His situation obviously caused considerable embarrassment to Council (11 May 1939).[42] Macintosh was the nominee of Lord Nuffield for the Chair of Anaesthetics which he had endowed in the University of Oxford. The reasons for this nomination included Nuffield's own experience as a patient who had personally experienced Macintosh's skill as an anaesthetist, and the ability of the great industrialist as a shrewd judge of men.[14,15] The minor specialist hospital appointments which Macintosh had in London at the time of his appointment, and which he had not held for the requisite period in any case even when added to the two years he had already spent as Professor since 1937, did not qualify him for the award of the Diploma without examination.[74] Robert Macintosh's appointment can not have been exactly popular with the well established teaching hospital anaesthetists in London at the time either; however, they had the good grace to nominate him for election to the Council of the Association at the Sixth Annual General Meeting on 29 October 1937.[42] It is to Macintosh's great credit, and typical of the man, that he sat and passed the examination for the Diploma of Anaesthetics in November 1939 shortly after the outbreak of the Second World War, at the same time as Freda Pratt, his assistant and co-author of *Essentials of Anaesthesia*.[72,75] One wonders whether the candidate or the examiners were put to the greater test!

The administration of anaesthesia and analgesia by nurses and midwives

The Association Council was naturally opposed to the administration of general anaesthesia by persons who were not medically qualified. Considerable concern was expressed when the matron of a nursing home offered her services as an anaesthetist in a circular letter. The Council, after considering the matter, called it to the attention of the Medical Defence Union and the BMA who took action (Council 15 December 1933 and the General Meeting 11 May 1934).[42]

Coroners also generally disapproved of the administration of anaesthetics by nurses and others who were not medically qualified.[76] It is, however, of interest that isolated instances of the employment of nurses as anaesthetists did not cease completely in the United Kingdom, particularly in East Anglia, until the nineteen fifties (A K Adams, Cambridge, C H M Woollam, Norwich, H Rex Marrett, Coventry: personal communications), and the administration of brief out-patient nitrous oxide "gases" by a nurse assisting a dentist was also not uncommon (author: personal experience as a patient).

The administration of analgesia by midwives to allay the pains of labour was, however, a different matter. It is to the credit of the Association of Anaesthetists that its Council took an enlightened view of this practice.[42] It should be remembered that, in the early nineteen thirties, domestic delivery by midwives was at its zenith. Later on, however, there was a tendency for domiciliary obstetrics for the lower income groups to pass from general practitioner control to local authority clinics and municipal and voluntary hospitals. This trend was further accelerated by the passage of the 1936 Midwives' Act.[8]

It was presumably in this context, and in the period of consultation preceding the passage of the 1936 Act, that Howard Jones, Honorary Secretary, introduced the following motion on the subject at the Second Annual General Meeting on 20 October 1933[42,77]:-

"That this General Meeting of the Association of Anaesthetists of Great Britain and Ireland views with concern any increase in the administration of anaesthetics by unqualified persons as a danger to the public; and hopes that if the practice is to be extended to midwives it will only be allowed under strict regulations and after adequate instruction".

It is noteworthy that the motion did not distinguish between general anaesthesia and analgesia. It is clear from the context, however, that it was the latter which was the main concern. Howard Jones stated that the issue had become critical because the suggestion was made that chloroform capsules should be authorised for use by midwives. These capsules consisted of a glass ampoule containing 4oz (120ml) of chloroform surrounded by a gauze cover; when the ampoule was broken the patient could inhale from the cloth. The capsules were given extensive trials.[77-79] Mennell reported that up to 129 had been used in one case![56] The capsules were never authorised for use by midwives but they were issued in the Second World War to provide temporary analgesia for extracting crew members from burning armoured fighting vehicles.[80] Howard Jones feared that the authorisation of the use of chloroform capsules for midwives might lead to the use of chloroform by them in other forms;[77] obviously this was quite a possibility as Mennell demonstrated his version of Junker's air-chloroform vaporiser at the 1933 Annual General Meeting and suggested that midwives might be authorised to administer chloroform.[42] R J Minnitt[81] of Liverpool gave what must have been one of the first public demonstrations of his apparatus for the self-administration of nitrous oxide air for the relief of labour pains at the same meeting. This apparatus ultimately provided the official and generally accepted solution to the problem of the use of analgesia by midwives for many years.[82] The use of a concentration of 10% oxygen in this, or any other anaesthetic context, would be considered inexcusable in the nineteen nineties, but it must be realised that the use of 7% to 10% oxygen mixtures was not unusual in general anaesthetic practice at that time, and little harm seems to have come of it.[10] The Minute Book shows that the Association of Anaesthetists worked with the British (now Royal) College of Obstetrics and Gynaecology and the Central Midwives Board before the technique was authorised for use by midwives in 1935.[42,83]

The Association of Anaesthetists continued to be concerned about the general level of instruction and the remuneration of anaesthetists who lectured to midwives for several years after the technique was authorised (Council 22 January 1937).[42,43] Hospital trials continued throughout the thirties but, despite the authorisation by the Central Midwives Board for the use of "gas and air" in 1935, it was not until after the Second World War that it was generally used in domestic practice.[8]

Coroners' inquests

Public and medical professional disquiet were aroused in the early thirties because of the unfair way in which some coroners conducted their inquiries, and their use of their ancient privileges to condemn or criticise individuals and organisations who had no legal means of defence or remedy.[84]

The concern was general but anaesthetists had particular grounds for complaint. Their dissatisfaction was expressed both in the *British Journal of Anaesthesia* and at the Second Annual Meeting in 1933.[42,85] They were unhappy, first, because many coroners invariably held inquests on every death under an anaesthetic, even when it could be attributed to the condition of the patient or surgical intervention; secondly a common verdict was that "the patient died from an anaesthetic given in a proper manner for a proper operation", even though the death might have been due to the patient's disease or condition, surgical shock or loss of blood; and thirdly, because the anaesthetist was invariably called to give evidence and rarely the surgeon, even when the death was due to a surgical mishap. The consequence of all these procedures was unfair publicity for the anaesthetist, with possible serious professional and financial consequences.[85,86]

A subcommittee to consider the matter was appointed at the Council Meeting on 15 December 1933. This was composed of Blomfield, (the Vice President),[2] Mennell (Honorary Treasurer)[3] and R E Apperly, a Council Member from the Middlesex Hospital, London.[87] Mennell reported, at the Third Annual General Meeting on 31 October 1934, that he had had correspondence with Sir Russell Scott, the Permanent Under-Secretary of State at the Home Office and with two of the under-secretaries who had "seemed sympathetic", and had agreed to forward copies of Council Subcommittee recommendations to the Ministry of Health.[42] This correspondence was doubtless one of the factors which prompted the Home Office to take action. Sir John Gilmour, the Home Secretary, announced in Parliament on 29 January 1935 that he had decided to appoint a committee to inquire into the conduct of coroners' inquests.[88]

Magill[65,66] was coopted on to the "Coroners Subcommittee" of the Association on 8 February 1935 (probably because he "knew somebody") and agreed to seek an interview with Sir John Gilmour.[42] Sir John announced that Lord Wright would chair the Committee of Inquiry and gave the names of its members on 28 February 1935. The terms of reference were to be "to inquire into the law and practice relating to coroners, and to report what changes, if any, are desirable and practicable".[89] Magill reported to Council on his interview with the Home Secretary on 22 March 1935. The President (Featherstone)[1] wrote to the Home Office asking that the Association of Anaesthetists should give evidence to Lord Wright's Committee. Featherstone, Mennell and Magill reported to Council on 5 July 1935 that they had been interviewed by the Committee of Inquiry for over 3½ hours and had also presented written evidence. Magill had entertained Featherstone and Mennell to lunch at the Savoy after the session.[42,90]

The report of the Committee on Coroners was published on 7 February 1936.[86] The section on Deaths under Anaesthetics was very satisfactory. The report repeated the evidence of the Association and then recommended that although "the Registrar-General's regulations require registrars to report to the coroner any deaths after an operation, necessitated by injury, or under an anaesthetic, or before recovery from the effects of an anaesthetic", such deaths "should not be regarded as violent or unnatural simply because an anaesthetic was given or an operation performed"; in these circumstances the coroner should have discretion to dispense with an inquest or necropsy if he was satisfied that "the operation has been performed and the anaesthetic given with reasonable care", but, in taking his decision, he must "be obliged to have regard to any views expressed by the relatives". If the coroner required a necropsy a pathologist from outside the hospital should perform it; if however the coroner did not require a postmortem the hospital should be informed, so that an examination could be made for scientific purposes. The general section of the report also states:-

"...the Committee strongly condemns the tendency of some coroners to animadvert upon the conduct of persons who come under their notice. A man has at law a right to preserve his reputation unassailed, but the coroner enjoys absolute privilege for any defamatory remarks he may make".[86]

Featherstone was certainly correct, when he emphasised, in presenting the report to Council at the Fifth Annual General Meeting on 30 October 1936, that the Committee of Inquiry, which had made extensive use of evidence provided by the Association representatives, showed in its report that it had been "much influenced by that evidence".[42]

Other business 1932-1939

The General Medical Council Curriculum Committee were persuaded to alter their requirement for the instruction of undergraduates from "a minimum of 10 anaesthetics administered under supervision" to "a course on theoretical and practical instruction in the administration of anaesthetics" (Council 3 April and Annual General Meeting 30 October 1936).

The British Journal of Anaesthesia was suggested by Mennell as being suitable for formal association with the Association of Anaesthetists at the Council meeting on 20 December 1935, but this was resisted by the Editor,

Joseph Blomfield, who pointed out that the meetings of the Association were already fully reported.[42] This confirms the reputation amongst his contemporaries of Blomfield's sturdy independence so far as both the editorial and business management of the *British Journal of Anaesthesia* were concerned!

There is, however, a rather ambiguous minute for the meeting of the Council of the Association of Anaesthetists of 23 September 1938. A tentative proposal was made to reduce the subscription from £1 to 10s (1996: from £35 to £17.50)! This was presumably in view of the satisfactory financial position of the Association. It was decided not to take any action; one of the reasons given for this was the possibility of reducing (subsidising?) the subscription which anaesthetists paid to the *British Journal of Anaesthesia*. Confirmatory evidence that all may not have been entirely well with the finances of the *Journal* at that time is suggested by the fact that on 11 May 1939 the Council of the Association voted £25 (1996: £867) as a donation to the *British Journal of Anaesthesia*, after Blomfield stated that his Editorial Board would welcome a donation.[42]

The construction and colour coding of medical gas cylinders was one of the few matters concerning equipment with which Council concerned itself in the prewar period.

A very early project of Featherstone's[1] was the promotion of the manufacture of light weight "Vibrac" steel gas cylinders; a topic which he introduced at the first Annual General Meeting on 28 October 1932. He cooperated in the ensuing year with Dr C M Walter, Research Engineer of the Birmingham Gas Company, Colonel Walker of Vickers-Armstrong, and Colonel Thomas of the Home Office and, at the Second Annual General Meeting on 20 October 1933, he was able to report that the cylinders had been authorised as gas containers for anaesthetic work.[42] These cylinders ultimately became the standard pattern, but this took many years because they were very much more expensive than those originally in use.

The Association of Anaesthetists appears to have taken independent action about a colour code for "cylinders, reducing valves and rubber tubing leading therefrom". A Subcommittee was appointed consisting of C Langton Hewer of St Bartholomew's[91] and M D Nosworthy of St Thomas'.[92] Their original recommendations were reported to the Sixth Annual General Meeting on 29 October 1937, but these were subsequently revised by Council on 18 February 1938 to conform more closely with those already used in the United Kingdom by the principal manufacturers of anaesthetic apparatus of the day (Coxeters, British Oxygen Company, A Charles King and Imperial Chemical Industries). Langton Hewer was not altogether happy because the colours finally chosen were different from those used in foreign countries (Council 23 September 1938) but Council nevertheless accepted them.[42] This code was subsequently in operation in British spheres of influence until 1952 when another attempt to reach international agreement was made.[93,94] The United Kingdom colours of 1938 and 1952 are compared below. Full international agreement has never been achieved.

Medical Gas	**1938**	**1952**
Oxygen	Black with white top	Black with white top
Nitrous oxide	Black	French blue
Carbon dioxide	Green	Grey
Oxygen with Carbon dioxide mixture	Black with green top	Black with grey and white shoulder quadrants
Cyclopropane	Silver with red top	Orange

Clinical questions were not generally considered to be within the remit of the Association except in answer to specific inquiries.[90] Council did, however, advise J Glover, Senior Medical Officer to the Board of Education that the use of chloroform and chloroform mixtures in Local Authority children's tonsillectomy clinics was undesirable except for individual children in very exceptional circumstances (Council Meeting 16 March 1934).[42]

The discussions on the use of nitrous oxide and oxygen by midwives had medicopolitical consequences. These have already been considered.

Summary: the early years 1932-1939

Harry Featherstone, the Founder President, and by then the Honorary Secretary, of the Association of Anaesthetists of Great Britain and Ireland must have felt well satisfied with the achievements of the Association at the conclusion of the Council meeting on 11 May 1939.[42] The meeting had gone

Summary: the early years 1932-1939 61

smoothly. Discussion had been mainly about routine matters. It was true that a number of problems were not yet resolved, but progress was being made by continued discussion and diplomacy. There was no doubt, however, that the Association of Anaesthetists had firmly established itself as the political voice of the specialty of anaesthesia in the United Kingdom, to which government, other public bodies, and specialist anaesthetists themselves turned for guidance, and that was something for which Featherstone was modestly both proud and thankful.[90]

An exciting new departure for the Association had also been considered at that May 1939 meeting. This was a projected joint scientific meeting sponsored in conjunction with the Section of Anaesthetics of the Royal Society of Medicine and the BMA under the Presidency of Professor (Sir) Robert Macintosh.[14] This was to be organised to follow an International Congress of Anaesthetists which was to be held in Paris in the July of the following year (1940). The ambitious proposal was for a meeting in London on Friday and Saturday the 19 and 20 of July with a Dinner on the Friday hosted by the Association of Anaesthetists, a meeting in Oxford on the Monday 22 July, and further papers at the BMA meeting in Birmingham on the 23, 24 and 25 July 1940.[42]

So much for "the best laid schemes o'mice an' men"![95] Before July 1940 France had fallen to the German war machine and Lieutenant Colonel Harry Featherstone[1] had resumed his distinguished military career, and had been evacuated from Boulogne by sea under heavy bombardment (Appendix A); meanwhile the Association of Anaesthetists of Great Britain and Ireland found itself with new tasks and heavy responsibilities. The Association and its members rose magnificently to the occasion.

5

War and Peace

3 September 1939 to 31 December 1948

"This is not the end......,
It is perhaps the end of the beginning"

Winston Churchill (1874-1965)
Speech at the Mansion House 10 November 1942

The Executive Officers

Presidents:-	Z Mennell (1938-1941)[1]
	A S Daly (1941-1944)[2]
	A D Marston (1944-1947)[3]
	J Gillies (1947-1950)[4]
Honorary Treasurers : -	H S Sington (1938-1941)[5]
	Z Mennell (1941-1947)[1]
	B Johnson (1947-1950)[6]
Honorary Secretaries : -	J Blomfield (1939-1941)[7]
	A D Marston (1941-1944)[3]
	W A Low (1944-1948)[8]
	G S W Organe (1948-1952)[9]

Editor of *Anaesthesia*:-C Langton Hewer (1946-1966)[10]

War and peace, and reform in post-war Britain

The dates 3 September 1939 to the 31 December 1948 mark out a period of dramatic change in the history of the United Kingdom. Six years of total war, fought on many fronts world-wide, were followed by several years of austerity; during this period a start was made at home, both in repairing the physical ravages resulting directly from the conflict, and in laying the foundations of a new social order. The ambitious aim was to abolish the worst consequences of poverty, and to ensure equal opportunities for all; in particular, the reform of the social services was to include a National Health Service (NHS) available free at the point of use to everyone regardless of income.[11-13]

The end of the war in 1945, first with Germany and her allies and then with Japan, did not represent a dramatic watershed before which the national effort was totally dedicated to the defeat of the enemy and after which undivided attention was given to reconstruction, or rather to rejuvenation and reform. The planners did not aim to put the clock back to the start of the war in 1939, but to create a greatly improved environment and new social conditions. Britain also still had vast commitments abroad. Some reduction in the armed services was possible, but a large civil service and military force was still required both for administering India and the colonies, and to enable her to play her part in policing the British Empire, as well as for the military occupation of Germany and Austria. The nature of the armed services began to change in character after 1945 however. The mature, comparatively young but experienced middle-aged men who had willingly been recruited for the global war, were rapidly demobilised. They were replaced by youthful conscript National Servicemen who had grown up during the conflict;[14] at the same time, as experienced specialists in the medical services returned to civilian life, they were replaced by recent graduates with the minimum of postgraduate training, or even none at all as there was not as yet a statutory year of provisional registration.

The origins of the National Health Service

Serious planning for the development of British social services had actually begun in the darkest days of the war. The public had been encouraged by the 1942 report of Sir William Beveridge on "Social Insurance and allied services", although it is said that the coalition government of the day were less enthusiastic![11,12,15]

The health care recommendations of the Beveridge Report (1942) ultimately became the blueprint for the NHS which was introduced with great tenacity and skill by Aneurin Bevan, the Health Minister in the postwar Labour Government. The main elements for the provision of an integrated health care scheme existed in 1939 before the outbreak of the Second World War, but their administration was chaotically divided between several central and local government authorities, the voluntary hospitals, and other charitable and independent organisations.[11,12]

The Emergency Medical Service (EMS) was the result of extensive prewar planning accelerated by the narrow escape from war at the time of the Munich crisis at the end of 1938.[11,16,17] The EMS scheme came into being at the outbreak of war in September 1939. It was organised on a Sector (Regional) basis. The initial aim was to provide a large number of emergency beds in city centres for the immediate care of civilian air raid casualties by evacuating routine and convalescent patients to hospitals in the periphery in safer areas; by reason of its country-wide organisation however, which involved the mobilisation of all acute hospitals both voluntary and municipal, the EMS became, in effect, a National Hospital Service. The EMS could certainly not have been so quickly embodied except by the exercise of the near dictatorial emergency powers assumed by the wartime government. The report on the Public Health Service after six years of war stated: -

"From a heterogeneous collection of over 3000 medical institutions of various grades under a variety of systems of administration, upwards of 1000 hospitals, well equipped and efficiently staffed, as far as the shortage of man and woman power would permit, had been welded into a homogeneous hospital service".[16]

Three important services organised by the Medical Research Council also came into being in parallel with the EMS.[11,12] These were destined to have inestimable benefits both during the war and in the peace which has followed. They were the Public Health Laboratory Service, the Hospital Laboratory Service, and the Civilian Blood Transfusion Service.

Things could never be the same again. The EMS structure was retained after the end of the war in 1945 and ultimately formed the Regional basis of the NHS in 1948.

The great increase in emergency trauma occasioned by the war made it necessary to recruit salaried anaesthetists for the EMS hospitals.[11,12,17,18] Many older general practitioner anaesthetists and others unfit for service in the armed forces (especially those with the Diploma in Anaesthetics) took up wholetime specialist posts with the EMS, which ultimately led to Consultant appointments in the NHS after the war. One such was a future President of the Association of Anaesthetists J Alfred Lee.[18] The first edition of the "anaesthetists' bible", Lee's *Synopsis of Anaesthesia* appeared in 1947 at the conclusion of his service with the EMS.[19] The book has now run to eleven English editions (ten with Lee as the sole author or as co-author) and numerous foreign language and pirated versions.[19] The contribution of the EMS to the war effort was greatly undervalued. Few honours were awarded to its staff after the war although they gave devoted care to their patients and worked very long hours. They were also sometimes under aerial bombardment, and certainly a number of them saw more action than many of those who joined the medical branches of the armed services! They also had at times to endure the suspicion sometimes engendered in the minds of the uninformed, because they were not in uniform, although amongst their patients were many soldiers, sailors and airmen in special military wards.

The Association and civilian medical organisation in the Second World War

The minutes of the first ("emergency") Council Meeting held on 27 October 1939 contain two items relating to the wartime administration of the civilian medical services.[20]

The Chairman of the Central Emergency Committee of the BMA had written in reply to a letter from the President of the Association of Anaesthetists (Mennell) looking with favour on the inclusion of an anaesthetist on his Committee, but the Secretary of the BMA had written rather deprecating the possibility. Once again the BMA seemed to look both ways like the god Janus!

The President (Mennell),[1] the Honorary Secretary (Blomfield)[7] and the Honorary Treasurer Harold S Sington (Honorary Anaesthetists to the Hospital for Sick Children, Great Ormond Street)[5] also wrote a letter to the Ministry of Health advocating the appointment of a "representative adviser" in anaesthetics.[20]

There is a report in the Council meeting of 13 August 1940 that a "satisfactory arrangement" had been made with the "Medical War Committee". The names of the committees are confusing but amalgamation probably occurred in the interests of efficiency. Mennell[1] (in his last report before handing over the Presidency to Lieutenant Colonel Ashley Daly[2] at the Annual General Meeting 28 October 1941) states that he has attended every meeting of the Central Medical War Committee as the Association representative and, in the Annual Report for 1943, Brigadier Ashley Daly[2] informs us that Mennell (then once again the Honorary Treasurer)[2] was a member of the Grading Committee of the Central Medical War Committee.[20] This was an important appointment; it enabled Mennell to give guidance on the award of "specialist" and "graded" status to anaesthetists who deserved such distinctions and to them alone. Mennell reported at the Annual General Meeting on 28 October 1941 that he had caused a sensation at a Central Medical War Committee by pointing out that "some flagrant misfits" had been appointed as specialist anaesthetists in the EMS at the beginning of the war on thei own personal assessment alone.[20]

It is clear that the Association of Anaesthetists of Great Britain and Ireland was the only recognised authority for anaesthesia on the civil side in the United Kingdom during the Second World War, and that much of the credit for this must go to Zebulon Mennell, first as President and then once again as Honorary Treasurer.[1]

The Association and anaesthesia in the Armed Services 1939-1945

The vast expansion in the medical branches of the armed services made necessary by the outbreak of the Second World War was achieved initially by an influx of experienced civilian practitioners of all grades and disciplines, who took over the clinical care of the soldiers, sailors and airmen. Crowns, pips, and rings descended like confetti on the shoulders and sleeves of the cadre of promoted regular and senior reserve medical officers; they took on administrative staff appointments and the command of hospitals and other medical units. The army, for example, had "only five regular medical officers with the Diploma in Anaesthetics, only two of whom were employed in their specialty at the outset of war, and even these were transferred to administrative posts after a few months".[21] Featherstone, the founder President and a senior officer in the Territorial Army Reserve, spent the war in command of a hospital ship and other units and not as an anaesthetist.

A very important item of business was conducted at that first ("emergency") meeting of Council after the outbreak of the Second World War on 27 October 1939.[20] This was to approve a report of correspondence which was to have a profound effect on status of anaesthetists during and after the war. Mennell[1] (the President) had received a letter from "an authoritative military source" inquiring "what constituted the status of a specialist anaesthetist". The reply which Mennell had dispatched on his own initiative was endorsed by Council. It read : -

"In reply to your letter to me as President of the Association of Anaesthetists, the answers to your questions are as follows: -

(a) Any anaesthetist on the staff of any London or big Hospital included in the Cambridge list [Chapter 3] should be considered a specialist.

(b) As regards the small London and Provincial Hospitals, many of the anaesthetists employed at these hospitals are General Practitioners and I do not think they come in to this category.

(c) Any man who has got the specialist DA [Diploma in Anaesthetics] can be safely considered a specialist."[20]

This is the first time that Council equated the possession of the DA with specialist status other than by reason of a teaching hospital appointment; previously, and for several years afterwards, the Association declined to accept the DA alone as a qualification for full membership; as recently as 1 June 1937, Council had not felt able to insist that candidates for hospital appointments should have passed the DA examination.[20] Mennell's action ensured that those who were properly qualified with the Diploma should take their place as specialists with the rank of Major, Squadron Leader or Lieutenant Commander in the Armed Services. It is fortunate that he acted when he did ahead of the Council meeting. Featherstone tells us that the date that the military authorities decreed that specialists including anaesthetists should be gazetted as Majors (or the equivalent in the other services) was 13 September 1939.[22] It is noteworthy that Transfusion Officers did not achieve recognition as specialists until after the cessation of hostilities in 1945, despite their universally acknowledged skills in resuscitation and pre-operative selection in the special resuscitation wards which they controlled.[23] It is interesting too, that, in the multiple casualty military situation in the 1939-1945 war, the work of the anaesthetist was largely confined to the operating theatre in the larger hospital units, whereas in postwar practice, the very essential pre-operative functions of the transfusion (resuscitation) officer specialists have been largely taken over by anaesthetists.

The position with regard to the higher direction and support of anaesthetists in the Army and the Royal Air Force (RAF) at the beginning of the war was not at all satisfactory. Anaesthetists in both these services had come under the jurisdiction of the Directors of Surgery in peacetime and, in addition, there was a policy, particularly in the RAF, of avoiding training medical officers as specialists devoting their time solely to the administration of anaesthesia.[21,24] Neither service had appointed civilian consultants in anaesthesia before the war, and much of the available equipment was archaic and based on the concepts of the Great War 1914-1918.[21,24]

Daly[2] tells us that, because of the absence of a civilian consultant or military adviser "a large number of officers with few or no credentials were created specialists in the early days of the [Second World] War!"[21] It was fortunate that Ashley Daly, who had served as a medical officer in the Great War 1914-1918, joined the Royal Army Medical Corps (RAMC) again at the beginning of the war and was posted as a specialist Major to the headquarters' hospital at Millbank, London; from this position he was able to provide unofficial advice. He was appointed Adviser in Anaesthetics to the War Office in February 1941 as a Lieutenant Colonel, and thereafter was able to do a great deal to upgrade anaesthesia and the status of anaesthetists in the Army. He was later promoted to the rank of Brigadier as Consultant in Anaesthesia to the Army.[21,25]

Professor (Sir) Robert Macintosh, who had been a Royal Flying Corps pilot in the 1914-1918 war,[26] was appointed civilian consultant to the Royal Air Force (RAF) in May 1941, and he accepted a commission as an Air Commodore in the RAF as its Consultant in the following October.[24] Thereafter he tirelessly raised the standards of anaesthesia in the RAF to a high level. He also held a watching brief over the affairs of the Royal Navy.

Brigadier Daly[2] was President of the Association from 1941-1944, Air Commodore Macintosh[26] was a Council Member, as were several other serving officers including Major Vernon Hall, a future President; together with Mennell[1] in the civilian Central Medical War Committee, the Officers of the Association of Anaesthetists certainly had a very considerable influence.

The Army and the Royal Air Force had similar training systems. Advisers were appointed in every command throughout the world. They conducted short courses and arranged attachments for young anaesthetists under their supervision at base hospitals. These trainees then went as "graded specialists" to the Field Surgical Teams and Casualty Clearing Stations. A number of these trainees managed to pass the examination for the Diploma in Anaesthetics during their training, and many of them became civilian Consultants when the British National Health Service came into being in 1948.[25]

Special mention must be made of the organisation of anaesthesia in the Indian Army.[27] The subcontinent had a Consultant Adviser of its own. This was Brigadier Harold K Ashworth, originally from Manchester and later of Charing Cross Hospital London, an enthusiastic reserve officer of long standing and a Member of Council of the Association from 1934-1937.[28] Five outstanding advisers (originally majors, later lieutenant colonels) were responsible for the supervision and training in the various Indian regions. They were William S McConnell [29] and T A B Harris [30], both of Guy's Hospital, London, R E Pleasance [31] of Sheffield, Vernon F Hall of Kings College Hospital, London, and Victor A Goldman of the Eastman Dental Clinic, London. Ashworth and McConnell were Founder Members of the Association and Harris, Pleasance and Hall were prewar Members. Goldman was not a Member before the war, presumably because his hospital appointments did not meet the original peculiar requirements (Chapter 3), but he became a

Member during the war and a Fellow in 1950 when various changes had been made in the regulations. Vernon Hall was to become President of the Association and he and Goldman have subsequently been elected to Honorary Membership. Vernon Hall ultimately achieved the rank of Brigadier as Director of Anaesthesia in India and South East Asia on the staff of Lord Louis Mountbatten. He has written a fascinating account of the activities of the Army Anaesthetists in India and South East Asia.[27] Each adviser ran courses to produce graded specialists and visited, assessed, and encouraged the anaesthetists in the field for whom he was responsible; as a result of highly organised team work, 216 clinical anaesthetists were in post in India by the end of the war in 1945; amongst them was Philip Helliwell, later Consultant at Guy's Hospital, London and President of the Association. The RAF medical field commitment in India and the Far East was naturally rather more limited, but they too supplied Mobile Field Hospitals in which specialist and graded anaesthetists played their full part.[32]

Many graded anaesthetists found themselves in Field Surgical Teams (FSTs) in all theatres of war. These small units had two or three officers - a surgeon and an anaesthetist and, optionally, a transfusion officer - and five or six other ranks. Their function was to be attached flexibly to larger units (Field Hospitals or Casualty Clearing Stations) to augment their surgical potential as the military situation demanded. Some of these units were specialised (e.g. maxillo-facial or neurosurgical FSTs). In the early part of the war tradition demanded that the surgeon should command the unit, whether or not he was junior or senior as an officer or a specialist relative to the anaesthetist. It was found later that, while an inexperienced surgeon could usually rise to the occasion with the aid of an experienced anaesthetist, the reverse was more difficult and command was given to "the officer most suited by seniority and temperament". Anaesthetists undoubtedly gained greatly in status and respect from other disciplines during the war when the great value of their work was realised.[27] This had important consequences in its negotiations which preceded the establishment of the NHS in the immediate postwar period.

Reference should be made to the use of specially trained nurses, orderlies and others to assist in monitoring patients under anaesthesia in mass or multiple casualty situations or even during routine work. Nurses and orderlies were so trained and used in the Second World War[24,33] as also in later conflicts.[34,35] Macintosh[26] was a strong advocate of this practice; in his opinion:-

"....a single anaesthetist could be better served if assisted by well-trained orderlies than if assisted by an occasional medical officer, particularly when large numbers of casualties have to be treated".[24]

Macintosh tells us that, after the Normandy landings in 1944, at the RAF Hospital at Halton, one skilled medical anaesthetist was able to deal with 38 major casualties in 10 hours "using simple apparatus with the help of trained orderlies".[24] There is no doubt that this is true, but there is a wealth of difference between the nurse or orderly supervised by a physician anaesthetist and the nurse or orderly nominally supervised by the surgeon. The Association of Anaesthetists has several times in its history had to ward off suggestions that the British tradition of physician anaesthetist should be modified. One such challenge caused deep concern to the Council of the Association in August 1940, in the run up to the introduction of the British NHS and on several subsequent occasions.[20,36] The citation of such circumstances as outlined above is unjustified as an argument for nurse anaesthesia as Macintosh later pointed out (see below).[37]

The Royal Navy had somewhat different medical problems to the other armed services in the Second World War.[37] Anaesthesia in base hospitals reflected contemporary clinical practice but, as Surgeon Commander Woolmer[38] pointed out, in those days before helicopter evacuation to larger vessels or shore establishments was available, the single medical officer in a small fighting ship could only use the simplest of techniques. He also tells us that, so stringent were the demands of man-power that, it was not found possible to organise courses of instruction for more than ten medical officers during the war years, though others were given extempore instruction in techniques best suited to the conditions.[37] Surgeon Commander Ronald F Woolmer wrote a short but valuable monograph *Anaesthetics Afloat*;[39] after the war he became the first British Oxygen Professor of Anaesthesia at the Royal College of Surgeons in England in 1959. He had a brilliant and innovative mind, but died prematurely at the age of 54 years.[38]

Clinical Anaesthesia 1939-1949

The introduction of curare to modern anaesthetic practice is usually dated from the publication of the classic paper by Harold Griffith[40] and Enid Johnson of Montreal, Canada in 1942.[41] This was not the first time that intravenous curare had been used for muscular relaxation in anaesthesia,[42] but neither was Morton's seminal demonstration of ether anaesthesia in 1846 the first use of general anaesthesia, or the use of ether as an anaesthetic.[43] The important facts are that Morton's demonstration established general anaesthesia as being a practical proposition; in the same way Griffith and Johnson's paper led to the general acceptance of the use of curare, first in the form of the Squibb preparation Intocostrin, and then as d-tubocurarine chloride. There the parallel ends however. Griffith's curare was much more slowly accepted than Morton's ether. Curare had in fact practically no influence on the techniques employed during the Second World War 1939-1945. Woolmer states that "curare was used in one Royal Naval Hospital"[37] and it is not mentioned at all in Daly's and Macintosh's reports on anaesthesia in the Army and RAF respectively.[21,24] Griffith and Johnson did not, of course, employ curare with respiratory paralysis and controlled respiration either. They used it as an adjuvant in the spontaneously respiring patient, and seem to have been mildly surprised that they did not encounter respiratory depression in their first twenty-five cases. They attributed this to the fact that pharmaceutical purification had eliminated the respiratory depressant effect of curare![41]

It has become customary also to date the development of the modern paralysis and controlled respiration technique from the publication of the paper presented by Gray and Halton of Liverpool to the Anaesthetic Section of the Royal Society of Medicine on 1 March 1946.[44] Perusal of this communication, however, and of the report of the discussion which followed it, shows that, though truly a "milestone" as the title of the paper implies, the Liverpool team had at that stage not completed their journey. Two of the three techniques described in the 1946 paper are examples of "lissive" anaesthesia employing curare with spontaneous respiration. Controlled respiration, though frequently employed in the third technique, is only used as necessary; moreover the speaker tells us that the antidote *physo*stigmine has only been used on two occasions, "and that they were not impressed with its action".[44] A more advanced technique is described in Gray's paper in 1949; by then controlled respiration and the use reversal with the newly introduced *pro*stigmine was routine.[45] There is no doubt that, in the period covered by this chapter (1939-1948), the use of curare was limited and used almost exclusively as an adjuvant to anaesthesia for the spontaneously respiring patient.[46-49] General acceptance of the use of obligatory controlled ventilation with tubocurarine, and the other neuromuscular blocking agents which were subsequently developed, did not revolutionise the practice of anaesthesia until the early nineteen fifties,[49,50] as the present writer knows from personal experience.[49]

Clinical anaesthesia during the Second World War 1939-1945 in civilian and military base hospitals was a continuation of the progress achieved between the two world wars. There were, however, obvious logistic difficulties in terms of the availability of apparatus, compressed gases and drugs in mobile field units. The possibilities were reviewed in anticipation of war in an Editorial (presumably by Blomfield[7]) in the *British Journal of Anaesthesia* of July 1939.[51] Chloroform is condemned, the possible value of the use of intravenous barbiturates is considered, but with regard to the question of whether or not it would be appropriate to use them for shocked patients is left open; regret is also expressed that cyclopropane, with its many advantages is not likely to be available in forward areas.[51]

The greatest advantage which the anaesthetist of 1939-1945 enjoyed over his predecessor of the Great War of 1914-1918, was not in fact the advent of new anaesthetic techniques or agents, but the benefit bestowed by the development of efficient means of blood volume replacement and advances in chemotherapy, particularly the introduction of penicillin. It was now appreciated that acute wound shock was primarily due to overt or sequestered loss of circulating blood volume, and efficient technical apparatus and adequate supplies of blood and dried plasma were available for replacement.[23,52-55] The way in which the world-wide military and civilian transfusion services were organised deserves the highest praise.[23]

Intravenous barbiturates were widely used. They were administered by intermittent injection or continuous infusion alone, or in combination with light inhalation anaesthesia with ether and/or nitrous oxide. The portability of the apparatus (a syringe and needles) particularly appealed to anaesthetists under field conditions.[21,24,37,55] The often repeated statement that, as a consequence of the use of thiopentone and hexobarbitone, a great many hypovolaemic casualties died at Pearl Harbour in December 1941 after the Japanese air raid has certainly been exaggerated. Perusal of the short article by Halford in *Anesthesiology*, upon which this legend is based, suggests that thiopentone was administered to some of the earlier hypovolaemic casualties in inappropriately large doses, and that they succumbed either to respiratory obstruction or hypotension; later casualties were anaesthetised with open drop ether.[56] The same issue of *Anesthesiology*, in which Halford's article appears, includes a case report of the successful use of continuously administered incremental thiopentone to a patient with a large chest wound whose blood loss was at least partially replaced during the operation.[57] There is also a very common sense editorial,[58] and, incidentally, an article extolling the virtues of intravenous morphine.[59]

Draw-over apparatus, reviving the use of air with or without supplementary oxygen, as a carrier gas, was developed by Macintosh[26] and his colleagues at Oxford for use in the field (the Oxford vaporiser for ether and the ESO vaporiser for chloroform for airborne forces); 2700 Oxford vaporisers were manufactured by Lord Nuffield at Cowley motor car works.[60] This was the first time that an accurately calibrated, thermo-compensated anaesthetic vaporiser was combined with the means of assisting or controlling respiration. Oxford vaporisers gave valuable service in many parts of the world during the Second World War.[21,24,32,37,61]

Trichloroethylene was reintroduced into anaesthesia in 1941 by Christopher Langton Hewer[10], a Council Member of the Association and the future founder Editor of the Association journal *Anaesthesia*.[62,63] It was hoped that it would prove to be an inexpensive, less toxic, and non-flammable replacement for chloroform; unfortunately its use under service conditions was limited. This was because it was best employed as a supplement to nitrous oxide and oxygen for anaesthesia, but could not be used in the closed circuit with soda lime with which it formed toxic products, and this made it wasteful of limited gas supplies.[21] Its powerful analgesic properties later enabled trichloroethylene to be used in midwifery in the nineteen fifties and sixties using air draw-over vaporisers without the patient becoming unconscious. Trichloroethylene was also a very useful analgesic if used in this way for such procedures as major wound and burn dressings.[35] It was also used very successfully in the Tri-service draw-over apparatus in combination with halothane by the British Army in the Falklands Campaign in 1982,[64] but its manufacture has now been discontinued because of a fall in demand..

Research by the Nuffield Department at Oxford during the Second World War

The development of portable vaporisers by the Oxford Department has been mentioned already. Another piece of practical research led to the introduction of the Macintosh laryngoscope in 1943.[60,65] This is now the instrument universally preferred by anaesthetists world wide.

The collaboration of Air Commodore Macintosh[26] and Squadron Leader E A Pask[66] in a series of experiments connected with anoxia at altitude, artificial respiration, and the use of life-saving apparatus, is an amazing story of superlative courage and fortitude.[67] Pask became a member of the Nuffield Department in February 1940 but left to join the RAF Institute at Farnborough. Pask was frequently the subject of the investigations. He was anaesthetised by Macintosh, had apnoea induced by curare (an early use of the drug) and was flung into a swimming pool while unconscious as well as being parachuted into the North Sea.[60] Macintosh subsequently remarked that this was probably the only time that the author of a successful MD thesis was unconscious with his head under water at the time of the experiments upon which it depended.[67] The appointment as an OBE with which Pask was gazetted in 1944 was scarcely adequate acknowledgement for his outstanding bravery.

Pask became the first Professor of Anaesthetics in the University of Durham at Newcastle upon Tyne after the war and was Honorary Treasurer of the Association from 1960 until his sudden and premature death in 1966.[66] He himself was awarded one of the first John Snow Silver medals in 1946 and the Association Certificate of Honour has been named after him.[68]

The business of Council 1939-1948

The first meeting of Council after the outbreak of hostilities on 3 September 1939 was the "emergency" meeting held on 27 October at the rooms of the President Dr Zebulon Mennell at 149 Harley Street. This was also the first meeting of Council since 11 May 1939.[20]

The long gap must have been occasioned by the 1939 summer holiday season followed by the disruption resulting from the outbreak of war on 3 September 1939, and the consequent reorganisation of the British medical profession into its new role in the medical branches of the armed services and the civilian Emergency Medical Service. The October 1939 Council meeting was held in the atmosphere of the "Phoney-War". The British Expeditionary Force, including the redoubtable former President and Honorary Secretary Major Featherstone, was in the process of establishing itself in the defensive positions of a sector of the Maginot Line in France, and the expected major air attacks on cities in the United Kingdom had not materialised. It was a time of unnatural quiet, uncertainty, and gloomy foreboding.[69]

The meeting of 11 October 1939 first took several emergency administrative decisions; the 1939 Annual General Meeting should not be held; the Officers and Council should remain in Office for the ensuing year with Blomfield[7] acting as Honorary Secretary in the place of Featherstone, who was on active service; there being £616.0s.3d (1996: £21,375) in the bank the £1 (1996: £35) subscription was placed in abeyance for one year (or credited if paid by Banker's Order); action in cases of emergency was delegated to Council with a quorum of three members.[20]

The vitally important business of this meeting with regard to specialist status and representation on the wartime professional advisory committees in the armed services and the EMS has already been considered. The Council concluded by resolving that "an account of the meeting should be circularised to all Members of the Association wishing them all the best of luck and a happy and early issue to all their troubles".[20] Blomfield[7] also inserted a factual report of the meeting in the *British Journal of Anaesthesia*.[70]

According to the minute book Council only met twice more (on 13 August 1940 and 10 June 1941) before the next Annual General Meeting on 28

October 1941 (there being no Annual General Meeting in 1940). Reports were received that satisfactory arrangements had been made for representation on the "Medical War Committee", and to the effect that the rank of Major (and its equivalent in the Navy and RAF) would be granted to specialists who met the qualifications specified by the Association of Anaesthetists and to them alone. The main business of the meeting however, was to initiate a response to an advertisement for nurses to train as anaesthetists which had been inserted in the *Nursing Times* by the authorities of Addenbrooke's Hospital, Cambridge and replies to subsequent correspondence (see below).[20]

It is not surprising that there were only two Council meetings between August 1940 and October 1941. These were dark days indeed for the United Kingdom; by October 1941 France had fallen, there had been severe air raids on British cities, Greece and Crete had been evacuated, the Germans had almost reached the gates of Moscow, Major John Challis of the London Hospital,[71] Major W Stanley Sykes of Leeds (1894-1961),[72] Founder Member of the Association, and Major Geoffrey Steel (1900-1970)[73] a Member of the Association, were prisoners of war, and the United States had not yet joined the Allies. The President, Zebulon Mennell,[1] and his Officers may not have met formally as a Council but they had been very active on behalf of the membership of the Association, as the Report to the 1941 Annual General Meeting clearly demonstrates. Mennell's work as a member of the Central Medical War Committee, and (looking to the future post-war period) of promised representation on the BMA Reconstruction Committee, the inauguration of which was certainly an act of faith at that time, was reported. The Secretary of the Conjoint Examination Board had written asking if some of the regulations relating to eligibility to sit the Diploma in Anaesthetics should be relaxed. Mennell had replied that there would be no change, and added that, on the contrary, if there were to be any change, the regulations should be made more severe. There obviously was still great concern amongst senior anaesthetists, that the standards for full specialist status (and consequent higher military rank) should be maintained. The question of the nurse anaesthetists had been resolved satisfactorily and a number of letters had been written about the remuneration of anaesthetists and petrol coupon allowances. Offers of anaesthetic apparatus had been received from the United States and arrangements were being made for acceptance. The subscription to the Royal Medical Benevolent Fund had been renewed, (this had been a commitment of the Association of Anaesthetists from its earliest days and still is today), a payment was made to the Red Cross for books supplied to anaesthetists who were prisoners of war, and it was suggested that surplus deposit money was transferred to National Saving Certificates. Major Featherstone raised the matter of extended membership at this meeting for the first time (see below)[20].

Mennell[1] certainly thoroughly deserved the vote of thanks, which the meeting passed with acclamation, before he handed over the Presidency to Ashley Daly in 1941.[2] Mennell once again became Honorary Treasurer and thus the emergent wartime military and civil leaders of the specialty held the two senior positions in the Association of Anaesthetists. Archibald Marston,[3] of Guy's Hospital, an astute medical politician, joined the team as Honorary Secretary. He was destined to be the next President of the Association, to play a vital part in the negotiations leading up to the inauguration of the National Health Service, and to be the first Dean of the Faculty of Anaesthetists of the Royal College of Surgeons of England when it was formed in 1948.[74] Harold Sington,[5] the retiring Honorary Treasurer, who had been a Royal Naval Surgeon in the Great War, had resigned because he had gallantly joined the RAMC in defiance of all the regulations; as his obituary says he had "utterly refused to take 'no' for an answer"![5]

The Council met regularly after the Annual Meeting of 1941. First they looked after the interests of anaesthetists throughout the war and celebrated both the victory in 1945 and the centenary of Morton's first successful public demonstration of ether anaesthesia at the Massachusetts General Hospital in 1846; then they led the specialty into the NHS with equal status with other specialties. This itself was no mean achievement (see below).

The Membership issue

Major Featherstone, back after his escape from France with the British Expeditionary Force, was in a determined mood at the 1941 Annual meeting. He wished to ensure that Service anaesthetists should be included under the wing of the Association of Anaesthetists.[20,22] He recognised that the limitation of Ordinary Membership to 150 anaesthetists who were on the staff of university teaching hospitals was far too narrow. He therefore proposed that

Consultant and Graded anaesthetists in the armed forces should be eligible for membership of the Association as Service Members.[20] Featherstone's proposal was passed "after considerable discussion". The majority which the resolution commanded is not recorded, but it was agreed that its content should be considered fully by Council and "applied if deemed practical". This proposal does not seem to have been popular with some of the members of Council. The matter was debated again at its meeting on 28 January 1942, at which Featherstone was not present. The possibility of an Associate Membership (presumably not just exclusively for Service Members) was considered and, once again, the matter was deferred for consideration at the next General Meeting.[20] The need to accommodate fully trained anaesthetists who did not meet the selective criteria for Ordinary Membership (Chapter 3) was recognised, but at the same time there was a determination to maintain exclusiveness for the specialists in teaching hospitals.

There was no intermediate General Meeting and Featherstone although Vice President did not attend the other three Council meetings in 1942. He reappeared at the Annual General Meeting of 28 October 1942 however. He asserted that he was not in favour of an Associate Membership and made an even more radical proposal than in 1941 which was seconded by Ivan Magill;[20,75] this was to the effect that all those who had obtained the Diploma in Anaesthetics and devoted 50% or more of their time to anaesthesia should be admitted as Ordinary Members without a limitation in numbers. This obviously alarmed the Officers. A counter proposal by Mennell for Associate Membership was defeated, and Featherstone's proposal twice resulted in a hung vote (nine against, nine for, and two abstentions). The President, (Ashley Daly) pointed out that a two thirds majority was required to alter the rules and, after a proposal by Major Stanley Rowbotham[76] to limit the concession to all practising specialist anaesthetists for the duration of the war only, the matter was referred back to Council. The Gordian knot was cut by R J Minnitt of Liverpool[77] at a Council Meeting on 2 December 1942. He proposed a Fellowship (or Senior Fellowship for those who had retired) for those who met the old narrow criteria, and Ordinary Membership for other specialists. The idea of a "Fellowship" specifically related to anaesthesia obviously appealed to the old guard! A General Meeting endorsed the proposal on 10 February 1943 (17 votes for and 3 against) and Ordinary Members were granted equal voting rights, and, on 1 April 1943, it was agreed that any two Fellows could propose a new Ordinary

Member to Council for approval (interestingly "for the time being"). Publicity was to be left to individual Fellows to circulate details of the new rules amongst their colleagues! The new rules were commended by Ashley Daly, President at the Annual General Meeting on 28 October 1943; in doing so, he paid a graceful tribute to Featherstone's persistence, a tribute which Featherstone appreciated![20,22] The requirement that a Fellow should hold a teaching hospital appointment was dropped in 1946. Fellowship was thereafter to be awarded on seniority and merit. Victor Goldman suggested to Council on 6 May 1949 that the category of Fellow should be merged with that of Ordinary Member but this was not finally achieved until 1963 (Chapter 7).

Honorary Fellows

The Association elected six Honorary Fellows during the period 1939-1948. Sir Francis Shipway, KCVO,[78] then the only living anaesthetist to have been honoured with a knighthood, was elected at the 1942 Annual Meeting, three more were elected at an intermediate General Meeting on 10 February 1943, these were H Bellamy Gardner a pioneer anaesthetist of Charing Cross Hospital who died shortly after election,[20] Colonel Beverly C Leech[79] of Regina Saskatchuan (at that time Assistant Director of Medical Services, 2nd Canadian Division) and Lieutenant Colonel Ralph M Tovell[80] Canadian born Director of Anaesthetics at Hartford, Connecticut (who was serving as Adviser in Anaesthetics to the American Forces in Europe). The fifth Honorary Fellow of the 1939-1948 period was elected at the Annual General Meeting on 2 October 1943; rather surprisingly it was J F W Silk,[81] the founder of the original Society of Anaesthetists in 1893, who had been elected as Honorary "Member" at the first Annual General Meeting in 1932. It is not clear whether this had been forgotten or whether it was considered appropriate to change his title from "Honorary *Member*" to "Honorary *Fellow*" under the new rules; unfortunately Silk died one month after his election. Sir Alfred (later Lord) Webb-Johnson,[82] President of the Royal College of Surgeons of England over the period of the negotiations which preceded the introduction of the NHS, was elected in 1945; by then Sir Alfred had already shown a supportive interest in the discussions about the status of anaesthetists in the new service and had arranged for the then President of the Association (Marston) to sit on the Council of the Royal College of Surgeons of England.

The confidence which the Association placed in Webb-Johnson was not misplaced (see below).

Nurse anaesthetists

Reference has already been made to the problem of nurse anaesthetists earlier in the present chapter. The controversy flared up again as the result of an advertisement placed in the *Nursing Times* on 6 July 1940 by the Board of Governors of Addenbrooke's Hospital, Cambridge. This was for a sister to act as a nurse anaesthetist.[20,83] The Council of the Association of Anaesthetists met in emergency session on 13 August 1940. A letter was concocted addressed to the Board of Addenbrooke's Hospital, and its text was released to the Editors of the *British Medical Journal*[84] and the *Lancet*[85] The letter is signed by Mennell[1] (the President) and Blomfield[7] (as Acting Honorary Secretary) but a list of the names of all the members of Council is added in a footnote. The text expresses "grave misgiving" at the action of the Board of Addenbrooke's Hospital which it believes to be "injurious to public welfare". A recent decision of the Canadian Courts is also cited. this had the effect of making the nurse anaesthetist in Canada illegal.[84-88] Letters were also sent to the Medical Defence Union and to Professor J A Ryle, Regius Professor of Physic at the University of Cambridge, after a Council Meeting on 10 June 1941.[20]

Mennell referred to the "correspondence which the Council started in the lay press" at the Annual General meeting on 28 October 1941.[20] He reported that the outcome of the affair had been satisfactory. Addenbrooke's had agreed not to appoint any more "sister anaesthetists", and he also had in his possession letters from the Medical Defence Union, the Secretary of the Royal College of Nursing, the Secretaries of the BMA and its local Cambridge branch, a copy of a clause in the Medical Act and a letter from the *Lancet*, all of which supported "our contention"; presumably the phrase "our contention" meant that the training and employment of nurse anaesthetists was undesirable, as is recorded in a statement by the Royal College of Nursing, quoted in the *Lancet*.[89]

All this was indeed "satisfactory", but as Mennell also mentioned at the 1941 Annual General Meeting, as a result of Council's action in copying its original letter to Addenbrooke's to the *Lancet*[85] and the *British Medical Journal*[84], considerable correspondence had been provoked in those medical journals and this had spilled over into the lay press.[20] It would not be appropriate to reference all the letters which appeared in the *Lancet* (Volume 2, 1940 and Volume 1, 1941) and the *British Medical Journal* (Volume 2, 1940 and Volumes 1 and 2, 1941). One can not agree however with Mennell's contention that the replies to the Council letter were "voluminous and rather silly". Many of the letters, not all written by anaesthetists, were favourable to medical anaesthetists, although the ironic letter from J E Elam, a General Practitioner (Honorary Anaesthetist at Barnet) published in the *British Medical Journal*[90] was misunderstood by a surgeon and had to be explained subsequently.[92] Elam's' actual views were more succinctly expressed in his letter to the *Lancet*![93] He contends that many General Practitioners, who had held resident appointments and were anxious to practice as anaesthetists, were denied access to hospital practice by surgeons who "see to it that surgery.... is going to be the only specialty in their district";[93] whatever the truth of this, however, no amount of sabre rattling about the essential benefits of specialist anaesthesia could possibly disguise the fact that Visiting or Honorary Anaesthetists, especially those in General Practice were often unable to supply a comprehensive service for emergency anaesthesia (Chapter 2).[94]

One can have sympathy with the surgeon who frequently received messages to the effect that the Visiting Anaesthetist could not attend with the result that the anaesthetic had to be administered by an untrained, newly qualified House Surgeon or physician attempting to use the more complicated techniques which had been introduced since the Great War. It can be readily understood why surgeons who frequently found themselves in such situations might favour the training of nurse anaesthetists who would be always available in the hospital.[95] The solution adopted by a number of hospitals by 1940 had been to appoint Resident Anaesthetists who had had house appointments as anaesthetists in teaching hospitals.[96] F B Parsons, the Honorary Secretary of the Medical and Surgical Staff of Addenbrooke's Hospital published his reply to the Association's open letter of protest[84,85] *in the British Medical Journal*[97] and the *Lancet*.[98] He first points out that five of the eight (General Practitioner) Honorary Anaesthetists in the hospital had been called up to serve in the armed forces at the same time as the number of beds at the hospital had been increased to meet civilian needs. He then goes on to say that Resident Medical Anaesthetists had been recruited in the past, but that satisfactory applicants had either been few, or had had only the minimum amount of training required by the medical undergraduate curriculum of "London Hospitals", and were consequently unsatisfactory because of their inexperience. He also rather pompously draws attention to the fact that "the Central Medical War Committee, in their circular D.77 of July 1940, have asked all hospitals as far as possible to give house appointments to the newly qualified in preference to more experienced applicants".[97,98] J F Rickards, at that time Resident Anaesthetist at the Royal Berkshire Hospital, Reading, joined in the correspondence to point out that Addenbrooke's only offers £130 per annum (1996: £4,400) whereas at the Royal Berkshire there was no difficulty in securing a medical man with the necessary experience at a salary of £250 (1996: £8,500) per annum[96] (in those days, when young medical graduates married later than they do now, both these salaries would be, of course, plus keep). The Royal Berkshire Hospital had had a long tradition of having Resident Anaesthetists; the first being appointed in 1903.[99] (Sir) Geoffrey Organe (President of the Association 1953-1956) was one of them in the mid-thirties;[9] he stated off the record that he, too, accepted the appointment because it paid better than was the case at other hospitals (personal communication)!

Council considered a protest to the General Medical Council again on 1 March 1945, after it had been reported that an apparently healthy patient anaesthetised by a nurse anaesthetist had died. It was decided not to take any action, however, out of consideration for the position of the United States Army Hospitals operating in the United Kingdom who routinely employed nurse anaesthetists.[20]

It is still not illegal for nurses or others who are not medically qualified to administer anaesthesia or to perform surgical operations in the United Kingdom! The veterinary surgeons are better protected - unless properly licensed a citizen can only operate on or anaesthetise an animal if he or she actually owns it. The last attempt to promote legislation on the subject was made by Sir Frederic Hewitt (anaesthetist to St George's Hospital, London) early in this century,[100] and indeed in at least one hospital in the United Kingdom there were nurse anaesthetists into the nineteen fifties! It has been emphasised earlier in the chapter however that the possible use of trained nurses or technicians to monitor, or even anaesthetise, patients under the direct supervision of a physician anaesthetist may be an acceptable British practice in certain unusual circumstances[24,33,101] as it is routine in other countries.[34,101-104] The practice of a nurse or other nonmedically qualified person administering anaesthesia under the nominal supervision of the surgeon is however unacceptable. Professor Sir Robert Macintosh,[26] whose attitude on the subject of nurse anaesthesia has been misunderstood in the past, made his position quite clear in an excellent letter to the *Lancet* during the 1940 controversy,[104] and also in 1962[105] when the issue had again been raised.[106] It is possible that physician-directed nurse anaesthesia might have developed in the United Kingdom if the architectural tradition in prewar British hospitals had been different and operating theatres had been grouped together in suites or units as in the United States or Scandinavia, instead of having single theatres widely dispersed on a large site to suit the convenience of individual surgeons.

A first headquarters for the Association

Meetings of Council in the early days were held at the rooms of Mennell in Harley Street, and following the election of Marston[3] as Honorary Secretary, his rooms were also used. Ashley Daly, as President began to use accommodation at the house of the Royal Society of Medicine at 1 Wimpole Street. Secretarial assistance was provided by the personal secretaries of one or other of the officers. A Miss Olive was thanked and given a wedding present of five guineas (1996: £180) on 15 October 1937 and the work of a Miss Williams was acknowledged in the minutes in 1944, otherwise the names of the ladies who acted as the secretarial staff of the Association of Anaesthetists in this period are not recorded.[20]

A proposal from the Secretary of the Royal College of Surgeons of England inviting the Association of Anaesthetists to join some of the surgical societies in a scheme to form a Joint Secretariat, was received by Council on 22 July 1943. The accommodation available was at 45 Lincoln's Inn Fields adjacent to the Royal College of Surgeons. There was an "excellent room" for the secretariat and a room leading out of it which could be used for Council meetings. The Association was to pay £150 (1996: £4,500) per annum, to include a share of the salary of the secretarial staff, light, heat, insurance of the contents, telephone and committee and office teas. It was certainly a generous offer which Council accepted, and it provided the Association with the privilege of using the official address of the Royal College of Surgeons of England.[20]

The new secretariat opened on 25 March 1944 and the retiring President Ashley Daly[2] was able to report that "the new arrangements were working admirably" at the Annual General Meeting held at the Royal College of Surgeons of England on 25 October 1944.[20]

The transfer of the Association to Lincoln's Inn Fields marked the beginning of a period of close and fruitful collaboration between the Association and the Royal College of Surgeons of England in which Archibald Marston[3] was to play a leading role.

The coat of arms of the Association

Ronald Jarman[107] of the Royal Marsden Hospital reported to Council on 24 February 1944 that he had persuaded a Mr Leslie Gamage to donate £150 (1996: £3,300) to enable the Association to apply for letters patent for a grant of arms. This was a forerunner of the large sums which Jarman later raised for research and educational projects, both for the Association of Anaesthetists and for the Royal College of Surgeons of England.

The grant of arms was dated 12 February 1945 "in the 9th year of the reign of King George VI". The full achievement of the arms granted to the Association of Anaesthetists is described in Appendix B; in the United Kingdom the granting of the right to bear arms to a corporate body is a significant step in the recognition of its status by the establishment.

Preparation for the National Health Service

The British NHS, which came into being on 5 July 1948, was not, as is sometimes popularly supposed, the creation of the postwar Labour government which was somewhat unexpectedly elected in 1945, after the cessation of hostilities with Germany and Italy but before the defeat of the Japanese. It was, as has already been intimated in the earlier chapters, the climax of a gradual process initiated by the Lloyd George Insurance Act of 1911.[11-13] The imaginative part which the BMA played in planning a national health service both before and during the Second World War is often conveniently forgotten by politicians. This culminated in the setting up of the Medical

Planning Commission at the time of the darkest days of the war in 1940. This body included all the Royal Colleges as well as the medicopolitical left wing. The report of the Commission in 1942 foresaw many of the features ultimately incorporated in the structure of the NHS in 1948, including cover for the whole population, the national administration of hospitals, part time hospital consultants and payment by capitation fee for general practitioners.[108] The introduction of the NHS stemmed immediately from the general report on the social insurance services chaired by Sir William Beveridge, which was published on 2 December 1942 under the wartime coalition government.[109] Much early work on the scheme was done under the Conservative Health Minister in that coalition, Sir Henry Willink. All parties realised that the health service, particularly the hospital service, needed reorganisation.[11-13,110]

The Beveridge Report stated axiomatically that no satisfactory scheme of social security can be devised unless certain assumptions are accepted. These included the vital Assumption B:-

"Comprehensive health and rehabilitation services for the prevention and cure of disease and restoration for capacity for work, available to all members of the community".[11]

Beveridge stressed that his plan required "a health service providing full preventative and curative treatment of every citizen without exception, and without an economic barrier at any point to delay recourse to it". He believed, however, that the colossal task of organising such a scheme lay outside the scope of his report; however, Beveridge did say "the possible scope of private general practice will be so restricted that it may not appear worthwhile to preserve it;" these were chill words indeed for the General Practitioners of those days!

Perusal of reports and literature of the time reveals that an extraordinary feature of the events which preceded the inauguration of the NHS on 5 July 1948, was how many major problems of terms and conditions of service remained to be directly negotiated with the BMA, even after the passage of the Health Service Bill in 1946;[111] for example the Presidents of the Royal Colleges of Physicians, Surgeons and Obstetrics and Gynaecology asked quite fundamental but unresolved questions in their open correspondence with the

Labour Minister of Health, Aneurin Bevan, published on 11 January 1947.[111-113]

Bevan was a firm but approachable man and a pragmatist who realised that it was essential to "get the cooperation of the medical profession and of all health workers because without that co-operation the scheme was bound to fail".[113] He kept his fundamental objectives in mind (universal coverage of the population and the inclusion of all hospitals both municipal and voluntary in a single scheme under state control), but he made a number of major concessions which, after much huffing and puffing, ultimately received the cooperation of the BMA and the medical profession.[11,12,113]

It is neither practicable nor is it necessary to detail the give and take of the negotiations between the profession and the Minister of Health, but the final outcome was a deal which was very satisfactory for both the public and the hospital service, but perhaps, not so good for General Practitioners.[11,12] It is true that some members of the profession foresaw with gloomy foreboding the long term dangers of centralised bureaucracy and ministerial control, which did not begin to bite until the costs of running the service began to outstrip the money available in the nineteen seventies, and which have brought such unhappiness in the eighties and nineties;[113] but the immediate effects on the hospital service were markedly beneficial. Voluntary hospitals, which had struggled to maintain their income by private donations, had money to spend; hospital services within each district, previously divided between the municipal and voluntary sectors, were united and nationalised; the dreaded local authority control of hospitals was avoided; Consultants were given seats on the management committees, and they were awarded a salary scale on which they could live with reasonable comfort, with a distinction award system to reward excellence; and the right to practise privately, both inside and outside NHS hospitals, was preserved to provide the jam on the bread and butter. The influence of general practitioners over Consultants due to the financial aspects of the referral system was thus reduced (or abolished altogether if the consultant took a wholetime contract), and it was still further diminished because there was to be a 'firm' system with Registrars and House Surgeons in all hospitals similar to that which had previously only been found in the teaching hospitals; this was instead of the alternative, at one time considered, of the use of general practitioners to assist consultants in the hospital service.[11,12] The annual gross rates of pay finally accepted for the various grades are interesting[11] (approximate 1996 purchasing power in brackets): -

Consultants, (Wholetime figures, part-time *pro rata* on a notional half day basis).
£1,700 (£30,600) rising in ten years by increments to £2,750 (£49,500). Distinction awards A £2,500 (£45,000), B £1,500 (£27,000), C £500 (£9,000).

Senior Hospital Medical Officers. (A permanent sub-consultant specialist grade of which a great deal more will emerge later).
£1,300 (£23,400) rising in ten years by increments to £1,750 (£31,500).

Senior Registrars.
£1,000 (£18,000) rising by three increments to £1,300 (£23,400).

Registrars.
£775 (£13,950) first year. Thereafter £890 (£16,000).

Senior House Officers.
£670 (£12,100), plus keep.

House Officers.
£350 (£6,300) 1st year, plus keep. £400 (£7,200) 2nd year, plus keep.

It is probable that most specialist anaesthetists covertly or overtly favoured the introduction of the NHS with its prospect of an improved and more regular income without reliance on the surgeon, always provided equal status with other specialties could be achieved. It is interesting that, as early as 1935, Gilbert Brown,[114] the first President of the Australian Society of Anaesthetists, after returning from a visit to the United Kingdom, shrewdly observed:-

"Already a few men [in the United Kingdom] have resigned an honorary appointment at a teaching hospital for a paid one at a county council hospital. This appears to be the thin edge [sic] of the wedge in the payment of doctors for hospital work. It is realised

that this may mean the socialization of medicine and the problems this entails, yet it seems to a large number of doctors that the time has come to abandon the honorary system."[115]

The vital question that concerned specialist anaesthetists in the immediate postwar period was not whether there should be an NHS, that was a foregone conclusion, but whether they would be accepted as full and equal specialist Consultants, and, if they were so accepted, how would Consultant Anaesthetist status be defined?

The Association of Anaesthetists minute book and Annual Reports of the period (1941-1948) indicates that the Royal Colleges and Government bodies were rather more willing to assist anaesthetists to obtain Consultant status than was the BMA with its large General Practitioner membership, many of whom administered anaesthesia. There are also indications that General Practitioners were willing to undercut specialist anaesthetists in the private sector as well as with local authorities who remained in control of hospitals in the interim period before introduction of the NHS, (10% of the surgeon's fee instead of 20% for qualified specialists recommended by the Association).[20]

The Association of Anaesthetists played a major part in the negotiations between the Government and the profession. Its officers were invited members from the start in 1942 of the combined Committee on the Beveridge Report formed by the Royal Colleges of Surgery in England, Physicians of London and Obstetricians and Gynaecologists. The Association was also invited to send an observer to the Council of the Royal College of Surgeons in 1944 and, after modifications of the Charter of the College in 1947, to send a coopted member; Archibald Marston[3] was the Association representative and ultimately took his seat as Dean of the newly formed Faculty of Anaesthetists in 1948.

The Association of Anaesthetists gave evidence by invitation to the Goodenough Committee of the Ministry of Health on academic staffing and teaching in medical schools and, in this connection was instrumental in establishing a Committee of Representatives of the Honorary Anaesthetists of the London Teaching Schools in 1947. This was dissolved, however, when responsibility for matters concerning teaching was handed over to the Faculty when it was established in 1948. The Association was also represented on the

Central Medical Academic Council and gave evidence in 1946 to the Committee chaired by Sir William Spens, Master of Corpus Christi College Cambridge, on the remuneration of the medical profession in the forthcoming NHS.[20]

The attitude of the British Medical Association to anaesthetists remained somewhat ambivalent however. Its Officers and Council repeatedly asserted that all Consultants should have equal remuneration, but they nonetheless maintained that the number of anaesthetists that could be considered to be of Consultant rank was limited. The anaesthetists' case was weakened by the fact that there were not enough specialist anaesthetists available in the United Kingdom to be responsible for all anaesthetics in all hospitals, and that many General Practitioners continued to administer most of the anaesthetics outside the great cities. The original official estimate of the number of anaesthetists required was 4 to 6 Consultants per million population. The estimate of the Association of Anaesthetists in 1946 was 20 per million.[20] That would mean that the requirement for Consultants would be about 1,000 in England and Wales (population 50 million), 100 in Scotland (population 5 million) and 20 in Northern Ireland (population 1.6 million). The active membership of the Association (Ordinary Members and Fellows) was 308 in 1948. The ratio of consultant anaesthetists to population was about 40 per million in 1992, but it must be remembered that anaesthetists are now concerned with Intensive Care and other responsibilities outside the theatre.

The successive committees of the BMA concerned with reconstruction and planning for the NHS took evidence and received memoranda over the years, but found excuses for not having the Association of Anaesthetists actually represented on the Committees.[20] The BMA insisted, in the end, that only by the formation of a new body (an "Anaesthetists' Group") within the BMA structure itself could representation for anaesthetists be received on the Special Practice, Medical Planning, Consultants and Specialists and other important committees, and through them on the Council of the BMA itself. The BMA Anaesthetists Group was founded in 1946 with the Association of Anaesthetists having two representatives, including a seat on the Committee of the Group (Council Minute of 5 April 1946).[20] It was fortunate for anaesthetists that in subsequent negotiations W Alexander Low[8] played a leading part in the business of the Group. The successor to the Group

Committee in 1998 is the Anaesthetists Subcommittee of the Central Committee for Hospital Medical Services on which the Association provides the Chairman and has four representatives. The Group itself has been disbanded.

The position of the local authorities was an added complication to the negotiations between the Government and the medical profession. This was because the decision to exclude local authorities from the administration of the NHS in favour of centralised control at Ministry level was not promulgated until late in the preparatory period.[11,12] Negotiations on pay and conditions in relation to municipal and county hospitals had, therefore, to be continued meanwhile. The local authorities, in their bid to be given control of the NHS, obviously had the intention of introducing new staffing structures and terms and conditions of service in hospitals which would be applicable if they were to be in charge of the NHS. Middlesex County Council for example published new proposals for medical staffing and pay in the county service in December 1945;[116] in these they proposed that departments of anaesthetics "would be staffed by an experienced senior anaesthetist holding a diploma, a less experienced chief assistant also holding a diploma, as well as resident and house anaesthetists". They asserted that: -

"Since anaesthetics is a limited specialty, the salary scale is put somewhat lower than that of a general physician and surgeon, and it is recommended that a senior anaesthetist should receive £1,000 (1996: £21,000) rising to £1,400 (1996: £29,400)."[116]

Surgeons and physicians were to receive £1,200 to £1,800 (1996: £25,200 to £37,800). This proposal was strongly resisted by the Association of Anaesthetists through the BMA who agreed that all Consultants and Specialists should receive the same scale of remuneration.[20]

The BMA set up a special committee during 1946 to make proposals for the revision of the scale of sessional fees for part-time Consultants in local authority hospitals. Marston[3] as President and Low[8] as Honorary Secretary were asked to attend.[20] The Chairman of the Committee reiterated that all

Consultants should receive the same remuneration per session - the suggestion was five guineas for two hours (1996: £108). He went on to say, however, that the question had been raised as to whether anaesthetists were eligible to receive such a fee; he asserted that opposition to the recognition of anaesthetists as specialists had come both from surgeons and anaesthetists themselves (presumably the last reference was to the attitudes of General Practitioner anaesthetists without Diplomas who were, at that time, trying to keep a foothold in the hospital service). The Committee Chairman further stated that it was "certainly not the intention" that every practitioner who undertook anaesthetic sessions should receive the full fee. The Association of Anaesthetists were then asked to submit a definition of the qualifications required for the acceptance of a specialist anaesthetist as a Consultant (Council Minutes 13 March 1946).[20]

The definition of a Consultant in anaesthesia was, in fact, requested from the Council of the Association of Anaesthetists several times by various bodies which were debating and negotiating terms and conditions of service of medical practitioners before the introduction of the NHS. The answer given did not vary and was as included in the Minutes of Council of 13 March 1946[20]:-

> *"The Council of the Association has considered the criteria which should be adopted for the recognition of Consultant status in the NHS."*

> *"Realising that the only true definition of Consultant and specialist status is the fact that he is recognised as such by colleagues in the locality or hospital in which he works, the Council is of the opinion that this should be the chief criterion. It is also recommended that:-*

> *(a) He should have the Diploma in Anaesthetics of the Conjoint Board of the Royal College of Physicians of London and Surgeons of England.*

> *(b) He should have been in practice in the specialty for at least 5 years.*

> *(c) He should be on the full staff of a recognised hospital as an anaesthetist.*

"The Association has accepted the criteria laid down by the Royal Colleges for future Consultants. It will be remembered that one of these is that the Consultant shall be engaged whole-time in the specialty. Some who should be recognised as Consultant Anaesthetists at the present time may, however, have other duties, but it is essential that the major portion of their time should be devoted to the specialty."

"The Council wishes to draw attention to the fact that, on its recommendation, the examining Board in England has recently doubled the period which must elapse after qualification before a candidate may sit the Diploma in Anaesthetics, so as to bring it into line with other diplomas".

This is a comprehensive definition. It confirms the Diploma in Anaesthetics as an important factor in the definition of a Consultant, and the last paragraph was an effort to confirm the status of the Diploma as an acceptable higher qualification. The purpose of the penultimate paragraph was to protect the status of eminent anaesthetists like Mennell[1] who were also General Practitioners. Future aspirants to Consultant status would, however, be required to devote themselves exclusively to the practice of anaesthesia. The Achilles' heel of the definition is the statement in the second paragraph. It was probably intended to protect the interests of senior anaesthetists who, not having a teaching hospital appointment, had not been entitled to be granted the Diploma without examination following its introduction in 1935. It was unfortunate, however, that the wording seemed to give it precedence over the specific requirements labelled (a), (b), and (c).

Most specialists of reasonable seniority in disciplines other than anaesthetics who had a higher diploma of one of the then established Royal Medical Colleges of Physicians, Surgeons or Obstetricians and Gynaecologists were graded as Consultants almost automatically on the introduction of the NHS, whereas those specialist practitioners who did not have such a qualification, of which there were a considerable number in the former local authority hospitals, were placed in the lesser grade of Senior Hospital Medical Officer (SHMO). Former General Practitioner physicians, surgeons and obstetricians in possession of higher diplomas usually gave up general practice altogether and were accepted as Consultants in the new Service, whereas many of those without such qualifications gave up their specialist practice and continued in the NHS solely as General Practitioners thereafter.[113] A smaller number of General Practitioners both with and without specialist diplomas opted to combine general practice with SHMO status. It was unfortunate that, in the early days of the NHS, a considerable number of established anaesthetists, who had passed the Diploma in Anaesthetics (DA) and were on the staff of recognised hospitals, were graded as SHMOs. This may have been because local opinion in their hospitals refused to accept anaesthetists as being of equal status to other specialists (a course of action as unfortunately suggested in the second paragraph of the definition promulgated by the Association of Anaesthetists), or because the DA was not considered to be equivalent to the medical and surgical diplomas. The Association protested vigorously and the President John Gillies[4] of Edinburgh reported at the Annual General Meeting in October 1948 that a considerable number of injustices had been ironed out.[117] This had been achieved either by revision of the grade of individuals or by their successful application for newly advertised consultant posts. The upgrading of the Diploma and the establishment of the Faculty of Anaesthetists (see below) undoubtedly played an important part in securing favourable decisions.

The SHMO problem persisted for many years however.[117-120] It is true that only a few of those with the DA remained permanently in the grade but many SHMOs without the DA felt aggrieved that they were asked to take Consultant responsibility without Consultant status; in the end those with Consultant obligations received supplementary pay but were generally denied consultant status.[120] This was a compromise that was not entirely acceptable to those concerned but, in retrospect, it does not seem to be unreasonable that those who did not pass the original DA, or had not been awarded the Fellowship of the Faculty of Anaesthetists should not be granted Consultant status.

Sir Alfred Webb-Johnson Bart takes a hand

Anaesthetists should be ever grateful to Sir Alfred (Lord) Webb-Johnson, President of the Royal College of Surgeons of England 1941-1949[82] for the altruistic interest he took in their welfare and status during the critical negotiations which preceded the introduction of the NHS in 1948. It was also particularly fortunate that his friendship with Archibald Marston[3], and the latter's coincident Presidency of the Association of Anaesthetists, enabled the two of them to collaborate closely during this critical period. There can be little doubt that the unprecedented invitation extended to the Association to send a representative to sit on the Council of the surgeon's College, which has been mentioned above, was initiated by Webb-Johnson himself.

This was only a beginning; Webb-Johnson was invited by Marston to address the Council of the Association on 11 April 1947.[20,121,122] He supported the concept that anaesthetists should be regarded as equal in status for remuneration in the new NHS, as had been the case during the Second World War both in the armed services and in the civilian Emergency Medical Service. He believed, however, that this equality could only be achieved if anaesthetists continued their wartime interests outside the operating theatre in peacetime in such areas as pre- and postoperative care, resuscitation, blood transfusion and oxygen therapy.

Webb-Johnson's immediate concern was that the Diploma in Anaesthetics (DA) was of too low a standard to be certain of acceptance as a higher qualification which would automatically be considered to be adequate for an anaesthetist to be accepted as a Consultant in the NHS. Time was short, the quickest solution would be to upgrade the existing DA to include a primary examination in basic sciences as soon as possible, and to found a Faculty of Anaesthetists within the Royal College of Surgeons. The Faculty could then award its Fellowship both to the more senior holders of the original DA who held higher positions in teaching hospitals, or who, by their attainments or merit were entitled to it, and to those who passed the new upgraded DA in the interim. It was a bold plan, but rapid and decisive action was needed; even then, as has been recorded earlier, its adoption did not entirely avoid the initial grading of a number of potential consultant anaesthetists as second class specialist SHMOs Far greater injustice might have ensued if the immediate intention to upgrade the then existing DA had not been expressed; or the Association of Anaesthetists had waited for a Faculty to be established which could then institute its own Fellowship by examination.

The introduction of the two-part DA and the FFARCS

Dissatisfaction with the 1935 DA as a qualification for full specialist status was not new. There was a justified feeling of inferiority when it was compared with the higher diplomas of the Royal Colleges of Physicians and Surgeons. A gloomy 1941 editorial in the *British Journal of Anaesthesia*,[123] almost certainly written by the editor himself, Joseph Blomfield,[7] is entitled "the struggle upwards". It suggests that anaesthetists can not hope to be accepted as equal specialists unless they aspire to a higher diploma of one of the Royal Medical Colleges or a university doctorate in medicine (MD). Blomfield was himself an MD. Webb-Johnson's homily acted as a stimulus however. A high level subcommittee was nominated immediately after his address, the Council of the Association of Anaesthetists sought discussions with the Conjoint Board without delay, and Marston was able to announce that the new regulations for the two-part DA would be effective from 1 January 1948 at the Annual General Meeting on 30 October 1947.[20]

The new examination was still in the hands of the Conjoint Board but its regulations had been the result of recommendations made by the Council of the Association of Anaesthetists.[124] The examination was to be in two parts. Part 1 could be taken by medical graduates after holding an appointment as a House Surgeon or House Physician for six months in a recognised general hospital (there was still no compulsory preregistration house officer year). The examination would consist of written and oral parts and cover physiology, pharmacology and clinical pathology with special reference to anaesthesia, and anatomy as applied to anaesthesia and analgesia. Part 2 could be taken twenty-four months after qualification after passing Part 1 and holding a resident or whole-time post in anaesthesia for not less than 12 months. The examination was to be written, oral, and clinical and the subjects of the examination were to be:- anaesthesia and analgesia, including preoperative and postoperative treatment and clinical medicine and surgery "so far as it concerns these treatments". A broad synopsis of the subject matter required was published at the same time as the new regulations.[125]

The Association of Anaesthetists had thus promoted an examination comparable with and modelled on the Fellowship of the Royal College of Surgeons of England (FRCS). The first examination under the new regulations took place in November 1948. The *British Journal of Anaesthesia* published a resumé with details of the questioning in the oral examination; a liberty which probably would not be permitted nowadays![126] Eighty-two candidates presented for Part 1 and 17 passed (21%), and 108 candidates entered for Part 2 of whom 36 passed (33%). The article comments:-

"The examination was most impressively conducted in a most fair and pleasant manner. It can not be said, however, that the knowledge of the candidates was satisfactory. Many of them made it all too clear that they had not properly prepared themselves for the examination, and some were unable to answer questions which a fifth year student could have tackled with confidence".[126]

Surely this comment could have been written by the Chairman of the Board on several occasions in the nineteen eighties and nineties when the low pass rates in today's examinations have been questioned!

The Association of Anaesthetists handed over its role of adviser to the Conjoint Examination Board to the Faculty of Anaesthetists when it came into being in 1948. The two-part DA became the model for the diploma of the Fellow of the Faculty of Anaesthetists of the Royal College of Surgeons of England (FFARCS) introduced at the November examination in 1953, after a clinical examination with living patients had been added to Part 2 of the examination. Responsibility for the FFARCS examination was then vested in the Royal College of Surgeons of England, while the DA reverted to the status of a Conjoint diploma to be taken after approximately one year of training in anaesthesia. All those who had passed the DA in two parts, or passed the original DA and were established consultants in the NHS by the end of 1955 were granted the Fellowship after payment of the appropriate fee. There were a few hard cases, but the rapid expansion of the anaesthetic services of the NHS, coupled with the time that had elapsed which had enabled considerable regrading of unfairly designated SHMOs to take place, meant that these were reduced to a minimum.[127] Responsibility for the FFARCS and the award of the diploma were delegated to the Faculty by the College of Surgeons in 1983 and the examination became the Fellowship of the College of Anaesthetists (FC Anaes) in 1988 and the Fellowship of the Royal College of Anaesthetists (FRCA) in 1992.

The basic two-part form of the examination (consisting of a Part 1 or "Primary" in basic sciences and Part 2 or "Final" in clinical anaesthesia and related aspects of medicine and surgery) continued with only minor modification until 1985, when a three-part examination was introduced. Part 1 was a vocational examination based on the old Conjoint Board Diploma which had been taken over by the Faculty in that year, and was considered to have relevance to promotion in the training grades of the specialty and to practice in developing countries; Part 2 consisted of a multiple choice paper and an oral examination in physiology and pharmacology, and the Part 3 or "Final" was a searching examination covering the whole field of applied basic science, clinical anaesthesia, intensive care, and related medicine and surgery. The status, standards, and responsibilities of the specialty of anaesthetics have certainly come a long way since the Association of Anaesthetists promoted the inauguration of the first Diploma in Anaesthetics in 1935! Success in the Part 1 FRCA examination plus the completion of two years training (one of which must be in the United Kingdom) entitled the candidate to apply for the Diploma in Anaesthetics which was granted by the College of Anaesthetists. The Royal College of Anaesthetists has however made fundamental changes in the examination structure in 1997, amongst which is the discontinuation of the Diploma in Anaesthetics and reversion to a two-part FRCA examination.

The Association petitions for a Faculty of Anaesthetists

Sir Alfred Webb-Johnson's suggestion of the creation of a Faculty of Anaesthetists within the Royal College of Surgeons of England was also quickly acted upon. A subcommittee was appointed on 18 July 1947. Negotiations with the Royal College of Surgeons of England were initiated, and a Special General Meeting of the Association of Anaesthetists was held on 6 February 1948 at which 75 Members and Fellows were present.[128] The new President John Gillies[4] was in the Chair.

Marston,[3] the Immediate Past President addressed the meeting in what was obviously a persuasive and effective speech. The functions of the Faculty would be training and the promotion of research. The Faculty would have direct representation on the Committee of Management of the DA; hitherto the Association of Anaesthetists, not being a constituent part of the Royal Colleges of Surgeons or Physicians, could only send memoranda to the Board of Management - though it must be said that, on the whole, these had been acted upon by the Conjoint Board.[124] The institution of a higher diploma would be considered. There would also be direct input into the General Medical Council, the Central Midwives' Board and the General Nursing Council. Marston attempted to pre-empt criticism by comparing the situation which he envisaged to a carriage drawn by four horses, the Association of Anaesthetists, the Faculty, the Royal Society of Medicine Section and the BMA Group. His statement that "the Association would continue its activities unchanged" could not bear close scrutiny however; after all its responsibilities with regard to education, the examination, and recently increasingly frequent requests to nominate assessors to attend appointment boards of NHS consultants,[20] would be handed over to the Faculty.

Some reservations on these lines were expressed by both Mennell[1] and Featherstone who were both now elder statesmen and no longer members of the Council of the Association of Anaesthetists. Mennell[1] was concerned lest the Association of Anaesthetists might become a mere advisory body to the Faculty, and Featherstone remarked gloomily that he had only driven a coach and four once, but he had driven a pair of horses frequently, and, even in the latter case, it was quite difficult to get them to pull together![128]

George Edwards[129] of St George's Hospital, London then moved the following resolution:-

"That this meeting is in favour of the proposal that the Association of Anaesthetists should apply for the formation of a Faculty of

Anaesthetists within the Royal College of Surgeons of England".[128]

This motion was seconded by the Honorary Treasurer of the Association of Anaesthetists, Bernard Johnson,[6] in so doing he made the somewhat unnecessary observation that there was nothing to prevent the Royal College of Surgeons creating a Faculty of Anaesthetists without consulting the Association of Anaesthetists. How often has one heard gratuitous remarks of this kind (often erroneous) made in committees in an attempt to force an issue? Johnson need not have been concerned; in the event the resolution was carried unanimously.[128]

Rapid action followed. The Faculty met for the first time on 24 March 1948.[130] Twelve of the twenty anaesthetists on the original Faculty Board were also on the contemporary Council of the Association of Anaesthetists including all the Officers. Marston[3] (the Immediate Past President of the Association of Anaesthetists) became the Dean, Bernard Johnson[6] (the Honorary Treasurer) became Vice Dean, and Gillies[4] (the President), Low[8] (the Honorary Secretary), and Hewer[10] (the Editor of *Anaesthesia*) became founder Board Members; moreover the majority of the remaining members of the Board had served on the Council of the Association at one time or another; one of these was Katherine Lloyd-Williams, CBE, Consultant Anaesthetist and Dean of the Royal Free Hospital, the first lady to serve on both the Association Council and the Faculty Board.[131,132] The influence of the Association of Anaesthetists was assured - for the time being at any rate!

The journal *Anaesthesia*

Previous chapters have emphasised the important part which the independent *British Journal of Anaesthesia* (*BJA*) played in the development of anaesthesia in the United Kingdom, both in the nineteen twenties, when it was virtually the only medicopolitical mouthpiece of the specialty, and in the thirties after the establishment of the Association of Anaesthetists in 1932. The reputation for playing his cards close to the chest of Joseph Blomfield[7] its second editor (1930-1948), both as an editor and proprietorially, has also been noted. Attempts to enlist the *BJA* as an organ of the Association of

Anaesthetists were resisted by Blomfield in 1935, but a request from him for a donation to its funds from the Association in May 1939 suggests that all was not well with the financial status of the *BJA* at that time (Chapter 4).

The Second World War and the period of austerity which followed it resulted in a shortage of paper and hit medical publication hard. It is therefore difficult to distinguish whether the causes of the erratic publication of the *BJA* and its diminution in size and content, between the outbreak of war in 1939 and the second and last (4th) issue of Volume 18 published in July 1943, were chiefly general or specific to the journal.

Prewar the volumes of the *BJA* had followed the unusual pattern of running from No 1 in October of one year to No 4 in July of the next. Volume 17 consisted of 175 pages in 4 issues beginning October 1939 and ending July 1941. There were no October 1941 or January 1942 numbers and volume 18 runs from No 1 in March 1942 to No 4 in July 1943; thus only four issues appeared over a period of two years (there being once again no October number in 1943). Volume 19 begins with the January 1944 (No 1) number and ends with July 1945 (No 4), which was the last issue in that year. It is, however, recorded in the Association minutes of 1 February 1945 that a message of sympathy was sent to Blomfield who had recently undergone a "severe operation".[20]

Blomfield[7] ended his term of Acting Honorary Secretary of the Association of Anaesthetists in place of Featherstone in October 1941. He continued as a Council Member until the Annual General Meeting on 2 October 1943, but his last attendance is recorded as being on 22 July 1943. It is therefore significant that the initial proposal for "an official journal of the Association" was made by Victor Eades Vessell, Honorary Anaesthetist to the Royal Northern Hospital, London, at the 1943 Annual General Meeting. A lengthy discussion followed with contributions amongst others from Mennell,[1] Langton Hewer,[10] Jarman,[107] and Organe.[9] The tenor of their remarks is not recorded, although it may be assumed that there was considerable dissatisfaction with the recent performance of the *BJA*, but there was some reluctance to compete with it. A subcommittee was appointed, composed of

Langton Hewer[10] as Chairman, Eades Vessell and Jarman.[107]

The subcommittee reported to Council on 24 February 1944 and a resolution was passed approving the policy of publishing an official journal "to start as soon as practicable".[20] This was easier said than done!

Restrictions on paper during the Second World War were very severe. Ronald Jarman[107] was active in exploring a number of avenues but even he could not find a source of supply; meanwhile Christopher Langton Hewer[10] accepted the post of Editor of the proposed new journal *Anaesthesia* on 1 March 1945 and began a tenure of office which was to last until 1966. It was not until after the end of hostilities with Japan in August 1945 that Hewer was able to report to Council on 6 December 1945 that the controls on paper had been "so much relaxed that it would be possible to start a new journal at any time". Various options were considered; these included publication through the BMA, publication through the Royal College of Surgeons, independent publication using a printer, and even the purchase of the *British Journal of Anaesthesia*! Independent publication was chosen on 7 February 1946 using the facilities provided by George Pulman and Sons Ltd of Thayer Street, London W1. R Blair Gould[133] of the Hospital for the Diseases of the Throat, Golden Square, London was appointed Subeditor, and John Gillies[4] became "Scottish representative".[20]

The first issue (the only number in Volume 1) appeared on 1 October 1946 in time for the centenary celebrations of Morton's first public demonstration of ether anaesthesia on 10 October 1846. This first number contained just 42 23cm x 14cm pages and its circulation was about 500. *Anaesthesia* was destined to appear quarterly until 1973; thereafter the frequency of publication was gradually increased to twelve issues per year in 1980.[134]

The first number began with a foreword by Sir Alfred Webb-Johnson,[82] the then President of the Royal College of Surgeons of England. He stressed the potential value of *Anaesthesia* in making "British teaching and records of discovery and achievement available for the medical profession throughout the world". Langton Hewer's editorial which follows, emphasises the scientific functions of the journal; but he goes on to stress that *Anaesthesia* is the journal of the Association of Anaesthetists of Great Britain and Ireland and must therefore have a political role. The editor then mentions the contemporary anxiety about the negotiations concerning the status of anaesthetists as the "appointed day" (1 July 1948) for the inauguration of the National Health Service approached. It is natural, in view of the centenary of Morton's seminal demonstration on ether in 1846[43] that there should be two historical articles. The first of these is Featherstone's account of the foundation and development of the Association;[135] the second by the reigning President of the Association of Anaesthetists, Archibald Marston, is on the four British pioneers (Hickman, Simpson, Snow and Clover) who were shortly to be commemorated on a plaque to be unveiled by the then Princess Royal (HRH Princess Mary) at the Royal College of Surgeons in Lincoln's Inn Fields.[136]

The scientific contents of the first number include contributions on curare (the great talking point in 1946), local analgesia for abdominal operations, pre- and postoperative care, the effect of the war on American anaesthesia, and a contribution on the import of extrasystoles detected by palpation during anaesthesia as a morbid prognostic sign. There are also some abstracts of current literature. The "Association News" section gives the programme for the centenary celebrations.[136]

There are no statistics in this first number of *Anaesthesia* and, like many journal of that era, there are deficiencies in production which would not be acceptable today, including the erratic, and sometimes inaccurate or incomplete, citation of references; despite the shortcomings, however, the pages of the first number of *Anaesthesia* are packed with interest and information. It certainly must have had a considerable impact in 1946.[136]

The journal *Anaesthesia* and the *British Journal of Anaesthesia*

It might have been expected that some graceful acknowledgment of the role that the *British Journal of Anaesthesia* had played in the development of anaesthesia in the United Kingdom would have been made either in the Foreword or the Editorial of the first number of *Anaesthesia* in 1946, but this was not the case. In fact the reverse is true; both the Foreword and the Editorial almost imply that *Anaesthesia* is first in the field. Webb-Johnson in his foreword, says "It is fitting that the country (sic) which made such valuable contributions in the early days of anaesthesia [Great Britain and Ireland] ..... should be represented in the medical literature", and Langton Hewer writes, "it has become obvious for some time that the rapid advance in all types of anaesthetic and analgesic technique requires fuller and quicker expression than can be provided in the overloaded columns of the general medical press".[136]

Many references have already been quoted in this and previous chapters to both the *British Journal of Anaesthesia* and *Anaesthesia,* and more will naturally be made in the subsequent text; it is therefore appropriate to trace briefly the subsequent history of the two journals and their inter-relationships at this stage, even though these matters are, strictly speaking, outside the time span of this chapter.

The *British Journal of Anaesthesia*, after the lean years which have already been mentioned, appeared twice in 1946 and twice in 1947. These four numbers published over two years constitute Volume 20, 1946-1947. A significant announcement entitled "Future policy" appeared as the editorial to the January 1948 number. It states that a meeting of the Board of the *BJA* had been held (which is said to have been a rare event during Blomfield's editorship!); however, be that as it may, the Board had decided "to solicit the cooperation of the Heads of the Departments of Anaesthesia in several universities and schools of medicine" in order to "heighten its [the *BJA*'s] authority and to widen its circulation". The Board is listed on the cover of that number of the *BJA*: only Blomfield himself has an appointment at a London teaching hospital, the others are leading anaesthetists from Liverpool, Leeds and Glasgow (two from each city), and one each from Edinburgh, Aberdeen, Manchester and Sheffield. None of the Board Members were currently Members of the Council of the Association except John Gillies of Edinburgh[4] who had become President in October 1947; however, whatever the ins and outs, the following minute of the Association Council for 2 April 1948[117] was a sad ending, if only for the time being, to the intimate relationship of the Association of Anaesthetists and the Editors and Board of the *BJA*:-

"The President said that he felt it was anomalous for him to serve on the editorial boards of both anaesthetic journals and that he was resigning from the Board of the British Journal of Anaesthesia. He considered that it was undesirable that any Officer or Member of Council of the Association should be on the Board of the BJA".[117]

Blomfield died in November 1948 and tributes were paid to him both in *Anaesthesia*[7] and the *BJA*.[137] T Cecil Gray (then Reader at Liverpool) and the veteran E Falkner Hill[138] of Manchester were appointed joint Editors.[139,140] The *BJA* was immediately revitalised and has never looked back. The first issue under the new Editors contained Professor (Sir) Robert Macintosh's[26] paper on "Deaths under anaesthetics;" this was one of the most forthright articles on what is now called "medical audit" that has ever been written.[141] The *BJA* resumed quarterly publication from January 1950, it came out every two months in 1954 (Volume 26), monthly in 1955 (Volume 27), and has published 2 volumes each year since 1989. *Anaesthesia* increased its frequency of publication rather more slowly - from four to six times each year in 1973, to nine times in 1976, to ten times in 1977 and has appeared monthly from 1980 onwards.

The proprietors of the independent *British Journal of Anaesthesia* offered to present the journal to the Faculty of Anaesthetists with a view to it becoming the official organ of that body in 1949 shortly after its formation in 1948. The close relationships of the Faculty to the Association at this stage of development is exemplified by the fact that, though the Faculty was prepared to accept the offer, it declined to do so if the Association of Anaesthetists "had no objection". The Association certainly did have objections but its Council seriously discussed the possibility of amalgamation, and a joint committee was formed with the Faculty at the Council meeting of 2 December 1949. The matter was discussed further at Council meetings on 2 December 1949 and 3 February, 5 May, 7 July and 6 October 1950, but the project was finally abandoned on 1 December 1950 with negotiations in deadlock.[117] This was apparently because of financial and constitutional legal difficulties as well as because Pask believed that competition was essential and threatened to start another journal if the *British Journal of Anaesthesia* and *Anaesthesia* amalgamated.[142] Both journals published Editorials announcing that both the proposal for amalgamation and the possibility of the *BJA* becoming the official organ of the Faculty had been abandoned by mutual consent. The Editor of *Anaesthesia* believed that "friendly rivalry" between the two journals would be beneficial, wished the *BJA* well and looked forward to "a spirit of friendliness and cooperation" between the journals.[143] The Editors of the *BJA* emphasised the "extraordinarily close cooperation and spirit of mutual assistance" which existed between the various bodies representing the specialty.[144]

The possibility of the amalgamation of *Anaesthesia* with the *BJA* was discussed again during 1959. This was after the accounts of the Association of Anaesthetists, presented at the 1958 Annual General meeting at Southport had shown an excess of expenditure over income for the first time in its history. This was mainly because of an apparent fall in the income generated by *Anaesthesia*, but this decrease was subsequently shown to be actually due to the timing of payment of subscriptions to the journal.[20] Serious negotiations were conducted with Messrs Sherratts, who were, at that time the publishers of the *BJA* (Council minutes 6 February, 5 June, 3 July and 18 September 1959).[117] The project was once again abandoned partly because Professor Pask[66] (Honorary Treasurer) and others believed that competition between the two journals was both healthy and desirable (personal communication T C Gray) and also because amalgamation would necessitate a rise in the Association subscription from two pounds ten shillings (1996: £31) to five guineas (1996: £65.50) instead of the three guineas (1996: £37.50) which was then being proposed, because the *BJA* cost more to publish than *Anaesthesia*. Agreed statements appeared in *Anaesthesia* and the *BJA*. These were identical except that the *BJA* version incorrectly gives the date of the AGM at Southport as 1959 instead of 1958.[144,145] The statement concludes that the Council of the Association considered that, "in the absence of unanimous enthusiasm", it was undesirable to proceed further with the proposed amalgamation and hope is expressed that "both journals will go from strength to strength and remain worthy of the high standard of the specialty in this country",[145,146] The two journals have generally fulfilled this promise.

Anaesthesia has remained the official journal of the Association of Anaesthetists. It has, perhaps, tended to lay emphasis on, and to attract articles on, clinical anaesthesia and it carries announcements and reports related to the business of the Association and its membership. It has, however, been relieved of this last duty to a considerable extent since the introduction of the separate publication *Anaesthesia News* in 1987. The Editor of *Anaesthesia* is an Officer of the Association but he enjoys complete editorial freedom (except for the very occasional restraint over political matters!). The Editorial Board reports to Council but is empowered to conduct the business of the journal independently, subject only to financial constraints.

The *BJA*, while not neglecting clinical matters, has tended to stress the scientific basis of anaesthesia. It has, however, also indulged in political editorials over major issues from time to time. These have included the SHMO controversy of the nineteen fifties which has already been mentioned, and the "College question" in the seventies and eighties (Chapter 8). The *BJA* became the official journal of the College of Anaesthetists in 1990 (this time without the need for the specific approval of the Association of Anaesthetists!). The agreement between the journal and the Royal College provides for the absolute editorial freedom of the *BJA* as well as a very considerable degree of financial independence for the Board which is now a charitable institution.[147] The *BJA* is largely relieved of the need to carry administrative material on behalf of the College because of the concomitant publication of the *Newsletter of the Royal College of Anaesthetists*.

Postwar Research Fellowships

The Association of Anaesthetists was able to sponsor research in the immediate postwar period largely due to the activities of Ronald Jarman[107] as a fund raiser. The British Oxygen Company (BOC) contributed £500 (1996: £10,000) per year, George Weston Holdings made a covenant for £1,000 (1996: £20,000) per year for seven years and the Ciba Foundation gave a donation of two hundred and fifty guineas (1996: £5,250).[117]

Edith Gilchrist (later Consultant Anaesthetist to the Royal Free Hospital, London) was appointed as the first Research Fellow on 28 February 1945 to study obstetric analgesia and the advantages and disadvantages of carbon dioxide absorbers. She began work at the Royal Free Hospital on 1 August 1945 but resigned in June 1946.[20] A research grant of £50 (1996: £1,000) for 6 months was made to Bernard G B Lucas (later Consultant Anaesthetist, University College Hospital) on 5 April 1946, and then on 19 July 1946 it was announced that Philip Helliwell (a future Consultant to Guy's Hospital and later the President of the Association of Anaesthetists from 1973 to 1976) had been awarded a Research Fellowship. He began his highly successful work on the use of trichloroethylene in obstetrics on 1 October 1946 and A M Hutton,[148] another future Guy's Consultant, joined Helliwell as a Research Fellow. They each received £500 as salary and £150 as expenses (1996: £10,320 and £3,100). The investigation was a model of its kind for the time; it involved both clinical trials and animal experimentation to determine placental transfer.[149,150] The animal work was carried out with sheep and goats at the Buxton Browne Farm of the Royal College of Surgeons of England. Helliwell later informs us that, unfortunately in those days of rationing in the United Kingdom, the meat resulting from the experiments was not edible due to contamination with trichloroethylene![151]

Education

The Association of Anaesthetists had always been very wary of entering the field of education. It had always regarded the holding of scientific meetings as the prerogative of the Section of Anaesthetists of the Royal Society of Medicine (RSM). Attitudes were changing however, and many felt that the single monthly meeting of the Section in London was inadequate provision; at the Council meeting on 1 February 1945 Bernard Murtagh[152] of Birmingham proposed that the Association should hold clinical meetings both in London and in the provinces. The response of Council was to determine "to arrange something on these lines" in time for the Annual General Meeting in October 1945. The result was that a programme of the famous series of films prepared by the Westminster Hospital Department of Anaesthesia in collaboration with Imperial Chemical Industries (ICI), was shown after the tea break which followed the Annual General meeting at the Royal College of Surgeons, Lincoln's Inn Fields on 25 October 1945. They included "How not to do it", "Spinal anaesthesia" and "Respiratory and cardiac arrest". The first Annual

Dinner of the Association was held that evening at the Royal College of Surgeons. The next morning clinical demonstrations were arranged by three future Presidents of the Association - Ronald Jarman[107] at the Cancer (now Royal Marsden) Hospital, W Derek Wylie at St Thomas', and (Sir) Geoffrey Organe, and F W Roberts (1910-1970) of the Middlesex Hospital, and afterwards of Hobart, Tasmania (Council Minutes 4 October 1945).[153] The programme was greatly appreciated (Council 6 December 1945).[20]

The Association was also asked to arrange a course of postgraduate lectures at the Royal College of Surgeons in 1947 and 1948 in anticipation of the foundation of the Faculty; the list of lecturers reads like a roll of honour of the immortals (four future Presidents of the Association of Anaesthetists, three future Deans and two Vice Deans of the Faculty, and at least four future John Snow Medalists).[153]

Miscellaneous matters

It is not possible to record all the many other matters which were considered by Council of the Association of Anaesthetists during the period covered by this chapter but some of these should be mentioned. Close cooperation was maintained with the Royal College of Obstetricians and Gynaecologists and the Central Midwives Board over obstetric analgesia and the training and examination of midwives in the use of nitrous oxide and oxygen. The long and fruitful collaboration between the Association and the British Standards Institute, which continues to the present time, was also initiated in this period over the question of the care and use of oxygen cylinders, and the famous Nosworthy punched record card was introduced and promoted.[20]

The centenary of ether anaesthesia celebration 1946

Morton's first public demonstration of ether anaesthesia at the Massachusetts General Hospital, Boston, USA on 16 October 1846[43] was commemorated in style by the Association.[122,154,155] This was before the inauguration of the Faculty but the Association of Anaesthetists, the Section of Anaesthetics of the Royal Society of Medicine, the Royal College of

Surgeons of England and other organisations joined forces to present a fascinating programme.

The Section of the History of Medicine of the Royal Society of Medicine held a meeting on 16 October 1946. The speakers included Barbara Duncum PhD, who had collaborated with the Nuffield Department of Anaesthetics at Oxford to produce her classic text on the history of inhalation anaesthesia,[156] and Joseph Blomfield.[7] Later in the day Lord Moran, President of the Royal College of Physicians opened an exhibition of historical anaesthetic equipment at the Wellcome Medical Museum.

The Association's own celebrations were held on 30 and 31 October 1946. Archibald Marston,[3] the reigning President, gave a talk on the wireless on the morning of Wednesday 30 October, and, in the evening, Her Royal Highness Princess Mary, the Princess Royal, unveiled the plaque to the British pioneers in anaesthesia in the Hall of the Royal College of Surgeons.[157] Marston delivered his paper on the lives of the pioneers on this occasion.[158] The plaque displays the arms of the Royal College of Surgeons of England and the Association of Anaesthetists. The cost was born by Mr A J Whitehead (another patient of Jarman's?). The unveiling ceremony was followed by a buffet supper at which the President and Council of the Royal College of Surgeons were hosts. The museum of historical anaesthetic equipment, which the anaesthetic instrument manufacturer A Charles King of Devonshire Street had collected, was also exhibited; this collection was bequeathed to the Association on the death of Charles King in 1966 (Chapter 7).[154,155]

On Thursday 31 October clinical demonstrations had been arranged for members at a number of London university teaching hospitals on the lines of those introduced at the time of the 1945 Annual General Meeting.[154,155]

The 1946 Annual General Meeting of the Association took place in the afternoon of 31 October. The three anaesthetists who had been decorated for their services during the Second World War were presented with the Association's newly introduced John Snow Medals of Honour. The exploits of Lieutenant Colonel Harry Featherstone, OBE the Founder President, and of the intrepid research worker Squadron Leader E A Pask, OBE have already been described. Major Leslie G Morrison was a young Edinburgh consultant who had been awarded the Military Cross for gallantry. The record states that the citations were received amid great enthusiasm. Marston was also invested with the Presidential Badge of Office for which the Fellows of the Association had subscribed at the same meeting.[155,157]

The Annual General Meeting was followed by the first Annual Dinner of the Association of Anaesthetists held in the Great Hall of Lincoln's Inn which is adjacent to the Royal College of Surgeons. Wesley Bourne attended from Canada and speeches were made by Marston,[3] Sir Alfred Webb-Johnson,[82] John Gillies[4] and Charles Hill, Secretary of the BMA. The Editor of *Anaesthesia* records "that dignity, erudition, wit and sarcasm were nicely blended"![155]

The Section of Anaesthetics of the Royal Society of Medicine held a meeting the next day (Friday 1 November). Sir Gordon Gordon-Taylor the Immediate Past President of the RSM held a reception. This was followed by the Presidential Address of the incoming President of the Section of Anaesthetics, Stanley Rowbotham, who delivered a "profusely illustrated" lecture on "A hundred years of anaesthesia".[155]

A Dinner and Dance was held at the Dorchester on Saturday 21 December.[154]

The centenary of the introduction of chloroform 1947

Edinburgh celebrated the introduction of chloroform in 1847 by Sir James Young Simpson with as much elan as London had marked the Anniversary of the introduction of ether the year before.[159] John Gillies,[4] the reigning President of the Association of Anaesthetists and the newly appointed Director of the Edinburgh Department of Anaesthesia, was largely responsible for the arrangements. Gillies read a paper before the Royal Medical Society (the oldest in the world), Simpson relics were displayed, and there was a scientific meeting to which Professor (Sir) Robert Macintosh[26] contributed. There were also demonstrations of "most methods of anaesthesia (except chloroform)" as the recorder of the event archly remarks in *Anaesthesia*.[159]

A pleasing feature of the celebrations was that Honorary Doctorates of Laws of Edinburgh University were conferred on the Founder President Harry Featherstone, and Sheriff T B Simpson, grand-nephew of Sir James Simpson.[159]

Summary September 1939 to December 1948

The winds of change in the form of the Second World War and the establishment of the British NHS had wrought a revolution in the affairs of the specialty of anaesthesia. The Association of Anaesthetists, in its turn, had seized the opportunity and responded with pragmatism, ingenuity and determination. It had markedly influenced the destiny and development of the specialty. The organisation itself had expanded from an elite and exclusive coterie of just short of 150 university teaching hospital anaesthetists, to an active membership of 670 Fellows and Members who were now bringing specialist anaesthesia to every District in the new NHS, whether metropolitan, provincial or rural.

The Association of Anaesthetists, with the assistance of leading surgical colleagues, had put its own academic house in order by being the motivating force behind the upgrading of the Diploma in Anaesthetics to a level at which it could be assimilated as one of the Fellowships of the Royal College of Surgeons of England; and it had gone on to petition for a Faculty within the College to authenticate the change under Royal Charter.

The service which the specialty had rendered to the country in the Second World War and the postwar changes in its academic status, had earned it equality with other disciplines, but nonetheless considerable effort had been required on the part of the Association of Anaesthetists to ensure its position within the NHS as an equal specialty.

There were now four bodies dealing with different aspects of the affairs of British anaesthesia. One of them (the Anaesthetic Section of the Royal Society of Medicine) continued as it had, and has, always done, to provide a forum for erudite scientific discussion within its own house, a medical library second to none, and valuable club facilities. The other two (the Group within the BMA and the Faculty within the Royal College of Surgeons of England) had been formed, after active promotion by the Association of Anaesthetists, to look after the political and academic interests of the specialty respectively.

What then could be considered to be the future role of the Association of Anaesthetists at the end of 1948? First it enjoyed one great advantage over the other bodies, it remained totally independent, and thus could continue to receive and discuss the aims and aspirations of individual rank and file anaesthetists and to channel its conclusions to the BMA and the Faculty, and the world at large; secondly it could continue to assist and advise individual members and groups of anaesthetists; thirdly it was poised to develop its research and educational activities, and thereby provide opportunities for scientific discussion and social intercourse among anaesthetists at a national and local level; fourthly, in the next decade, it was destined to play an important part in the development of international relations, and lastly, by carefully husbanding its financial resources the Association of Anaesthetists was potentially able to make very considerable funds available for research and development when they have been most required. The Association of Anaesthetists of Great Britain and Ireland was certainly able to enter the nineteen fifties with confident anticipation.

6

Consolidation and Progress

1 January 1949 to 31 December 1959

"Progress is not an accident,
but a necessity......
It is part of nature."

Herbert Spencer (1820-1903) *Social Statistics*

Officers

    Presidents: -   J Gillies   (1947-1950)[1]
                             W A Low (1950-1953)[2]
                             G S W Organe (1953-1956)[3]
                             T C Gray (1956-1959)
                             R Jarman (1959-1962)[4]

    Honorary Treasurers: -   B Johnson (1947-1950)[5]
                             T C Gray (1950-1955)
                             V F Hall (1955-1960)

    Honorary Secretaries: -   G S W Organe (1948-1952)[3]
                             R P W Shackleton (1952-1956)[6]
                             A J W Beard (1956-1960)[7]

    Editor of *Anaesthesia*:-   C Langton Hewer (1946-1966)[8]

The brave new world of the nineteen fifties

The population of the United Kingdom entered the nineteen fifties in a spirit of hope and determined optimism. It is difficult to convey to those who are too young to have experienced it, the extent of the feeling of euphoria and faith in the future that gripped the country at that time, despite what was a very gloomy political and economic atmosphere.

The Second World War was over but the British economy was in tatters. The immediate post-war period was a time of shortages and austerity in the victorious European countries as well as in those that had been vanquished; in Britain petrol rationing ended in 1950 but food rationing became even more severe for a time and continued until 1954. Maintenance work on buildings, hospitals, public utilities, industrial plant and transport had been minimal during the war years and civilian industrial development negligible. Extensive bomb damage accentuated the prevailing decrepitude and disrepair. There were as yet no motorways and few dual carriageways, the steam locomotives and rolling stock of the railways were worn out and outmoded, central heating in private houses was an unusual luxury, coal and coal gas were still the main domestic and industrial fuels, there was no clean-air policy, and chimneys belched forth pollution; as a consequence "pea-soup" fogs in London and the associated deaths from acute respiratory disease were not unusual.

Despite the dreary conditions there were a number of favourable factors which stimulated a general air of optimism however. Social barriers had been broken down by the war and new skills learned, and there was virtually full employment. This was partly due to the need for reconstruction, but also, it is true, because industrial automation as we know it had not yet fully developed. The United Kingdom also still needed to maintain large military forces and civilian services to police and administer its colonial empire.

The moral and financial burden occasioned by the needs of the dependent British overseas possessions was indeed formidable. The colonies, like those of other European states were clamouring for independence. This was conceded to the majority of them during the fifties and early sixties, but the British Government, unlike some other European administrations, endeavoured to suppress terrorism before handing over to the newly independent authorities. Large civilian and armed services had to be maintained to preserve peace and fight "actions in aid of the civil power" in many parts of the world, including Palestine (divided but independent in 1948), India and Pakistan (1947), Sudan (1956), Ghana (1957), Nigeria (1960), Cyprus (1962), Malaya and Kenya (1963) and Aden (1967); in addition troops were required for the support of the United Nations in Korea and in the abortive Suez campaign which followed the nationalisation of the Suez Canal by the Egyptians in 1956. The bulk of the rank and file and the junior officers engaged in such actions on the ground were youthful conscript National Servicemen. They acquitted themselves well, as did the slightly older but inexperienced recently qualified National Service medical officers who supported them.[9-11] The Consulting Surgeon to the Far East Land Forces wrote of the Malayan campaign:

> *"Any report of war surgery in Malaya would be incomplete without a tribute to all ranks of the Army Medical Services........... Despite constant shortages of staff and long hours of work their efforts have been tireless........ In particular we have been indebted to the junior surgeons and anaesthetists without whom it would have been impossible to carry on".*[11]

The experience to which the present author was subjected as a junior medical officer in the RAMC was not unique. He found himself in the position of being the only anaesthetist in North Malaya (civil or military) from 1950 to 1952, after a total civilian training of 6 months as a House Officer Anaesthetist in a teaching hospital, and he was, in addition, "the specialist in skins and venereal diseases" (with no experience or guidance except from an experienced Corporal and a general medical textbook!) A future Dean of the Faculty of Anaesthetists, John Nunn, was filling a similar role as an anaesthetist in the Colonial Service in the neighbouring Crown Colony of Penang at the time!

The Festival of Britain and the Exhibition of London's South Bank in 1951 heightened expectations for future prosperity, and the ladies startled their menfolk by discarding the austere but practical "coat and skirt" of the war years and appearing in the neo-Edwardian "New-Look".

His Majesty King George VI had been held in high esteem by his subjects, but his death in 1952, followed by the Coronation in 1953 of the young Queen, and the conquest of Everest by a British Commonwealth team, seemed to promise a second Elizabethan age.

There was certainly determination amongst both politicians and the population to make Britain the leader of the world in scientific, technical and industrial development. British inventiveness made a fine start in the immediate postwar period with innovations such as jet and turboprop aircraft engines, the Comet jet airliners, the first computers, and in atomic power but, by the end of the decade, the lead was in the process of being lost to other nations. Not for the first or last time, the United Kingdom, having suffered all the teething troubles of being first in the field (such as the Comet airliner disasters), was forced to stand by and watch other countries make commercially successful developments based on British research; either because of enormous financial power as was the case with the USA; or because autocratic governments allowed the bulk of their populations to live in comparative poverty while money was concentrated on dramatic developments such as space exploration, as happened in the USSR; or because nations such as Germany, which had had their industrial base destroyed in the war, re-equipped from scratch and introduced progressive management instead of trying to build on prewar technology in the face of outdated industrial practices, as was often the case in Britain.

These nationalistic considerations apart however, the nineteen fifties was a decade of truly amazing scientific advance for mankind. The key to the rapid development was, undoubtedly, the science of electronics. The decade began in the days of the early cumbersome computers based on the thermionic valve, progressed with the introduction of transistors, and ended on the threshold of further circuit miniaturisation with the microchip, and it began when inter-continental air travel was a novelty experienced by comparatively few, and ended with space exploration presaged by the launch of the first space satellite by the USSR in 1957.

Medicine and Surgery in the nineteen fifties

Medicine is an international discipline. Equipment and drugs may be patented and their costs may escalate and cause frustration, but, on the whole, the professional expertise required to operate apparatus and to administer therapy is freely disseminated amongst medical men - indeed there is often almost unseemly haste to claim the priority of being the first to employ and publish papers about a new discovery! The medical developments of the fifties, like those in science generally, and not least those in anaesthesia, were as dramatic and revolutionary as in any decade, or perhaps in any century in history.[12] Many of these developments directly influenced the nature of the practice of anaesthesia and brought fresh challenges for the specialty.

Antibiotics, tuberculosis and other infections. The only antibacterials generally available at the end of the Second World War were the sulphonamide group of antimicrobials and the antibiotic penicillin, but gradually many antibiotics were produced from various fungi or synthetically and put on the market.

The first of these was streptomycin which was introduced by Walksman and his colleagues in 1944.[13] This marked the beginning of the conquest of the scourge of tuberculosis when it came into general use in the early nineteen fifties. Resistant strains appeared, but combinations with paraaminosalicylic acid (PAS) and isonicotinic acid hydrazide (isoniazid) reduced this eventuality.[14]

A great deal of the work of the thoracic anaesthetist in the early fifties consisted in the administration of general and local anaesthetics for various procedures connected with tuberculosis (thoracoplasty, lobectomy, etc). Other thoracic operations were undertaken for the treatment of carcinoma of the lung and for closed cardiac procedures such as mitral valvotomy. The scene had changed considerably by nineteen sixty; carcinoma was still a problem of course, but surgery for tuberculosis was no longer required, and open cardiac surgery was becoming established.

Other antibiotics, including synthetic derivatives of penicillin, were introduced in the sixties and helped to make surgery and anaesthesia safer; amongst them were the broad spectrum agents chloramphenicol, neomycin and the tetracyclines.[15]

Poliomyelitis was still a dangerous and disabling disease in nineteen fifty. The **poliomyelitis** epidemic in Copenhagen in 1952 was the occasion when Bjorn Ibsen (later Chief of Anaesthesia at the Kommunehospital), working with Professor H C A Lassen, very successfully substituted manual positive pressure ventilation via a tracheotomy for the then standard method of management with negative pressure ventilation using tank or cuirass respirators.[16] This event revolutionised the management of respiratory failure in general and led ultimately to the establishment of intensive care units and the involvement of anaesthetists as a subspecialty. It also encouraged the introduction of mechanical ventilators into clinical anaesthesia.

Poliomyelitis itself was not destined to be a significant cause of respiratory failure for much longer in the developed world however. Jonas E Salk of the University of Michigan devised a vaccine which was given a nationwide trial in the United States in 1954, and Albert Sabin developed an attenuated oral vaccine a few years later; in the year before Salk's vaccine was commercially available (1955) there were 55,000 cases of poliomyelitis in the United States; in 1987 there were under 200 cases.[12,17] There were approximately 7,500 cases in the United Kingdom in the epidemic of 1947, 310 were treated in negative pressure respirators and 93 of these would subsequently require permanent ventilatory support,[18] fifteen years later poliomyelitis was a rare disease.

Kidney dialysis was first used successfully by William J Kolff in the Netherlands in 1945 using heparin for anticoagulation and cellophane as a filtration membrane.[19] Others improved and modified the apparatus and the procedure became well established by the mid nineteen fifties.

Renal transplantation using an identical twin as a donor was first undertaken in Boston, Massachusetts by Murray in 1954[20] but, though a number of attempts at homographs were made using total body irradiation for immunosuppression, the really successful application of the procedure had to await the use of steroids and other immunosuppressive drugs; a development based on research in the United Kingdom by Medawar and his colleagues which they published in 1951.[21,22]

Intravenous fluid therapy was beginning to be fully appreciated as an intraoperative adjunct to maintaining the patient's condition during surgery and in the postoperative period by 1950. This was both the result of wartime experience of the importance of the maintenance of the intravascular volume (Chapter 5) and a better understanding of salt and water balance.[23,24] There were, however, still a few older surgeons who regarded the putting up of an intravenous infusion, and still worse the administration of blood, as a thinly veiled hint that their surgery was causing more blood loss than was strictly necessary!

Cardiopulmonary resuscitation. Internal defibrillation of the arrested heart was developed by Kouwenhoven and his colleagues of the Johns Hopkins Hospital, Baltimore in the nineteen thirties.[25] The first successful internal defibrillation in man was reported by Beck of Cleveland, Ohio in 1947.[26] The technique was well understood in the United Kingdom by the mid-fifties and alternating current internal defibrillators were available in the operating rooms of major hospitals.[27] External cardiac compression was not yet developed however. The only available method was direct internal cardiac compression after the chest had been opened, or through the diaphragm from the peritoneal cavity. This was not encouraged outside the operating theatre in the United Kingdom, but in the USA at that time (1956) the modern practitioner in any discipline was expected to be able to open the chest and employ expired air respiration, which had recently been reintroduced,[28] and internal cardiac compression if a sudden cardiac arrest occurred. Kouwenhoven and his colleagues fortunately continued their investigations and described both external cardiac compression and external defibrillation in 1960.[25,29] This made cardiopulmonary resuscitation much more practical and generally acceptable.

Cardiac surgery. There had been isolated instances of closed digital and instrumental dilatation of the mitral valve in the nineteen twenties both in Britain[30,31] and in the United States,[32] but modern cardiac surgery really began in 1948 with reports of successful cases of dilation of the mitral, pulmonary and cardiac valves by, amongst others, Brock in the United Kingdom and Bailey in the United States.[33,34] These developments were parallel with the introduction of the new anaesthetic technique of neuromuscular paralysis, light anaesthesia and controlled ventilation (Chapter 5),[35] and were well established in British practice by the early fifties.

The introduction of open heart surgery techniques in Britain followed closely developments in the United States throughout the decade. Surface hypothermia and cardiac arrest, for the closure of atrial and ventricular septal defects, was introduced about 1953.[36,37] The first successful cardiopulmonary bypass operation was undertaken by Gibbon of Philadelphia in 1953 after prolonged research,[36,38,39] and by 1960 open heart surgery was well established on both sides of the Atlantic.[36,39]

The sterilisation of instruments and syringes. The sterilisation of surgical instruments at the start of the decade was largely effected by boiling, but by 1960 autoclaves were in general use in the United Kingdom. Delicate equipment such as cystoscopes and instruments with sharp cutting edges, including scalpels, were immersed in various chemical fluids or treated in formaldehyde cabinets. The question of the sterilisation of glass and metal syringes was however a problem throughout the decade. This was both because of the danger of transmission of hepatitis B and the inherent dangers in the administration of spinal (subarachnoid) anaesthesia.[40,41] Hot air ovens were recommended and considered to be better than autoclaving because of the need for the steam to penetrate in the latter case.[42] Chemical sterilisation and storage of syringes in spirit was the norm at the start of the decade, but many hospitals set up syringe services later on.[43] General Practitioners continued to use immersion in spirit well into the sixties. The eighteenth edition of Pye's Surgical Handicraft, published in 1962, still describes dissolving a tablet in heated water in a spoon as the standard method of preparing a morphia injection.[44] Disposable prepacked items sterilised by ethylene oxide gas were destined to revolutionise the use of syringes in the early sixties but were not generally available in the late fifties.[43,45] Younger anaesthetists who have not had to practise with non-disposable syringes with badly fitting plungers and blunt resterilised needles, have been denied a stressful and sometimes humiliating experience! Red rubber infusion giving sets and needles and cannulae for the administration of intravenous infusions were also re-usable until at least the mid fifties; their use often gave rise to venous thrombosis and pyrogenic reactions.

Clinical anaesthesia 1948 to 1958

Clinical anaesthesia in the operating theatre developed to full maturity in the nineteen fifties. The decade began with the gradual introduction into anaesthetic practice of neuromuscular blocking agents and the realisation that essential patient oxygenation in major cases could be best maintained by controlled ventilation of a paralysed patient,[35] moreover this procedure produced the best surgical conditions in terms of muscular relaxation and reduced blood loss, not least by avoiding hypercarbia.

These great benefits could not be obtained without risk if fatalities were to be avoided unless the anaesthetist improved his skills and professionalism. The fundamental fact that controlled or assisted ventilation was essential if the respiratory muscles were partially paralysed was not at first always appreciated; nor was the importance of reversal of nondepolarising muscle relaxants with neostigmine.[46] Many new intravenous drugs also had side effects which were potentially dangerous unless they were used skilfully; for example thiopentone is a cardiodepressant and essentially dangerous unless titrated carefully taking into account the physical and pathological condition of the patient, and tubocurarine produces hypotension by ganglion paralysis and must also be treated with respect, particularly in the hypovolaemic patient.

Monitoring during anaesthesia. The introduction of muscle relaxants and paralysis and controlled respiration techniques also created a need for more careful monitoring. When all patients breathed spontaneously the heart was automatically monitored. The anaesthetist at least knew that, if the patient was breathing the heart was beating; on the other hand the patient on controlled ventilation might well be dead. The writer does, however, remember a staff nurse of this period who believed that it was not possible for a patient on a mechanical ventilator to die!

Mechanical ventilation itself brought with it other hazards; for example disconnection became a most dangerous event, whereas previously the disconnection of a spontaneously respiring patient from an anaesthetic machine merely meant that the level of anaesthesia became lighter.

Electronic monitoring was, however, in its infancy at the beginning of the decade and the wizardry made possible by transistors and silicon chips was in the future. The electrocardioscopes were crude and temperamental and the potential hazard of cardiac arrest due to electrocution because the circuits were not isolated was unrecognised. The basic guides were the colour of the blood in the wound, the intermittent application of the finger to the pulse, observation of chest or lung movement, the "feel" of the reservoir bag (handing the patient over vicariously to the mechanical ventilator was at first a cause for considerable anxiety), noninvasive sphygmomanometry or the oscillometer and, if one were very advanced, various pulse meters based on the carbon microphone. These were often home made. It is a curious fact that, despite its rightful popularity in North America, the use of the chest stethoscope has never caught on in Britain, except perhaps in paediatric practice.

Open heart surgery, right at the end of the decade, brought with it more sophisticated monitors and the invasive measurement of arterial and venous blood pressure; even so the early monitors, still dependent on the thermionic valve, were monolithic pieces of apparatus!

Postoperative recovery. Open heart surgery, bringing with it a need for mechanical ventilation and careful monitoring in the postoperative period, was also to stimulate interest in the sixties in the provision of recovery rooms.[47,48] These were pioneered for general surgery by a few enthusiasts in the United Kingdom in the late fifties and still earlier in North America.[48-50]

Spinal subarachnoid anaesthesia enjoyed considerable popularity in the United Kingdom in the nineteen forties for abdominal and lower extremity procedures, although the reasons for the hypotension which it caused were not well understood, and the dangers of aortocaval compression in obstetrics were not yet appreciated.[51] The popularity of the technique plummeted in the United Kingdom for almost two decades after 1953 however. This followed the trial of the action for negligence in the "Wooley and Roe" case in which at least two, and possibly three, patients on the same operating list developed paraplegia following subarachnoid anaesthesia.[52,53] The cause of the damage was attributed to contamination of either the contents of the ampoules following chemical sterilisation, or more probably of the syringes and needles which were boiled in a steriliser previously "descaled" with the aid of a chemical[53] and the case against the anaesthetists was dismissed.[52,53] A suspicion remained amongst anaesthetists however, that the possibility existed that the spinal local anaesthetic solutions themselves might occasionally cause neurological damage, as was suggested by some eminent neurologists at the trial.[52,53]

Lumbar and caudal extradural anaesthesia. Extradural techniques gained popularity in the nineteen fifties particularly for gynaecological surgery but continuous lumbar extradural (epidural) analgesia was not yet used for analgesia in childbirth.

Caudal (sacral) extradural block for obstetrics had been introduced in the United States in the forties and was already very popular there by the fifties.[54] Galley advocated the technique in *Anaesthesia* in 1949[55] but it never became popular in the United Kingdom except, perhaps, to a very limited extent in private practice. The reason for this difference was probably due to the fact that there was a high forceps rate under caudal analgesia and, whereas obstetric deliveries were almost exclusively conducted by medical practitioners in the United States, in the United Kingdom most normal cases were managed by midwives, many of them in the patients' own homes. British obstetricians of that era were apt to look upon the high forceps rate in the USA with derision, and to teach that the sacral extradural technique was inherently dangerous. The comparison was not reasonable however; in those days "forceps" in the United Kingdom often meant the strenuous intervention of mid-level forceps, not the gentle lift off the perineum practised in the United States!

Advances in pharmacology in the fifties

It seemed to many British anaesthetists by the mid fifties that, so far as anaesthesia for major surgery was concerned, the pinnacle of development had been reached with the adoption of the light anaesthesia, muscle relaxant and controlled respiration technique - "the big syringe and the little syringe".[56] Attention consequently turned to measures designed to maintain or improve the physical status of the patient during surgery; for example by mechanical ventilation and the control of fluid balance,[57] and the provision of better operating conditions for the surgeon. The latter included measures designed to reduce haemorrhage during neurosurgery, plastic surgery and microsurgery of the ear. There were, however, gaps in the pharmacopoeia at the start of the decade; for example the quickest method of securing rapid recovery in the dental surgery and outpatient department was still the combination of nitrous oxide and asphyxia, a short acting muscle relaxant for endotracheal intubation had yet to be developed, and the long established but most used local anaesthetic procaine was slow in onset and its potency was diminished by heat sterilisation. All of these problems were at least partially solved by the dramatic development of new pharmacological agents before the end of the decade, but there were also false trails and enthusiasms.

"Controlled" hypotension, designed to reduce surgical bleeding almost completely, occupied much space in the journals and discussions of the early fifties. It is incontrovertibly fortunate that the attempt to minimise bleeding by reactive vasoconstriction, resulting from haemorrhage from elective arteriotomy,[58] was quickly superseded by the more logical concept of hypotension following vasodilation brought about by the paralysis of the sympathetic nervous system. This objective was first achieved by the alarming, but apparently successful, "total" spinal technique (in which, at times, the only signs of life were spontaneous respiration and palpation of the apex beat [59,60]), and then by the use of the ganglion blockers. The first of these were pentamethonium (C5)[61] and hexamethonium (C6);[62] they were shortly followed by the introduction of the more controllable pentolinium,[63] trimetaphan (Arfonad) and phenacyl homatropinium (Trophenium).[64]

Pethidine, (USA Demerol) the first totally synthetic analgesic, had been in use for some years[65] as a general analgesic and in obstetrics, but, in the early nineteen fifties, it found a new use as an intravenous supplement to nitrous oxide and oxygen anaesthesia.[66,67] This was particularly valuable before the introduction of halothane. It also provided a method of facilitating intubation by obtunding laryngeal reflexes which was useful before succinylcholine was introduced.[68] The advent of both halothane and succinylcholine are considered below.

The phenothiazines chlorpromazine (Largactil) and promethazine (Phenergan) were first used in anaesthesia by Laborit and Huguenard in France in 1951.[69] These drugs are notable as one of the first psychokinetic drugs capable of altering the patients' mood and mental attitude without necessarily producing sedation, and they were first used orally by psychiatrists and for pre- and postoperative sedation. They came into prominence in the early fifties, however, because of the use of chlorpromazine in combination with promethazine and pethidine (the so called 'lytic cocktail') as a basal anaesthetic in the first Indo-Chinese war.[70] This had both real and alleged advantages under field conditions, particularly in the control of the autonomic system. Various forms of the technique were used in clinical anaesthesia and these were well reviewed by Dundee in 1954.[69] Anaesthetists in the United Kingdom were sceptical however. The accepted legitimate uses of the phenothiazines were summarised in an editorial in *Anaesthesia* in 1955.[71] These were chiefly for the control of anxiety, as an anti-emetic and, possibly, to promote cooling by vasodilation in the surface hypothermia technique then in use both in cardiac and neurosurgery.

Neuromuscular blocking agents. The mechanisms by which the muscle relaxants produced their effects at the neuromuscular junction were not properly understood at the start of the nineteen fifties but, by 1960, the distinction between depolarisers and non-depolarisers had been defined. Several synthetic non-depolarising agents were produced in the fifties but only gallamine triethiodide (Flaxedil), introduced in France by Bovet[72] and to British practice by Mushin,[73] has stood the test of time.

Succinylcholine. The depolarising agent decamethonium enjoyed a spell of popularity,[74,75] but revolutionary progress was made when succinylcholine (Scoline) became available.[75,76] Here, for the first time, was an agent of rapid onset, which produced profound relaxation for intubation but from which recovery was rapid, enabling spontaneous respiration to be resumed.

Succinylcholine still "enjoys widespread popularity (in 1998) despite its many untoward side effects and the introduction of several short-acting alternatives".[77] It is of interest that one "complication" which at first caused widespread concern was its "all or nothing" action compared with curare. The writer recalls the consternation of two very senior Consultants who decided to "try out" the "new" muscle relaxant which had just become available in 1952. Both these eminent gentlemen employed tubocurarine merely as an adjuvant while their patients breathed spontaneously. Great was the dismay when this particular patient ceased to breathe altogether after a cautious dose of half that recommended by the manufacturer; there was still greater relief when the patient started to breathe again after two or three minutes!

Halothane (Fluothane), a powerful nonirritant inhalation agent from which recovery was rapid was, without doubt, the most exciting discovery of the nineteen fifties. It was the product of painstaking research by Suckling[78] and Raventos[79] in the laboratories of Imperial Chemical Industries (now Zeneca). Their research was a deliberate attempt to develop a new nonexplosive agent which would supplant ether, chloroform (when still used), and trichloroethylene. The agent rapidly gained popularity after its clinical introduction in 1956, almost concurrently by Johnstone of Manchester[80] and Bryce-Smith of Oxford,[81] despite what was then considered to be its exorbitant cost. One benefit, amongst many, was that it was now possible to administer an anaesthetic to an outpatient, from which rapid recovery was possible, without hypoxia. The side-effect which halothane had of producing hypotension also proved useful in controlling surgical haemorrhage and, to some extent supplanted the intravenous hypotensive agents. Halothane, because of its potency, also made it necessary to introduce accurate calibrated temperature controlled vaporisers (including the first British Fluotec) into continuous flow anaesthesia, in place of the simple uncalibrated glass Boyle bottles previously in use - a further cause of confrontation about cost with supply departments! The honeymoon between anaesthetists and halothane was brief but idyllic, the ideal volatile agent seemed to have been found before complications such as possible liver damage[82] and the occasional initiation of malignant hyperthermia[83] were appreciated; despite these concerns however, and given their rarity, most anaesthetists felt able to live with this easily administered agent, at least until other less toxic inhalation anaesthetics were introduced in the nineteen seventies and eighties.

Methohexitone (Brietal) was introduced in the United States in the same year as halothane (1956)[84] and underwent trials in the United Kingdom in the late fifties,[85] but it did not come into general use until the early sixties. It was the first intravenous agent from which recovery was rapid and safe enough to be considered for general use in British outpatient departments and dental surgeries.

Lignocaine (Xylocaine), the first amide local analgesic, was introduced into clinical practice by Gordh in 1949.[86] It rapidly replaced procaine which had led the field since its use was described by Braun in 1904.[87] The two chief reasons for this remarkable revolution in local anaesthetic practice were its rapid onset and its stability when sterilised by heat. It was however considerably more toxic than procaine. Those who used the drug rapidly learnt, sometimes the hard way, that a great deal more respect had to be paid to ensuring that stipulated maximum safe dosages were not exceeded than was the case with procaine!

Academic anaesthesia 1949-1959

Professor (Sir) Robert Macintosh, as head of the Nuffield Department of Anaesthetics in the University of Oxford, was the only Professor of Anaesthetics in Great Britain at the beginning of 1949, but John Gillies[1] had been elected Simpson Reader in Anaesthetics in Edinburgh in 1946, W W Mushin[88] Independent Lecturer and Director of Anaesthetics at the Welsh National School of Medicine at Cardiff in 1947 (Professor 1953), and Edgar Pask[89] became Reader in Anaesthetics at the University of Durham Medical School at Newcastle upon Tyne in 1948 and Professor a year later; both Mushin and Pask were former members of Macintosh's Nuffield Department at Oxford. T Cecil Gray had been appointed Reader in Anaesthetics at Liverpool in 1947 and was elected Professor in 1959, and Ronald Woolmer, Head of the Department of Anaesthetics at the Royal College of Surgeons of England in London, was also elected to the British Oxygen Company (BOC) endowed professorial chair at the surgeons' College in 1959.[90]

University departments under Readers or Senior Lecturers were established at Belfast (J W Dundee, later Professor),[91] at Glasgow (A C Forrester, later Professor), at Leeds (R B Harbord), at Bristol (first under Ronald Woolmer and then under Professor J Clutton-Brock[92]), and at the, not yet "Royal" Postgraduate Medical School, Hammersmith, London (J P Payne, who later succeeded Woolmer as Professor at the Royal College of Surgeons of England) during the nineteen fifties.

The NHS in the fifties

Sir Reginald Murley in his book '*Surgical Roots and Branches*' has referred to the fifties and sixties as the "vintage years" of the NHS.[93] He is probably right! The fundamental deficiencies in the old system had been addressed but the structure and dedication of the hospital staff was retained.[93-95] The funding provided by central government was adequate in terms of the technology of the period. The former voluntary hospitals no longer had to rely on bequests and flag days, and municipal hospitals were freed from the nationally uneven provision by local government. The combination of voluntary hospitals and municipal hospitals under a single District, Regional and National administration rationalised the system, and remuneration for work done by senior and junior medical staff for the NHS had been introduced at rates that were not unreasonable in the late forties. Consultants were given the choice of combining NHS with private practice, both in private wards within the NHS and in privately run "nursing homes" outside it. Consultant anaesthetists in particular benefited from having Consultant status and a basic salary which did not depend on the goodwill of their surgical colleagues and competition from referring general practitioners (Chapter 4).

There was one other important factor. The essential structure of the former voluntary hospital administration was retained at District level.[93-95] The new NHS had the benefit of the dedication to the primary objective of care of patients of the staff (medical, nursing, administrative, domestic and service) which was traditional and vital in the previous system. Hospital Management Committees were largely composed of the same public spirited laymen and senior medical men who had raised money and managed the hospitals prior to 1948,[95] although they were now relieved of the former duty and often somewhat irked by the restrictions imposed upon them by the Regional Boards to which they were now responsible. Hospital Secretaries supervised all aspects of administration and supply in each hospital, often with the aid of a single personal secretary, and were not averse to coming out of their office to investigate problems on the spot! The Matron was a highly respected figure who devoted herself to the care and comfort of the patients in the widest sense, and was a frequent visitor to the hospital wards. The ill-famed Salmon Report on nursing was a long way in the future (Chapter 7),[96] and senior nursing sisters were proud to spend their whole career in both the practice and supervision of bedside care in the wards (where it should be stated their influence on the prescriptive therapy of the medical profession was considerable because of the very high degree of respect and trust between the two mutually symbiotic professions). Sir Reginald Murley in recalling these early days wrote in 1990:-

> *"When we look back on it all now..... we recognise these as the vintage years of the NHS. Everyone worked with enthusiasm, and pay disputes and militant unionism were unknown. One hates to misuse, or overuse, the word 'dedication' but only an organisation with truly dedicated staff could have operated so well under government near monopoly and centralised bureaucracy... Even those who had harboured serious doubts about the nationalisation of medicine were puzzled by the seeming smoothness with which the system surely operated. But as had been so surely predicted...... this was the lull before the storm."*[93]

The reason for this "lull before the storm" which lasted until the mid sixties is not far to seek with hindsight. It was simply that the costs of technological medicine and inflation were only just beginning to rise in the fifties and expenditure on the NHS was still within the means of the National Treasury. The independent Guillebaud Committee on "the cost of the National Health Service"[97-99] reported that, in real terms, the amount expended on the NHS in 1945-1950 had not risen by 1954-1955, and that:-

> *"any charge that there has been widespread extravagance in the National Health Service, whether in respect of spending money or the use of manpower, is not borne out by the evidence".*[98]

The Committee concluded further that only very minor changes were necessary in the structure of the service.[98,99] The storm, when it came in the seventies and eighties was precipitated by the realisation by the Government of the day that the cost of a comprehensive service entirely free at the point of use had outstripped the ability of the Treasury to pay for it. This has resulted in several attempts at reorganisation of the Service by successive governments of all parties in the seventies, eighties and nineties, in a thinly disguised but useless attempt to demonstrate that the gap between funding and spending is due to the inefficiencies of its active clinical staff, and not to a fundamental deficiency in financial provision.

Medical manpower, management and remuneration were the cause of considerable difficulty in the fifties however. There is no doubt that General Practitioners were badly treated initially when the NHS was introduced, both from the point of view of remuneration and practice conditions, but the unexpectedly generous Dankwert's award of 1952 did much to alleviate their position.[97] This was, incidentally, the first and only occasion when any Government has agreed to submit a claim for increased medical salaries to arbitration by a High Court Judge!

Established hospital doctors were much less discontented than General Practitioners with their conditions of service in the early years of the decade.[97] Dissatisfaction developed however; this stemmed from a cause which has dogged the relations between the profession and Government throughout the history of the NHS, namely the disproportionately large number of training posts in relation to the inadequate number of consultant appointments.[97,100,101] Early on the situation was very grim indeed as a result of clumsy regulations introduced in 1951 in an attempt to bring the number of Senior Registrars into line with the expected Consultant vacancies. The solution adopted was, not to increase the number of Consultant posts, but to limit the tenure of Senior Registrar appointments to three years. Much anxiety was caused before new regulations were introduced in 1953 providing for the retention of time expired Senior Registrars.[102] Nonetheless, in some specialties, a large number of very well qualified Senior Registrars were held in that grade for inordinately long periods. Many others with specialist qualifications opted for General Practice at this time with the result that there was gross overloading of application lists, and a great many others emigrated to the United States, Canada, Australia and New Zealand - countries that were, at that time, underdoctored and open to British graduates with minimal formality.[103-105] The words of a popular wartime army song of the nineteen forties headed one report on the subject in 1962: - "You'll get no promotion this side of the ocean, So cheer up my lads. Bless 'em all"![105] The specialty of anaesthesia was less affected than those of surgery and medicine because of the initial expansion in Consultant Anaesthetists at the start of the NHS, but secondment to the United States for a year became fashionable and the BTA ("Been to America") an advantage in obtaining a teaching hospital consultant appointment.[106]

A fortuitous event which hastened the establishment of anaesthesia as a postgraduate, rather than an undergraduate, study was the introduction 1 January 1953 of the compulsory provisional registration year after obtaining a medical qualification, under the Medical Act of 1950. Anaesthesia was not listed as a medical or surgical appointment for the provisional registration year and, consequently, all House Anaesthetist posts were upgraded to Senior House Officer appointments. Medical and surgical House Officers also began to refuse to administer anaesthetics in the Casualty Department and elsewhere (Council Minutes 7.7.61),[107] and, as a result few practitioners who entered General Practice after their provisional registration year, were prepared to become General Practitioner Anaesthetists.

The business of the Association 1949-1959

The foundation of the Faculty of Anaesthetists in 1948 and the inauguration of the NHS in the same year changed the tenor of business conducted by the Association of Anaesthetists. The Faculty had taken over the responsibility for matters concerning the examinations and the supervision and standards of training, including the postgraduate lectures for trainees which had been inaugurated by the Association of Anaesthetists. The extent of the changes in the standards and methods of remuneration of anaesthetists that came about with the inauguration of the NHS was such an improvement on the previous position that, except in employment not covered by the NHS salary and in the private sector, Council was more concerned with ensuring that the status of individual anaesthetists was such that they were able to enjoy the rewards of Consultant rank when this was appropriate.

The division of responsibility between the various organisations of anaesthetists was apparent rather than real, however. This was because of the very considerable overlap between membership of the Council of the Association of Anaesthetists, the Board of the Faculty and the Committee of the BMA Anaesthetists' Group; for example the Annual Report of Council for 1954-55 states that "ten members of the Council serve on the Board of Faculty and five on the Anaesthetists' Group Committee, and the President of the Association [(Sir) Geoffrey Organe][3] is Chairman of the Group Committee and represents it on the Central Consultants and Specialists Committee." The Council Minutes indicate that there were occasional discussions about the division of responsibility,[107] but it is not to be wondered at that it was stated that "the Liaison Committee (between the three organisations) has not met during the past year but the policies of the three bodies have been in accord"! Additionally from 1949 onwards, following a resolution of Council on 27 October 1948, the Dean of the Faculty, the Adviser to the Ministry of Health and the President of the Section of Anaesthetics of the Royal Society of Medicine were coopted to Council as observers (Annual Report 1950). The Council of the Association was already then, as it still is, the central clearing house for discussion of the affairs of the specialty.[107] *Anaesthesia,* the journal of the Association also assumed the role of disseminating information about the activities of the Association itself, the Faculty and other organisations and societies, which had been previously filled by the *British Journal of Anaesthesia.*

The Council of the Association concerned itself specifically with giving evidence to committees of inquiry (both directly and through the BMA), with the grading of individual anaesthetists in the NHS, and the promotion of research and what is now (in 1998) termed "medical audit"; the assessment and standardisation of equipment; the considerable extension of international relationships amongst anaesthetists which took place in the fifties; recommendations regarding fees in private practice; advice to and the support of individual anaesthetists; and finally, towards the end of the decade, it began to enter the field of the continuing education of its clinically active Fellows and Members. This last development provided for a need to which the Section of Anaesthetics of the Royal Society of Medicine, with its smaller membership, was not fully able to respond because of an increased demand. The increased need for educational activities was undoubtedly partly due to the fact that the anaesthetists' livelihood was no longer dependent on private fees for individual cases leaving them free to attend meetings. All these activities were accompanied by the promotion of the social fellowship for which anaesthesia, as a specialty was, and is still, renowned.

The administrative structure and organisation of the Association of Anaesthetists

The headquarters of the Association of Anaesthetists remained at the Royal College of Surgeons of England in Lincoln's Inn Fields, London throughout the nineteen fifties as an integral part of the Joint Secretariat (Chapter 5).

The beginning of the Presidency of John Gillies,[1] was marked by the start of a new Minute Book containing more ordered typewritten accounts of Council meetings,[107] and the fifties saw an increasing sophistication in the way the affairs of the Association were conducted.

Standing committees were established to which business of Council was delegated. The Council Minutes for 2 January 1959 lists the following committees and Chairmen[107]:-

Apparatus	W D Wylie
Deaths associated with anaesthesia	G Edwards[108]
Editorial Board	G S W Organe[3]
Finance Committee	R P W Shackleton[6]
Research	E A Pask[89]
Appeals (for Research funds)	R Jarman[4]
Annual Meeting	R Jarman[4]
Advisory	W W Mushin

The nature of the last named committee calls for comment. It served a very different purpose from the Advisory Committee of the Association in 1998 which corresponds to the Cabinet in British Parliamentary government, and is charged with sorting out, debating, and presenting matters for consideration by the full Council. The Advisory Committee of the fifties and sixties considered constitutional matters and dealt with the many personal problems, usually concerning terms and conditions of service posed by members from all over the world. In many cases they succeeded in improving the lot of the individual concerned.[107]

Fellowship and Membership

The requirement that Ordinary "Fellows" of the Association of Anaesthetists should hold teaching hospital appointments (Annual Report

1945) was dropped during 1946 (Annual Report 1946). Candidates for Fellowship after 1946 were required to hold the Diploma of Anaesthetics of the Royal College of Physicians and Surgeons (DA) and to be actively engaged in teaching anaesthetics at the university schools of medicine, or to be specialising entirely in the practice of anaesthetics and to hold hospital appointments approved by Council, or to be engaged in full-time research in subjects related to the theory and practice of anaesthesia. Members were not required to hold the DA but merely had to have professional interests predominantly in anaesthetics.

The introduction of the Fellowship of the Faculty of Anaesthetists of the Royal College of Surgeons of England (FFARCS), and the appointment of many with that diploma to consultant status, reduced the need for a distinction between Fellows and Members of the Association of Anaesthetists. Victor Goldman suggested as early as 1949 (Council Minutes 6.5.1949)[107] that the division into Fellows and Members should be abolished, but this idea was rejected out of hand at that time. Consumer resistance developed to paying the additional fee required for elevation to Association Fellowship status in 1955, however, when a number of Members either declined or ignored the invitation of Council to become Fellows and:-

> *"Members of Council were concerned that there should have been any rejections of the Fellowship and felt that the policy previously followed had possibly been wrong" (Council Minute 3 November 1955).*[107]

The categories of membership were reviewed pragmatically and the following solution was adopted (paraphrased from Council Minute 1 June 1956. Annual Reports 1956 and 1957 and an Editorial in the April 1957 number of *Anaesthesia*):-[109]

> *Ordinary Fellows* would be elected from amongst registered medical practitioners predominantly engaged in the practice of anaesthetics.
>
> *Members* would be elected from amongst registered medical practitioners who practised anaesthetics but not as a predominant interest.
>
> *Associate Members* would be elected from amongst registered

medical practitioners (usually Registrars or Senior House Officers) who were training in anaesthetics.

The categories of *Senior Fellows* ("elected from amongst Ordinary Fellows who had retired from medical practice"), *Corresponding Fellows* elected from anaesthetists of established position who practised outside the British Isles, and, of course, *Honorary Fellows* (distinguished persons whether medically qualified or not or whether anaesthetists or not), were retained.

The latter three categories were not required to pay a subscription and an allowance was made for the £1 (1996: £12.50) entrance fee which existing Members who were elected as Fellows had already paid. The new entrance fee was three guineas (1996: £39) and the annual subscription, including the journal *Anaesthesia*, £2.50 (1996: £31).[109]

The significance of these imaginative changes was considerable. The inauguration of the NHS 'with its emphasis on specialist cover and trainee career staff in all hospitals' had meant the end of the elitism of the teaching hospitals, even though the consultants in the latter establishments were generally respected as the leaders of the specialty. An Editorial in *Anaesthesia*[109] commented that for the first time all medical practitioners interested in anaesthetics could now join the Association of Anaesthetists. Ordinary Membership or Fellowship was definitely confined to medical practitioners. No mention is made of academic qualification even for the Fellowship category; this reflected confidence that insistence that the possession of the FFARCS was a necessary qualification as a key to Consultant Status in the NHS was generally insisted upon, but accepted that Senior Hospital Medical Officers (SHMOs), who probably only had the DA, could be Ordinary Fellows also, as indeed could Senior Registrars and even Registrars who had obtained the FFARCS. Those General Practitioners who retained anaesthetic appointments in hospitals or who administered general anaesthetics in dental surgeries were also eligible to be drawn into the fold. Provision was also made for the first time for inclusion of trainees as Associate Members; for the moment they did not have voting rights but they were not required to pay an entrance fee when they became eligible for promotion to Fellowship. Corresponding Membership remained a minor mark of recognition short of Honorary Membership which the Association of Anaesthetists could bestow on well known "established" anaesthetists from overseas.[109]

These changes resulted in an increase in the numbers enrolled in the Association and in the nominal proportions of new-style Members and Fellows, and meant that all practising senior specialists in the United Kingdom and Ireland were eligible for Fellowship of the Association, whether they were Consultants or SHMOs.

Comparison of the Annual Reports for 1956 and 1958 demonstrates the effect of the changes. There were 10 Honorary, 23 Corresponding, 24 Senior and 431 Ordinary Fellows, and 617 Members in 1956 (total membership 1105), and 10 Honorary, 29 Corresponding, 25 Senior, 619 Ordinary Fellows, 433 Members and 74 Associates by 1958 (total membership 1190). The total membership at the end of the decade was 1228, of which number 654 were active Ordinary Fellows practising in the United Kingdom and Ireland, 411 were Members and there were 94 Associates in training (Annual Report 1959).

Associate Fellowship was yet another category of membership with no voting rights which was added at the Annual General Meeting in 1959.[107] This was for "registered medical practitioners *and others* who are interested in anaesthetics but not engaged in the medical practice of anaesthetics". The list of Members bound with the Annual Report of 1959 lists only one Associate Fellow. This was a Dr Papantonopoulos of Athens who had both medical and dental qualifications and whose application for membership had given rise to considerable discussion at Council meetings during 1959. The 1960 list of Members adds a dental practitioner, a veterinary surgeon from Nyasaland and Barbara M Q Weaver of the Department of Veterinary Surgery of the University of Bristol who was to become an Honorary Member of the Association.

The removal of a name from the List of Members

The Council Minutes of 3 January 1958 state that the name of J Bodkin Adams "must [sic] be removed from the List of Members as he was no longer included in the General Medical Register".[107] This recalls a well publicised legal case. Bodkin Adams had been acquitted of murdering his patients but had been subsequently struck off the Register for offences connected with dangerous drugs; in actual fact his name had not been included in the List of Members circulated with the Annual Report since 1956.

Association Honours 1949-1959

Honorary Membership (or Honorary Fellowship as it was known at the time) was bestowed on eight eminent anaesthetists during the period covered by this Chapter. Five of them were ageing pioneer members of the Association mentioned in preceding chapters who were past or near retirement age (Ashley Daly and Sir Ivan Magill in 1956, Henry Featherstone in 1957, and John Gillies and Archibald Marston in 1959). Sir Robert Macintosh (1892-1962) was also elected in 1959; he was younger and was to be active in the affairs of the specialty of anaesthesia for another 10 years, but his dominant position as the head of the first professorial department of anaesthesia in the United Kingdom at Oxford, his distinguished wartime career, and his knighthood which had been gazetted in 1955, made him a very worthy recipient. The other two Honorary Members to be elected were Canadians, both from Montreal. Harold Randall Griffith, Chief of Anaesthesia at the Montreal Homeopathic Hospital, who introduced the use of curare as a muscle relaxant to modern anaesthesia became an Honorary Fellow in 1953. Wesley Bourne of McGill University received the honour in 1955; he was the first Canadian Professor and Chairman of the McGill University Department of Anaesthesia and Griffith described him in an obituary as "A light that has illuminated the whole field of anaesthesiology for fifty years".[110]

John Snow Medals. The acknowledged doyen of British anaesthetists Zebulon Mennell was presented with the fourth John Snow Medal at the Annual General Meeting in 1948.[111] Nobody had contributed more to the early development of the Association or to the organisation of the civilian anaesthetic services during the Second World War. Four John Snow Medals were awarded in the nineteen fifties; all of them in 1958.[112] Two of the recipients were Past Presidents of the Association (John Gillies and Archibald Marston). The others were Sir Ivan Magill and Robert J Minnitt from Liverpool, the pioneer of the use of nitrous oxide for obstetric analgesia in 1935.

Status and remuneration

The Senior Hospital Medical Officer (SHMO) grading controversy was considered in Chapter 5. Some injustices were perpetuated well into the nineteen fifties. The Association of Anaesthetists was active in achieving regrading to Consultant status for many suitably qualified specialists in England, Wales, and Scotland, but the Northern Ireland Hospitals Authority remained stubbornly adamant that Consultant status in the NHS could only be granted to anaesthetists if, in addition to the Diploma in Anaesthetics (DA), they had also proceeded to the MD degree or had obtained the diploma of Fellowship of one of the Royal Colleges of Surgeons (FRCS) or Membership of a college of Physicians (MRCP) (Annual Report 1950).[113] This was despite the upgrading of the DA to two parts. The Association made representations. Dr H H Pinkerton[114] of Glasgow went over to Belfast to assist in presenting the case of the Northern Irish anaesthetists (Council Minutes 6 April 1951), but the problem was not finally resolved until 1954 after the examination for the two-part DA had been translated into one for the Fellowship of the Faculty of Anaesthetists in 1953.[115,116] The Northern Ireland Hospitals Authority then recognised the FFARCS as a suitable qualification for Consultant status even though the differences between the examination for the two-part DA and that for the FFARCS were minimal. The Irish Medical Association recommended at about the same time that specialist anaesthetists should be paid at the same rate as physicians and surgeons in the Republic of Ireland, where, of course, the writ of the NHS did not run (Council 23 July 1954).[107] It is, incidentally, an interesting reflection on the status accorded to the new qualification of the FFARCS, even amongst anaesthetists themselves, that, in Council Minutes and contemporary reports in *Anaesthesia,* senior anaesthetists who were honoured by being elected to the Fellowship of the Royal College of Surgeons, were immediately designated as "Mr" instead of "Dr", thus adopting the style traditionally employed by surgeons in the United Kingdom and Ireland; for example, "Mr" Magill, "Mr" Marston and "Mr" Daly![107]

The shortage of Consultant posts which has been mentioned earlier in this chapter concerned the Council of the Association of Anaesthetists throughout the decade (Annual Reports 1954, 1955, 1956, 1957, 1958);[117] unlike many of the other specialties there was also a lack of Senior Registrar posts, and thus, at times, even though there was an overall shortage of

Consultant posts there was a deficiency of appropriately graded candidates for promotion for those vacancies that were available. The Council submitted a memorandum in 1954 to the Joint Consultants' Committee (JCC) which is composed of representatives of the Royal Colleges and the BMA, which had come into being under the Chairmanship of Sir Lionel Whitby who had previously been President of the BMA. (Sir) Geoffrey Organe[3] was one of the delegation which met the representatives of the Ministry of Health in 1955. A marked improvement was secured by the end of 1956; Consultant posts in anaesthesia in England and Wales had been increased from 688 to 748 between 1954 and 1955, and Senior Registrarships from 48 to 67. Thirty five of the Senior Registrar posts were in teaching hospitals, 31 in non-teaching hospitals and one, which was held by the present writer, was the first to rotate between a Teaching and a District General Hospital. The 1956 Annual Report to Council welcomed the increase but noted that "the number of Senior Registrars is appreciably below what we consider desirable if an adequate number of consultants are to be trained". There were 2116 Consultants in post in 1989[118] and 368 Senior Registrars in September 1988[119] and even these numbers were still too low. Council also produced memoranda on the subject to the Royal Commission on the Remuneration of Doctors and Dentists in the NHS (Annual Report 1957) and to the Joint Working Party on Medical Staffing Structure in the Hospital Service under Sir Robert Platt the President of the Royal College of Physicians (Annual Report 1958). The Platt Committee again recommended increases in consultant establishments when it reported in 1961.

Dental Anaesthesia

The administration of outpatient anaesthetics to NHS patients in dental surgeries was and still is a service for which additional NHS fees are payable. Concern about the adequacy of these fees has been a preoccupation of the Association of Anaesthetists from the inception of the NHS up to the present time. The fifties were no exception. Discussions were held with the British Dental Association (BDA) and the BMA without a satisfactory unanimity being reached (Annual Reports 1949 and 1950). Low (the President Elect of the Association) reported to Council on 31 March 1950 that the President of the BDA had stated at a meeting that, "the NHS fee laid down was one paid to the dentist for the waste of his time while the anaesthetic was given" and, by inference, it was up to an arrangement between the dentist and the anaesthetist as to how much of the fee was passed on to him! This was unfortunately a true statement of the position. Low confirmed that "he believed that the Ministry had no statutory powers to pay a fee to the anaesthetist".[107]

Council appointed a committee under the Chairmanship of R P W Shackleton, to consider various aspects of dental anaesthesia.[107] This committee asked the Faculty of Anaesthetists to inquire into the amount and quality of training in outpatient anaesthesia in medical and dental schools (Annual Report 1959). Further hard fought negotiations were to take place during the next thirty years (Chapters 7-9).

Fees for private patients in NHS hospitals

A particular issue was the scales and limitations of fees for patients undergoing treatment in the private wings of hospitals taken over by the NHS. A subcommittee prepared the following recommendations which were forwarded to the Joint (Whitby) Committee set up by the Royal Colleges and the BMA and were copied to the Ministry of Health. They proposed that for the administration of the anaesthetic, preoperative examination of the patient and one routine postoperative visit fees should be as follows (paraphrased from the Council Minute at 7.1.1949)[107]:-

1. Minor surgical procedures except where such procedures involve possible obstruction of the airway:- 3 guineas (1996:£54)

    All other anaesthetics:- 5 guineas (1996: £90)

2. An additional fee of $2^{1}/_{2}$ guineas (1996: £45) shall be pay able for one of the following complicating factors, and a further $2^{1}/_{2}$ guineas for two or more:-
    (a) an operation lasting more than $2^{1}/_{2}$ hours
    (b) the severity of the operation
    (c) the site of the operation (e.g. involving possible obstruction of the airway) and,
    (d) the condition of the patient as it effects the anaesthetic risk.

3. Where the anaesthetist is called upon to attend the patient in a consultant capacity, or to take part in the diagnosis or

treatment of the patient, any procedure he undertakes should be paid for on the same basis as any other consultant.

The largest possible fee for an anaesthetic would therefore be 10 guineas (£1996: £180).

The response of the BMA to this proposal was disappointing. The Annual Report of the Association of Anaesthetists for 1949 states that:-

"The schedule of fees issued by the Ministry of Health was considered to be most unsatisfactory and an amended schedule had been sent to the Ministry and the Joint (Whitby) Committee based on the principle that the anaesthetists' fee should not be in relation to that of the surgeon, but should be related to the anaesthetic given and not the operation. Various complicating factors in connection with the patient should raise the fee from one category to another. It is understood, however that the BMA are pressing for the whole schedule to be withdrawn and a maximum fee of 75 guineas only specified."

This fee would be equivalent to £1,340 in 1996 terms, and it must therefore represent the maximum fee chargeable by any specialist including the surgeon in the private wards of NHS hospitals. The Association's suggested schedule was therefore very modest. The 1957 Annual Report and the Minutes which preceded it[107] record a change of attitude on the part of the BMA negotiators:-

"A memorandum on the scale of fees charged to private patients.... approved by Council has been very favourably received by the Anaesthetists' Group of the BMA and forwarded by that Committee to the Central Consultants' Committee".

Annual General Meetings and Dinners 1949-1955

The tradition of holding an Annual Dinner following the Annual General (business) Meeting at the Royal College of Surgeons of England in Lincoln's Inn Fields became firmly established. This followed the first dinner held in 1946 during the celebrations in honour of the centenary of Morton's seminal ether demonstration at the Massachusetts General Hospital (Chapter 5). The dinner was held at Claridge's Hotel from 1947 to 1955, apart from 1949, when it was at the Savoy Hotel' and 1954, when it was in the "beautiful new Great Hall" of the Royal College of Surgeons of England which had been rebuilt after wartime bombing. The reports in *Anaesthesia* indicate that these were convivial affairs and that they increased in sophistication as the years went by. Presidents, Masters, and Deans of learned and Royal Societies, together with Ministers of the Crown and Senior Civil Servants graced an expanding guest list, and many laudatory and thinly disguised medicopolitical speeches were made.[120] The Association of Anaesthetists had by now become a well recognised body of importance in the medical world. It was certainly fulfilling the last of the official objectives of its founders in 1932 to encourage and promote cooperation and friendship amongst anaesthetists in addition to its medicopolitical activities.

The 1955 Annual General Meeting and Dinner

It was significant that the 1955 Annual General Meeting at the Royal College of Surgeons, Lincoln's Inn Fields in November was timed to precede immediately the scholarly Faculty Frederic Hewitt lecture by M H Armstrong Davison of Newcastle upon Tyne entitled "Ut non percipiatur dolor" ("in order that pain may not be felt").[121-123] This was the first occasion when the Annual General Meeting of the Association was combined with an academic lecture, albeit with the cooperation of the Faculty. The 1955 Annual General Meeting itself was important because it included a proposal by the President (Geoffrey Organe)[3] that the 1956 Annual General Meeting should be accompanied by the Association's own scientific sessions and coincide with both the Frederic Hewitt Lecture of the Faculty and the Presidential Address at the Royal Society of Medicine.[107] The customary Annual Dinner was held at Claridge's in 1955.[124]

The 1956 Annual Meeting

President Organe's proposal was acted upon. Professor Pask,[89] who was not at that time a member of Council, was coopted. It is interesting that, as at its preliminary meeting in 1932, Council was still anxious that the Association of Anaesthetists should not compete with the Section of Anaesthetics of the Royal Society of Medicine in choosing its own scientific programme. The Minutes (6.1.1956, 6.7.1956 and 5.10.1956)[107] record that there was a good response to the invitation to submit papers for presentation but regretted that only five could be chosen. These were delivered by Francis Baker of Dartford on "The effect of pethidine and nalorphine administered to women in labour"; by J D Robertson of Edinburgh on "Some experimental and clinical aspects of the action of anaesthetics on circulatory dynamics"; by J W Dundee, then of Liverpool, on "Adjuvants in the relief of chronic pain"; by L A Boeve of Leiden, Holland on "The risk of ventricular fibrillation hypothermia", and by J P Payne, then of the Postgraduate Medical School, Hammersmith on "The effects of carbon dioxide on muscle relaxation produced by succinylcholine". This 1956 meeting at the Royal College of Surgeons extended over two days.[124] It included a session at which the above lectures were presented, the Annual General Meeting at which T Cecil Gray took over the presidency from Geoffrey Organe,[3] the 1956 (Faculty) Hewitt Lecture on "Artistry and science in anaesthesia" by Ronald Woolmer[125] (the newly appointed Director of the Research Department of Anaesthetics at the Royal College of Surgeons), a session on anaesthetic practice in relation to operating room construction, the Presidential Address to the RSM Section of Anaesthetics by Kathleen Lloyd-Williams[126] of the Royal Free Hospital, London, and the Annual Dinner, also at the Royal College of Surgeons which was followed by dancing![124]

The Silver Jubilee Meeting of the Association 1957

The Silver Jubilee of the Association (1932-1957) was celebrated with considerable panache between Wednesday 4th and Saturday 7th of December 1957 once again at the Royal College of Surgeons.[127-130] The redoubtable Ronald Jarman[4] was the Chairman of the Jubilee Meeting Committee and Cyril F Scurr was responsible for a first class scientific programme.[131]

Jarman once again showed his flair for organisation and obtaining sponsorship as he had done on so many previous occasions. A trade exhibition, for which A Charles King, the apparatus manufacturer, was responsible, was introduced for the first time. This raised £1,000 (1996: £12,500) and in addition further donations of £900 (1996: £11,250) were made towards the expenses of the meeting from various sponsors (Council Minutes 7.12.1956, 1.2.1957, 7.6.1957, 5.7.1957, 13.10.1957, 1.11.1957). "Nearly five hundred anaesthetists registered at the meeting including a number from the Continent, Canada and the United States".[128]

Henry Featherstone, the Founder President (1932-1935) must have been well pleased as he took the Chair at the first scientific session at 9.45 am on 5 December 1957.[131] All the aims and objectives which he had envisaged were now in the process of being fulfilled, including the first of them - "the promotion of the study of anaesthetics and their administration".

Twenty five papers were delivered. Speakers from abroad included Ritsema van Eck from The Netherlands, Francis Foldes of the USA (a future President of the World Federation of Societies of Anaesthesiologists - WFSA), and from the United Kingdom many who were already, or were to become prominent leaders of the specialty in Great Britain. John Nunn (Dean of the Faculty 1979-1982) gave the first paper on "carbon dioxide tensions during anaesthesia" and others on the programme included J P Payne (BOC Professor 1963-1988), C F Scurr (Dean of the Faculty 1970-1973 and President of the Association 1976-1978), W W Mushin (Professor at Cardiff 1954-1975), John Dundee (Professor at Belfast 1957-1987 and Dean of the Irish Faculty 1970-1973), James Robertson (Professor at Edinburgh 1968-1982), Frankis T Evans (Dean of the Faculty 1955-1958), C W Suckling, the chemist who synthesised halothane, and Michael Johnson of Manchester who was one of the first to use it clinically in the year before the Jubilee Meeting, and the physicists who have devoted their professional lives to anaesthesia, H G Epstein in Oxford and W W Mapleson of Cardiff. It is noteworthy that all the contributions were related to the administration of anaesthesia for surgery, and that there was one paper on the organisation of a syringe service. The involvement of anaesthetists in intensive care and the advent of presterilized disposable syringes and related items were still in the future![127-131]

The registrants were also able to attend the (Faculty) Frederic Hewitt Lecture for 1957 by M D Nosworthy,[132] of St Thomas' Hospital, London, on "Pseudo-science and modern anaesthesia"[133] and Henry K Beecher, the first Professor of Anaesthesia at the Harvard Medical School in Boston, Massachusetts, addressed a meeting of the Section of the Royal Society of Medicine, held specially at the Royal College of Surgeons, on "Studies of the effects of drugs on mental states".[128]

The social round included a cocktail party of welcome to overseas visitors, a cocktail party given by the Faculty of Anaesthetists, a "buffet-dance" at Londonderry House, Park Lane and, of course, the Annual Dinner in the Great Hall of the Royal College of Surgeons.[127,128] The latter was a splendid "white tie and tails" affair! The toast of the Association was proposed by the Minister of Health, Mr Derek Walker-Smith, and brought a noteworthy reply by the President T Cecil Gray in which he paid tribute to Harry Featherstone and Ivan Magill and reviewed the achievements of the Association since 1932.

The registration fee for the Meeting was £2 (1996: £25), the dinner cost 2 1/2 guineas per head "including wines" (1996: £33), and the Buffet-Dance (including supper) 3 guineas (1996: £39).

The 1958 Meeting at Southport in Lancashire

Professor Pask[89] had suggested in 1948 that:-

"the Annual Meeting..... should be held in the provinces, perhaps at a seaside town, lasting two days at which scientific papers would be given, films shown and manufacturers invited to exhibit". (Minutes of the 1948 Annual General Meeting 27.10.1948).[107]

It took ten years for this suggestion to be acted upon.

The 1958 Annual Meeting was organised by the reigning President, T Cecil Gray and his Liverpool colleagues at a hotel in Southport, Lancashire. This departure from tradition proved popular and the event was "extremely well attended".[134,135]

There was a preliminary meeting on the morning of Thursday 30 October 1958. This consisted of closed circuit television demonstrations of Liverpool anaesthetic techniques at the Tate Hall of the University of Liverpool by courtesy of Messrs Smith, Kline and French Laboratories Ltd.

The Annual Meeting proper was held at The Prince of Wales Hotel, Southport and continued through Friday 31 October and Saturday morning 1 November 1958. There were, for the first time, all the features of the present day Annual Meeting of the Association - the civic cocktail party and mayoral welcome, the Annual General Meeting, the John Snow Memorial Lecture, the scientific sessions, a trade exhibition and the Annual Dinner. There was also a dinner-dance.[135]

The John Snow Memorial Lecture of 1958 was the first to be presented. It had been reported to Council on 7 March 1958[107] that the Board of the Faculty of Anaesthetists had decided that its Joseph Clover and Frederic Hewitt lectures would in future be presented in alternate years at the time of the Annual Anniversary Meeting of the Faculty in the Spring; in future, therefore, neither lecture would coincide with the Annual Meeting of the Association in the autumn. Dr Langton Hewer[8], Editor, proposed that, as 1958 was the centenary of the death of John Snow ,the first professional anaesthetist, it would be appropriate for the Association to initiate a lecture in his memory. It was immediately agreed:-

"that a John Snow Memorial Lecture should be given annually for four years; after 1961 the advisability of holding the lecture at longer intervals should be considered. The Officers were given power to invite a lecturer for 1958 [and], that a fee of fifty guineas [1996: £630] plus expenses should be given".[107]

The John Snow Memorial Lecture has been delivered every year since 1958 with the exception of 1968; in 1968 the Annual Scientific Meeting of the Association was not held because it would have been overshadowed by the Fourth World Congress of Anaesthesiologists held in London that year with the Association acting as host Society. The fee for the John Snow Lecture is now (1998) £1,000.

The first John Snow Memorial Lecturer was George Edwards[108] of St George's Hospital, London. He gave a well researched biographical presentation entitled "John Snow MD (1813-1858)".[136]

The scientific programme was once again concerned only with the administration of anaesthesia for surgery. All the contributors were already, or were destined to be, well known.[137] There was a reasoned terminal plea for the retention of chloroform in the anaesthetist's armamentarium for certain specific indications[138] by M H Armstrong Davison (1911-1970)[139] of Newcastle upon Tyne, one of the remaining protagonists of the agent, a paper by

J B Wyman, Consultant Anaesthetist and later Dean of the Medical School of Westminster Hospital, London, on cardiac arrest reflecting the practice of the time (thoracotomy and internal defibrillation), a communication on controlled ventilation in neurosurgical anaesthesia by S Galloon, then of University of Wales, Cardiff (a subject of controversy at the time),[140] and academic papers from other established university departments in London, Newcastle upon Tyne, Manchester, Belfast, and Glasgow.[137]

The 1959 Annual Meeting at Stratford upon Avon

The 1959 meeting was held at hotels in Stratford upon Avon. It was attended by over 300 anaesthetists amongst whom were registrants from Denmark, Iran, Malaya, the Netherlands, Portugal, South Africa and Sweden and followed the pattern of the 1958 meeting.[141,142] Ronald Jarman[4] succeeded T Cecil Gray as President at the Annual General Meeting and the scientific programme[143] included a contribution on anaesthetic methods in animals from the veterinary anaesthetist Barbara Weaver. There were also lectures on the now almost forgotten technique of profound hypothermia for cardiac surgery by David Benazon, the then novel concept of antanalgesia by John Clutton-Brock[92] of Bristol, and a paper by Leslie J Wolfson of the Birmingham Accident Hospital (1908-1980)[145] on the contemporary management of the full stomach in trauma (this was before Brian Sellick described his now well known manoeuvre of oesophageal compression in 1961).[146] Wolfson was a much loved colleague and early enthusiast for massive blood transfusion after major trauma and extensive burns. He was the subject of a well deserved, but none the less touching, tribute from one of his surgeons after he died in 1980,[147] in addition to his official obituary.[145]

International relations in the fifties

It is true that British anaesthetists had not ventured far from the operating theatres by the mid nineteen fifties, but British anaesthesia had nonetheless achieved a high reputation internationally. The independent status of British physician anaesthetists, which had resulted from the introduction of the NHS, and had given them equality with other medical and surgical specialists, was the envy of their colleagues in other countries and, in some instances, this is still the case today. The technological expertise of British anaesthetists was also highly respected, as indeed it had been before and during the Second World War. Europe looked to British anaesthesia for inspiration and instruction in the postwar period, and they did not look in vain.

The Association of Anaesthetists and the Faculty together were also able to assist and advise the Australasians whose problems were organisational rather than technical, and the British became leaders in the establishment of the WFSA.

Relationships with the United States were cordial and mutually respectful. There were academic centres of excellence in the USA at that time, such as Ralph Water's Department at the University of Wisconsin, which surpassed anything in the world in terms of organisation of facilities for teaching and research,[148] but the standards of clinical anaesthesia nationwide in the USA left much to be desired and the status of the anesthesiology as a specialty was not high.[106] There was, moreover, considerable reluctance to adopt the curare and controlled respiration technique. Beecher and Todd, with all the authority of the Department of Anesthesia at the Massachusetts General Hospital, Boston, had pointed the finger at curare itself as a cause of death in anaesthetic practice after a retrospective study, without recognising that the real culprit was the use of curare without controlled ventilation.[149]

The problem of the coexistence of nurse and technician anaesthesia under the nominal direction of the operating surgeon, and the shortage of trained anesthesiologists also compounded the problem in the USA.[106,150,151] Certain senior British anaesthetists were reluctant to accept the true situation however, apparently for fear of upsetting their American colleagues![152]

Some idea of the spread of international cooperation amongst anaesthetists, as well as the influence of British anaesthesia, can be gathered by studying the membership lists circulated with the Annual Reports at the beginning and the end of the decade. Selective election to Corresponding Fellowship was the only category of membership of the Association open to specialist anaesthetists practising outside the United Kingdom and Ireland at that time. There were just nine Corresponding Fellows in 1949 (five from Australia, one from Canada, one each from Sweden and Denmark, and one from Lebanon); by 1959 there were 32, including 14 from Europe (two each from Sweden, Switzerland, France, West Germany, and one each from

Denmark, Finland, Portugal, Holland, Austria and Romania), six from the United States and one from Canada, four from Australasia, four from the Indian subcontinent and three from South America.

The authority of the Faculty of Anaesthetists was paramount in the United Kingdom in matters concerning international standards of training and practice and reciprocity of qualifications, and it enjoyed close relations with its sister Colleges and Faculties in Australasia, Ireland, Canada and South Africa and with the United States Board of Specialty. The Association on the other hand, with its broader and more flexible constitution, had become the usual vehicle for conducting international relationships in the scientific, cultural and medicopolitical fields.

The Association of Anaesthetists became a founder member of the WFSA in 1955 and of the United Kingdom Committee for the World Health Organisation (WHO) in the same year (Annual Report 1955); from then on Annual Reports record official attendance by one or other of its Officers or Council Members at the increasing number of European and overseas Congresses held by the various national and regional societies, most of which were inaugurated or reinvigorated in the nineteen fifties. Financial provision was made for Officers acting as official representatives at foreign meetings (Council Minutes 5 June 1959).[107]

The influence of British anaesthesia in Europe

The specialty of anaesthesia in continental Europe was a very early stage of development at the end of the Second World War;[153-156] as Sir Geoffrey Organe[3] wrote in 1985:-

> *"The centenary of the introduction of ether anaesthesia*
> *was celebrated in 1946. During that long period advances in general*
> *anaesthesia were almost wholly confined to the English-speaking*
> *world: to the United States and Great Britain with its dominions and*
> *colonies. The system prevailing in continental Europe, whereby a*
> *Professor of Surgery was responsible for the activities of his*
> *department actively discouraged any specialisation; anaesthetics*
> *were administered by junior doctors, nurses and even porters under*
> *the direct control of the surgeon..... During the next five years there*

was a tremendous upsurge of interest in anaesthesia among doctors, many of whom had trained abroad.."[156]

An early and very successful example of the part that British anaesthetists played in assisting in the training of European anaesthetists after the Second World War was the year spent in Yugoslavia by Patrick Shackleton.[6] This was initially with a British plastic surgery team.[157] Shackleton introduced endotracheal anaesthesia and taught the first Yugoslavian physician anaesthetists. "He changed the course of Yugoslavian anaesthesia from pure layman empiricism to a professional art and science". [157] Shackleton continued to take an interest and visit his trainees who regarded him as the "Grandfather of Yugoslavian anaesthesia"! Shackleton's work was extended by Russell Davies[158] of the Queen Victoria Hospital, East Grinstead.

The Association of Anaesthetists also arranged for two young British anaesthetists to assist the Professor of Surgery at the University of Utrecht in training Dutch doctors as anaesthetists (Annual Reports 1946, 1947 and 1948). Many other British anaesthetists participated in the spread of the knowledge of modern anaesthesia to Europe in the postwar period,[159] and a considerable number of pioneers were trained in the United Kingdom.[160] Ritsema Van Eck of Groningen, Holland paid tribute to the part British anaesthetists had paid in training European doctors in a speech at the Association Silver Jubilee Celebrations in 1957 when he, rather quaintly, thanked them "for teaching us to use our nice new guns".[128]

The Anaesthesiology Centre Copenhagen was founded on a Danish initiative by the World Health Organisation in 1950, and continued until 1976.[161] It played a vital part in the development of World anaesthesia. It trained 220 Danes, 205 from 26 other European countries, and 118 from Africa, Central and South America, the Eastern Mediterranean, Southeast Asia and the Western Pacific. Instructors and lecturers came from many parts of the world, including in particular the United States and the British Isles. Ronald Woolmer[90] was at the Copenhagen Centre for a year (1951-1952) and the list of others who gave of their time and expertise includes many whose names figure prominently in the history of British anaesthesia and the Association (Sir Robert Macintosh, Sir Geoffrey Organe,[3] T Cecil Gray, Patrick Shackleton,[6] John Beard,[7] John Zorab, Harry Churchill-Davidson,

Gordon Jackson Rees, Phyllis Edwards and Cedric Prys-Roberts.[161]

The special relationship of British and Australasian anaesthesia

Gwen Wilson devotes a generous amount of space to the relationship between British and Australian anaesthesia in her admirable book *Fifty Years* written to celebrate the Golden Jubilee of the Australian Society of Anaesthetists (1934-1984).[162] Australian anaesthetists of the nineteen thirties faced many of the same problems as those in Great Britain (inferior status, unremunerated work in public hospitals; and reliance on the goodwill of their surgical colleagues for private work to provide an income). The small population of Australia in relation to its immense size resulted of necessity in a much more broadly based membership of the Australian Society of Anaesthetists from the beginning than was the case in the early days of the Association of Great Britain and Ireland, as well as division into State sections. Another difference was that, from the start, the Australian Society had a scientific programme at its meetings in addition to conducting medicopolitical business. There was no other forum for scientific discussion other than a Section at the Annual meeting of the Australian branch of the British Medical Association (the Australian Medical Association (AMA) did not separate from the London based BMA until January 1951).[162]

It was fortunate that Z Mennell (the Treasurer of the Association of Anaesthetists) had been invited to speak at the Annual meeting of the BMA parent body which was held in Melbourne in 1935 at which anaesthetics had a shared Section with pharmacology and therapeutics, because he was also able to speak at the first Annual General Meeting of the Australian Society of Anaesthetists which had been arranged to follow immediately the BMA meeting.[162]

It has already been recorded that Mennell's rather conservative lecture on "Ether is not dead" was not particularly well received, but his invitation to affiliate the new Australian Society with the Association of Anaesthetists of Great Britain and Ireland was accepted with acclaim (Chapter 4). This resulted in the election of Corresponding Members (later Fellows) from the Australian States. The Australian Society therefore turned to the United Kingdom, with its recently established Diploma in Anaesthetics for training and advancement of the specialty rather than to American based institutions such as the International College of Anaesthetists which had, in fact, also made an approach to the Australian Society in 1936.[162]

A comparative worldwide study of the functions and varying fortunes of societies of anaesthetists on the lines of that conducted by Betcher and his colleagues for the American based societies[163] would fill many pages but has no place in this volume. The Australian Society certainly had a stormier passage than the Association of Anaesthetists of Great Britain and Ireland in its earlier years. Its problems included such matters as affiliation, disaffiliation and reaffiliation with the BMA, and later with the Australian Medical Association, as well as temporary strained relations with the Faculty of Anaesthetists of the Royal Australasian College of Surgeons over representation in negotiations with the Australian Government.[162] The Australasian Faculty was inaugurated in 1952 at the request of the Australian Society with the immediate objective of initiating a Fellowship in Anaesthesia,[162] as had been the case in the United Kingdom.

The Second World War was instrumental in raising the status of the Association of Anaesthetists of Great Britain and Ireland, but the Australian Society almost became a casualty of the War and required all the ingenuity and tenacity of its dedicated Honorary Secretary, Geoffrey Kaye,[164] to revive it.[162]

The Australian Travelling Scholarship. There was however one activity conducted in the name of the Australian Society of Anaesthetists during the war years which had an important sequel:-

"Dr A D Morgan of Sydney, recalling the hospitality of English colleagues [in prewar years], and reading of the stringency of food rationing in Britain arranged for the Australian Society to send food parcels to AAGBI for distribution amongst its members."[162]

Three hundred and twenty six such parcels were received by the end of 1949 (Annual Report 1949); as a result Council, at its meeting on 10 June 1949, as a token of appreciation, decided to recommend to the Annual General Meeting that £500 free of tax (1996: £8,500) be voted to finance a travelling scholarship for an Australian anaesthetist under 40 years of age to visit and work in the principal centres in the United Kingdom.

This gesture was greatly appreciated by the Australian Society. They chose Frank Leventhal, a Resident Anaesthetist at the Sydney Hospital, who arrived by sea with his wife in December 1950. He proved to be a most appreciative and well liked ambassador for the Australian Society. His letters to John Barker, the Honorary Secretary of the Australian Society, not only express his enthusiasm, but contain much information of interest about the current practice of anaesthesia in the United Kingdom in the early nineteen fifties. It is a source of sadness that Frank Leventhal, who was so highly regarded in both this country and in Australia, died prematurely in 1960 after a long illness.[162]

Overseas visitors to the Australian Society of Anaesthetists. The prewar visit of Zebulon Mennell in 1935 and its outcome has already been mentioned. Sir Robert Macintosh, a New Zealander by birth, combined a private visit to Australasia with attendance at the Australian Society of Anaesthetists' Annual Meeting in Sydney in 1951, and subsequently visited and lectured in the other State capitals of Melbourne, Adelaide and Perth. He stimulated great enthusiasm and, as a result of this resounding success, Mary Burnell, visiting London, persuaded Bernard Johnson,[5] the reigning Dean of the Faculty, to come to Australia in 1953 when she was President; once again his lecture tour was greatly appreciated. The Australian Society officially inaugurated its Overseas Visitors programme in 1955 when John Gillies[1] was invited; since then many British anaesthetists who have served as Officers or Members of Council of the Association of Anaesthetists of Great Britain and Ireland have savoured the exhausting but pleasurable hospitality of the Australian Society (Geoffrey Organe[3] 1957, William Mushin 1959, Cecil Gray and Derek Wylie 1961, Gordon Jackson Rees 1963, Cedric Prys-Roberts 1973, Michael Rosen and Gordon McDowall 1975, Stanley Feldman 1981, F Richard Ellis 1983, and John Nunn in 1984). A further token of the friendship between the two bodies was the presentation by John Nunn of a Presidential Medallion on behalf of the Association of Anaesthetists of Great Britain and Ireland to the Australian Society during the latter's Golden Jubilee Celebrations in 1984.[162]

The International Congresses in London and Paris in 1951

These two international congresses are important in the history of world anaesthesia because they created an opportunity for physician anaesthetists to make the initial moves to the foundation of the World Federation of Societies of Anaesthesiologist.

The 26th Congress of Anesthestists of the International Anesthesia Research Society and the International College of Anesthetists, 3-7 September 1951 in London[165-167] was the well established routine meeting of the related North American-based International Anesthesia Research Society and the International College of Anesthetists, for which the Association was asked to be joint hosts. These two bodies had both been founded by F H McMechan of New York.[163] The Members of the Council of the Association of Anaesthetists were cautious when first invited to participate because of possible financial implications, but the Annual Reports and Minutes gradually reveal a growing enthusiasm for the project (Annual Reports 1950 and 1952, Council Minutes 3.2.1950, 7.7.1950, 31.3.1951, 1.6.1951).[107] In the end the event was a considerable success[167] and Ronald Jarman[4] (once again the organising genius) was able to hand over a profit from registration and other fees.[166] £232.9s.6d (1996: £3,800) was paid into the Research Funds of the Association (Council Minutes 5.10.1951 and 2.5.1952).[106,167] The programme, dominated as it was by British contributors, must have impressed even the Americans![165]

The International Congress of Anesthesiology 20-22 September 1951 in Paris was convened by the Société Française d'Anesthésie et d'Analgésie.[168] Its proximity to the London Congress enabled the Americans to cross the Atlantic in style by the Cunard Liner *SS Samaria* and return by the *SS Caronia*, taking in some sight seeing between the two Congresses (44 days for an exclusive charge of approximately £300 (1996: £4,950)!).[165]

The foundation of the WFSA in 1955

The explosive spread of interest in anaesthesia was world-wide; indeed the First Latin American Congress had already taken place in Buenos Aires.[156,169-171]

The foundation of the WFSA in 1955

The initial suggestion for an international society of anaesthesiologists came from the Société Française d'Anesthésie et d'Analgésie who proposed that the organisation should be based in Paris. The Council of the Association of Anaesthetists first considered the French invitation to a preliminary discussion on 5 May 1951 in Paris on 6 April 1951.[107] The minutes state that the general feeling of Council members was that "France was not the country to initiate an international society" but nonetheless it was decided that the Association should send Katherine Lloyd-Williams (1896-1973),[172] who spoke fluent French, as an observer to the meeting. The reason for this apparently cool reception of the French proposal is not far to seek; both the President, the Treasurer, and the majority of the members of the French Society were surgeons.[156]

World anaesthesia at that time was divided into four groups according to the state of its development:-

The British sphere of influence, in which physician (if not yet entirely specialist) anaesthesia was the norm, included the United Kingdom and the British Dominions of Australia, New Zealand, Canada and South Africa, India and the British Colonies and Dependencies as well as the Republic of Ireland.

The United States: where academic anaesthesia was of a high standard and progressing rapidly despite the nurse anesthetist problem, and where an international organisation had already been founded in the nineteen twenties.[163]

The Scandinavian countries: which, with their smaller populations and pragmatic approach, were fast developing their own particular, and highly successful, brand of physician and physician-directed nurse anaesthesia. This combined elements of British and American professional philosophy. They had also already founded their own Research Society.[174-178]

Anaesthetists in the other European countries, notably Germany and France, were still dominated by the surgeons,[153-160] and consequently the continental European societies felt the urgent need to be included in any proposed international organisation.

The influence of the independent Far East countries of Japan and China could be discounted as their anaesthesia was in an embryological state of development with the assistance of varying degrees of British and American influence.[179-181]

Archibald Marston,[182] as Dean of the Faculty, having consulted the President of the Royal College of Surgeons of England, expressed the view that the Faculty should not have a direct connection with the proposed International Society (Council Minute 6.7.1951).[107] This left (Sir) Geoffrey Organe,[3] who was at that time Honorary Secretary of the Association of Anaesthetists, free to proceed to sound out international opinion on the French proposal. The Scandinavian Society lent its support to the views of the British Association (Council Minute 6.7.1951).[107]

An informal international meeting was held in London on 6 September 1951, during the Congress of the International Anesthesia Research Society, under the Chairmanship of the Canadian Harold Griffith[183] who also represented the International Anesthesia Research Society (IARS). Those present were anaesthetists from Australia, Belgium, Brazil, Canada, France, Holland, Italy, New Zealand, Portugal, Spain, Sweden, the United Kingdom and Ireland (represented by Gillies,[1] Jarman,[4] Magill,[184] Organe[3] and Katherine Lloyd-Williams[172]) and the Section of Anaesthetics of the American Medical Association (AMA) and the American Society of Anesthetists (ASA).

The proceedings of this meeting were reported to a Special Meeting of the Council of the Association of Anaesthetists the next day (7.10.1951)[107] by John Gillies.[1] He stated that the general view of those present at the meeting had been that the whole matter should proceed "slowly and carefully" but, (predictably) a few continental European societies felt that action should be taken soon following the French lead. Some hostility had been expressed by the representatives of the North American-based IARS, who considered that they had done reasonably well in the international field for many years past. It was pointed out to them, however, that the IARS had little influence in Europe, that the activities of the IARS were confined to holding an Annual Congress and publishing a journal, and that its objectives would have to be widened medicopolitically if it were to act as a proper international society. John Gillies reported that there was a considerable majority against the proposal for the creation of a Paris-based organisation along the lines put forward by the French, which would include surgeons and others interested in anaesthesia, and that there was a danger that anaesthetists might split into two groups "English speaking and European". The President of the Association of Anaesthetists, Alexander Low,[2] then revealed that he had correspondence with Jean Delafresnaye, the Secretary for the Council for the Coordination of International Congresses of Medical Sciences (CCICMS) which was sponsored by UNESCO (United Nations Educational Scientific and Cultural Organisation) and the World Health Organisation (WHO). This body had already been consulted by the French. A number of questions had been asked by the CCICMS, to which the Council of the Association of Anaesthetists proceeded to frame replies. The crux of these was that the proposed international society should be a federation of national societies of anaesthetists, that professional medically qualified anaesthetists should have a majority among members of the society, that *all* members of the executive committee and *all* Officers of the proposed International Society should be medically qualified anaesthetists. It was agreed that Katherine Lloyd-Williams[172] (Council Member 1947-1950) and (Sir) Geoffrey Organe[3] should actually represent the Association at the Paris meeting rather than be present as mere observers (Council Minute 7.10.1951).[107]

The delegates returned from Paris well pleased with the results of the discussions during the Congress, in which they had taken a leading role on behalf of the Association of Anaesthetists (Council Minute 5.10.1951).[107] The representatives of the 32 nations present at the Paris Congress had decided that the international organisation should be in the form of a federation of national societies governed by an executive of physician anaesthetists . The function of the organisation would be "to assist in the development of anaesthesia throughout the world by means of international congresses and other activities". An Interim Committee had been formed and it had been decided that an international congress sponsored by the Organisation would be held in 1955.[169,185]

The Interim Committee consisted of Harold R Griffith[183] of Canada as Chairman, Alex Goldblat of Belgium as Secretary, John Gillies[1] of the United Kingdom and Ireland, Torsten Gordh of Sweden, and Jacques Boureau of France[169] (although earlier reports give the name of P Huguenard as the French representative).[185] This list of names is notable for the absence of representation from the largest society of anaesthesiologists - the American Society of Anesthesiologists (ASA) of the United States. The Association of

Anaesthetists of Great Britain and Ireland thus came to play the predominant role in the organisation of the WFSA. The ASA, in fact, remained officially outside the organisation until the Second World Congress of Anaesthesiologists in Toronto, Canada in 1960. Griffith tells us that the traditional isolationism of the USA came to the surface and many members of the ASA "doubted the wisdom of foreign entanglements".[169] Griffith was, however, a prominent member of both the IARS and the ASA. The IARS kept a close eye on the development of the WFSA. The IARS would not have been acceptable as an international society even if it had been able to extend its influence worldwide, because of its constitution based on individual membership under the Board of Governors; it did, however, give considerable encouragement and financial support to the Interim Committee. It is probable that without the contributions it made towards the travelling expenses of the members of the Interim Committee the whole project might have petered out.[156,169]

The low profile adopted by the American Society left the Association of Anaesthetists of Great Britain and Ireland in a position to play the dominant role in the framing of the Constitution of the Federation (Annual Reports 1953, 1954 and 1955).[107,156,169] The membership of the Interim Committee expanded around its original nucleus at its meetings in Brussels and The Hague in 1954 and 1955; in addition to John Gillies,[1] Low,[2] Organe[3] and Shackleton,[6] who 'together represented the British Association', anaesthesiologists from Holland, Belgium, Germany, Italy and Australia, as well as representatives of the IARS and individuals from the USA also took part in the discussions. The draft constitution was an excellent one. It is based on a general assembly of all member societies delegating the conduct of affairs to an Executive Committee. It ensured that each member society, however small, still had a voice in proportion to its membership in the General Assembly but, at the same time provided that the "two largest societies" would always each have one representative on the Executive Committee.[156,169]

The First World Congress of Anaesthesiologists was held at Scheveningen in the Netherlands from 5-10 September 1955.[186] This event was a spectacular success; it was attended by approximately 1,200 registrants including members and their families, from 34 countries of whom 212 came from Great Britain and Ireland (Annual Report 1955).

The inaugural meeting of the General Assembly of the World Federation of Societies of Anaesthesiologists (WFSA) was held on the last day of the 1955 World Congress "amidst almost universal acclaim".[186] The first 26 official member societies were Argentina, Australia, Austria, Belgium, Brazil, Canada, Chile, Colombia, Cuba, Denmark, Finland, France, the German Federal Republic, Great Britain and Ireland, India, Israel, Italy, the Netherlands, Norway, Portugal, Spain, Sweden, Switzerland, South Africa, Uruguay and Venezuela; many of the member societies from these countries had only recently been formed. The American Society of Anesthesiologists still held itself aloof, but joined at the Second World Congress of Anaesthesiology in Toronto, Canada in 1960, together with the societies of Ceylon, Czechoslovakia, Greece, Hong Kong, Japan, Korea, Mexico, New Zealand and the Philippines. The further expansion and development of the WFSA has been described by Zorab[170] and by Howat.[187]

Harold Griffith[183] (Canada) was elected as the first President with Vice Presidents from the Netherlands, Belgium, Germany and Cuba. (Sir) Geoffrey Organe[3] (at that time President of the Association of Anaesthetists of Great Britain and Ireland) was elected Secretary-Treasurer "with acclaim", and both John Gillies[1] and Patrick Shackleton[6] became members of the Executive Committee together with single representatives from Argentina, Australia, Austria, Belgium, Brazil, Canada, France, Italy, the Netherlands and Sweden.

Members of the Association have played a vital and important part in the development of the WFSA. The contribution of (Sir) Geoffrey Organe[3] was outstanding. He was first the seemingly tireless and peripatetic Secretary-Treasurer in the difficult early years (1955-1964), and then the President (1964-1968). His term of office culminated in the outstandingly successful Fourth World Congress in the Festival Hall in London at which the Association of Anaesthetists was host Society under the presidency of Patrick Shackleton.[6] Other Members of the Association who have played a leading part in the affairs of the WFSA have included Douglas Howat (Chairman of the Executive Committee 1976-1980) and more recently, John Zorab (Secretary General 1980-1988 and President 1988-1992).[170,187] At the present time (1998), Michael Vickers (President of the Association 1982-84) is President of the WFSA having completed a successful term as Secretary-General, and Michael

Rosen (President of the Association 1986-88) is Treasurer.

The Association and the Regional Societies of the United Kingdom

The suggestion that "Regional Societies in the specialties might help to spread knowledge and promote friendship" has been attributed to Aneurin Bevan, the Minister of Health at the time of the discussions preceding the inauguration of the Health Service;[188] if this is really so it was a further example of the perspicacity of that enlightened politician. The Anaesthetics Section of the RSM continued to provide a national forum for anaesthetists from teaching hospitals all over the United Kingdom and, in the nineteen fifties, many of them made long journeys by train to attend each first Friday in the month throughout the lecture season. These RSM meetings were usually crowded with anaesthetists working in London and in the district general hospitals of the home counties anxious to glean the latest information about new concepts and techniques from academics from all over the United Kingdom and elsewhere. The practical difficulties in the way of attendance at RSM meetings of rank and file consultants from the distant provinces in a shortage specialty such as anaesthesia were very considerable. There was certainly a need for Regional Societies in Great Britain and Ireland which would be prepared to organise scientific and social meetings at a local level which would obviate the need for travelling to London except on special occasions. The Scottish Society of Anaesthetists was founded in 1914, and is indeed probably the first national society in the world. The Liverpool Society of Anaesthetists, had also been founded before the Great War, but most Regional Societies came into existence in the late forties and early fifties at the time of the inauguration of the NHS. This was at a time when specialist anaesthesia was becoming established in the provinces. One of the first to be founded after the Second World War was the Manchester and District Society of Anaesthetists in 1945. This Society subsequently merged with the Manchester Medical Society as its Section of Anaesthetics in 1950.[189] The very successful Society of Anaesthetists of the South Western Region based in Bristol, which has published its own journal *Anaesthesia Points West* since 1968, was founded in 1947,[188,190] and many others followed. In the early years of the NHS the Regional Societies indulged in some medicopolitical activity *vis-a-vis* their Regional Boards; but nationally this function was soon largely taken over by the Association of Anaesthetists itself, and it also continued to advise individual members; at a local level the Regional Anaesthetists' Subcommittees took over the local advisory and political roles, once they came into existence.

The Council considered the question of its relationship with the emergent Regional societies as early as 7 January 1949 (Annual Report 1949). It was recognised that these new organisations were filling the potential need for continuing education, in which even the Association of Anaesthetists itself was not yet ready to take part. It was agreed, however, that formal affiliation with the Association would be constitutionally difficult. It was also pointed out that the journal *Anaesthesia* was already giving publicity, and reporting the activities of, the Regional meetings. It was decided that "the Honorary Secretary should write to the various Regional Societies, stating that the Association officially recognised them, expressing appreciation for their work, and informing them that the Association would be pleased to consider any problems of national interest which they might like to submit," and this is still the relationship which exists at the present time. *Anaesthesia* has handed on the important function of publicising and reporting the activities of the Societies to *Anaesthesia News*, the in-house publication of the Association of Anaesthetists, since it was first published in 1987. This role is important both concurrently and archivally.

In 1957 Council decided to publish a list of the Regional Societies and their Officers with the Annual Report. Fourteen English, three Scottish and one society each from Wales, Northern Ireland and the Republic of Ireland are listed in the 1959 Annual Report at the end of the decade - though, perhaps it was scarcely tactful to include the national societies of Scotland, Ireland, and Wales under the general title of "List of Provincial Societies of Anaesthetists"!

Provision for the support of Research 1949-1959

The first two Research Fellows of the Association of Anaesthetists (Philip Helliwell and Michael Hutton) completed their work (Council Minute 10.6.1949)[107] and published their final report at the beginning of the decade[191] (Annual Report 1949) but, despite the success and importance of their project, no more Research Fellows were appointed during the period 1949-1959. This circumstance seems to have been both due to a paucity of suitable applicants and a desire to allow funds to accumulate so that a better salary and conditions could be offered (Council Minutes 3.2.1950 and 7.7.1950 and Annual Report 1950). The salary offered in 1950 to a candidate who was required "to possess the DA or a University science degree" was only £700 to £800 (£,11,900 to £13,500: 1996) plus an unspecified grant towards expenses "if necessary"![192] It must be remembered also that the Consultant grade in anaesthesia was rapidly expanding at that time and the possession of the two-part DA was practically a ticket for early promotion (Annual Report 1954).

Council concentrated on the conduct of its own pioneer projects of the investigation of deaths associated with anaesthesia, explosions and the use of heroin in anaesthetic practice (see below), and the support of individual research by providing grants for the purchase of equipment, materials and experimental animals by anaesthetists already in salaried appointments[193] (Council Minutes 7.3.1952, 4.12.1953 etc[107] and Annual Reports 1949-1959). Applications for grants were carefully assessed before being accepted or rejected - especially when Pask[89] was the Chairman of the Research Committee (Council Minutes 3.7.1959!)[107]

A grant to the appeal for the proposed Faculty of Anaesthetists Research Department Endowment Fund of £1,000 was made following a Special General Meeting of the Association on 5 March 1954. This would be the equivalent of about £13,800 at 1996 values and was the first donation made to the appeal. It was received with gratitude by the Faculty, and the "essential community of purpose of the Association and Faculty" was expressed in an exchange of letters[194] between the President of the Association (Geoffrey Organe)[3] and the Dean of the Faculty (Bernard Johnson).[5] It must be admitted, however, that the decision to make this donation was not made without some Members of Council expressing reluctance to donate such a large sum (Council Minutes 5.2.1954!)[107] The Research Department at the Royal College of Surgeons of England came into being in 1957.

The Research Accounts were considerably augmented during the fifties and charitable Trusts were created to facilitate management and distribution. Ronald Jarman[4] was, as usual, active as a fund raiser. The Annual Reports

1949-1962 (the end of the final year of Jarman's Presidency 1959-1962) tell a dramatic story.

The "Research Fund" was included in the general balance sheet of the Association in 1949. The balance in hand of the Fund at the beginning of that year was £1,315 (1996: £22,350) and the sole income was an instalment of a gift of £650 (1996: £11,050) from George Weston Holdings. The only items of expenditure were final payments to the two Research Fellows for salaries and expenses totalling £956.50 (1996: £16,260) and the cash in hand at the end of the year was £999 (1996: £16,980). The only income from investment which the Association had as a whole was £6 (1996: £102) odd from a Post Office Savings Bank Account.

A separate legally constituted Research Trust was established in November 1955 by transfer of the cash from the old fund. The Trustees were John Gillies,[1] T Cecil Gray, and Geoffrey Organe[4] (Annual Report 1955). The assets of the Trust by the end of the first financial year (30 June 1956) were £2,075 (1996: £28,500). The only donation received was one of £350 (1996: £4,725) from the British Oxygen Company. Expenses in connection with the "Deaths associated with Anaesthesia" and "Heroin" inquiries (see below) had been paid out as well as the £1,000 (1996: £13,800) mentioned above to the Royal College of Surgeons of England Anaesthetic Research Department Fund. The Trust did not have any investments.

The circumstances of the Research Trust had improved by the end of 1959, predominantly as the result of a Silver Jubilee appeal launched in 1957 (Annual Report 1959). Donations (by covenant and otherwise) amounted to £532.50 (1996: £6,400); the Trust's investments (valued at £3,584 (1996: £43,000)) had brought in £186 (1996: £2,330) and, because of trust status, there had been a tax rebate of £5.75 (1996: £70). The "Deaths associated with Anaesthesia" inquiry had cost £19.75 (1996: £330) and research grants and travelling expenses totalling £180 (1996: £2,200) had been made.

A new fund - the Research and Education Trust - with a broader remit was instituted in 1959 on the eve of Jarman becoming President; the trustees were Jarman himself,[4] Vernon Hall and Patrick Shackleton.[6] A vigorous appeal was started and the Research and Education Trust was allowed to accumulate with only administrative expenditure until 1962, while the Research Trust was used as the routine vehicle for grants. The accounts in the 1962 Annual Report show an income from donations and covenants to the Research and Education Trust of £2,671.25 (1996: £29,400) and £126 (1996: £1,386) interest from investments with a market value of £21,043 (1996: £231,500) recovered in tax rebate. This represented a truly magnificent achievement during Jarman's[4] Presidency. Amongst the contributors over the years to the Research Trust and the Education and Research Trust had been (Annual Reports 1956-1962):- British Oxygen Company, the African Manganese Company, Abbott Laboratories, Imperial Chemical Industries, May and Baker, Roche Products, Lloyds and Lloyds Brokers, the Wellcome Foundation, G D Searle and Company, Eli Lilley and Company, Ore Sales and Services, and Thomas Stevens and Sons. There were also a number of private donations, ranging from £5.25 (1996: £64) to a magnificent £15,000 (1996: £182,000) from Mr G Antony Vandervell in 1960.

The two Trusts continued to be in existence until 1969 but the assets and liabilities of the Research Trust were gradually allowed to dwindle and the remaining balance was finally transferred to the Research and Education Trust on 30 June 1969.

Deaths associated with anaesthesia

The involvement of the anaesthetists in the investigation and open discussion of the cause of death in the perioperative period has a long history. The investigation of the "chloroform controversy" in the second half of the nineteenth century and the first decade of the twentieth century was an early classic example.[195,196]

The Association became involved from its earliest years, not only from a desire to learn the truth, but also as a reaction to an attitude of the general public, the press, and some coroners that resulted in many perioperative deaths being labelled as "deaths *due* to anaesthesia" when it was patently obvious that, though "*under* anaesthesia", the demise of the patient was due to the patient's own condition or surgical intervention (Chapter 4).

The Association of Anaesthetists may be justly proud of being one of the earliest specialist organisations to attempt to audit the outcome of its practice.

It began its first formal investigation into "deaths associated with anaesthesia" in 1949.[197,198] This was initiated by a letter to Council from George Edwards[108] of St George's Hospital, London (Council Minute 3.12.1948)[107] soon after the introduction of the NHS. He pointed out that in the former London County Council (LCC) Hospitals, in addition to the coroner's investigation, it had been the practice for Medical Superintendents to prepare a confidential report on deaths under, or immediately following, anaesthesia for consideration by a special subcommittee of the LCC medical services meeting in camera. This subcommittee made recommendations with regard to practice from time to time. Edwards went on to say that Senior Administrative Medical Officers (SAMOs) in some Regions of the NHS were attempting to institute a similar scheme. Edwards believed that any such scheme should be undertaken nationally, and suggested that a committee consisting of interested parties, including the Ministry of Health and the Association, should be formed to consider the best method of investigating deaths occurring under anaesthesia and, where indicated, to make recommendations of a general nature. Council considered George Edwards' proposal at some length. There was general agreement that such an investigation would be valuable, but there was opposition to the inclusion of representatives of the Ministry of Health in the preliminary committee. Council therefore set up a subcommittee consisting of Alexander Low,[2] Bernard Johnson,[5] Katherine Lloyd-Williams[172] and (Sir) Geoffrey Organe[4] to advise Council. Events moved rapidly during 1949. A voluntary reporting scheme was instituted and every effort was made to secure confidentiality. A standard form for reports was prepared and approved by Council, a campaign was mounted to ensure that as many anaesthetists as possible were aware of the scheme both by publication in the journal *Anaesthesia* and by direct mailing,[197,198] and a subcommittee consisting of George Edwards[108] (Convener), H J V Morton[199] of Hillingdon Hospital,[199] Edgar Pask[89] and W Derek Wylie was appointed to consider the reports (Council Minutes 7.11.1948, 10.6.1949, 8.7.1949). The Annual Report presented at the Annual General Meeting on 3 November 1949 records that the scheme was in being, and that the SAMOs of Regions which had begun their own investigations had agreed that the scheme should be on a national basis conducted by the Association of Anaesthetists.

Morton[199] presented an interim assessment based on the first 100 of 200 reports which had been received at the Annual General Meeting in 1950.[200]

Sixty two of the cases were deemed to be wholly or partly due to anaesthesia, and seventeen of these had died from the inhalation of gastric contents following regurgitation after the use of a thiopentone induction with or without curare, and a further nine from an overdose of thiopentone in which a muscle relaxant (doubtless curare with its hypotensive effect) had been given at the same time. It was clear that the use of newer agents and techniques of intravenous induction and neuromuscular paralysis were not completely understood and had brought with them their own complications. It was small wonder that there were frequent pleas for a return to spontaneous respiration with nitrous oxide, oxygen and ether![198,201,202]

There was considerable concern about the number of deaths attributable to regurgitation and vomiting at this time. It must be remembered that curare was being used freely in 1951, but the short acting muscle relaxant succinylcholine had not been introduced for intubation, and Sellick's description of the manoeuvre of cricoid pressure, for obstructing the oesophagus and reducing the danger of regurgitation, was a decade into the future.[146] Contrary to the belief of some examination candidates today, however, "crash" or "rapid sequence" induction was already being practised using thiopentone and curare with a 20° foot down tilt.[202,203] The Committee had collected 43 cases out of the 350 reports received by October 1951[203] and, as a result, Morton and Wylie published a "frankly didactic" article on the subject.[204] This contains much sound advice. Inhalation induction with nitrous oxide, oxygen and ether was recommended when a full stomach is suspected; the respiratory tree being protected by laryngeal reflexes at the stage when active vomiting may occur.[204] The present writer was instructed as a novice anaesthetist in 1949 never to use curare before the patient had been intubated! An interim report on 400 cases was published in 1952 when regurgitation was still a major cause of death,[205] and the Committee decided that urgent communications were indicated on two further occasions before their major report was published in 1956.[206] The first of these was on fatal cases in which various deliberate hypotensive techniques had been used,[207] and the second on those in which it was considered that deaths were due to conditions in which "postoperative care was inadequate to meet the circumstances which arose."[208] Curare had been given to spontaneously respiring patients in a number of the cases without subsequent reversal with prostigmine.

The 1956 paper was published after 1,000 reports had been examined;[206] 598 of these were deemed to be directly due to the drugs or technique used for the anaesthetic. One hundred and ten deaths were considered to be due to aspiration (15 of them during Caesarean section or forceps delivery) but overdosage with thiopentone and inadequate blood volume replacement were also implicated. It was emphasised that the way in which the data had been collected (voluntary reporting which was known to be incomplete)[202] precluded:-

"the formulation of inferences with respect to the relative safety of agents and techniques and the various forms of fatality in the country as a whole.... In the great majority of the reports however, there were departures from accepted practice."[206]

This latter aspect of the conclusions was particularly emphasised in the accompanying Editorial in *Anaesthesia*,[209] but a well balanced leading article in the *British Medical Journal*[210] which praised the Association of Anaesthetists on its initiative, also included a paragraph on the inadequate conditions for post operative recovery facilities in British hospitals: -

"Too often the acute observer can see unconscious patients left unattended or in the case of a junior probationer [nurse], wards without the means of efficient suction, powerful drugs given without enough thought for their pharmacological effects or outmoded techniques used".[210]

A number of letters appeared subsequently in the correspondence columns of the *British Medical Journal* (1956; Volume 2). These mostly re-emphasised the points made in the report, but they included a letter from Massey Dawkins[211] of University College Hospital, London. This drew attention to the fact that the latest statistic available of 562 deaths associated with anaesthesia for England and Wales in 1953 was the lowest since 1925 at a time when operations were less numerous and extensive.[212] There was also a strongly worded criticism of "the miserably inadequate theatre accommodation in many of our hospitals" by (Sir) R S Murley, who was to be President of the Royal College of Surgeons of England from 1977 to 1980.[93,213] Murley asserted that:-

"a number of the misadventures to which your leading article refers would be avoided if hospitals were provided with adequate theatre suites and ample recovery rooms".[213]

This was indeed a perspicacious comment from a surgeon in 1956 at a time when the need for postoperative recovery rooms in British hospitals was only just beginning to be generally appreciated even by anaesthetists.

It is also interesting that the same volume of the *British Medical Journal*, (1956; Volume 2) contains an article by A R Hunter[214] describing the then mysterious condition of "neostigmine resistant curarisation".[215] This also gave rise to a considerable amount of correspondence. This was a condition which undoubtedly had its origin in the effect of carbon dioxide accumulation, acidosis and gross electrolyte imbalance on the prolongation of neuromuscular blockade into the recovery period, particularly in patients with pre-existing impaired respiratory function;[216] it had almost certainly contributed to death in a number of the cases described in the report on deaths by the Association of Anaesthetists.

Reports on deaths associated with anaesthesia continued to be sent into the Association of Anaesthetists after the 1956 report[206] although they were not so energetically solicited. O P Dinnick of the Middlesex Hospital, London, then Honorary Secretary of the Association, reviewed a further 600 reports in 1964.[217] It is possible that the 1956 report had had an effect on practice, as almost certainly had the introduction of succinylcholine for relaxation for intubation and the popularisation of the cricoid pressure manoeuvre.[146] Aspiration after regurgitation had now been replaced by the conduct of anaesthesia and surgery in the face of a pre-existing low blood volume as the cause of death which was most often identified (209 cases).[217,218] It is evident that the lessons learnt in the Second World War were being forgotten in peacetime when massive haemorrhage was less frequent! The second factor which was reported frequently was underventilation during anaesthesia and failure to re-establish respiration at its conclusion after the use of muscle relaxants (74 cases). These patients were often known to have been in gross electrolyte imbalance or fluid depletion which should have been restored pre-operatively; a diagnosis of "neostigmine-resistant curarisation" was often made in many of these cases.[215-217] Regurgitation was now ranked third of the most frequently reported causative factors (48 cases).

These important pioneering reports of data collected with a great deal of persistence and care were echoed in the more structured inquiry into "Mortality associated with anaesthesia" conducted by the Association and published by the Nuffield Provincial Hospital Trust in 1982,[218] the subsequent Confidential Enquiry into Perioperative Deaths (CEPOD) and the ongoing "National Confidential Enquiry into Perioperative Deaths" (NCEPOD) conducted by the anaesthetic and surgical Associations and a number of Royal Colleges and their Faculties (Chapter 8).

The use of heroin

The monograph on heroin (diamorphine) was omitted from the 1953 *British Pharmacopoeia* in response to pressure from the Expert Committee of the WHO on drugs liable to produce addiction, which had already succeeded in banning the drug in more than 50 countries. A leading article in the *British Medical Journal* generally welcomed the action of the editors of the *British Pharmacopoeia*.[220] It also suggested that there would be "the most respectable precedent for Government authorities should they decide on the revolutionary step of making the use of the drug illegal in Britain".[220] This suggestion provoked only one letter of protest.[221] Things were different after 28 April 1955 when the Government announced that it was placing a ban on the manufacture and export of heroin after 31 December 1955 and, at the same time, continuing the prohibition of imports of the drug which had been in effect for many years.[222] This announcement placed a virtual ban on the prescription of the drug. The parliamentary statement caused a furore amongst the members of the British medical profession, both from the point of view of the alleged unique properties of the drug, and also because of the interference with the jealously guarded freedom of the practitioner to prescribe. Letters of protest filled the correspondence columns of both the *British Medical Journal* and the *Lancet* (*British Medical Journal* 1955 volumes 1 and 2 and 1956 volume 1, and *Lancet* 1955 volumes 1 and 2) and the British Medical Association passed resolutions and made representations.[223] The proposed ban on the manufacture of heroin in the United Kingdom was withdrawn on 26 January 1956, but the prohibition of both import and export was retained.[224] Heroin thus survived in British practice, particularly for use in the control of pain in terminal cancer and, in due course, in the nineteen eighties, as an extradural and intrathecal narcotic (Chapter 8).[225]

The attention of the Council of the Association was drawn to the impending ban on heroin by a letter from J P Payne who asked if the Association had been consulted (Council Minute 16.9.1955).[107] The Minutes state that:-

"It was pointed out that heroin was not regarded as an important drug in anaesthetics but it was regretted that the Association had not been consulted in this matter as heroin was used in anaesthesia in neurosurgery".[107]

A letter from another member was received by Council on 6 January 1956 suggesting that the Association of Anaesthetists should investigate the opinions of practising anaesthetists on the question of heroin. A subcommittee was formed consisting of T Cecil Gray (Liverpool), W W Mushin,[88] and H Bruce Wilson (Aberdeen). The investigation was to be financed by the Research Trust.

The investigation took the form of a questionnaire circulated to all the Fellows and Members of the Association resident in the United Kingdom. The Subcommittee reported to Council on 1 February 1957, and the results of the inquiry were published in the April 1957 issue of *Anaesthesia*,[226] and commented upon by a subsequent Editorial in *Anaesthesia*.[227] The response rate was 72% (887 questionnaires were sent out, 639 replies were received). Two hundred and forty three respondents used heroin (38%) in their practice and, of these, 138 regarded the drug as irreplaceable. The Editorial noted that at that time (1957) there were only 54 registered heroin addicts in the United Kingdom![227]

Explosions in operating theatres

Ether and cyclopropane were still favourite agents throughout the fifties. W Alexander Low[2] was concurrently President of the Association and President of the Section of Anaesthetics of the Royal Society of Medicine; on 1 December 1950 he delivered a comprehensive Presidential Address to the Section on "Fires and explosions connected with anaesthesia".[228] The report of the address must have come to the attention of the Home Office, as

Low reported to the Council of the Association on 2 February 1951[107] that he, and other representatives of the Section, had been invited to a meeting with "Dr Swann of the Home Office and Mr Powell and Mr Davis, the newly appointed safety electrical engineers for the National Health Service, with a view to investigating this problem and issuing directives". Low had pointed out that this was more a matter for the Association of Anaesthetists. The Association Council therefore appointed Morton[199] and Woolmer[125] to represent the Association. They had a further meeting with the Ministry of Health and the Home Office officials (Council Minute 6.4.1951).[107]

There followed protracted negotiations to set up a joint committee with the Ministry of Health to investigate the problem of explosions in operating theatres. These were obviously occurring sufficiently often to give cause for concern; the Ministry of Health issued a memorandum on the subject independently (Council Minute 1.6.1951)[107] and an Editorial in *Anaesthesia* mentions that "the recent series of explosions in operating theatres has focused attention on this problem which has exasperated anaesthetists for many years".[229] The Association of Anaesthetists was concerned that expensive alterations were being carried out to operating theatres without there being adequate guidelines as to the specification of such matters and the resistance of operating theatre floors (Council Minute 3.10.1952),[107] and also that anaesthetists were perhaps using more lethal anaesthetic drugs such as chloroform unnecessarily, because they feared the use of ether under any circumstances in the X-ray Department (Council Minute 6.4.1951).[107]

The Association formed a joint committee with the Medical Defence Union in 1952 (Annual Report 1952), but this was disbanded when the Ministry of Health finally appointed a Working Party with strong representation from the Association of Anaesthetists (Archibald Galley (1909-1986) of Kings College Hospital London, Low,[2] Marston[230] and Morton[199]) (Annual Report 1953).

The Working Party reported in 1956.[231] Their report was well received:[232] a leading article in the *British Medical Journal* stated:-

"This report.... can be welcomed as the first authoritative, sensible, helpful, topical and readily understandable communication on this

matter from official sources that has appeared in Britain".[232]

The report contained many recommendations and detailed technical data on essential antistatic precautions (including the use of antistatic rubber). There was also an up to the minute mention of the introduction of nonflammable halothane in that year (1956). This was, of course, to lead ultimately to a permanent solution to the problem; even so, the possibility of explosions was a concern to the Association into the early seventies.[233]

A Charles King and the Museum of the Association of Anaesthetists

Charles King, designer and manufacturer of anaesthetic apparatus, was a remarkable man who played a leading role in the development of modern anaesthesia as well as in the history of the Association.[234,235]

Charles King served his apprenticeship as a practical engineer before the Great War and, after a brief period as a salesman for a general medical supply company, he served in the British Army in France in the Great War. King managed to open his own medical supply business after the Great War and, having borrowed £100 (1996: £2,200) from an uncle, he purchased the lease of a shop at 34 Devonshire Street, London W1. This was adjacent to Harley Street and Wimpole Street with their consulting rooms and nursing homes. He obtained the franchise for the United Kingdom sales of the American McKesson apparatus[195] at the suggestion of Francis P de Caux of St Bartholomew's Hospital, London,[236] and proceeded to modify it at the latter's request.[235] Thus began King's association with the specialty of anaesthesia as a manufacturer and supplier of anaesthetic apparatus which nearly became a monopoly in the United Kingdom at one stage between the two World Wars. King developed apparatus in collaboration with many leading anaesthetists including Sir Ivan Magill,[184] Robert Minnitt (1890-1974),[237] whose original nitrous oxide analgesia apparatus for midwifery was based on the McKesson machine (Chapter 4), and Victor Goldman; but he would also with great kindliness lend an ear to the inventive aspirations of less well known and more junior anaesthetists and often manufacture their brain children to his own financial detriment. Number 34 Devonshire Street (and later number 27 after number 34 was destroyed by a landmine during an air raid in 1941) became a place where anaesthetists could have a cup of coffee and meet and talk to their friends and with Charles King and his staff.[238] King also built up an excellent library of anaesthetic textbooks and journals at his premises and formed a museum of historic equipment. Ralph Waters described his shop as a "Mecca for anaesthetists".[234] This happy situation continued until King retired in 1953 despite amalgamation with the firm of Coxeter in 1926 and a take-over by the British Oxygen Company in 1939.

Charles King became a recognised world authority on modern and historic anaesthetic equipment. He was highly respected by anaesthetists for his expertise and unfailing friendliness and willingness to assist them. He became an Honorary Fellow of the Section of Anaesthetics of the Royal Society of Medicine and of many overseas societies.[234]

W Stanley Sykes[239] suggested at the Annual General Meeting in 1935[240] that the Association of Anaesthetists ought to make a collection of historic anaesthetic equipment. This suggestion was before its time however; Sykes received a rather stuffy reply from the Chair to the effect that the Royal College of Surgeons of England already had an excellent collection, and anyone who was able to do so could add to it if they wished (Annual General Meeting 1935).[240] The implementation of Sykes' suggestion of a museum collection for the Association had to wait until 1953 when Charles King donated his collection of historic apparatus to the Association on his retirement. The Charles King Collection of Historical Anaesthetic Apparatus was formally received by the President of the Association at a sherry party on 6 March of that year (Council Minutes 4.2.1953).[107] The Collection continued to be housed at 27 Devonshire Street, however, under the eye of King's friend and successor, James Juby, until the shop was closed on the expiry of its lease in the early sixties. M H Armstrong Davison[139] of Newcastle upon Tyne was appointed as the first Curator of the Museum in 1956 (Council Minutes 2.3.1956 and 1.6.1956)[107] and, after prolonged negotiation, the Collection was housed in show-cases at the Royal College of Surgeons of England in Lincoln's Inn Fields, where the Association of Anaesthetists still had its headquarters in the Joint Secretariat. Charles King lived just long enough to see this accomplished.[235]

The display of the Collection was improved by Kenneth Bryn Thomas (1917-1979)[242] of Reading who succeeded in arranging for the provision of new show-cases. These were capable of accommodating the whole Collection in the Professorial Department of Anaesthesia at the Royal College of Surgeons of England. Bryn Thomas also published an inventory of the Collection in Anaesthesia in 1970,[243] and an authoritative book on *The Development of Anaesthetic Apparatus,* based on the Charles King Collection in 1975.[195]

The Collection continued to be housed somewhat inadequately in the Royal College of Surgeons until it was transferred to the Association's own building at 9 Bedford Square in 1986; since then it has been augmented and displayed in a series of imaginative exhibitions in its own accommodation within the building.[235]

The Association and the British Standards Institution

The Association of Anaesthetists formed its own Standing Apparatus Committee (initially composed of Organe,[3] Macintosh[244] and Edwards[108]) in 1948 (Council Minutes 27.10.1948),[107] when it was informed that no committee of the British Standards Institution (BSI) had yet been set to deal with anaesthetic apparatus. The Association subsequently readily accepted an invitation to join the BSI when it was invited to do so in 1950 (Council Minutes 1.12.1950),[107] and thus began the long and fruitful collaboration between the two bodies.

The Association had already given an opinion to the BSI on rubber gloves (Annual Report 1949) and international standardisation of colour codes and non-interchangeable couplings for medical gases (Annual Report 1950 and Council Minutes 1.12.1950).[107] The negotiations with regard to the colour codes of medical gases finally reached the stage of international agreement in 1952 (Annual Report 1952); as has been the case with many international agreements however, both before and since, the British immediately complied with the new regulations, others did not, (Council Minutes 16.9.1955)[107] and, as recorded in Chapter 4, full international consensus has never been achieved! Eight Members of Council visited the British Oxygen Company Filling Station at the end of 1955 (Council Minutes 6.1.1956)[107] and found the non-interchangeability arrangements for filling gas cylinders with different gases "entirely satisfactory".

Memorials to John Snow (1813-1858)

The monument over the grave of John Snow,[136,245] the first professional and scientific anaesthetist, was originally erected in the Brompton cemetery, London, shortly after his death in 1858. It was restored in 1895 at the expense of Sir Benjamin Ward Richardson, his contemporary as a physician and as an anaesthetist and his original biographer and friend. The inscription was renovated in 1938 "by members of the Section of Anaesthetics of the RSM and anaesthetists in the United States of America". The memorial stone was wrecked in an air raid in April 1941.[246-248] This condition was brought to the attention of the 1949 Annual General Meeting;[246] a subscription was raised and the monument was restored at the cost of £160 (1996: £2,900) (Council Minutes 6.10.1950, Annual Reports 1949, 1950 and 1958).

The centenary of the death of John Snow was commemorated on 6 June 1958 by the laying of wreaths on his grave by the President of the Association of Anaesthetists, the Dean of the Faculty and the Presidents of the Sections of Anaesthetics and Epidemiology of the RSM; Snow's work on the water-borne transmission of cholera being his other outstanding contribution to medical science.[246] The inauguration of the John Snow Memorial Lecture in the same year has also been noted earlier in this Chapter.[136]

The development of the Association between 1949 and 1959

This chapter on the development of the British specialty of anaesthesia and the Association of Anaesthetists itself between 1 January 1949 and 31 December 1959 not only covers a period when many new drugs were introduced and the modern techniques of anaesthesia as we know them today were evolved, but also the decade at the end of which the Association of Anaesthetists emerged in its present form.

The expansion of British anaesthesia is reflected in the increase in Membership of the Association; in 1949 there were 692 United Kingdom Fellows and Members, 9 Corresponding Fellows from overseas and 7 Honorary Fellows; by 1959 there were 1182 United Kingdom Fellows, Members and Associates, 34 Corresponding Fellows and 12 Honorary Members. The introduction of the category of Associates, mostly anaesthetists in training, is significant; it represents the beginning of a process which led to the establishment of the definitive group in 1967 (Chapter 7).

The Association of Anaesthetists, having given up its responsibility for the training and examination of anaesthetists to the Faculty, consolidated its position as the authoritative voice of anaesthetists on clinical and medicopolitical matters during the fifties. Another important development was the extension of the Annual General Meetings to include scientific sessions of topical interest to established and trainee anaesthetists alike, as well as enjoyable social programmes which promote the good fellowship and unity of the specialty. The Association had also established a firm financial base and put aside considerable funds for research, as well as conducting its own seminal investigation into deaths associated with anaesthesia.

The hesitation shown by the United States had resulted in the Officers of the Association of Anaesthetists playing the leading part in the establishment of the World Federation of Societies of Anaesthesiologists. British anaesthesia was consequently highly respected, particularly in Europe.

The next decade was to see another important and far reaching development - the extension of the remit of physician anaesthetists outside the operating theatre, first into postoperative recovery units and then into the field of intensive care and pain therapy (Chapter 7).

Expansion

7

Expansion

1 January 1960 to 31 December 1969

"Honour the physician with the honour due to him for the uses ye may have of him"

The Apocrypha *Ecclesiasticus* Ch XXXVIII.vi

Executive Officers

Presidents:-	R Jarman (1959-1962)[1]
	V F Hall (1962-1965)
	H H Pinkerton (1965-1967)[2]
	R P W Shackleton (1967-1969)[3]
	A J W Beard (1969-1971)[4]
Honorary Treasurers:-	E A Pask (1960-1966)[5]
	A J W Beard (1966-1969)[4]
	D D C Howat (1969-1974)
Honorary Secretaries:-	H J V Morton (1960-1963)[6]
	O P Dinnick (1963-1966)
	P J Helliwell (1966-1968)[7]
	Aileen K Adams (1968-1970)
Editors of *Anaesthesia*:-	C Langton Hewer (1946-1966)[8]
	R Bryce-Smith (1966-1972)
Chairmen, Junior Anaesthetists' Group:-	A A Spence (1967-1969)
	J C Simpson (1969-1970)

National and international turbulence in the sixties

The violent episodes which preceded the granting of independence to some of the former territories of the British Empire were over for the most part by 1960 (Chapter 6); consequently the Union flag was ceremonially hauled down in the majority of former dependencies without major incident in the earlier years of the decade.[9]

The principal international role of the United Kingdom in the sixties was in Europe as a member of the North Atlantic Treaty Organisation confronting the Soviet Block Warsaw Pact countries in the cold war, symbolised by the erection of the Berlin Wall in 1961. The decade was one of great violence and lawlessness elsewhere in the world (Vietnam, Cuba, the 'wind of change' in Africa, the Congo, the Nigerian Civil War, the Chinese cultural revolution, race riots in the United States and the assassination of Martin Luther King and President Kennedy). It is true that these events had some repercussions on British internal politics but, despite being a nuclear power, the United Kingdom would not, indeed could not, intervene.[9]

The economic situation of the United Kingdom was precarious throughout the decade. Great Britain was divested of its Empire, but not yet integrated commercially into Europe nor able to export to the self-sufficient United States. Oil was not discovered under the North Sea until 1965. Industry was bedevilled both by archaic attitudes on the shop floor and traditionalist management. Alternating Conservative and Labour Governments employed increasingly desperate financial control in the face of mounting inflation, rising unemployment, industrial strife and low productivity. Looking back the only gleam of light which penetrated the encircling gloom was the triumphant victory of the English side in the World Football Championship in 1966.[9]

Some progress was made in improving road and rail transport (the last steam train on British Rail was withdrawn in 1966) but the flame of entrepreneurial enterprise kindled in the nineteen fifties was sadly diminished in the sixties; for example the nascent British lead in aeronautical engineering was lost (the revolutionary TSR2 fighter project was cancelled, even the supersonic *Concorde* (note the French spelling) which first flew in 1968 was an Anglo-French enterprise and probably commercially ahead of its time), and the last large scale achievement of Britain's once great shipbuilding industry, the Queen Elizabeth II, had breakdowns on its early voyages which made it an international laughing stock. The Exploration of Space was left to the United States and Russia; the first animal orbited the earth in a space capsule in 1961, closely followed by the first man (USSR), the first communication satellite was put in space in 1962 (USA), and the first man landed on the Moon in 1969 (USA).[9]

The social revolution of the sixties was dramatic and far reaching. Some enlightened domestic measures were introduced (for example the abolition of the death penalty for murder, the introduction of drinking and driving legislation, and the liberalisation of betting) but, by and large, it was a period of social unrest exacerbated by the repeated attempts to control pay in the face of inflation and rising personal expenditure. There were ugly and prolonged strikes, and the increase in terrorism in Northern Ireland resulted in 1968 in the deployment of troops to keep the peace for the first time since the nineteen twenties.

The worldwide protest of youth against authority did not pass Britain by. Students and other young people, often with some justification, began to feel that they had rights which were being denied them. The situation was aggravated by the general economic stringency and the possibility of atomic nuclear attack. The result was an exaggerated, and sometimes unthinking, condemnation and rejection of accepted values, and indulgence in uninhibited behaviour and sexual licence facilitated by the introduction of the contraceptive pill. It was not that the protesters were entirely selfish or oblivious to the needs of others. They believed passionately in good causes. The Campaign for Nuclear Disarmament and other peace movements, as well as many organisations vociferously demanding equal rights for ethnic and sexual minorities and the inhabitants of the Third World, and action on environmental pollution, etc, originated in the nineteen sixties; unfortunately, however, their protests were often, though not always, accompanied by demands that others (including that universal provider "the Government") should take action, rather than they themselves. Some universities and colleges witnessed scenes of ugly and sometimes violent protests by students often supported by avant-garde academic staff.

Young doctors were more responsible, but they too began to feel that the traditional autocratic structure of the medical profession was unacceptable, and to press for representation on the bodies which determined the conditions of their training and employment.[10]

The "swinging sixties" were certainly a wild and exciting time! The advent of the pop music of groups like the Beatles, the accompanying uninhibited dances, outlandish dress fashions, including the astonishingly revealing miniskirt in those days before tights were universally preferred to stockings, unusual hairstyles, and the use of hallucinogenic drugs, were symptomatic of the search for freedom of expression.

The new attitude to sexual morality was encouraged by the marketing of the first contraceptive pill in 1961[11] and later by the Abortion Act of 1967.[12] It is interesting to reflect on the contrast between the "Getting Married" affair of 1959 and the attitudes in 1998 to pre- and extra-marital sex. The "Getting Married" controversy arose when the British Medical Association (BMA) rather cravenly withdrew the fourth edition of the popular *Family Doctor* pamphlet in response to protests from the public and the profession. The offending article was headed "Is chastity outdated?" and merely stated *inter alia* that "one woman in every three in this country admits to premarital intercourse" and that "one bride in every eight is already having a baby at the time of her wedding".[13,14] Times change!

The Abortion Act, which (Sir) David Steel piloted through Parliament in 1967, has been liberally interpreted and has, to all intents and purposes, resulted in "abortion on demand" in the United Kingdom, despite theoretical restrictions.[12,15] It is difficult not to believe that some young women having their third or fourth abortion do not regard the procedure as an alternative to efficient contraception.

Medical practitioners and nurses who object on the grounds of conscience are exempted from participation in abortions under the Act, but it is indeed fortunate for the smooth running of operating lists, that most anaesthetists regard the Act as a liberal and enlightened measure despite the *volte-face* of the age old traditions of the medical profession which stretch right back to the Oath of Hippocrates.[15,16] The concurrence of anaesthetists is all too often assumed in this context nowadays, whereas, before the Act, on the rare occasions when an abortion was legal and justified, they were invariably specially consulted. The right of an individual anaesthetist to decline to anaesthetise for abortions has on the whole been respected, but refusal has sometimes caused difficulties with colleagues, and occasionally with Consultant Appointment Boards, even though questions as to whether or not an individual will or will not anaesthetise for abortions are officially forbidden (Annual Report 1976).

The Abortion Act has thrown a considerable strain on the resources of the NHS.[10,12] Anaesthetists who are in favour of male and female sterilisation, for which separate payments have been made since 1974, but against abortion, are placed in a particularly embarrassing position. The recent introduction of some Health Authorities of separately funded and remunerated abortion operating lists under the provisions of the 1991 reorganisation of the NHS is to be applauded. Those who wish to do so may now be able to demonstrate their genuine conscientious objection by leaving it to their colleagues to draw the additional remuneration.[10,12]

Developments in medicine and surgery 1960-1968

Fundamental research in the nineteen sixties in genetics, immunology and chemotherapy, both for infectious disease and in the treatment of cancer, laid the foundations for considerable clinical advances in the seventies and eighties;[15] and the acceptance by the medical profession that smoking caused lung cancer and was harmful to health in other ways, was a vindication of painstaking epidemiological research.[17]

Renal and hepatic transplants. The survival time of transplanted kidneys increased considerably as immunosuppressive drugs and techniques improved.[18] The first liver transplant was reported by Starzl and his colleagues from Denver, Colorado, in 1963[19] and the first hepatic transplant in the United Kingdom took place in 1968.[20]

Cardiac surgery also developed rapidly accompanied by the advent of implantable pacemakers and improved monitoring. This was particularly true in the field of valve replacement.[21,22] Professor Christian Barnard of Cape Town, South Africa undertook the first cardiac transplant in 1967.[23] The first British transplantation took place in 1968[24] amidst considerable surgical publicity.[25] The euphoria engendered by this event was not entirely shared by anaesthetists or the profession at large however (see the correspondence columns of the *British Medical Journal* 1968, Volume 2)! These early cases were premature. Surgical technical expertise and enthusiasm had outstripped the science of immunology, and, by the mid nineteen seventies, few cases were being undertaken.[26] The Chief Medical Officer of England wrote to surgeons in 1973 urging caution and advised the Government against the provision of special resources for cardiac transplantation until the scientific foundation of the procedure was clarified.[27] This was a cautious, but undoubtedly wise, decision. The pause has been followed by the very considerable progress that has been made in the eighties, after the rejection problem had to some extent been ameliorated.

Other procedures. Vascular surgery, particularly in the field of the treatment of aortic aneurysms[28] and portal hypertension,[29] was becoming more ambitious, as also were orthopaedic operations such as prosthetic hip replacement.[30]

All these increasingly more major operations brought new challenges for the anaesthetist in the management of the seriously ill patient and the treatment of massive blood loss and other complications, including fat embolism and hypotension following the use of methylmethacrylate cement in hip replacement.[28-33] The contributions which anaesthetists made to the satisfactory outcome of such procedures, before, during and after the operation were not always acknowledged![34] Anaesthetic skills of a different and more delicate order were required to ensure the success of microsurgery of the ear, eye and later for the re-attachment of limbs.[15]

Clinical anaesthesia 1960-1969

Mechanical ventilation during the muscle relaxant and light anaesthetic technique became the accepted choice for abdominal and thoracic surgery in the sixties. New and more practical ventilators were introduced including the original Manley workhorse.[35] The "educated hand" still had its devotees however![36]

Conversion to the pin-index system for medical gas cylinders was undertaken in 1967 (Council Minutes 7.7.67), thus eliminating the hazard of interchangeability and contributing considerably to patient safety.

The new muscle relaxants alcuronium (Alloferin)[37] and pancuronium (Pavulon)[38] were introduced in to clinical anaesthesia in the nineteen sixties to join tubocurarine and gallamine (Flaxedil). They were a welcome addition to the range of non-depolarising neuromuscular blocking agents.

Fentanyl and neuroleptanalgesia. There was a renewed interest in intravenous techniques for the maintenance of anaesthesia which was accentuated when doubts about the hepatoxicity of halothane developed.

combined the newly developed analgesics phenoperidine and fentanyl with the butyrophenone droperidol, one of the new psychoactive drugs which so revolutionised psychiatric treatment in the nineteen fifties and sixties.[39] The technique never really caught on in the United Kingdom or the United States but it was, and still is, popular in Scandinavia and Continental Europe. Short-acting fentanyl (phentanyl) has remained in the British anaesthetists' armamentarium as an important analgesic adjunct to general anaesthesia.

Diazepam (Valium), the successor to the original oral benzodiazepine tranquilliser chlordiazepoxide (Librium), was introduced in the nineteen fifties as an oral anxyolytic and premedicant drug. It became available for intramuscular and intravenous injection in 1966 and was used both to induce anaesthesia and as a sedative - especially as a cover for local anaesthesia.[40,41] Diazepam did not survive as an induction agent in British practice however as recovery tended to be prolonged.

Propanidid (Epontol) was an interesting short-acting intravenous induction agent which was introduced into the United Kingdom in 1964.[42] It was rapidly destroyed in the body and had advantages for short outpatient procedures; unfortunately it earned a reputation for causing allergic reactions and, though these were rarely fatal, it was withdrawn by the manufacturers in 1984.[43]

Methoxyflurane (Penthrane) was a non-flammable inhalation agent used extensively in the United States because of its safety, until its renal toxicity was demonstrated,[44,45] but it was never popular in the United Kingdom because of its odour and the slow induction and recovery which characterised its use. It was a good analgesic and had a brief period of popularity in obstetrics in sub- anaesthetic concentrations.[46]

The azeotropic mixture of two parts halothane to one part ether was an attempt to modify the cardiodepressant effects of halothane and provide analgesia.[47] An azeotropic mixture of halothane and methyl-n-propyl ether (Neothyl), an anaesthetic introduced in the nineteen fifties, was also tried.[48,49]

Bupivacaine (Marcain) is a long-acting local anaesthetic, which was used in clinical practice in the United Kingdom for the first time in 1968.[50] Its introduction was a milestone in the development of local anaesthesia, especially as its pharmacological properties made it a natural choice for the expanding use of epidural anaesthesia in obstetrics.[51]

The pharmacological harvest from the sixties was not large in terms of continuing use, but it produced pancuronium, fentanyl and diazepam and, right at the end of the decade, bupivacaine which was to facilitate a revival in the use of local anaesthesia in the United Kingdom in the seventies.

Complications of anaesthesia

Some of the most dreaded complications of anaesthesia were first recognised, or more fully researched, in the nineteen sixties.[52] They included the possible suppression of the adrenal cortex by corticosteroid drugs,[53,54] the toxic effects of halothane and other agents on the liver,[55-57] malignant hyperthermia,[58-59] and the dangers of administering anaesthesia to patients with sickle cell anaemia and thalassaemia.[60] The problems associated with sickle cell anaemia became particularly prominent in the United Kingdom due to postwar Afro-Caribbean immigration. The fear of precipitating complications such as these has sometimes led to unnecessarily exaggerated precautions being taken by anaesthetists; for example routine use of courses of large doses of cortisone and hydrocortisone to cover patients who had been on corticosteroid therapy in the past, and were consequently thought to be suffering from adrenal suppression, was found to be generally unnecessary.[53,54] The main consideration in the management of all these problems is to know about the possible danger to the individual patient; forewarned is forearmed! The corollary, which some learnt the hard way in the sixties, is that pre-operative visiting and assessment is an essential part of the anaesthetic process.

Halothane toxicity. The implication that halothane might be responsible for hepatic damage began to cause concern in the sixties.[55,56,61] Many anaesthetists seemed to refuse to believe that so apparently perfect an agent could possibly be so flawed. Considerable research was instituted. The consensus appears to be that the complication exists but is rare, that adequate oxygenation is essential if the complications are to be avoided, and that double exposure is dangerous.[56,57] Halothane was also implicated as one of the more likely triggers of malignant hyperthermia[59] and finally, at the very end of the nineteen sixties, the possible teratogenic and abortifacient consequences of the chronic exposure to halothane of operating theatre personnel began to be considered and, in turn, caused considerable concern in the nineteen seventies.[62]

Awareness during surgery. The muscle relaxant, paralysis, and controlled ventilation technique was taken to its extreme in the early sixties; hyperventilation with unsupplemented nitrous oxide and oxygen was often the only anaesthetic provided. It was therefore inevitable that the problem of awareness began to be a cause for concern, especially during Caesarean section when higher concentrations of oxygen were administered.[63,64]

The contamination of nitrous oxide with the higher oxides of nitrogen during the manufacturing process in September 1966 caused two deaths and widespread disruption of surgical practice in the United Kingdom while cylinders were withdrawn and tested.[65] The astute diagnosis made after the initial cases and the subsequent prompt action taken by Professor Clutton-Brock[66] of Bristol undoubtedly avoided a much greater tragedy.[65]

Cardiopulmonary resuscitation

The introduction of combined expired air respiration with external cardiac compression and defibrillation by Kouwenhoven and his colleagues in Baltimore revolutionised the treatment of cardiac arrest both in the operating theatre and outside it.[67,68] The advantages of the technique were immediately apparent to most surgeons and anaesthetists, particularly those concerned with cardiac surgery.[69] Anaesthetists played a leading part in establishing cardiac arrest teams within hospitals[70-72] and promoting the concept of teaching the new techniques of immediate first aid to nurses, paramedical personnel and the public at large.

This development was not without initial scepticism on the part of some cardiologists and others; it only took a few successful cases to convince the doubters however! The work in Brighton of the Consultant Anaesthetist Rex Binning[73] should be particularly remembered in popularising the technique for general use.[74] The simplest manoeuvres relating to care of the airway were not always understood at the time, even by emergency services. A newspaper photograph of a suicide victim associated with the notorious political Profumo scandal in 1963, depicted an unconscious patient being carried on a stretcher by ambulance attendants, supine, with his unsupported chin depressed in a position of actual or potential airway obstruction (personal recollection)!

Intensive care and the physician anaesthetist

It can be seen with hindsight that there was a certain inevitability both in the rapidity in which intensive care developed in the nineteen sixties, and in the emergence of anaesthetists into their present dominant role as consultants in charge of intensive care units (ICU) in the United Kingdom, to the point where 85.5% of ICUs are administered by anaesthetists (Association of Anaesthetists 1988 figures).[75,76]

The term "critical care" is sometimes used as a synonym for intensive care, but "critical care" covers any situation in which the survival of a patient depends on at least a one to one ratio of medical, nursing or paramedical relationship with the patient, and can include, for example, anaesthesia for surgery, and basic and advanced life support in the first aid situation.[77] Here we are concerned specifically with the development of ICU units within a hospital which are set aside to provide "a service for patients with potentially recoverable disease who can benefit from more detailed observation and treatment than is generally available in standard wards and departments".[75,78] There have been attempts to distinguish between "intensive *care* and "intensive *therapy"* on the grounds that "therapy" implies active intervention,[79] but the two terms are generally used synonymously. "Intensive care" is possibly the better term as it covers both active therapy and complex but nonetheless passive monitoring.

"Respiratory Units" were one of the forerunners of ICUs. They originated because of the desirability of concentrating poliomyelitis patients who required mechanical ventilation with negative pressure tank respirators. A number of such units were established in the United States by respiratory and contagious diseases physicians in the nineteen forties and early fifties because of the prevalence of poliomyelitis in that country.[80] Bower and his colleagues in Los Angeles used a positive pressure device to assist the negative pressure produced by the tank respirator. This unit reduced the mortality from bulbar poliomyelitis from 90% to 20%.[80, 81]

Relatively few "respiratory units" for the short term treatment and long term management of paralysed poliomyelitis patients in tank respirators were established in the United Kingdom, but the unit at the Western Fever Hospital in London was a notable exception. The use of the negative pressure "iron lung" in most hospitals was in the hands of general physicians who usually attempted to employ it only as a treatment of last resort. Resident Anaesthetists were called only to undertake laryngoscopy and suck out saliva from the respiratory tree of the patients. Intubation was often forbidden by the physicians. Those who lived through this era remember it only as a nightmare!

The use of intermittent positive pressure ventilation (IPPV) by the anaesthetist Ibsen, in support of the physician Lassen, in the 1952 poliomyelitis epidemic in Copenhagen revolutionised the treatment of patients with respiratory paralysis.[80,82,83] The Oxford Respiratory Unit was founded in 1953 by the neurologist J M K Spalding in association with the anaesthetist Alexander Crampton Smith.[84] Sir Robert Macintosh, who had shown an early interest in the management of respiratory failure in poliomyelitis in 1938 was of course still the Nuffield Professor of Anaesthetics at that time.

The Oxford unit developed Ibsen's technique using mechanical IPPV, although the use of the negative pressure respirator was not entirely abandoned.[85] The incidence of poliomyelitis declined after the discovery of the Salk vaccine in 1955,[86] and the treatment of other paralytic diseases with IPPV took its place. These included polyneuritis, tetanus, chest injuries, myasthenia, barbiturate poisoning, status epilepticus and polymyositis.[84,85]

Special mention should be made of those units which had a particular interest in the treatment of tetanus which still had a significant incidence in Great Britain in the fifties and sixties.[88-91] The anaesthetists expertise with muscle relaxant and IPPV techniques was particularly useful.[88-91]

IPPV became the accepted technique for the treatment of respiratory failure by the early sixties. Anaesthetists were often called upon to ventilate mechanically the cases which occurred intermittently in the wards of general hospitals in far from satisfactory conditions.[84,88] This state of affairs often resulted in a lower rate of survival than was possible, particularly in the absence of trained nursing staff; by the mid sixties many hospitals had profited by bitter experience and concentrated their patients in dedicated units.[70,71,92]

Intensive care units (ICUs) with a brief to treat those patients who need "detailed observation and treatment" but not necessarily mechanical ventilation, as well as those who required IPPV, did not evolve solely from Respiratory Units however. Another route was as a development of postoperative recovery wards, both general[93,94] and specialised; in the latter case particularly for those patients who required IPPV and special management following cardiac surgery.[95,96] Surgeons and physicians soon found that their severely ill patients could receive better care from expert nurses under supervision of anaesthetists in the Recovery Rooms. The presence of these cases was considered as a compliment to the recovery ward staff in the early days, but the resulting congestion often led to a demand from all sides for a separate properly staffed ICU to be provided.[92]

Physician anaesthetists were, and are, particularly suited to take charge of ICUs both by training and temperament. They have the necessary skills for the management of the acutely ill patient; in the ICU, as in the operating theatre, they are concerned with life support and patient comfort while specific therapy is administered, or, in the case of some patients in the ICU, the disease burns itself out. Anaesthetists are moreover, used to looking after other people's patients, and acquire the diplomatic tact necessary to cooperate with colleagues in other disciplines as part of their stock in trade![77,93]

The future pattern of intensive care in the United Kingdom was discernible by the end of the sixties, and some specially designed units were being established, usually by conversion of existing accommodation.[77,92,98] Coronary Care Units (CCU), rightly under the care of cardiologists, were beginning to separate from the general ICU. The function of the CCU is one of monitoring and the prevention of cardiac arrest rather than the treatment of its effects following resuscitation.[92,99,100] It was also generally agreed that short-term recovery units, and some longer term specialist recovery units such as those for postoperative cardiac and neurological surgery, were better separated from the general ICU. Paediatric intensive care units had also been established in the major children's hospitals.[101]

The Ministry of Health gave its encouragement to the establishment of ICUs as early as 1962[102] and in 1967 the BMA published the report of a working party on intensive care. This was chaired by Dr E M Moran Campbell (Physician at the Royal Postgraduate Medical School), and anaesthetists were represented by G T Spencer of St Thomas' Hospital, London (as Deputy Chairman) and D B Benazon of Bournemouth.[78] An appendix to the report gives very interesting details of 17 established ICUs at that time. Anaesthetists were in charge in 7 units, physicians in 5, a surgeon in one, and a surgeon and an anaesthetist, shared the responsibility in another; the medical responsibility had not been decided in the other three units.[78]

The Ministry of Health was also interested in a general concept of "progressive patient care" (PPC) as practised in some hospitals in Scandinavia and the United States as early as 1962.[102] PPC is "the systematic grouping of patients according to the degree of illness and dependence on the nurse rather than by classification of disease or sex." Three degrees of cases within the acute hospital (intensive, intermediate, and self-care) and two outside it (rehabilitation or long term, and home care) were recognised.[77,92,102] PPC was seen by some as an attempt to ensure that the one to one nurse patient ratio required for the ICU was provided with the minimum effect on global cost and without expanding the nursing work force.[72,92] The concept of PPC evoked considerable discussion but made little progress in British hospitals.[77,102]

Despite official support the establishment of ICUs and the participation of anaesthetists in their management was not achieved without controversy.[77,79,100,104-7] Some Hospital Administrators saw the development of ICUs as unjustifiably expensive. Administrative nurses looked with horror on the round the clock provision of one nurse for one bed in a mixed sex unit, and often failed to understand why the duties in the ICU could not be assigned to any registered nurse, however inexperienced in the technological details of life supporting apparatus.[77] Clinicians in charge of patients also sometimes found it difficult to bring themselves to hand over the management of their patients, even if they retained overall clinical control.[104] Others doubted whether ICUs were necessary and believed that ordinary ward staff could easily learn and be familiar with the specialist equipment involved.[79] Mushin and Lunn,[105] while accepting the suitability of anaesthetists for work in ICUs, believed that the anaesthetist should only be involved in a consultative capacity lest the specialty be deprived of their services in the operating theatre; such a situation may have been successful in some instances, but there is no doubt that, in others, it resulted in the anaesthetist being relegated to the technical functions of intubating the patient and adjusting the ventilator. Many ICUs were set up by individual anaesthetists working in their own time without sessional allocation; sometimes they became professionally isolated from their fellow consultant anaesthetists for so doing,[108] but they usually had the support of the junior members of their departments,[92] who began to look forward to obtaining consultant appointments with a substantial element of intensive care.[106] The situation gradually became regularised however. It became clear, in the majority of hospitals in the United Kingdom, that the anaesthetist was a clinician with the necessary clinical expertise who was best able to take charge of the new ICUs and whose department was large enough to provide round the clock junior staff cover; as retirement vacancies occurred and new consultant anaesthetist appointments were made, more and more jobs were advertised requiring "an interest in intensive care". Anaesthetists, too, were willing to accept the position that the physician or surgeon retained nominal clinical responsibility for his patient in the ICU, but happily, truth to tell, as they became more and more confident in the ability of their anaesthetist colleagues, they were usually content to leave matters in their hands.

Anaesthetists had thus filled a gap in the British medical services, and became the majority specialty in intensive care, at first almost automatically as an extension of their responsibilities in the operating theatre, but later with an enthusiasm that was to be expected from a young and rapidly developing specialty. The Intensive Care Society (ICS) was founded in 1970 on the initiative of Alan Gilston, Consultant Anaesthetist to the National Heart Hospital, London.[109] Intensive care in the United Kingdom and the ICS remains overtly multidisciplinary, however; in the nineteen eighties the Royal College of Physicians, the Royal College of Surgeons of England and the Faculty of Anaesthetists began an initiative designed to define acceptable cross-over training programmes in intensive care for senior trainees in all three disciplines.

Monitoring in anaesthesia and intensive care

The twin developments of open heart surgery and ICUs focused attention on minute to minute monitoring and recording of cardiovascular and pulmonary function. Editorials in the *British Medical Journal* and *Anaesthesia* reporting on a Symposium held by the Faculty of Anaesthetists early in 1970 summarised the status of monitoring at that time.[110,111]

Attempts to replace the bedside nurse in the ICU by centralised electronic monitoring, which were actively promoted during the early and mid sixties, were generally discredited by the end of the decade. Monitoring was obviously important but for its own sake as a guide to patient management both in the ICU and in the operating theatre.[111,112] There were still major difficulties, however; particularly in the reliability of sensors and transducers at the interface between the apparatus and the patient,[111,112] and some of the potentially dangerous hazards of electronic monitoring and invasive procedures were only just beginning to become apparent;[112-115] for example the quintessence of electrical safety was still considered to be the provision of a common earth[112] rather than the isolation of the patient circuit, the value of which was not really appreciated until the beginning of the next decade.[113,114]

The two developments which contributed most to monitoring in the sixties were sophisticated electrode monitoring techniques for blood-gas and pH measurement[116] and the invasive but relatively simple technique of central venous pressure (CVP) measurement, often with the aid of a saline manometer.[117,118]

The diagnosis of death

The combination of the development of transplant surgery and the improvement in cardiopulmonary life support techniques in ICUs inevitably caused growing concern about the diagnosis of death during the sixties.[119,120] The Conference of the Royal Colleges and their Faculties (including the Faculty of Anaesthetists) issued their carefully researched and considered guidelines in 1976, on which British practice has been confidently based ever since.[121] There was a considerable storm in the medical and lay press as late as 1980 however after an ill-judged *Panorama* programme on television. The argument raged round the question as to whether electroencephalographic evidence was pertinent or necessary before brain death could be diagnosed, as was the case in the United States and certain other countries. A great deal of public disquiet was caused by the controversy, and the transplant programme was markedly affected. Leading articles appeared in both the *British Medical Journal*[122] and *Lancet*[123] and much detailed correspondence followed. The diagnostic procedures as they concerned anaesthetists were well summarised in an Editorial in *Anaesthesia* by J F Searle, Consultant Anaesthetist, Exeter, in 1981.[124]

The treatment of chronic pain

Some British anaesthetists were involved in the treatment of chronic pain in the nineteen forties and fifties and even earlier. This was chiefly because of their expertise in the techniques of using local anaesthesia to block peripheral nerves and inject local anaesthetic agents into the subarachnoid and extradural spaces of the patients referred to them by surgeons, neurologists and other physicians.[84,125,126] Interest quickened in the nineteen sixties and more formal pain clinics were inaugurated.[126-129] The Group which became the Intractable Pain Society in 1971 (since 1990 The Pain Society) was formed in 1967 on the initiative of Mark Swerdlow (Consultant Anaesthetist to Salford Royal Hospital and the Hope Hospital, Salford) who became its first President. There were 281 formal pain clinics operating in the United Kingdom by 1991 (excluding hospices for the terminally ill); over 94% of these are run by anaesthetists, very often working single handed (Swerdlow personal communication 1992). The multidisciplinary approach involving physicians, psychiatrists, psychologists and surgeons as well as anaesthetists, which has developed in the United States and Australia,[130] was not until recently a feature of British practice.[127-129]

The professional attitude to chronic pain relief has changed considerably especially since the promulgation of Melzack and Wall's gate theory of the psychosomatic modulation of pain in 1965.[131,132] Treatment involves psychological and spiritual counselling and the use of many drugs that are now available for modifying mood and mental attitude as well as the use of analgesics and stimulation produced analgesia. The blocking of nerves by local anaesthetics and neurolytics is becoming much less an essential part of chronic pain management, especially in the treatment of chronic pain of nonmalignant origin.[128-131]

The wisdom of the involvement of the anaesthetist in the overall management of patients suffering from chronic pain has been challenged.[133] It is certainly true that the continuing care of patients, perhaps over several years, is foreign to the philosophical temperament of many anaesthetists. Their expertise is essentially in the acute treatment of patients in the operating theatre or the ICU. Chronic pain therapy is not a field that is to the liking, or perhaps even within the competence, of many anaesthetists; as John Lloyd (formerly Director of the Oxford Regional Pain Relief Unit) has emphasised, "there is now no longer any place for the occasional dabbler in pain management".[129] Those anaesthetists who have felt drawn to enter the field as a major interest have, however, shown considerable aptitude for the work and now dominate the subspecialty in the United Kingdom. It may be that the contacts which anaesthetists have with so many disciplines in their day to day practice help those members of the specialty who are involved with pain relief services in Great Britain, to assume successfully the role of "practitioners" in pain clinics.[134]

Interest in the establishment and expansion of pain therapy, including the effective treatment of postoperative pain, has increased considerably in the eighties and nineties. Advertisements for consultant anaesthetist appointments which include sessions in pain relief (nowadays both acute and chronic) are appearing with increasing frequency in the medical journals.

The thalidomide tragedy and the Medicines Act

Thalidomide (Distaval) was introduced in Germany in 1957 and subsequently widely prescribed in the United Kingdom, Australia and Japan. The drug was regarded as a safe sedative particularly in pregnancy. It was considered to be safe because, although overdose induced deep sleep, it rarely if ever resulted in a fatality. In 1961 unequivocal evidence was reported in Germany and Australia that thalidomide was causing fetal abnormalities in the long bones of the arms and legs (phocomelia).[135] The drug was withdrawn by the Distillers Company, the United Kingdom distributors, in December 1961.[136] It is estimated that over 10,000 children were probably affected worldwide.[135]

It is almost incredible but true that, prior to the thalidomide tragedy, the prevailing medical opinion was that the human embryo or fetus were immune to this sort of pharmacological "environmental perturbation". This despite the fact that it had been known since 1941 that the rubella virus could cause malformation.[135] The devastating thalidomide tragedy had two major consequences; firstly it stimulated research into both normal fetal development and the possible effect of drug teratogens, and secondly it led directly to the Medicines Act of 1968, and the establishment of the Medicines Commission and the Committee on the Safety of Medicines (CSM) in 1972. The CSM now rigorously applies regulations governing research, clinical trials and the licensing and introduction of new drugs in the United Kingdom. Its activities are on similar lines to those of the Food and Drugs Administration (FDA) in the USA which has been in existence since shortly after the Second World War. Prior to 1972 research and investigation of the safety of new drugs in Great Britain depended on the pharmaceutical industry itself. The controls necessarily slow down the introduction of new drugs and greatly increase the expense of marketing. This is rightly the price of safety. Research and evidence presented in the United Kingdom has to be repeated for the FDA in the USA however, and *vice versa*; and some countries still do not have regulatory bodies even today; perhaps sometime in the future an international body, possibly under the auspices of the United Nations or WHO, will facilitate the exchange and acceptance of information.

The National Health Service 1960-1968

The honeymoon period engendered by the apparent new found financial freedom in the NHS, both in terms of the provision of hospital revenue and in professional remuneration, began to become less happy during the sixties. One of the assumptions of the Beveridge Report on which the concept of the NHS was built was that of "a health service which will diminish disease by prevention and cure..... and, as a consequence of this development, a reduction in the number of cases requiring [the use of the service]".[137]

The danger of such a palpably false premise was recognised early in the history of the NHS. Frangcon Roberts, a radiologist of Addenbrooke's Hospital, Cambridge wrote these prophetic words in 1949:-

> *"I believe that through ignorance and miscalculation in its preparation the cost of the Health Service has been grossly underestimated.... In the twentieth century, civilisation is faced with*

a threat unique in its history, the existence of more ill-health than it can afford, due not to any temporary calamity but paradoxically to the advance of civilisation itself. Society has opened a new Pandora's box, releasing new diseases of its own creation and with them innumerable new methods of treating all the diseases which it cannot cure" [138]

The sixties opened hopefully enough with far-sighted reports both for the building of new hospitals (virtually none had been commissioned since 1949) and for the remuneration of doctors and dentists.[10,139-141]

The Hospital Plan for England and Wales was promulgated by Enoch Powell, the then Minister of Health, in 1962. It owed much to the BMA report published in the *British Medical Journal* in 1959, and it supported the concept of large centrally based District Hospitals.[10,139,140] A good deal of hospital building did, in fact, take place during the sixties but was curtailed during the financial crises in the early seventies. This left a number of NHS Districts with new buildings they could not open for lack of funds, or which had to be used for purposes for which they were not originally intended, because of failure to complete all the phases of the individual hospital plans. Another unsatisfactory development was the creation of isolated obstetric blocks which cause grave difficulties to overstretched departments of anaesthesia.

The Royal Commission on Doctors' and Dentists' Remuneration (Pilkington) Report was published in February 1960.[10,141] Inflation had already eroded the value of the pay of the profession. The Pilkington award was well received by hospital doctors although there were some reservations by General Practitioners, and it was accepted and implemented. Specimen percentage increases and actual resulting salaries on appointment were House Officer 59% to £675 (1996: £8,200), Senior Registrar 36% to £1,500 (1996: £18,200), and Consultant 21% to £2,550 (1996: £30,900).

The average rise for general practitioners was 22.8% to £2,672 (1996: £32,400). A Consultant without a distinction award would rise to £3,900 (1996: £47,300) after 10 increments. Actual salaries for the equivalent appointments in 1996 would be House Officer £13,000; Senior Registrar £21,185; Consultant £39,930 to £46,390. Average General Practitioner £40,010.[141-144]

The monetary award was welcome but a still more important and far reaching proposal in the Pilkington Report was for an establishment of a Review Body for doctors' and dentists' pay to make annual recommendations.[141-144]

The Review Body was appointed in 1962 and made its first report in February 1963. This was an across the board increase of 14%. This was considered to be reasonable for hospital doctors but caused uproar amongst General Practitioners who were determined to alter the mechanism by which the overall award was distributed amongst them (the "pool system"), and to reduce what was called the "differential" between total career-long earnings of Consultants and General Practitioners (figures of £117,000 (1996: £1,345,500) and £79,000 (1996: £908,500) were quoted at the time). The details of the ensuing dispute between General Practitioners and the Government have no place in this history; suffice to say that it led to threats of resignation from the service, the promulgation by the BMA of the "General Practitioners Charter" in 1965,[144] and a differential salary award for the profession in 1966 (33% for General Practitioners but 10% for Consultants!).[10] It was unfortunate however that, immediately after agreement was finally reached with the Government in 1966, one of the "pay pauses" characteristic of the time was imposed; as a result of the delay caused by the General Practitioner dispute the whole profession, hospital doctors as well as General Practitioners, irretrievably lost the benefit of six months of the increase.[10]

The Charter for Hospital Doctors issued by the BMA in 1966 summarised many of the deficiencies of the hospital service in buildings, in equipment, and in the terms and conditions of service of its medical workforce, and suggested possible solutions; but it had less practical impact than the General Practitioners' Charter.[10,145,146] Some idea of the frustration prevalent in the Hospital Service can be gauged from the first paragraph of the Charter:-

"Never before have hospital doctors been so disenchanted with the conditions under which they are called upon to practice. In the eighteen years since the National Health Service was inaugurated there have been a long series of inquiries into its major problems. There was the Spens report on remuneration, the Guillebaud report on cost, the Royal Commission on remuneration, the Platt report on

medical staffing, the Porritt report on the medical services in Great Britain and, finally the reports of the Review Body...... Despite all these investigations frustration has mounted, the tide of emigration has risen to a flood, and resentment at Government indifference to medical problems has reached a critical point. Discontent is rife not only amongst junior staff but amongst young consultants too. In less than twenty years the Governments of this country have reduced a noble profession to a state of seething unrest."[146]

The whole situation was aggravated by the financial crisis into which the United Kingdom was plunged at the time and a shortage of hospital manpower at a junior level which was felt particularly acutely in the developing clinical service specialty of anaesthesia. The general shortage was chiefly the result of a serious miscalculation concerning medical school intake by the Willink Committee which reported in 1957.[10] There was also an increasing "flood" of emigration of disillusioned younger British doctors including Consultants, as was suggested in the preamble to the Charter for Hospital Doctors quoted above, but this was balanced by considerable medical immigration into the United Kingdom, particularly from the Indian subcontinent. The Platt Report on the "Medical Staffing Structure in the Hospital Service" estimated that, even by 1960, one third of the 9,543 junior doctors employed in British Hospitals had qualified outside Great Britain;[147] by the end of the decade the proportion was undoubtedly larger still.

The general feeling of gloom was echoed in a bitter Editorial in *Anaesthesia* in 1967.[148] Needless to say little positive action was taken by the Government on the Charter for Hospital Doctors. It is to the credit of hospital medical staff that day by day and month by month much clinical progress was achieved in the sixties despite the prevailing financial stringency. Those who were keen enough, and knew the ropes, and the right people in the hospital administrative hierarchy to contact, could by-pass the inefficient bureaucracy and obtain equipment and other benefits for their patients by a combination of stealth, tub-thumping and persuasion. It was fortunate that they did!

Hospital doctors' remuneration. The purchasing power of the pound fell by over 30% during the period 1960 to 1970 but the pay of hospital doctors was not increased proportionately. The BMA Council reported in 1968, "the basic consultant rate of remuneration is now standing at a totally unrealistic level".[10] The Government delayed the publication of the Review Body's report in May 1970 in the face of an impending general election and then, after disclosing its contents under pressure from the BMA, declined to honour the 30% award to both Consultants and General Practitioners and referred the claim to the Prices and Incomes Board. The Review body, which was chaired by the greatly respected banker Lord Kindersley, resigned *en bloc*. The BMA organised protest action including undated resignations from the NHS, and asking general practitioners to refuse to sign National Insurance sickness certificates (75% of them complied). The Labour Government was defeated in June 1970 but, even then, though the Review body was reinstated, the new Conservative administration declined to honour the award in full (General Practitioners and junior hospital doctors received 20%, Consultants on appointment the full 30%, but more senior Consultants only 20%).[10,149]

A "New Deal" for medical officers in the Armed Forces

Call up for National Service ended in 1960 and all conscripts were discharged by 1963.[150] The British Medical Association Council reported in 1961 that:-

"In 21 years of conscription 27,000 doctors were recruited into the Forces, and the [medical] recruitment committees dealt with an enormous number of application for deferment. The Council considers that the recruitment committees succeeded in striking a very fair balance between the competing claims of the Forces and the Civil medical service..."[10]

The demobilisation of the very experienced medical men who had served throughout the Second World War shortly after the cessation of hostilities in 1945 considerably reduced the specialist expertise available in the Armed Forces. The policy of deferment for postgraduate training of a proportion of medical graduates was consequently an important factor in ensuring the provision of basic specialist services in the postwar period.

The regular combatant senior officers of the "Big Army" were naturally keen to have done with National Service by the end of the nineteen fifties to enable them to return to the close knit regimental family atmosphere of prewar professional soldiering;[10] however, they and the mandarins of the Ministry of Defence do not seem to have anticipated the vital gap that would be created when the continuous and automatic supply of compulsorily recruited National Service doctors dried up. It was apparently not appreciated either that medicine had moved on; the day of the general purpose military "surgeon" was ended and specialisation was the order of the day. The Council of the Association of Anaesthetists was aware of the problems of anaesthetists in Her Majesty's Forces and, in February 1961, it was decided to coopt to Council one of the Advisers in Anaesthetics to the Services in rotation for two year periods. This is a valuable custom which has continued. Colonel (later Major General) K F Stephens was the first Adviser in Her Majesty's Forces to be coopted (Council Minutes 6.2.1961 and Annual Report 1961).[151]

It was not however until December 1961 that a deputation from the BMA met the four Defence Ministers.[10] Events moved surprisingly rapidly. A new deal was worked out both with regard to pay and the status of the medical professional specialists in the Forces. Lieutenant General Sir Alexander Drummond,[152] Director General of Army Medical Services 1956-1961, an otorhinolaryngologist by training, was closely concerned with improving the lot of specialist medical officers. He was determined that specialists in the Armed Forces should be, and be seen to be, the equal of Consultants in civilian life. He worked closely with the Royal Colleges and the Armed Services Consultant Advisory Boards (ASCAB) with both civilian and military membership were established to vet applicants for Consultant status in the Services. The anaesthetists' ASCAB was at first combined with that of the surgeons but, since the early seventies, it has become independent.

The "new deal" meant that, for the first time anaesthetists and members of certain other specialties were able to progress to the military rank of full Colonel (or the Royal Navy or RAF equivalent) on a length of service basis while still practising as specialist clinicians; previously promotion for anaesthetists above major meant transferring to administration except in the unique case of the single "Adviser" in the specialty. It had taken the Armed Services a very long time to accept that a Military Hospital might be commanded administratively by a Lieutenant Colonel when the specialists working in the Unit might be full Colonels and thus senior to him! Recruitment to the Armed Forces improved as a result of these reforms but it fell off for a time between 1966 and 1969 during the recurrent Governmental "pay standstills", which, as has already been noted, characterised fiscal policy in the late sixties. The incoming Conservative Government established a Review Body for Service pay in 1970. An increase of 38% for Service doctors was recommended and implemented in 1975. Recruitment again improved thereafter.[10] There were some anomalies in the military system however; for example in the army the senior general physician, general surgeon, pathologist, psychiatrist and general practitioner were classified as "Directors" and usually became Major Generals, while the senior members of other specialties, including anaesthesia, only achieved the rank of Brigadier as "Advisers". Two anaesthetists have become Major Generals in administrative appointments, but, so far, none have held the Office of Director General of Army Medical Services. Surgeon Rear Admiral D A Lammiman, and Surgeon Rear Admiral A L Revell, former consultant anaesthetists, and members of the Association, both became Directors of the Royal Naval Medical Service, and Tony Revell has subsequently become Vice Admiral and Surgeon General of all the Defence Services; this is the highest rank that can be reached by a Medical Officer. The highest rank yet achieved by an anaesthetist in the Royal Air Force is Air Commodore. Promotion in the Territorial Army (TA) is open to all medical officers whatever their specialty but, above the rank of major, it remains tied to administrative appointments. There are obvious advantages to the Treasury in maintaining this pre-nineteen sixty state of affairs!

Academic anaesthesia 1960-1969

The quality and quantity of research in the British Isles had expanded considerably by the close of 1969. There were by then academic university departments headed by established or titular Professors at:- (in alphabetical order) Belfast (J W Dundee), Birmingham (J S Robinson), Bristol (J Clutton-Brock), Cardiff (W W Mushin), Dublin at the Royal College of Surgeons in Ireland (T J Gilmartin), Edinburgh (J D Robertson), Glasgow (A C Forrester), Leeds (D G McDowall), Liverpool (T C Gray), in London at the London Hospital (B R J Simpson), the Royal Postgraduate Medical School (J G Robson), Royal College of Surgeons (J P Payne) and Westminster Hospital (Sir Geoffrey Organe), in Newcastle upon Tyne (E A Cooper) and Oxford (under Alex Crampton Smith, Professor Sir Robert Macintosh having retired in 1965 after 24 years of distinguished service).[84] There was, in addition, the Division of Anaesthesia at the Medical Research Council Clinical Research Centre at the new Northwick Park Hospital in Harrow. This was under J F Nunn as Director who had been appointed proleptically and had held the post of Professor of Anaesthesia at Leeds from 1964 to 1968 in the interim. The University Department of Anaesthesia at Sheffield had also been established under J A Thornton who was to become Professor in 1970.

The Anaesthetic Research Society came into being in 1970, but it had its origins in the informal but select Anaesthetic Research Group formed in 1958 and had published the abstracts of its papers in the *British Journal of Anaesthesia* since 1964.[153]

Physics and anaesthesia. British anaesthesia has been fortunate in having several outstanding physicists as long serving members of its research departments, including H G Epstein of Oxford, D W Hill of the Royal College of Surgeons of England and W W Mapleson of the Welsh National School of Medicine

The business of the Association 1960-1969

The decade leading up to the very successful Fourth World Congress of Societies of Anaesthesiologists which was hosted by the Association of Anaesthetists in September 1968,[154] was a period of considerable development in its resources and professionalism and responsibilities of the specialty of anaesthesia.

The composition of Council in the sixties

Both the traditional hierarchical structure of the medical profession and the original organisational pattern of the NHS remained in being throughout the sixties. Teaching hospitals retained a direct and special relationship with the Ministry of Health until the reorganisation of 1974. The specialty of anaesthesia was led by a respected but relatively small elitist oligarchy based on the teaching hospitals; together they shared and overlapped in the control of the Council of the Association, the Board of Faculty and the Committee of the British Medical Association Anaesthetists Group. Council Minutes of 3 September 1965[155] record that the President (Vernon Hall of Kings College Hospital, London) and the coopted adviser to the Chief Medical Officer (Geoffrey Organe)[156] reminded Council of the various routes by which the

Association of Anaesthetists could exact its influence on the joint subcommittee of the three bodies "which was called when matters of policy were under discussion". Common policies concerning pay and conditions of service "could thus be passed through two channels, the BMA and the Royal College of Surgeons, to the Joint Consultants (Negotiation) Committee (JCC); on the other hand the views of the Association of Anaesthetists on matters of technical and general interest could and should be communicated directly to the Ministry of Health".[155]

It is interesting that, at the time, the Royal Colleges and their Faculties had a direct negotiating right over pay and conditions through their membership of the JCC. They surrendered this privilege in 1966 when doubts were cast on the legality of the arrangement because of the charitable status of the colleges, and the BMA thereafter assumed sole negotiating rights.[10] The BMA dissolved its Anaesthetists' Subcommittee in 1973 and its place was taken by the Anaesthetists' Subcommittee of the Central Committee for Hospital Medical Services (CCHMS) with increased representation of the Council of the Association of Anaesthetists and thus improved direct access to the negotiating machinery (Council Minutes 2.11.1972, Annual Report 1973).[155] The Council of the Association maintained, and still maintains, its influence in 1998 by cooption. Cooption was originally by name (in 1961 for example the Faculties of Anaesthetists' Deans of the Royal Colleges of England and in Ireland, the Adviser in Anaesthetics to the Chief Medical Officer, and one of the Advisers to the Armed Services were, specifically coopted), but in 1970 a permanent alteration to the Rules was made coopting the holders of these offices *ex-officio*.[155] The resolution to coopt specifically the President of the Anaesthetic Section of the Royal Society of Medicine seems to have been put into abeyance in the sixties - possibly because of the strictly non-political and academic nature of that body.

The Council of the Association of Anaesthetists remained a benign self perpetuating oligarchy throughout the nineteen sixties. The method of election had been inherited from the procedures of the RSM. Council itself nominated a list of suitable candidates to fill the necessary number of vacancies to the Annual General Meeting after an internal vote if this was necessary. There was one counternomination in 1959, and a postal ballot was held, but all the candidates nominated by Council in the sixties were elected *nem con*. Professor

Mushin (Cardiff) suggested that the method of election to Council should be changed in 1965 (Council Minutes 2.7.1965)[155] but it was decided not to take any action. It is to the credit of Council that a satisfactory geographical spread of membership was consistently achieved, and that the nonteaching university hospitals were adequately represented.

The agenda of Council 1960-1968

It is noteworthy that Council did not concern itself with the considerable political turmoil over medical NHS remuneration described earlier in this Chapter. This aspect was left to the Anaesthetists' Subcommittee of the CCHMS. The Ministry of Health has always maintained a policy of not negotiating salaries with specialist societies. This is an advantage as it has ensured the equality of basic remuneration for all specialties. This practice should be jealously guarded, but it has been threatened by the creation of locally negotiating Hospital Trusts in the most recent NHS reorganisation in 1991-1992; anaesthetists may be very vulnerable under these circumstances. Council in the nineteen sixties was, however, concerned with making its voice heard about additional sources of professional income, including private fees in NHS hospitals and elsewhere, fees for dental anaesthesia, and distinction awards (see below).[151,155]

Some of the issues which were debated and reported upon by Council in the sixties[151,155] have been adequately covered in Chapter 6; in particular the investigation of deaths associated with anaesthesia and the management and display of the Charles King Collection of Historical Apparatus.

The Categories of Membership of the Association

The title of "Fellow" of the Association of Anaesthetists was abolished by resolution at the 1962 Annual General Meeting on 9.11.1962.[151] The distinction between Ordinary Fellows and Ordinary Members, which had gradually become increasingly anomalous and unnecessary since the introduction of the Fellowship of the Faculty of Anaesthetists (FFARCS) diploma was consequently abolished and the two were merged as "Ordinary Members". The category of Honorary Membership (formerly Honorary

Fellowship) was, of course, retained in 1962 to provide recognition for "eminent persons" both medical and lay, as were the minor honours of Corresponding Membership (elected from "distinguished anaesthetists practising outside the British Isles") and Senior Members ("elected from Ordinary Members who have retired from practice"). The category of "Associates" for anaesthetists in training, which had been designated as "Trainee Associates" since the 1960 Annual Report, was renamed "Associates in Training" in 1962. All the above categories except Honorary Membership and Corresponding Membership were by definition only available to United Kingdom and Ireland Registered Medical Practitioners, but only Ordinary Members were allowed to vote at the Annual General Meetings and in elections for Council.

A category of Associate Member replaced Associate Fellow in 1962 (Annual Report 1962). This was "to be elected from registered medical practitioners *and others* not necessarily engaged in the practice of anaesthetics in the British Isles". The 1964 Annual Report made clear that the category of "Associates in Training" was restricted to those training in Great Britain and Ireland and that, if such a member moved permanently overseas, he would be recategorised as an Associate Member. Associates in training joined Ordinary Members as full voting members in 1970 (Annual Report 1970).

The seven Associate Fellows were transferred to the new category of Associate Member in 1962. They included two dentists (one practising in the United Kingdom and the other in Australia) and two veterinary surgeons (one from England and one practising overseas).

The words "and others" in the definition of Associate Member, and previously of Associate Fellow, caused some embarrassment to the Association in 1961 (Council Minutes 7.10.1961).[151] Several dental surgeons who were leading members of the Society for the Advancement of Anaesthesia in Dentistry (SAAD), applied for the then Associate Fellowship category and were rejected. This was at a time when relations between the Association of Anaesthetists and SAAD were somewhat strained. One particular bone of contention being the intermittent intravenous methohexitone technique which had begun to be employed by operating dental surgeons, with or without the assistance of trained non-medical staff (see below).

Council took legal advice about their right to refuse membership to dentists and then published the following statement in the Annual Report for 1964: -

"Some misunderstanding continues to persist about the qualifications for Associate Membership. This category is primarily for members permanently resident overseas, but also includes a few members who are not practising anaesthetists."

"Council has given very considerable attention to the possibility of admitting dental practitioners to this category and remains very eager to encourage advances in dental anaesthesia. However, bearing in mind that the first object of the Association reads .. the recognition of the administration of anaesthetics as a specialised brand of medicine it passed the following resolution: - The Association of Anaesthetists of Great Britain and Ireland does not undertake the responsibility of representing the interests of dental practitioners..... The election of dental practitioners is, at the present time, appropriate only in exceptional circumstances". (Annual Report 1964).

The application of another prominent member of SAAD was rejected in 1966 on the grounds that there were no exceptional circumstances (Council Minutes 3.6.1966).[155]

Further alterations were made in the rules at the 1968 Annual General Meeting. The Associate Member category was dropped and Overseas Membership was introduced. The Australian dental surgeon, who had been an Associate Member became an Overseas Member, and the single United Kingdom dentist and the three veterinary surgeons (all of them by then working in the United Kingdom) became Ordinary Members of the Association.[155] The Association reintroduced a nonvoting Associate category for dental surgeons and other nonmedical anaesthetists, which now includes at least one overseas nurse anaesthetist, in 1981, after the British medical and dental professions had to some extent buried their differences (Annual Report 1981).[158]

No further Senior Members were elected after 1972 and a decision was taken to discontinue the creation of Corresponding Members in 1976. This was after the Pask Certificate of Honour was instituted to be presented to "persons whom the Association wishes to honour from Great Britain and Ireland or from overseas" (Annual Report 1976).

The Association at the end of 1969 had a total membership of 2,229, compared with 1,228 in 1959. There were 16 Honorary Members (12 in 1959), 49 (34) Corresponding Members; 26 (23) Senior Members; 1,554 (1,055) Ordinary Members; 308 (0) Overseas Members; 276 (94) Associates in Training (Annual Report 1959 and Annual Report 1969).

Subscriptions to the Association

A Special General Meeting on 5 April 1968[155] authorised the first increase in subscription for 25 years (Annual Report 1968). The subscription for Ordinary Membership was raised from "two guineas" (1996: £19.00) to "five guineas" or £5.25 (1996: £47.25). The subscription for Associates in Training remained at £2 (1996: £18).

The position of retired members had been regularised in 1960. If they wished to be retired members who were not elected to the Senior Membership Category without voting rights but to continue to receive the journal *Anaesthesia*, their subscription would be £2 (1996: £18). The question of commuting to a Life Membership on retirement was also considered at that time but, as it was estimated that the subscription would have to be at least £20 (1996: £180), it was decided not to proceed further. (Council Minutes 1.7.1960).[151]

Association Honours 1960-1969

The John Snow Medal, then the Association's highest honour, was converted from a bronze to a silver medal in 1967; at the same time, a bronze medal for John Snow Lecturers was introduced and awarded retrospectively to previous lecturers (Council Minutes 8.9.1967).[157] Four John Snow medals were awarded to eminent retired British anaesthetists during the decade; to Christopher Langton Hewer[8] in 1967 on his retirement from the Editorship of *Anaesthesia* after twenty years in the post, to Professor Sir Robert Macintosh[159] of Oxford and Michael Nosworthy[160] of St Thomas' Hospital in 1967, and to Ronald Jarman[1] (President of the Association 1959-1962) in 1969.

Honorary Membership was bestowed on seven British anaesthetists whose achievements have already figured in this volume between 1960 and 1969, on a veteran Canadian anaesthetist in connection with the Second World Congress of Societies of Anaesthesiologists in Toronto in 1960, and on a non-medical benefactor of the Association. The new Honorary Members were E Stanley Rowbotham[161] (Magill's colleague in developing wide-bore tracheal intubation), the Canadian Harry J Shields[162] in 1960, E Falkner Hill[163] (Editor of the *British Journal of Anaesthesia*) and R J Minnitt[164] (pioneer of nitrous oxide analgesia for obstetrics), G A Vandervell Esq (benefactor), C Langton Hewer [8] (Editor of *Anaesthesia* 1946-1967), Ronald Jarman[1] (President 1959-1962, Katherine G Lloyd-Williams[165] (the first lady member of the Council of the Association of Anaesthetists and of the Board of Faculty), Frankis T Evans[166] (Dean of the Faculty 1955-1958) and Michael D Nosworthy[160] (pioneer thoracic anaesthetist) in 1968.

Professor E A Pask OBE

British and international anaesthesia and the Association of Anaesthetists of Great Britain and Ireland suffered a grievous and unexpected loss when Professor Edgar A (Gar) Pask died on 30 May 1966 at the age of 53 years.[167] He was at that time Honorary Treasurer of the Association and had already held office as President of the Section of Anaesthetics of the RSM and Vice Dean of the Faculty of Anaesthetists. He was one of the most outstanding scientists the specialty of anaesthesia has ever produced. His Second World War research, including dangerously courageous self experimentation in air-sea rescue techniques, have already been described and brought him appointment as an Officer of the British Empire (OBE) and one of the first John Snow medals awarded by the Association of Anaesthetists. It is no wonder that his appointment as the second Professor of Anaesthesia in the British Isles at the Medical School of the University of Durham, then at Newcastle upon Tyne, was universally acclaimed. The Association paid tribute to his name when they established the Pask Certificate of Honour in 1977 which *inter alia* is awarded for courageous conduct by anaesthetists in the face of danger.[168] He was indeed "a truly remarkable man".[167]

The Objects of the Association

A letter, which was received in 1965 from Henry E Pooler (1906-1977)[169] (Consultant Anaesthetist at Chesterfield Royal Infirmary and a former Member of Council), drew attention to the fact that the Objectives of the Association, as promulgated in the original 1932 Constitution of the Association were somewhat outdated and unsophisticated (Council Minutes 5.3.1965).[155] This was especially the case since one of the primary objectives, the establishment of a Diploma in Anaesthetics, had long since been achieved. The Objectives were therefore modified at the 1965 Annual General Meeting to read:-

(a) *"To promote the development and study of anaesthetics and their administration and to maintain the high standard of this branch of medicine."*

(b) *"To foster research into anaesthesia and allied subjects."*

(c) *"To encourage and support world wide co-operation amongst anaesthetists."*

(d) *"To represent and protect the interests of its members."*

(e) *"And to do such lawful things as may be incidental or conducive to the attainment of such objects."*[155]

These remain the objects of the Association in 1998 except that the words "and to.... medicine" in Object (a) were omitted as being redundant, when the organisation was incorporated under the Companies Act in 1985.

Administrative matters

The Secretariat of the Association of Anaesthetists remained part of the Joint Secretariat at the Royal College of Surgeons of England in Lincoln's Inn Fields; in the early nineteen sixties the Secretary allocated to the Association of Anaesthetists also looked after the orthopaedic and accident associations and shared a very small office with another secretary ("between their desks was the route to an inner office - so sitting beside her was a cramped and intermittent procedure; for all her work she had but one filing cabinet and one cupboard"; O P Dinnick, personal communication). Secretaries who served the Association of Anaesthetists under these difficult conditions, but whose services are minuted with appreciation in the Association Minute books and Annual Reports in the sixties were, Miss Joan Paternoster, who died unexpectedly in 1961 following a surgical operation,[170] Miss Diana Cresswell, Miss Elizabeth Duncan and Miss Shirley Yarnold.

There was a 36% increase in total membership (1228 to 1773) of the Association between 1959 and 1964 including a 238% (94 to 318) rise in Associates in Training. Council itself expanded by cooption from 19 to 26, and correspondence with sister organisations and government committees increased dramatically (Annual Report 1959 and Annual Report 1964). The Annual Scientific Meeting and exhibition was also becoming increasingly sophisticated and, in addition, from 1962 the Annual Registrar's Meeting also had to be organised (O P Dinnick, personal communication).

It is small wonder that successive Honorary Secretaries found increasing difficulty both in performing their executive duties, and in having their work translated into administrative action by the part-time secretaries; for example the compilation and printing of the Annual Report and Membership List became very much delayed in those precomputer days, and those for 1967 and 1968 were published together in 1969.

It is to the great credit of the Honorary Secretaries of the sixties and the ladies who assisted them that the show was kept on the road at all. An Assistant Honorary Secretary was elected at the 1964 Annual General Meeting, to ease the burden of the Honorary Secretary and with a view to becoming Honorary Secretary two years later. The period in Office of Honorary Secretary was reduced from three to two years at this time (though, of course, the total period in office as Assistant Honorary Secretary, Honorary Secretary and Immediate Past Honorary Secretary was actually thereby increased to four years.

Miss Joyce Baxter. Another most important step was taken in 1968. Miss Joyce Baxter became the first Administrative Secretary of the Association of Anaesthetists without responsibility to any other organisation. She continued to be accommodated for the time being within the joint Secretariat at Lincoln's Inn Fields until 1971, when the Association moved to its own self contained offices as tenants of the British Medical Association at Tavistock House. Joyce Baxter continued to look after the Association and its Officers and Council until 1973. The value of her efficient and benign reign, conducted with a quiet sense of humour cannot be overestimated; in a personal communication she tells us of her early experiences at the Royal College of Surgeons in Lincoln's Inn Fields : -

> *"The Association's affairs were carried out in half an office, with the President's Entertainment Fund (in other words gin) kept in the filing cabinet. The surroundings may have been modest but the Association's output most definitely was not. I never ceased to be impressed by the range of topics and issues on which the Association formulated views and presented evidence to official bodies".*

and she concludes : -

> *"I feel very privileged to have played a small part in the Association's history, and I look back on those five years [1968-1973] as the most enjoyable time of my working life. No one could have had more generous or considerate employers".*

The journal Anaesthesia

Anaesthesia had expanded from the 164 pages per year in 1947 (its first complete year of four issues) to 452 pages by 1960. Christopher Langton Hewer[8] of St Bartholomew's Hospital, London had been its Editor throughout this period, with Ralph Blair Gould[171] of the Royal National Throat Hospital as Assistant Editor. The Council Minutes are discrete but it is known that there was a feeling amongst the Officers and Council of the Association that the content and style of *Anaesthesia* was becoming rather old fashioned, although its clinical bias continued to commend it to many more senior members of the specialty. There had also been the question of the nominal accounting deficit in 1959 - an injustice which rankled Langton Hewer for several years afterwards (personal communication) - and also the abortive discussions about possible amalgamation with the *BJA* during 1959. Comparisons were also made with the *BJA* which had immeasurably improved in style and scientific content since its nadir in Volume 20: 1946-1947, moreover, the *BJA* was publishing twelve issues, in comparison with *Anaesthesia's* four, and provided the reader with 620 double column pages each year, against *Anaesthesia's* 450 single column pages.

It was decided that the Editorial Board should be considerably strengthened (Annual Report 1960). R P W (Patrick) Shackleton[3] of Southampton, a highly respected figure who was to be President of the Association from 1967 to 1969, took over as Chairman of the Board from (Sir) Geoffrey Organe (President 1953-56) and a strong panel of advisers was appointed; this panel included Professor Edgar Pask[167] and Professor (Sir) William Paton, Professor of Pharmacology in the University of Oxford. Sir William was a good friend and adviser to the Association for many years and was elected to Honorary Membership in 1980. Blair Gould[171] retired in 1960 and J Alfred Lee,[172] Southend-on-Sea, and Cyril F Scurr of the Westminster Hospital were appointed Assistant Editors.[173]

Anaesthesia gained considerably in reputation, format and scientific content thereafter in the period up to Langton Hewer's eventual retirement in 1966 after twenty years in the Editorial Chair.[174] The circulation in that time rose from 3093 in 1960 to "over 4000" in 1966, although it must be remembered that the captive circulation due to the increasing membership had also risen by 660. The publication of *Anaesthesia* is reported as incurring an annual loss in most of the Annual Reports in this period (a loss of £443 (1996: £4,975) in 1963 and of £393 (1996: £4,150) in 1964 but in 1965 it made a profit of £1,018 (1996: £10,500). These were not easy years for Hewer. It is known that his decision to retire in 1966 at the age of seventy was not taken lightly. He left active Editorship as *Anaesthesia* was gaining in stature and influence, and he paid tribute to the support he had received from Pat Shackleton[3] as Chairman of the Editorial Board in a moving letter in the Correspondence Columns of *Anaesthesia* when the latter died in 1977.[175]

There were also changes amongst the Assistant Editors in this period. Cyril Scurr resigned at the end of 1963 because of the pressure of other commitments, and Alfred Lee[172] followed at the end of 1964. Roger Bryce-

Smith of Oxford replaced Scurr and then succeeded Langton Hewer as Editor in 1966. Thomas B Boulton, then of St Bartholomew's Hospital, London, followed Alfred Lee, and ultimately took over from Bryce-Smith as Editor in 1973. (Sir) M K Sykes became an Assistant Editor when Bryce-Smith took up the Editorship in 1966 and made an especially important contribution over the next few years (Annual Reports 1963, 1964 and 1966).

The Association owes a tremendous debt of gratitude to Langton Hewer.[8] He became Founder Editor of *Anaesthesia* in 1946, when anaesthetic literature was largely based on empirical and clinical impression, and he saw his task through until it was firmly established on a scientific basis.

Roger Bryce-Smith later described the production of *Anaesthesia* during Hewer's and his editorships (1946-1972) as a "cottage industry". The Editor certainly shouldered an enormous burden in the early days. Hewer had neither office nor secretary when he began his editorship, and his principal hospital did not have a departmental office or secretary either (as was the rule rather than the exception even in London Teaching Hospitals at that time); in fact, throughout his editorship the majority of Langton Hewer's letters were personally typed on his own rather ancient machine. He was assisted by Mrs Prince, a part-time literary agent, from 1957-1965; her responsibility was the management of the distribution of the journal and the organisation of the advertisements (Council Minutes 5.3.1965).[155] Mr A W Mycroft, an invaluable free-lance technical adviser (Council Minutes 1.9.1972),[155] served the journal well from shortly after the first major re-organisation in 1960 to the second in 1972. Both Mrs Prince and Mr Mycroft worked from their homes. The Association of Anaesthetists has always retained its rights as the *de facto* publishers of *Anaesthesia*. The journal was *printed* by George Pulman and Sons Ltd of London from 1946 to 1962 and by H E Warne Ltd of St Austell from 1962 to 1972. It was *"published for"* the Association from 1972 to 1981 by Blackwell Scientific Publications of Oxford, and from 1982 to 1996 by the Academic Press (now W B Saunders) of London and returned to Blackwell Science in 1997.

Langton Hewer himself wrote 75 of the 80 editorials which appeared during his editorship.[176] Read consecutively these provide a fascinating overview of the scientific and political development of British anaesthesia over these twenty exciting years (1946-1966). Each new development and issue is examined carefully and its advantages, and disadvantages or pros and cons fairly considered, before a thoughtful, if usually conservative, conclusion is drawn. His last guest editorial in 1976, on the occasion of the thirtieth anniversary of the first publication of *Anaesthesia*, is a masterpiece. It demonstrates that, even at 79 years of age, he had kept up with the development of the specialty and preserved his quietly quizzical sense of humour.[176]

Langton Hewer remained associated with *Anaesthesia* even after his retirement; first as Advisory Editor (1966-1976) and then as Editor Emeritus (1976-1986). He was awarded a John Snow Medal and elected to Honorary Membership of the Association in 1966, and received the prestigious Eleventh award of the Henry Hickman medal of the Royal Society of Medicine in the same year. He was also a Faculty Gold Medallist and was thus one of the few people who have been honoured by receiving all three medals.[177]

The foundation of the Junior Anaesthetists' Group

The Association first made provision for the admission of anaesthetists in training as Associate Members in 1956. The concept of "courses for anaesthetists up to and including Senior Registrars" was first considered by Council on 4 October 1960[151] (Annual Report 1960). It was agreed that the meetings should be open to all junior anaesthetists, but that preference should be given to Trainee Associate members of the Association of Anaesthetists, who would also be entitled to travelling allowances from the Research and Education Trust Fund.

The first and very successful meeting was held under the guidance of Andrew Hunter,[178] Consultant and later Professor at the Manchester Royal Infirmary, on 30 March 1962 (Annual Report 1962). The Registration fee (including tea) was 5 shillings (1996: £3), accommodation (including breakfast) was at a "University Hostel" at 19s.6d (1996: £12) and the "informal dinner" cost £1.2s.6d (1996: £13); coffee was provided by the hospital.

A Registrars' meeting was held at Oxford in 1963 organised by Sir Robert Macintosh[159] and James Parkhouse, then First Assistant, with an attendance of 148 and a Dinner in Pembroke College (Annual Report 1963). There was an initial difficulty about finding a hospital to act as host to the meeting for

Registrars in London in 1964; but finally the offer of Guy's Hospital to hold a meeting limited to 80 people was accepted, with Michael Hutton[179] as organiser (Council Minutes 6.12.1963[155] and Annual Report 1964). The next year (1965) an especially successful meeting was held at Cardiff under the direction of Professor W W Mushin (Annual Report 1965).

The suggestion that an 'Associates in Training Section' might be formed came in the first instance from Rex Binning[73] of Brighton at the Council Meeting on 3 September 1965 towards the end of Vernon Hall's Presidency.[155] The initial stimulus was a desire to increase recruitment to the Association of Anaesthetists. The Association was, it is true, growing steadily in size (total Membership 1960, 1,317: 1963, 1,636: 1965, 1,872) but there was some concern that the expansion was not in proportion to the increase in the number of specialist and trainee anaesthetists in the National Health Service (O P Dinnick personal communication). A subcommittee was set up to examine the question of recruitment. The members of this subcommittee were Rex Binning,[73] Aileen Adams and Philip Helliwell.[7] The subcommittee reported to Council on 4 February 1966.[155] Its principal recommendation was that the formation of a Section of Associates in Training should be discussed at the forthcoming Registrars' Meeting in Southampton in April 1966, and further that it might have a committee of five members whose Chairman should be a coopted Member of Council.[155]

H H (Tony) Pinkerton,[2] the new President, informed Council on 8 May 1966 that the 1966 Registrars' Meeting, which had been held at Southampton on 15 and 16 April and had been organised by Pat Shackleton[3] and Douglas Pearce (Consultant Anaesthetist, Southampton), had been "enormously" successful, and, further, that the proposal to form a "Trainee Associates Group" was received with "much enthusiasm".[155] Council referred the matter to the subcommittee on Recruitment which reported on 3 June 1966.[155] The subcommittee proposed that a Steering Committee should be nominated with the objective of establishing an elected autonomous group to represent the junior staff with direct representation on the Council of the Association of Anaesthetists. This proposal was accepted and a nominated Steering Committee was appointed.[155,180,181] This consisted of:-

Alastair A Spence (Chairman). Senior Registrar in President Pinkerton's[3] Department at the Western Infirmary Glasgow, Scotland (subsequently

Professor of Anaesthesia in the University of Glasgow and, presently, in the University of Edinburgh, who was elected President of the College (now Royal College) of Anaesthetists in 1991).

John C Simpson (Secretary). Senior Registrar at Guy's Hospital London (later Consultant Anaesthetist, Royal Brompton and National Heart Hospitals).

Margaret L Heath. Senior Registrar at the Hammersmith Hospital (Royal Postgraduate Medical School), London (later Consultant Anaesthetist, Lewisham and North Southwark Health Authority, Vice President of the Association of Anaesthetists and Vice Chairman of the BMA Anaesthetic Subcommittee for Hospital Medical Services).

Geoffrey Hall-Davies. Senior Registrar, Birmingham and later Consultant Anaesthetist, United Birmingham Hospitals, and subsequently appointed CBE (Commander of the Order of the British Empire) and Honorary Surgeon to the Queen for his work in the Territorial Army Reserve.

Peter L Jones. Senior Registrar of the United Cardiff Hospitals (later Consultant Anaesthetist, University Hospital of Wales).

Rex Binning[73] Representative of the Council of the Association.

The trainee members of this subsequently very distinguished Committee were obviously chosen with great care with the objective of providing the maximum possible geographic representation of the countries and regions of the British Isles, but, curiously enough, no representative of the Irish, North or South, was nominated. This omission was not remedied until 1970 with the election of William H K Haslett, Registrar, Queens University of Belfast (later Council Member and Consultant Anaesthetist to the Ulster Hospital).[155,180]

The Steering Committee was elected *en bloc* as the first Committee of the "Associates in Training Group" during the outstanding Registrars' Meeting in Leeds from 13 to 15 April 1967 at which 180 members were present.[180] This event was organised by John Nunn who was at that time Professor at

Leeds. A draft Constitution was prepared, considered by Council, and approved at the Annual General Meeting of the Association in Belfast (5-7 October 1967). Alastair Spence took his seat as a coopted Member of Council on 1 December 1967 and the Constitution of the Group was endorsed at its Annual General Meeting held during the Registrars' Meeting at Bristol on 29 and 30 March 1968.[182] The scientific programme of this meeting was organised by Professor Clutton-Brock[183] (Council Minutes 1967 and 1968,[155] Annual Report 1967 and 1968). The 1969 meeting was held at the Royal Postgraduate Medical School, Hammersmith, London, with Professor (Sir) J Gordon Robson as host.

The Constitution of the Associates in Training Group was liberal[181] and its adoption in 1967 was a far sighted advance in the development of the Association of Anaesthetists. It enabled Associates in Training to have a voice in the affairs of the Association for the first time; before this they were neither represented on Council nor did they have a vote, either in the election of the Council of the Association or on any other matter at its Annual General Meetings. The only privileges they enjoyed were the right to join without payment of the customary entrance fee, the right to transfer to Ordinary Membership without payment of a further fee at the completion of their training (usually on appointment to Consultant status), and the receipt of the journal *Anaesthesia* (Annual Report 1966). The adoption of the Constitution of the Group of Associates in Training gave them direct representation on Council through their own elected representative, albeit at first as a coopted nonvoting member. The radical constitutional reforms passed at the 1970 Annual General Meeting of the Association under the Presidency of John Beard[4] entitled the Group to be represented on Council by two Members with full voting rights, and also bestowed full and equal voting rights at Annual General Meetings or, when indicated, by postal vote, on individual members of the Group (Annual General Meeting 27.1.1970).[155,180] The Group changed its title to Junior Anaesthetists' Group (JAG) in 1970, and the designation of "Associate Member" to "Junior Member" although the alteration was not made in the Annual Report until 1972. The name of the Group was again changed to "Group of Anaesthetists in Training" in 1991.[180] The Group very soon began to make its mark in the affairs of the Association in the first years of its existence. It successfully brought recommendations to Council on recruitment, study leave, the problems of married women, and proposed regulations for postgraduate training, which were already under discussion towards the end of the decade and which were to set the pattern of training for the next twenty years.[180]

The development of the representation of juniors within the specialty followed the general pattern of increased influence of younger people in the conduct of affairs, both in general and in the particular case of the medical profession. The BMA formed its Registrars Group Council in 1950 and this became the Hospital Junior Staffs Group in 1957. The BMA Junior Members Forum was established in 1958 and its Chairman became an *ex-officio* member of the Council of the BMA in 1961. There were further radical changes in 1967 and the influence of the junior doctor on the BMA representative body increased markedly from 1968 onwards.[10] These changes were not achieved by the BMA without considerable agitation and aggravation both from within that body and from external schismatic pressure groups such as the Junior Hospital Doctors Association.[10] The recognition of the rights of the junior members of the Association of Anaesthetists was achieved without rancour and in a civilised manner however; indeed the changes in the Constitution were initiated by Council itself. The writer recollects that some more senior Members of Council expressed reservations about the extent of the changes and, in particular the granting of equal voting rights to members of the JAG in 1970, but the diplomatic handling of the debate by the Officers won the day.

The Association of Anaesthetists has not had cause to regret the confidence which it has placed in its junior members. The Junior Anaesthetists' Group, now the Group of Anaesthetists in Training (GAT), has gone on from strength to strength and, by 1992 constituted nearly half of the voting membership of the Association (Annual Report 1992). GAT is the envy of trainee members of many other specialist societies. It is surely a happy coincidence that the Association itself and the Group of Anaesthetists in Training celebrated their respective diamond and silver jubilees in the same year (1992)! Elizabeth Spencer, the 1992 Chairman of GAT, has recorded the history of the Group in fascinating detail in an interesting monograph.[180]

The Platt Report and the Medical Assistant Grade

The Joint Working Party on Medical Staffing Structure of the Hospital Service was appointed by the Minister of Health and the Secretary of State for Scotland in 1958 under the Chairmanship of Sir Robert Platt (1900-1978), President of the Royal College of Physicians of London. Its Report was published in March 1961.[10,184,185] It was written against the background of a grave shortage of medical personnel, and in particular, of young medical graduates trained in the United Kingdom. This shortage had been aggravated by the miscalculations of the Willink Committee of 1957 after which the intake into medical schools had been reduced. The Report of the Royal Commission on Medical Education of 1968 (the Todd Report) estimated that by 1976 there would be a shortfall of some 10,000 medical practitioners.[10] The shortage of British Medical School Graduates particularly affected clinical service specialties like radiology and anaesthesia in which there was a considerable shortage in the Senior Hospital Officer (SHO) and Registrar posts. This meant that the possession of a Fellowship qualification, and subsequent promotion to Senior Registrar, often led rapidly to a Consultant appointment in those days before the additional hurdle of "accreditation" had been introduced. The position was different in the major "bed-owning" specialties (medicine, surgery and gynaecology), these continued to recruit well, but still had a considerable number of "time expired" or very elderly Senior Registrars.

The Platt Report confirmed the view that Consultants were the only hospital medical practitioners who were regarded as having the experience and training "to take full responsibility for the complete medical care of all patients within their particular specialties". The Report emphasised the need for the expansion of the Consultant grade but, at the same time, recommended that provision should be made for practitioners to assist Consultants both in the training (Registrar and Senior Registrar) grades, and in a new limited "Medical Assistant" subconsultant grade.[10,184,185]

The idea of a specialist subconsultant career grade of undetermined tenure was not received with enthusiasm by the profession![10,185] The SHMO controversy had left a bad taste even though most of the injustices had been eliminated (Chapters 5 and 6). This was not the first time either that a subconsultant career grade of specialists who were not in training had been proposed. The BMA's own Strachan Report of 1955 had originally made a number of suggestions which had engendered professional opposition. Its main recommendation had to be modified to a proposal for an intermediate career grade of indefinite tenure, which would not be a training grade nor have ultimate clinical responsibility for the treatment of patients, but would be for those preparing for a consultant appointment by active experience.[10,186] This proposal was not implemented.

The Platt proposal was for an intermediate specialist grade to assist Consultants who would retain the ultimate clinical responsibility for patients. This would be recruited from:-

1. The remainder of those in SHMO grades. These would presumably be those SHMOs without the higher diplomas of their Royal Colleges.

2. Senior Registrars who had failed to reach Consultant status. (There were still a few Senior Registrars at that time who had been promoted without higher diplomas, but it is doubtful if any Senior Registrar who was fully qualified for Consultant status would have been happy in this subconsultant grade especially if the proposed consultant expansion were about to take place).

3. Specialists who had aspired to higher appointments but had failed in the competition for advancement to Consultant but, by the time they had accepted this position they "had become so specialised that this, and their age, would prevent them getting work outside the hospital service".[184] (There were many Registrars in this category in anaesthesia particularly amongst medical immigrants, who were efficient clinical anaesthetists for routine work and who had the ability to pass the Diploma in Anaesthetics (DA) but did not seem to have the necessary academic expertise to proceed to the higher Fellowship (FFARCS) qualification. (The rationale for placing these useful practitioners in an adequately remunerated Medical Assistant Grade was obvious, particularly in a shortage specialty which

lacked recruits such as was the case of anaesthesia in the sixties. The Platt report stressed that over one-third of practitioners working in the training grade of the Hospital Service in the United Kingdom in March 1960 had qualified in medicine outside the United Kingdom, that 22% of the Registrars had entered the service of the NHS ten or more years previously, and that 48% of these were aged 37 or more.[184,185] The percentage given in these overall figures were undoubtedly less than those for anaesthesia at that time.)

4. General Practitioners working part time.[10,184,185]

The danger of creating a subconsultant career grade is, and always has been, that without rigid safeguards the Department of Health and its peripheral Health Authorities might attempt to enlarge it and include within it practitioners fully qualified to be Consultants, instead of creating new Consultant posts. Anaesthesia was, and unfortunately still is, especially vulnerable, particularly if projected expansions in the Consultant grade are not implemented, or are biased in favour of the major "bed-owning" specialties. The requirement for an increased Consultant establishment was stressed by the Platt Committee but the proposal was never fully implemented. Sir Thomas Holmes Sellors, at that time Chairman of the JCC and later President of the Royal College of Surgeons of England 1969-1972, in a carefully reasoned letter to the *British Medical Journal* in 1964,[187] demonstrated the impossibility of meeting the requirement of consultant expansion advocated following the Platt report from the Senior Registrars then in post; this apparently despite the undoubted glut of time-expired medical and surgical Senior Registrars and the lack of a defined minimum tenure of that grade at the time. Grey-Turner and Sutherland in their *History of the British Medical Association 1932-81*[10] give other reasons which have "frustrated consultant expansion over the years". They include "the cost of providing the necessary supporting facilities (such as theatre-time and laboratory back up) for each Consultant post; and the (unspoken) consideration of the reluctance of existing Consultants to see the limited sector of private practice invaded by an influx of new Consultants"! The present writer can honestly say, from his own observation, that the latter factor was not a major consideration in anaesthesia, though the trend was undoubtedly to be observed in the deliberations of some other specialties! The Council of the Association of Anaesthetsits has consistently pressed for an increase in Consultant Anaesthetist appointments (Council Minutes 2.3.1962).[155]

A great deal of discussion and negotiation followed the publication of the Platt Report. The prestigious and wide-ranging Porritt Report of the Medical Services Review Committee of the BMA was published in 1962.[10,188,189] It said of the Platt Report proposal for a Medical Assistant grade that "it is contrary to the traditions of the teaching and voluntary hospital system which has always encouraged independent responsibility of the patient. We view the proposal with much anxiety".[188] The specialist 'Assistant Medical Officer' had, however, been a fact of life in the old local authority hospital system before the NHS came into being, but the hierarchical structure of the NHS (the choice of which was largely that of the medical profession) was that of the old voluntary hospital (Chapter 4).

The Council of the Association of Anaesthetists first discussed the Platt proposals for the Medical Assistant grade on 2 March 1962, and a Memorandum for the guidance of members of the Association involved in the review of anaesthetic staffing, which was about to take place, was prepared by Professor T Cecil Gray (Council Minutes 2.3.1962 and 6.4.1962[151] and Annual Report 1962). This Memorandum has not survived but it is probable that the contents were similar to those expressed at the meeting on 2 March 1962. The view of Council was that there was little need for a permanent career grade under that of Consultant in anaesthesia *except part-time for general practitioners*. There was also concern lest the SHMO debacle would be repeated, and it was considered vital that, if appointed, Medical Assistants should work directly under Consultants in the same way as Registrars. It was moreover difficult to assess the use to which the grade might be put without information about the salary scale, but the proposed eligibility for acceptance into the grade after two or three years of experience was considered to be too short and a "minimal qualification" (presumably including the DA) should be laid down (Council Minute 2.3.1962).[152]

The Government response to the Platt Report was published in August 1964[190] and the consequent "guidance" to hospital boards (HM(64)94) was circulated by the Ministry of Health in the following November.[191] The Ministry accepted *inter alia* the need for limited Consultant expansion although the circular baldly states "adjusted figures will not be attainable......

for some specialties - e.g. anaesthetics....."[191] The Medical Assistant grade was to be introduced with effect from 1 November 1964. The remaining SHMOs who had not been upgraded were to be absorbed into the Medical Assistant category but would keep their title (SHMO) and existing salary scales; for those newly appointed to the grade the salary scale was to be £1,650 (1996: £18,000) rising by 14 increments to £2,910 (1996: £32,000). "No provision for part-time posts had yet been made".[191] The process proposed for converting a Registrar or SHO post to a Medical Assistant, or obtaining sanction for a new post, was quite complicated and bureaucratic. It involved applying to the Ministry through the Regional Board with Committees at every stage, with all the frustration and delay that such a procedure involves. Appointments were to be for two years in the first place and were thereafter renewable for an indefinite period of tenure. The appointments were also personal to the individual and the establishment had to be reviewed when and if the holder resigned before they could be readvertised.[190,191]

A leading article in the *British Medical Journal* expressed disappointment at the "halfway" response to the Platt Report and, in particular, was concerned about the limited proposals for expansion of Consultant and other grades, but it welcomed the end of the "distressing ailment" of the redundant time-expired Senior Registrars and of the SHMO grade.[192] The leading article also doubted (correctly) whether promotion from Medical Assistant to Consultant rank would be possible, despite the view expressed by the Ministry. The writer of the article did not believe that the salary scale for Medical Assistants would tempt many recruits away from general practice despite the fears expressed by the BMA General Medical Services Committee (GMSC). The article also noted that General Practitioners would be deterred from becoming part-time medical assistants until payment for hospital work had been removed from the calculation of the central "Pool".[192] This "Pool" system of remuneration meant that payments made to a few General Practitioners for undertaking hospital appointments would reduce the money available to be dispersed as incidental fees for service items for the majority[192] (see also below for the description of the iniquities of the "Pool" system for fees for the administration of dental anaesthesia).

The Association of Anaesthetists had always been in favour of the employment of suitably trained General Medical Practitioners in the hospital service on a sessional basis and concerned about the problems of married lady practitioners who had experience in anaesthesia and who wished to follow a part-time career in the specialty, while at the same time engaged in the equally important occupation of looking after the home and rearing children (Annual Report 1965 and Annual Report 1969). Council responded to the adoption of the Medical Assistant Grade by the Ministry of Health by revising its 1962 Memorandum (Council Minutes 2.7.1965,[155] and Annual Report 1965). There was now general agreement with the proposals but Council emphasised that those appointed to the grade should have had training in anaesthesia for a minimum of three years and have held Registrar posts for at least two of these years; furthermore Medical Assistants should only be allotted work considered to be equivalent to that suitable for the Registrar grade and should be responsible to a named Consultant. The Memorandum then went on to endorse the concept expressed in it that suitably experienced General Practitioners should be given part-time appointments as Medical Assistants; in this regard they were destined to be disappointed as, despite the expressed intention in the Ministry Circular, the grade was never widely operated upon a part-time basis.

The Medical Assistant (later renamed Associate Specialist) grade, though practically unknown in university hospitals, has served the specialty of anaesthesia well in the District General Hospitals, and has provided a career for a number of capable but less academically minded clinicians. The grade provides much needed cover at the Registrar level without overloading the training and promotion pathway to Consultant status. It is a pity that provision was not made to offer reasonably remunerated sessional appointments to medically qualified wives (later, in response to the Sexual Discrimination Acts called "Doctors with Domestic commitments or DDCs").

The Hospital Practitioner grade, limited to a maximum of five sessions per week, which was proposed in 1969 for General Practitioners "and other doctors such as married women who wanted part-time work in the hospital service" would have met the requirement for married DDC lady anaesthetists (many of whom were in possession of the FFARCS qualification), but it was not to be.[193] The sorry story of the negotiation between the BMA, on behalf of General Practitioners alone, and a dilatory Department of Health over the establishment of this grade can be read in the volumes and supplements of the *British Medical Journal* from 1971 to 1976, and is summarised in a leading article in the *BMJ* in November 1976.[193] Instead of being, as intended by its originators in 1969, a suitable part-time appointment for General Practitioners *and others including married women*, it emerged in 1975 as a well paid sessional grade with tenure for *principals* in general practice alone.[193,194] The approved annual scale of remuneration per session (£610 to £826: 1996: £2,720 to £3,680) was, in fact, more than more recently appointed Consultants were receiving if calculated on a sessional basis![193,195] Even Assistants in general practice with the FFARCS were excluded and, together with DDCs most of them were left in the poorly remunerated, annually renewable, Clinical Assistant grade. It is a sad story, and it is even sadder to have to relate that some of the leaders of the BMA General Practitioners were less than sympathetic to their less advantaged specialist colleagues![196] It is fortunate that the qualifications for admission to the Hospital Practitioner grade were set at a reasonably strict level and included the possession of the FFARCS but, nonetheless, some General Practitioners were appointed without this qualification because of a "grandfather" clause.[195,197]

Research and education

Reference has already been made to the financial management of the research and education funds of the Association of Anaesthetists up to 1969 and to the amazing facility for raising funds exhibited by Ronald Jarman.[1] The Minutes[151,155] and Annual Reports (1956-1966), during his time on the Council, record many donations both from commercial companies and individuals which he was instrumental in obtaining. Jarman certainly deserved the grateful tribute paid to him in the 1966 Annual Report.[198] The generosity of G A Vandervell Esq, who was elected to Honorary Membership of the Association in 1962, has also been noted. Jarman was also active in raising funds for the Royal College of Surgeons of England to which Mr Vandervell gave very substantial donations. The Association Council Minutes (22.9.1959 and 4.12.1959)[151] record a rather unusual transaction in which Jarman persuaded Vandervell to earmark £15,000 (1996: £18,000) of what must have been a very large sum which he had donated towards the endowment of the Chair of Pharmacology at the Surgeons' College, for transfer to the Association of Anaesthetists Research and Education Fund, which had just been opened with a view to replacing the former Research Trust. Comparison of the Annual Reports of 1959 and 1969 shows that, in real terms, the annual investment income available to the Association for research and education had increased between seven and eight fold during the ten years; that is £187 (1996: £2,350) in 1959 to £2,287 (1996: £20,600) in 1969, this was more than matched by an increase in the market value of the investment portfolios from which the income dedicated to these objectives was derived; that is £2,747 (1996: £34,300) in 1959 to £40,516 (1996: £365,000) in 1969.

Edgar Pask[5] was Chairman of the Research Committee from shortly after his election to Council in 1956 until his term ended in 1959. H J V Morton[6] (1910-1981), at that time Honorary Secretary, then took over, with Pask nominated as a member of the Committee although not a Member of Council (Council Minutes 4.12.1959)[151]. Pask, however, wrote to Council stating that he was unable to serve. He again became Chairman of the Research Committee when he was elected to the Office of Honorary Treasurer at the end of 1960, and chaired the Committee until his death in 1966, when Morton again took over. Morton served as Chairman until the end of 1969 when he in turn, having been a Vice President, ceased to be a Member of Council.

Pask[5] and Morton[6] together carefully husbanded the growing resources which were available. The rather ambitious putative objectives for the Research and Education programme of the Association were outlined in the 1958 Annual Report. These were:-

"*1. To provide grants for research when sufficient funds are not available from other sources.*

2. *To provide and equip laboratory accommodation.*

3. *To provide wholetime Research Fellowships.*

4. *To provide Student Fellowships both for overseas doctors in the United Kingdom and for United Kingdom doctors who wished to train in the Dominions or the United States.*

5. *To provide small sums such as £50 (1996: £640) or £100 (1996: £1,280) for apparatus; salaries to help technicians work outside routine hours, something in the region of £4 to £6 per week (1996: £50 to £75); to establish a full salary of a technician of £12 to*

£15 (1996: £150 to £190); to assist young anaesthetists to visit other centres in this country and to pay for their initial expenses."

All the grants in the early nineteen sixties came under objective No 5. Many young anaesthetists who have subsequently become leading research workers were aided by modest grants in this period. Each application for a grant was carefully and shrewdly assessed by Pask[5] and Morton[6] and their committee and a number were rejected as being insufficiently thought through or unsound. Reports for publication of the results in *Anaesthesia* were insisted upon. Pask[5] particularly was anxious to publicise the availability of modest grants to young research workers despite the need to build up funds to finance the more ambitious objectives outlined in the 1958 reports (Council Minutes 3.10.1958),[151] and the Annual Reports of the early sixties and notices in the journal *Anaesthesia*[198] drew attention to the availability of the grants.

Research Fellowships. It was not until 1966, however, that sufficient funds were available for the establishment of the first Research Fellowship since 1950. Alastair Spence, the first Chairman of the Associates in Training Group was appointed Association of Anaesthetists Steinberg Research Fellow in September 1966 with the aid of "very generous financial support" from Mr J Steinberg, another of Jarman's contacts (Annual Report 1966). Alastair Spence's brief was to study the problems associated with postoperative pain in the Department of Anaesthesia of the University of Leeds under John Nunn who was then its Professor. This was a fruitful association which lasted from September 1966 to December 1968. It resulted in several papers and a presentation at the Annual Scientific Meeting of the Association of Anaesthetists at Manchester in 1969.[199-201] Later in his career, Professor Spence demonstrated his continuing interest in postoperative pain relief (Chapter 9)! A second Research Fellowship was held from September 1966 to May 1968 by J A Bushman in Professor J S Robinson's Department at the University of Birmingham (Annual Report 1969).[202-203]

The 1969 Annual Report reviewed the research projects supported by the Association of Anaesthetists from 1965 to 1968 and the publications and presentations which resulted from them. The subjects covered reflect the leading developments of current practice of the sixties. They included hypotensive anaesthesia, acid-base disturbances, the assay of blood levels of lignocaine, electrical anaesthesia, closed circuit halothane, audiovisual aids, carbon dioxide response curves, and the seminal study by Plumpton, Besser and Cole of the indications for steroid cover during anaesthesia.[53,54]

Another aim of the 1958 proposals (Annual Report 1958) was to support overseas anaesthetists training in the British Isles, and several such anaesthetists were assisted during the sixties including Dr Casale of Zambia. Many travel grants were also made with the object of allowing British and Irish "anaesthetists holding temporary posts abroad to extend their experience and to present papers at important meetings" (Annual Report 1969).

It must also be remembered that the pioneering investigation into deaths associated with anaesthesia (Chapter 6) continued into the nineteen sixties. The calls on expenses from the research funds relating to this project were modest but the results were of considerable significance.

A donation to the Research Department of Anaesthetics at the Royal College of Surgeons. It can be deduced from the Association Council Minutes of 6 April 1962[151] that the Faculty of Anaesthetists were in some financial difficulty at the time. It was proposed that a donation of £1,000 (1996: £11,000) should be made for work on the pharmacology of muscle relaxants to the BOC Research Department of the Royal College of Surgeons of England under Professor Woolmer;[204] however, some Council Members expressed the view that a donation earmarked for the use of the Research Department of Anaesthetics (which was technically a department of the Royal College of Surgeons and not of the Faculty) might not help the Faculty in its financial difficulty. The matter was, therefore, "left on the table" until the next meeting of Council while further information was obtained. A satisfactory arrangement must have been reached because the Council Minutes of 6 July 1962[151] record laconically that the proposal to donate £1,000 (1996: £11,000) to the Royal College of Surgeons for the use of the Research Department of Anaesthetists was agreed. The reigning President of the Association (none other than that tireless fund raiser Ronald Jarman,[1] then announced that he had also received a donation of £2,000 (1996: £22,000) from Mr G A Vandervell for equipment which would be given to the Research Department "through the Association"

(Annual Report 1962).

It is interesting that it was during the tenure of Office of the then Dean of the Faculty (Professor W W Mushin 1961-1964) that the finances of the anaesthetists' Faculty and the surgeons' College were merged.

Association Prizes

The award of prizes for medical papers and essays specifically written for the purpose does not generally attract a large entry of presentations of an acceptably high standard. Medical practitioners are much more interested in having their work published in scientific journals without the intermediate step of submitting it for a prize in competition with other workers.

The Council of the Association made several attempts to use prizes to promote interest in the emergent specialty of anaesthesia in the sixties with generally disappointing results.

The unfortunate affair of the Dental Prize. A prize of no less than the large sum of 200 guineas (1996: £2,520) was offered in 1961 for the best essay on the subject of general anaesthesia for dental surgery (Annual Report 1960 and Annual Report 1961).[205] This was at a time when Council was greatly concerned to improve training in outpatient dental anaesthesia. Fourteen entries were received. The assessors, headed by Morton,[6] were agreed that none of these entries were of sufficient standard to merit the award of 200 guineas, but they recommended that four of the entries were of sufficient originality for each to deserve the award of an *ex gratia* recompense for out of pocket expenses of 20 guineas (1996: £252). This proposition was duly agreed (Council Minutes 7.4.1961)[151] but, unfortunately, some of the competitors chose to engage a solicitor to challenge this award. It was alleged that there was a breach of contract because only 80 guineas of the promised 200 guineas had been paid out. Counsel's opinion was taken and he agreed that the competitors had a case. The matter was settled out of court by the payment of a further 30 guineas (1996: £378) to each of the competitors who had received an *ex gratia* payment (Council Minutes 7.7.1961).[151]

The Research essay prizes were first offered in 1961 for papers based on research in anaesthesia or related subjects (Council Minutes 6.5.1960).[151] The winning papers would be published in *Anaesthesia*. It will be remembered that efforts were being made to upgrade the material in the journal at this time.

The pecuniary provision for three prizes each year was adequate (£100, £50 and £25: equivalent to £1,212, £606 and £303 at 1996 values) but there were few takers over the next few years. In 1963 Council regretfully concluded that no prize should be awarded in 1963 as none of the essays submitted was of sufficiently high standard (Annual Report 1964). Awards were again made in 1964 but "because the number of entries was disappointingly small" a change was to be made; from 1965 onwards one or more prizes of £100 (equivalent by then to £1,032 in 1996 terms) were awarded for papers published in *Anaesthesia*.[206] Prizes were awarded on this basis on the recommendation of the Editors of *Anaesthesia* over the next few years but the practice has gradually fallen into abeyance. There was never any evidence that any author wrote specifically for *Anaesthesia* in the hope of a prize!

The undergraduate essay prizes of £30 (1996: £310), for dissertations on a subject related to anaesthesia written by medical students training in Great Britain or Ireland, were instituted in 1965 (Annual Report 1965).[206] This award has continued with occasional interruptions (Annual Report 1973) up to the present time. Three awards of £100 each were made in 1992 (Annual Report 1992).

The Registrar's prize was instituted informally at the Brighton meeting of the Junior Anaesthetists' Group (JAG) in 1974.[207] It was inspired by a session of sparkling presentations by the local Registrars at the Annual JAG Meeting in Sheffield in 1973 entitled "Home Grown"; on that occasion a Yorkshireman's cloth cap was passed from speaker to speaker like a relay baton (author's recollection).[208] This monetary award (worth £200 in 1997) to the winner of this now popular and traditional competition at the Annual Meetings of the Group of Anaesthetists in Training, has been accompanied by the presentation of the President's Medal since 1985.[180]

Aid to "Developing Countries"

The terms "Developing Countries" and "Third World Countries" are usually applied to a group of independent nations which lack the resources to provide an acceptable standard of living for many members of their populations. The group includes many former colonial territories which have gained their independence from European powers since the end of the Second World War in 1945, as well as many other independent states which are unable to care properly for large sections of their populations, including the provision of adequate health services.

The transition from expatriate European rule to independent nationhood, while theoretically and intellectually desirable, has not been without pain for many former protectorates and colonial territories. It is easy for some politicians and sociologists in the nineteen nineties to condemn the past "exploitation" of the basic resources of these countries, but to conveniently forget the advantages of colonial rule. These benefits included stable and generally incorruptible civil government, the maintenance of law and order, the dedication of expatriate administrators, and the provision of scientific and technical expertise.

Earmarked funding by the colonial power has been replaced by, initially substantial, but often gradually diminishing, locally administered aid programmes, and a reduction of expatriate support and expertise. This change is not least apparent in the case of the health services in these countries, which often have to attempt to shoulder the burden of the traumatic consequences of civil war or the breakdown of law and order in addition to the normal provision of basic treatment and preventative medicine. It is moreover, often easier to define the problems and suggest remedies, than it is to obtain funding and to persuade proud but inexperienced, nationalistic, and bureaucratic regimes to accept and use the aid that is offered in the most effective and economic manner. Tackling the problem of promoting the benefits which an emergent medical specialty like anaesthesia can bestow, is sometimes very difficult indeed under such circumstances!

The need to train anaesthetists for anaesthetically underdeveloped countries was recognised soon after the end of the Second World War. The major contribution of the WHO Centre in Copenhagen in training physicians in anaesthesia from all over the world between 1950 and 1976, as well as the part which British anaesthetists played in its work, has already been described (Chapter 6); but it was not until the mid sixties that the Association began to consider seriously what part it should play in assisting the developing countries.

An exploratory meeting in 1964. The Council of the Association of Anaesthetists was alerted to the need to consider the need to train anaesthetists for the "Third World" in December 1963 (Council Minutes 6.12.1963)[155] and (Annual Report 1964). Pask[5] reported that he had received a letter from Aileen Adams (Consultant Anaesthetists, Cambridge) and John V Farman[209] who was then a Senior Registrar at Cardiff and later became a Consultant at Cambridge. Their letter stated that they were personally aware of eight people in the United Kingdom who had worked in Nigeria, Pakistan and India, and it went on to suggest that the Association of Anaesthetists might be interested in convening a meeting to help to decide what could be usefully taught in developing countries. Pask suggested that the question of preparing a textbook applicable to the work in such countries should also be discussed. Council voted the necessary expenditure and Organe asked that W D Wylie (then the Adviser in Postgraduate Studies to the Faculty), should also be asked to attend (Council Minutes 6.12.1963 and 7.2. 1964).[210]

The meeting was held on 14 March 1964. Pask reported to Council that eighteen people had attended "most of whom had spent a considerable time overseas" (Council Minutes 5.6.1964).[155] Three positive suggestions were made: -

1. That the Association should run an advisory bureau holding instructional material and prepared to advise on "equipment for remote areas".

2. The Editorial Board of Anaesthesia should be asked to produce a series of articles on "techniques of anaesthesia for people who work with little help and very little laboratory equipment".

3. That another meeting should be held.

A series of nine articles on "Anaesthesia in difficult situations" was subsequently published in *Anaesthesia* between 1966 and 1968 by the Senior Assistant Editor, T B Boulton with the cooperation of P V Cole (St Bartholomew's Hospital, London) and A H Gilbertson (Royal Liverpool Hospital). A number of subsidiary articles and supporting letters were also published in this period (*Anaesthesia* 1966; volume 21: 1967; volume 22: 1968; volume 23:1969). It has been reported that this series had an important impact in a number of developing countries and that it has subsequently been photocopied many times (personal communications).

A meeting on anaesthetic problems facing developing countries. John Farman[209] also held a successful meeting at Cambridge in June 1967, to which many interested parties contributed and which was reported in *Anaesthesia*.[211] It is known that one eminent British anaesthetist declined to chair a session because the summaries revealed that the question of the administration of anaesthesia by nurses was to be considered; surely a somewhat ostrich-like attitude in the circumstances!

The Anaesthesia Educational Research Foundation was established by Robert A Hingson who held senior anaesthetic appointments in several leading American universities and was ultimately Professor of Anesthesiology and Public Health Practice at the University of Pittsburg, USA (1968-1977).[212] Hingson was a tireless worker dedicated to promoting medical aid for third world countries. He became Chairman of the WFSA Action Committee in 1964, and, in 1965, developed the Anaesthesia and Educational Research Foundation with the objective of raising large sums of money to found training centres for anaesthesiology at suitable locations world wide. Large sums of money were in fact raised from anaesthesiologists, professional societies and industry, particularly, but not exclusively, from within the USA, and WFSA Training Centres were opened in Caracas, Venezuela (1966) and Manila, Philippines in 1970.[212,213] A proposed African centre has never materialised.

The attention of the Council of the Association was first drawn to Hingson's WFSA fund raising scheme by T Cecil Gray in January 1965. He referred to correspondence he had received suggesting a contribution of $10 to $50 from each physician specialist anaesthesiologist in the world to set up training centres in Asia, South America and Africa. Consideration of the letter was deferred until further information could be obtained (Council Minutes 8.1.1965).[155] Organe[156] (then President of WFSA) who had received another letter from Hingson raised the matter again in March 1965, but Council were unhappy with the apparently individualistic method of fund raising. It was resolved that the Honorary Secretary should write to the Secretary General of the WFSA (Professor Mayrhofer of Vienna) to express disquiet, and to ask who would be responsible for giving advice to developing countries (Council Minutes 5.3.1965).[155]

At the next meeting of Council the Honorary Secretary reported the receipt of a letter from the Australian Society of Anaesthetists which also expressed concern about the way the appeal was being conducted and its objectives (Council Minutes 7.5.1965).[155]

The Honorary Secretary reported the receipt of another letter from the Australian Society of Anaesthetists in December 1965. The Australian Society asked for further information about the attitude of the Council of the Association of Anaesthetists to Hingson's Committee. The letter also stated that they were raising funds for developing countries, but were undecided whether to send the money to Hingson or to control its use themselves (Council Minutes 3.12.1965);[155] in the event the Australian Society of Anaesthetists "Action Fund" was officially designated in 1971. It was used to fund a number of projects in the Asian-Australasian region, including specific support for the WFSA Training Centre in Manila which was established in 1970.[214]

The Australian letter triggered fresh discussion in Council. Geoffrey Organe[156] pointed out that Hingson had already raised $20,000 US (1996: £82,500 UK), and he suggested that the time had come for the Association of Anaesthetists to make a gesture and support for Hingson's objectives in establishing Training Centres. Organe went on to propose that a letter should be written to Hingson expressing support for his objectives but explaining that the funds available to the Association of Anaesthetists of Great Britain and Ireland were being used to fund its own commitments directly. He further recommended that information should be collected and recorded regarding the extent of the considerable commitment which anaesthetists in the United Kingdom already had, both in training anaesthetists for overseas and in rendering service in developing countries.[155]

A subcommittee was then set up "to collect detailed information on the extent of the United Kingdom's existing contribution to helping anaesthetists in developing countries". The report was to form the basis both for a reply to Hingson and for discussion relating to future action by the Association of Anaesthetists. The Australian Society were to be kept informed. Aileen Adams, who had been elected to Council in 1964, was appointed Convener, Organe[156] and Mushin were to be members, and there were to be powers to coopt. It is recorded that Council reminded the subcommittee that Pask[5] and Wylie (the Faculty Postgraduate Adviser) had an interest in the matter.

The report of the Subcommittee on Aid to Developing Countries was presented to Council by Aileen Adams in September 1966 (Council Minutes 2.9.1966) and the section dealing with the "Britain's Contribution" was published in *Anaesthesia* in April 1967.[215]

This comprehensive review begins with an historical perspective of Britain's provision of medical services in British Commonwealth countries, its traditional acceptance of undergraduate and postgraduate students in its own medical schools and the continuing close liaison with medical schools in the Commonwealth countries and, in some cases, the granting of British degrees and diplomas to graduates from those institutions. The continuing interchange of anaesthetists on an individual basis is emphasised and details are given of the resultant establishment of academic departments in such countries as India, Pakistan, Malaya, Hong Kong, West Indies, etc. Attention is also drawn to the contribution of British anaesthetists as instructors at the Copenhagen Training Centre (Chapter 6).

The report then goes on to give details of the facilities that were available in Britain in 1967 designed to aid the training of anaesthetists from developing countries. The Faculty of Anaesthetists provided (and still provides in 1998) the "crucial" services of the Postgraduate Adviser (by 1966 named the Bernard

Johnson Postgraduate Adviser in honour of the Second Dean of the Faculty (1952-1955) who died suddenly in 1959),[216,217] hostel accommodation, through the Mary Kinross Charitable Trust at Bernard Johnson House, and it also gave grants to overseas doctors already in the United Kingdom to enable them to extend their training by courses, lectures and visits to anaesthetic centres.

The Government was also very active in the sixties in providing generous aid for former colonies and dependencies. The subcommittee report estimates that in the years 1962 to 1966 the Ministry of Overseas Development had awarded training grants to 60 postgraduate anaesthetists from former colonies at an estimated annual expenditure of between £18,000 and £20,000 (1996: £180,000 to £200,000).

The first British Commonwealth Medical Conference had been held in Edinburgh in October 1965 in an atmosphere of enthusiasm, and the Minister of Health (Kenneth Robinson) announced proposals for expanded schemes for scholarships and fellowships for British Commonwealth postgraduates in the United Kingdom and others for subsidising teachers from the United Kingdom, in developing countries.[218] It is sad that these good intentions, which were engendered by the initial optimism of a new administration flushed with euphoria after a general election victory in 1964, fell far short of full realisation in the ensuing years as the economic plight of the United Kingdom worsened.

The educational facilities provided by the British Council in the sixties (including 196 libraries in 83 countries) are also mentioned in the Association Subcommittee report; sadly too these facilities have greatly diminished in recent years due to financial stringency.

The contribution of the Association of Anaesthetists in terms of indirect aid to developing countries was not large in the sixties despite its desire to analyse the problem and give moral support to anaesthetists working overseas. The 1968 Annual Report records, for example, that Aileen Adams represented the Association of Anaesthetists at a meeting of West African surgeons and anaesthetists and visited hospitals in Nigeria and Ghana. It should be remembered also that Council was devoting a great deal of energy to preparing to be host to the World at the 1968 Congress at which the developing nations and their problems were well represented.[219]

The position is summed up by the Council of the Association of Anaesthetists in the 1969 Annual Report:-

"The Subcommittee felt that the problems of educating sufficient anaesthetists in developing countries were well understood although far from being solved, but there was no unanimity about how to solve them. The Association was only one of the organisations attempting to play a part. One of the best ways it could help was through the journal [Anaesthesia], which was distributed free of charge to some new Societies and Anaesthetic Departments in the Commonwealth until such groups were able to be self-supporting. The Subcommittee was wound up and Dr Aileen Adams asked to hold a watching brief on this matter, in conjunction with the Faculty Postgraduate Adviser Doctor S A Feldman [of Westminster Hospital]."

The journal *Anaesthesia*, under its Editor Roger Bryce-Smith (Oxford), certainly played an important part in disseminating information of the right kind and providing a vehicle for communications for and about developing countries.[211,219,220,221] The Editor had the consent of the Editorial Board to authorise a number of copies for free distribution, particularly to countries with currency difficulties, and Corresponding Members in a number of anaesthetically underdeveloped countries also received complimentary copies.

Outpatient dental anaesthesia

The fees payable for the administration of dental anaesthesia for outpatient dental treatment by the public authorities had been a concern of the Association from its foundation, and especially so since the introduction of the NHS. It will be recalled that a subcommittee of the Association was appointed by Council in 1959 to consider the whole question of outpatient dentistry (Chapter 6); from then on concern about remuneration became a secondary consideration compared with the whole question of the safety of outpatient anaesthesia, training for medical postgraduates in dental anaesthesia, and the problem of whether or not dental surgeons, for whom training opportunities were limited, should continue to be allowed to administer anaesthetics. More rhetoric was expended in Council and elsewhere in the next decade and, more column inches printed in British medical and dental journals on this topic, than on almost any other single matter, not to mention the attention paid by the lay press!

The reasons for this controversial, and sometime acrimonious debate were both complex and deep seated. The bitterness which developed between some members of the medical and dental professions even resulted in an unusual, but in the end inconclusive, legal action for defamation lasting 35 days. This was brought by a dental practitioner over the personal alleged implications of the conclusions of a scientific article published by established medical research workers.[221-224] This action, up to 1972 at any rate, was the longest libel case in British legal history and found a place in the *Guinness Book of Records!*[225]

It is pertinent to consider the factors which led to this state of affairs, the echoes of which can still be heard in the nineteen nineties! The historic role of dentists in the introduction of modern anaesthesia in the mid nineteenth century, both in the United States and in the United Kingdom, is incontrovertible.[226,227] There is a legal myth that the law permits that literally anyone may administer anaesthesia to humans in the United Kingdom whereas only veterinary surgeons, licensed research workers, and, curiously, the owner, can anaesthetise an animal; however, after the earliest days, and leaving aside isolated attempts to introduce nurse anaesthetists, it had been generally accepted up to the nineteen sixties that in British practice the privilege was confined to medical and dental practitioners. This was on the basis that they alone were trained to do so in their undergraduate days by reason of the regulations imposed by General Medical and General Dental Councils.[228] The actual position was that medical practitioners administered anaesthesia for all surgical procedures both inside and outside hospitals, except that it was acceptable for dentists to give short inhalational anaesthetics for dental extractions in their own practices if they wished to do so. Many dental anaesthetics were therefore administered by general medical practitioners and only a limited number by Consultant Anaesthetists. The position within the medical profession with regard to undergraduate training in anaesthesia had changed by the nineteen sixties however. The emergent medical practitioner no longer regarded himself as competent to administer anaesthesia without further training after the completion of his year as a provisionally registered practitioner. A few years later, in 1980, when vocational training for General Practice was introduced, anaesthesia was not regarded as an acceptable first line module for vocational training programmes,[229] thus further discouraging a new generation of General Practitioners from seeking to obtain Clinical Assistant sessions or to practice as anaesthetists.

The inauguration of the NHS in 1948 had led to a greatly increased demand for conservative dentistry. There had therefore been a steady decline in the number of patients requiring general anaesthesia for exodontia.[230] and, by 1976, a large proportion of outpatient dental anaesthetics were being administered to children rather than to adults.[231] There were thus fewer cases available for the teaching of medical or dental students the art of outpatient dental anaesthesia. There was consequently no way in which a dental surgeon could be considered to be competent to administer general anaesthesia on qualification, and there were virtually no facilities for the systematic training of postgraduate dentists in anaesthesia. The only courses available were the weekend introductory courses organised by SAAD. Dental surgeons who wished to gain enough experience in anaesthesia could only obtain it by apprenticeship in multiple partner practice (comparatively rare in the sixties) or by trial and error.

The philosophy of dental practice itself had moved on however. It was no longer acceptable practice to extract the tooth of a nervous patient under the oblivion of general anaesthesia rather than attempt to preserve it with a filling. What was to be done for such patients? The majority of patients could be managed with local anaesthesia and sympathetic understanding, but there was a need for some form of pharmacological sedation for a minority if satisfactory dental work was to be carried out.[232] Hypnosis can provide a solution for a certain number of dentists and for certain patients, but it is often unacceptable or unreliable except when employed by a skilful practitioner with the requisite temperament.[233] The solution adopted and taught by Stanley Drummond-Jackson[224] (1909-1975), a Wimpole Street dental practitioner, was the "ultra-light minimal incremental methohexitone technique". It was this that sparked the greatest controversy both within the dental profession itself and with the medically qualified anaesthetists.

Drummond-Jackson[225] had used the early intravenous barbiturates (pernocton, nembutal and thiopentone) successfully in his practice since the thirties despite the disapproval of the medical establishment of the use of this group of drugs.[225,234,235] It was the introduction of the barbiturate methohexitone in 1956 which enabled Drummond-Jackson[225] to refine his technique. The theory behind the "ultra-light" technique was that the patient could be kept in the very light "sedation" stage of anaesthesia, at which there was lack of response to surgical stimuli and amnesia without complete loss of consciousness and consequent loss of the reflexes of the larynx, while the patient remained in verbal contact with the administrator. Drummond-Jackson[225] developed a highly sophisticated team approach to dentistry under his ultra-light technique assisted by at least one and usually two well trained dental nurses. One member of the team had responsibility for monitoring the patient, and the increments of methohexitone were often injected as instructed by the operator by one of the nurses into an indwelling intravenous line. Such a procedure obviously laid itself open to criticism as being undesirable as an "operator-anaesthetist" technique despite the very able assistance of the trained assistants.[236] Drummond-Jackson enthusiastically advocated this technique[237] and let it be said also that he had the initial support from several medically qualified anaesthetists; these included Professor (Sir) Robert Macintosh, who had himself used the intravenous barbiturates for dental anaesthesia against orthodox opinion in the thirties[235] and Jim (J G) Bourne of St Thomas' Hospital, London and the Odstock Hospital, Salisbury.[238,239]

Drummond-Jackson founded SAAD in 1957 with the object of imparting knowledge of his technique to fellow dental surgeons.[235] Many dentists attended weekend SAAD courses over the next two decades. It must be said, however, that, despite admonitions not to do so without further training, many of them went back to their practices and introduced the procedure without further instruction. The philosophic difficulty with the ultra-light technique was the claim that its practice always involved "sedation" rather than full general anaesthesia. There is no doubt that the ultra-light sedation stage of anaesthesia with the patient in verbal contact with the administrator during the operative procedure, exists, but the claim that this is invariably so can not be upheld. The therapeutic margin in terms of incremental dosage with methohexitone is so narrow that at some stage during many administrations the patient will be unconscious in a state of full general anaesthesia. This does not necessarily condemn the technique even if it is being practised by an operator working with skilled assistants, but it became politically important later when it began to be accepted that sedation techniques only required the presence of the operator besides his nursing assistants, whereas general anaesthesia demanded the presence of a second medical or dental practitioner.

The only other pharmacological sedation technique available at the time SAAD was founded in 1956 was the Jorgensen technique.[232] This involved very heavy sedation short of anaesthesia induced with increments of intravenous pentobarbitone, pethidine and hyoscine. The technique was popular in the United States where the cost of hospital admission to the patient encouraged quite major dentistry and oral surgery (impacted wisdom teeth, etc) to be undertaken in hospital dental outpatient departments. Recovery to normality was prolonged but the patient could relatively safely be taken home by his friends or relations to sleep the sedation off on the day of the operation (personal observations in the USA).

Death under anaesthesia in the dental surgery is an emotive subject and so it should be. The demise of an (often) fit young, or relatively young, person undergoing a minor operation is certainly a tragedy. There were no less than 22 such deaths in England and Wales in 1952, but by 1967 the rate had fallen to 4 to 6 per year.[240] Bourne analysed 37 outpatient dental deaths in 1966.[241] None of them had occurred during the conduct of ultra-light incremental methohexitone technique as described by Drummond-Jackson.[225,237] Bourne believed that the deaths he discussed were the result of cerebral ischaemia due to hypotension in the upright position; moreover, having reviewed the status of the administrators of the various anaesthetics concerned, he stated, "it is a fallacy to suppose that the tragedies of dental anaesthesia would end if only an end were put to the practice of the dentist giving his own anaesthetics".[241] There had in fact been no deaths before 1966 under the ultra-light methohexitone technique administered by the dental "operator anaesthetist".[237] Bourne published a review of a further 16 deaths connected with dental anaesthesia in 1970; only one of these occurred during the administration of intermittent methohexitone by an "operator-anaesthetist" in the upright position.[242] The practice of ergonomic dentistry with the patient supine using the intermittent methohexitone technique had been adopted by many users of intermittent methohexitone in the mid sixties.[243] A detailed survey of deaths associated with dentistry in England and Wales in the ten years from 1970 to 1979 was published by Coplans and Curson in 1982.[244] They showed that 55 deaths had occurred which could be wholly or partly attributed to general anaesthesia in outpatient practice (including General Community Dental clinics and Hospital outpatient departments), and they estimated that the incidence was 1 in 265,000 in 14,575,000 administrations.[244] The mortality resulting from longer administrations for conservative treatment and minor surgery was significantly higher than that for short administrations ($p < 0.01$). No particular technique was implicated as the cause of this higher mortality. The mortality rates calculated according to the professional status of the administrator were: second dentists 1:513,000, "doctors" (unspecified but probably mostly general practitioners) 1:263,000, and all operating dentists, whether using intermittent methohexitone or practising according to the Drummond-Jackson (SAAD) guidelines or not, 1:143,000. The difference between second dentists and operating dentists was just significant ($p = 0.05$).

Professional disagreement. It must be conceded that, with hindsight, there was little in these figures to justify the condemnatory line which the Association of Anaesthetists adopted towards its dental colleagues in the sixties.[245] It must be admitted, however, that Drummond-Jackson, though charming and generous in private life, was aggressive and challenging as a public speaker and writer, and provocative in his dealings with the medical profession.[225] His attitude stimulated the inevitable reaction, although it must be admitted that some medical anaesthetists indulged in ill informed criticism without taking the trouble to evaluate his personal expertise. The SAAD group close to Drummond-Jackson worked with highly trained assistants. They really studied their subject and developed a very high standard of team dentistry in well designed and equipped "operatories".[236,243] The problem was those dentists who, without training or adequate personal study, decided to "have a go" with the new techniques; as Jim Bourne wrote in 1973 when he withdrew his support for the operator anaesthetist : -

"It would seem that the much argued and widely publicised danger in the dentist giving his own anaesthetic has been exaggerated."

"Nevertheless I no longer support this practice. When doing so previously I stipulated, amongst other provisos that there should be in attendance at least two chairside assistants of suitable status and training and that the patient should be treated lying down. These provisos have not always been met and, fearing what I regard as inadequate care of the patient may be widespread, I now accept that there should be a second person present to give the anaesthetic."[245]

It must be admitted, however, that Bourne's advocacy of a technical paramedical grade, to take the chores of routine anaesthesia off the shoulders of the medical or dental anaesthetist in the operating theatre as well as in the dental surgery, was a less acceptable proposal![246]

The Dental Committee of the Association under the Chairmanship of Patrick Shackleton met three times in 1960 and, as already recorded, a prize of £200 (1996: £2,520) was offered for the best essay on the subject of general anaesthesia for dental surgery. The Committee, now under John Beard[4] (President 1969-1971) met only once in 1961, when the British facilities for postgraduate training in dental anaesthesia for dentists as well as medical practitioners were discussed.[151]

John Beard presented a very gloomy report about the work of the Committee in February 1963 (Council Minutes 1.2.1963).[151] He stated that cooperation in a joint committee between the Faculties of Anaesthesia and Dental Surgery about training had not proved to be easy and the Committee had fallen into abeyance. The question of a Diploma in Dental Anaesthesia was considered but not pursued, and further approaches to the dental profession were not thought to be worthwhile for the time being.

A symposium on the teaching of general anaesthesia was held at the Royal College of Surgeons, Lincoln's Inn Fields in April 1964.[247] It was organised jointly by the Faculty of Anaesthetists and the Wessex Regional Hospital Board (of which Shackleton[3] was a member) and it was supported financially by the Association of Anaesthetists (Council Minutes 6.9.1963).[155] The invited speakers and audience included specialist anaesthetists and oral surgeons and medical and general dental practitioners, amongst whom was Drummond-Jackson,[225] and other members of SAAD. A wide ranging discussion took place. The problems were clearly defined but, as might have been expected, there was little agreement about what should be done.[247]

Council had disbanded its Dental Anaesthesia Committee in December 1963 (Council Minutes 6.12.1963),[155] but the subject was again discussed in May 1965 (Council Minutes 7.5.1965).[155] This was because Ronald Green of St George's Hospital, London had written inquiring about the reaction of Council to a request he had received to teach dental postgraduates as Clinical Assistants; after considerable discussion Council passed the following resolution which was also included in the Annual Report for 1965:-

"This Council considers that a person who has not yet received a full medical training and therefore cannot properly assess the risks should not administer prolonged anaesthesia whether or not it includes intravenous or endotracheal techniques".

This policy was obviously designed to permit the teaching of short inhalation anaesthetics for exodontia to dental postgraduates, but to exclude intermittent methohexitone techniques for conservation. The Dental Subcommittee was also reconstituted at that meeting (Council Minutes 7.5.1965).[155]

The Joint Subcommittee of the Central Health Services Council Standing Medical and Dental Committees[248,249] was set up by the Ministry of Health in July 1965 in response to general professional and public disquiet about outpatient dental anaesthesia.[250-253] It was chaired by (Sir) Rodney Swiss (a general dental practitioner, then a member of the General Dental Council). The Subcommittee members included Archibald Galley[254] (1908-1988) of Kings College Hospital, London (Chairman of the BMA Anaesthetists' Group) and Professor Mushin of Cardiff (a Member of the Central Health Services Council), both of whom were coopted Members of the Association Council. The terms of reference of the Subcommittee were :-

"To consider the use of general dental practice and to advise :

(a) How far the administration of general anaesthetics for conservative treatment can be justified and

(b) *How far the administration of general anaesthetics for any purpose without the attendance of a second practitioner can be justified.*[205,248,249]

The Council of the Association of Anaesthetists received a letter informing it that the Joint Subcommittee had been constituted on 3 December 1965 (Council Minutes 3.12.1965).[155] The Dental Subcommittee of the Association, now under the chairmanship of Vernon Hall, immediately set about preparing written and oral evidence. A comprehensive memorandum was prepared by John Beard4 of the Royal Postgraduate Medical School, Hammersmith, Peter Dinnick of the Middlesex Hospital, London and Michael Coplans of St George's Hospital, London, and this was endorsed by Council at an Extraordinary Meeting on 7 January 1966[155] and summarised in the 1966 Annual Report; as things were to turn out the recommendations of the 1967 Report of the Joint Subcommittee were to closely resemble those of the Association of Anaesthetists in its evidence (Annual Report 1967).

The Joint Subcommittee of the Central Health Service Council took evidence from a number of organisations and individuals in the field of dental anaesthesia, both by invitation and in response to advertisements in medical and dental journals.[248,249] These included, in addition to the Association of Anaesthetists, the British Dental Association, the British Medical Association, the Faculties of Anaesthetists and of Dental Surgery of the Royal College of Surgeons of England, representatives of the dental schools of Great Britain and Ireland, SAAD, the Medical Defence Union and the Medical Protection Society, Victor Goldman of the Eastman Dental Clinic and Stanley Drummond-Jackson.[256]

There was extensive coverage and exhaustive correspondence on the subject of anaesthesia for outpatient dentistry with special reference to the intermittent methohexitone technique in the medical and dental journals while the Joint Subcommittee was deliberating, from July 1965, when it was appointed, until it published its report in May 1967 (*British Dental Journal* 1965: 119; 1966: 120 and 121; 1967: 122; the *British Medical Journal* 1966: 1 and 2; 1967: 1; *Lancet* 1966: 1 and 2; 1967: 1). Prominent among the numerous correspondents were Jim Bourne, Drummond-Jackson and Michael Coplans. There was also a controversial article in the *Daily Mail* extolling the virtues of the ultra-light intravenous technique (Council Minutes 1.4.1966)[155] and a parliamentary question about the safety of the intravenous intermittent methohexitone and its use in the National Health Service.[255]

The Joint Subcommittee Report (May 1967)[248,249,256] is a comprehensive if conservative document which must be read in the context of the time it was published. The value of methohexitone as an induction agent before inhalation anaesthesia was acknowledged, but there was "some anxiety" about the "ultra-light" technique because of the small therapeutic margin between the sedative and anaesthetic dosage. The report stressed that it should be "the sole responsibility of a trained and experienced administrator" and this consequently "necessitates the presence of a trained anaesthetist in addition to the operator". The report remarks also that a "varying degree of hypoxia may occur" if air alone is breathed and supplemental oxygen may be desirable. It is noteworthy that even those medical anaesthetists who lent support to the use of the 'ultra-light' methohexitone technique by dental surgeons at this time, were rarely able to convince their dental colleagues that, though the risk was small, the use of supplementary oxygen would be an additional safety factor. The intermittent incremental methohexitone technique was thus firmly placed in the category of general anaesthesia by the Joint Sub-Committee. Less convincingly the Jorgensen conscious sedation technique[232] was stated to have "a limited place" in the management of patients undergoing conservative dentistry as an alternative to general anaesthesia "but still has the dangers inherent in intravenous administration of barbiturates [for general anaesthesia]". The report does not include a reference to the intravenous use of diazepam, which was only just becoming available at that time.[232,257]

A table is included in the Joint Subcommittee Report summarising 51 deaths which occurred between 1959 and 1965 "with mention of dental anaesthesia". This had been compiled "from information supplied by the General Register Office". This list includes hospital inpatient cases. Methohexitone had been used for induction in three instances, but no deaths were recorded as having occurred during or after the administration of the intermittent methohexitone technique. The report also establishes by extrapolation that, in the NHS in England and Wales, in 1965 of 1,322,980 claims for payment for the administration of general anaesthesia, 22.6% were administered by the operating dental surgeon acting as his own anaesthetist (with or without the assistance of a nurse), 32.8% by a second dental surgeon acting as anaesthetist, 25.4% by medical practitioners without formal postgraduate training in anaesthesia, 12.5% by Consultant Anaesthetists and 6.7% by medical practitioners with special training in anaesthesia (for example those who had had a resident appointment in anaesthesia, and/or obtained the Diploma in Anaesthesia, before entering general practice). The figure of 12.5% for Consultant administrations, which does not include private practice cases, was larger than the 3% quoted in a report in *Anaesthesia* following a local survey undertaken in both private and NHS practice by the Yorkshire Society of Anaesthetists in 1961.[251]

The Joint Subcommittee, in consideration of its terms of reference, made four major recommendations. These were broadly consistent with the evidence submitted to it by the Association of Anaesthetists (Annual Reports 1966 and 1967) :-

1. That "ideally", all general dental anaesthetics should be administered by specialist anaesthetists trained in dental anaesthesia.

2. That dental and medical undergraduate training should deal with basic principles of general anaesthesia, and that much more postgraduate training should be available for general medical and dental practitioners pending the achievement of the ideal.

3. That the practice of the general dental practitioner acting as his own anaesthetist is to be deprecated.

4. That general anaesthesia for conservative dentistry can be justified only in certain classes of patients whose clinical condition requires it.[249]

A meeting of an invited audience consisting of medical "anaesthetists engaged in the teaching of dental surgery" to consider the report was jointly sponsored by the Association of Anaesthetists and the Faculty of Anaesthetists (Annual General Meeting 1967, Council Minutes 1.12.1967).[155,258,259] The recommendations of the Report were endorsed.

The approval in the Report[249] of a shift of emphasis from undergraduate to postgraduate training was an important step forward and consistent with the emergent views on medical education at that time, but the report did not suggest that an authorised list of trained dental anaesthetists should be instituted. The recommendation "deprecating" the administration of anaesthesia by the operating dental surgeon did not go as far as the Association of Anaesthetists' recommendation to discontinue the fee paid for the service from the NHS. This was in fact not achieved until 1983, at a time when a new Dentists' Bill was being considered by Parliament, after the General Dental Council issued its Guidelines effectively outlawing the operator-anaesthetist as distinct from the operator-sedationist.[260]

The British Dental Association (BDA) held a conference of representatives of all the major medical and dental organisations and colleagues concerned with general anaesthesia for dentistry on 25 May 1967.[261] The discussion at the meeting was based on a paper issued on the authority of the BDA shortly after the Joint Subcommittee Report had become available.[256,261] The dental establishment of the day rejected the concept that all anaesthetics should ultimately be administered by specialist (medical) anaesthetists as unrealistic and unacceptable. This is understandable. British dental surgeons had been shown to have an enviable safety record as anaesthetists in their own surgeries.[244,262] The other recommendations of the Joint Sub-Committee Report to the leaders of the dental profession were broadly acceptable. These included the deprecation of operator anaesthesia (except in emergencies for exodontia when a second medical or dental practitioner was not available to act as anaesthetist), the tacit acceptance that a dental surgeon on qualification could no longer be regarded as trained sufficiently to be capable of administrating general anaesthesia safely, and the implied very limited indications for the use of dental anaesthesia for conservative dentistry.

Evidence given to the Joint Subcommittee as to "the proportion of patients for whom general anaesthesia for conservative treatment was justified.... varied widely from 1% to (in the view of the minority) 95%. The majority thought it was justified in no more than 5%". It is assumed that the ultra-light technique is included under the category of 'general anaesthetic'.[249] This variation is not surprising. Dental practices having the facility to provide "anaesthesia" for conservative work naturally attract patients who need it, or think they do so, and referrals are treated from other practices.

It goes without saying that the SAAD practitioners were not happy with the report, especially with the inclusion of the ultra-light methohexitone technique under the heading of full general anaesthesia, and the consequent condemnation of it as an operator-anaesthetist technique.[263,264] A lively correspondence developed in the *British Medical Journal* (1967; volumes 3 and 4), the *Lancet* (1967; volumes 1 and 2) and the *British Dental Journal* (1967; volumes 122 and 123).

There were also other editorials and annotations generally welcoming the report of the Joint Subcommittee.[247,264] The Editorial in the *British Medical Journal*[248] did, however, pose the question as to whether "some [British] dental practitioners were making too little use of local analgesia for conservative dentistry", and went on to point out that, in other countries, such as the USA and Scandinavia, local analgesia was routine for pain relief for all types of dental surgery. The report of the Joint Subcommittee itself states that "enquiries in the Western European countries and the United States of America suggest that there was no general trend..... towards the use of intravenous anaesthesia for conservative treatment".[249] One conclusion upon which all parties were agreed was that there was inadequate provision for instruction in outpatient anaesthesia for dentistry for both dental and medical postgraduates. This was emphasised by the finding of the Joint Subcommittee that the participation of Consultant Anaesthetists in the public sector was only 12.5% of the administrations of general anaesthesia[249] and when other more localised investigations had quoted 3%[251] in Leeds and 0.6% (Dundee).[262] The overall provision for postgraduate teaching for dentists in 1966 in England, Wales and Scotland was estimated to be a total of 200 places per year on 3 to 5 day courses at the Eastman Dental Institute and the Medical Schools of Dundee, Sheffield, Aberdeen and Leeds and 240 places on SAAD courses.[253,262]

The Windeyer Committee was set up at the invitation of the Council of the Association of Anaesthetists in January 1968 to make recommendations on postgraduate training in dental anaesthesia (Annual Report 1968). It consisted of representatives of the Faculties of Anaesthetists and of the Association of Anaesthetists, and the British Dental Association under the Chairmanship of the radiologist Sir Brian Windeyer. Michael Coplans (Secretary 1970-1972) represented the Association of Anaesthetists and W Derek Wylie of St Thomas' Hospital, London the Faculty of Anaesthetists. The Minute Book indicates that Council kept in very close touch with the proceedings of the Committee. The short Windeyer Report was published in 1969 and was reproduced in full in the *British Dental Journal*.[266] It first defined the "ideal" postgraduate training in outpatient dental anaesthesia as including six months training in general medicine and six months in anaesthesia with attendance at "a special course devoted to the theory and practice of dental anaesthesia". It then recognised that "the present pattern of dental education....does not enable the dental practitioner to fulfil these criteria; finally a section made suggestions for "training in the immediate future"; this consisted of little more than the encouragement of the facilities which already existed (short courses and apprenticeship training in general dental practice). It must be recognised that the Windeyer Committee had an impossible task within the constraints of the time; they could do no more than recognise the difficulties and put down markers. It is small wonder that its critics dismissed the report as irrelevant.[267]

Conscious sedation. The two or three years either side of the publication of the Joint Subcommittee Report[249] in 1967 probably saw the maximum use of the controversial ultra-light methohexitone technique by operating dentists. The introductory paragraph of the Windeyer report makes significant acknowledgement of "the increasing interest in the use of sedative, analgesic and tranquillising drugs in outpatient dentistry" in which there was a "therapeutic margin unlikely to produce accidental loss of consciousness". The new elements in dental pain control had emerged between the publication of the Joint Subcommittee Report in 1967 and that of the Windeyer Committee of 1969 were the introduction of the sedative diazepam[232,257,268] and "relative analgesia" (the use of minimal and limited analgesic concentrations of nitrous oxide as described by Langa).[232,269] These techniques had a sufficient therapeutic margin between conscious sedation or analgesia and unconscious general anaesthesia, to be acceptable to informed medical opinion for use by dentists for conservation without the presence of a second dental or medical practitioner;[257] indeed it can be argued that the verbal psychosedative support of these pharmacological conscious sedation techniques by the operator (rather than by a second practitioner) is not only essential for their success, but also considerably reduces the dosage of the intravenous drug or the concentration of nitrous oxide required. The safety of these procedures is incontrovertible. Coplans and Curson, in their classic review of deaths associated with anaesthesia in the 10 years 1970 to 1979[244] state:-

> *"In the 10 year period it is deduced that over 2 million sedative and analgesic techniques were used of which 1.5 million were given by operating dentists. There was one recorded death.... but the relationship is a speculative one. The patient was given 16 mg of unsupplemented diazepam intravenously by the operating dentist at midday, and at 6.00 pm was killed in a road traffic accident while driving a motorcycle".*[244]

The Windeyer Report recommended that "the theoretical and practical aspects [of the use of sedative, analgesic and tranquillising drugs] should form an integral part of the dental undergraduate's curriculum. A pious hope which was accepted by Council of the Association of Anaesthetists on 7 July 1969[155] and approved by the other bodies composing the Windeyer Committee (Annual Report 1970), but it was not even partially implemented in dental schools until the nineteen eighties!

The Windeyer Committee was not a statutory body and no professional or governmental action resulted from its publication and endorsement by the four bodies concerned in 1969 (Annual Report 1970). The position with regard to the specific postgraduate training remained static for nearly a decade until the Wylie Working Party, composed of representatives from the same organisations as the Windeyer Committee, reported in 1978[270] meanwhile the use of general anaesthesia in outpatient dental surgery continued to decrease[231,271] as the nation's dental health improved and, at the same time, the use of sedative techniques, or conscious sedation for conservative work, increased.[231,244] The Department of Health did not regard sedation or general anaesthesia for conservation to be clinically necessary and declined to make an NHS fee available for its use, but in 1967 they consented to the dentist charging a private fee if the patient requested an "anaesthetic" even though the treatment itself was being funded by the National Health Service.[272]

The technique of ultra-light intermittent methohexitone continued to be administered and actively taught by Drummond-Jackson[225] and his colleagues in SAAD. They maintained the convention that, despite its narrow therapeutic margin, the ultra-light intravenous methohexitone technique was a technique of conscious sedation. The SAAD courses continued to be virtually the only nationally available postgraduate training for dentists in the United Kingdom. Drummond-Jackson died unexpectedly in 1975;[225] after that SAAD began to turn their attention to the more generally acceptable sedation techniques and gradually but reluctantly abandoned the teaching of the ultra-light method altogether in the early nineteen eighties.

Stanley Drummond-Jackson[225] deserves more credit than the members of the anaesthetic establishment were (perhaps are!) prepared to give him, but his confrontational stance did not help his cause. He demonstrated the inherent safety of the intermittent use of the intravenous barbiturates when cautiously and skilfully administered, and he brought a very considerable number of nervous patients within the orbit of conservative dentistry. How many of these could have been managed by other methods it is impossible to estimate. At the time of the introduction in 1956 of his ultra-light intermittent methohexitone technique however, it was the only satisfactory method available for handling such cases short of full general endotracheal anaesthesia but, by the time Drummond-Jackson died in 1975, intermittent methohexitone was beginning to be replaced by other conscious sedation techniques with a wider therapeutic margin, and not least by improved attention to sympathetic behavioural management (or "chairside manner") on the part of the dentist, the study of which had been stimulated anew by the development of pain control techniques.

It is interesting that that great pioneer physician anaesthetist Sir Frederic Hewitt promoted an Act of Parliament which would have ensured that only medical practitioners would have been permitted to administer anaesthesia. This Act would have undoubtedly become law if the outbreak of the Great War had not intervened in 1914.[273] The question may well be asked "would a great deal of friction between the medical and dental professions have been avoided by the passage of this Act?", or would the lawyers, and perhaps even Sir Frederic himself, have had difficulty in distinguishing between general anaesthesia and conscious sedation?

Fees for the administration of anaesthetics to NHS dental patients in General Dental Practice. Little progress was made during the sixties in improving either the fees or the iniquitous "pool" system under which they were paid in the NHS. The basic problem was that, from the inception of the NHS, dental anaesthetics, unlike all other anaesthetics, were considered to be dental "items of service"; moreover the operating dentist was paid a fee by the NHS for administering the anaesthetic himself in addition to that paid for the dentistry, provided the anaesthetic was considered to be "clinically necessary", whereas, if a medical anaesthetist was called in, the dentist was paid the fee which theoretically he shared with the anaesthetist. The convention mentioned earlier which enabled a private fee to be charged for sedation or anaesthesia if it was not strictly "clinically necessary", was deemed to apply in most cases,[272] in British practice, general anaesthesia could usually be regarded as essential in many cases of exodontia.

The basic fee per case for anaesthesia was not large; in the sixties it was about £1.50 (1996: £15) and by 1978, after rampant inflation (Chapter 8), it had only risen to £2 (1996: £6.50). The equivalent minimum 1935 National Insurance Fee had been "half a guinea" (£0.53) with a 1996 purchasing power of £20)! The dentist often kept back a small portion of the fee for overheads (after all his portion of the fee was subject to income tax and he probably supplied and maintained the anaesthetic apparatus as well as providing the nitrous oxide and oxygen). The anaesthetist, out of his share, had to pay income tax, his travelling expenses, the cost of supplementary drugs such as halothane and methohexitone and provide personal equipment for anaesthesia and resuscitation;[274] obviously if the dental surgeon collected a number of cases together for an anaesthetic session, attendance by a medical anaesthetist became more worthwhile.

> *"The level of the fee was fixed on the recommendation of the Dental Rates Study Group [of the Department of Health] but since its sole source was the 'Dental Pool' [a fixed annual government allocation out of which all dental fees were paid], any increase in anaesthetic fees would ipso facto have to be paid at the expense of some purely dental item of service".*[274]

The Association of Anaesthetists was concerned that this financial arrangement gave little incentive to the participation of Consultant Anaesthetists in the administration of anaesthetics in general dental practice, thus negating its express desire to improve standards; however, despite the fact that outpatient dental anaesthetics was an interest of the minority of Members of the Association of Anaesthetists, they were a significant and vociferous minority who persistently bombarded Council with correspondence and memoranda (Council Minutes 1963-1969).[155] The Officers and Council did their best by pressing the British Medical and Dental Associations, and through them the Department of Health, for a change. Numerous meetings were held between the professional bodies, and jointly with the Ministry of Health, but to no avail. The Annual Reports for the years 1963 to 1969 indicate increasing frustration. The 1966 Annual Report wryly comments "It is encouraging to learn that the Ministry [of Health] has now recognised that fees for dental anaesthesia are a matter of interest to the medical as well as the dental profession"; and included an attempted "withdrawal of service" from NHS practice by medical anaesthetists in 1977 however, the dispute was to carry over into the next decade (Chapter 8).[274,275]

Fees for private practice

Private fees, both within the private wings of NHS hospitals and in private nursing homes continued to be a source of concern to Council of the Association of Anaesthetists throughout the sixties. This was both with regard to the level of the fees and with discontent over the mechanism by which they were paid; to some extent this is still the case in the nineties (Annual Report 1992).[276]

A revised memorandum concerning the statutory scale of fees which might be charged in NHS Hospitals under the NIIS Regulations (Statutory Instrument 1953. No. 420) was submitted to the Ministry of Health, by the Association of Anaesthetists through the BMA, in 1964 (Annual Report 1964).[277] The new memorandum was an amended version of that prepared by (Sir) Geoffrey Organe[156] in 1956 (Council Minutes 5.7.1963 and 6. 9. 1963 and 5.6.1964).[155] The maximum fee which could be charged under the regulations in 1964 for a private anaesthetic for a *major* operation in an NHS hospital was seven guineas (1996: £73.50); this compared with ten guineas

(1996: £110) to a surgeon for a most *minor* operation.[277] Comparable figures in 1996 might be £200 for an anaesthetic for a major abdominal operation and £100 surgeon's fee for a minor procedure.[278]

The Statutory Scale for patients in NHS hospital private beds was abolished during 1966 however (Annual Report 1966); from then on the principal negotiations with the Provident societies were over their practice of allocating a single global sum for the fees for an operation to be divided between the surgeon and the anaesthetist, and leaving it to the surgeon to reach agreement with the anaesthetist about the percentage of the global fee which should reasonably be paid to the anaesthetist. Negotiations with the Provident Societies in the sixties "were unrewarding" (O P Dinnick personal communication). Negotiations with the surgeons can not have been easy either as, at that time, and for many years thereafter, they collected the whole fee and passed a percentage on to the anaesthetist; however, Archibald Galley[254] (Chairman of the BMA Anaesthetists' Group) reported to Council in May 1966 that it had been accepted that "if the anaesthetist and the surgeon agree to abide by any schedule of the Provident Societies, the anaesthetist's share of the fee should be five guineas (1996: £55) plus 20% of the surgeon's fee. This proposed fee was to include pre- and postoperative visits and the setting up of an intravenous infusion during the course of the procedure (Council Minutes 6.5.1966). The position in 1998 is still not satisfactory and has been further complicated by ruling of the Monopolies and Mergers Commission in 1994 concerning the list of guidelines fees for anaesthesia and surgery issued by theBMA (Chapter 9).[279]

Operating Theatre Technicians

R H Higgs, a senior Operating Theatre Technician (OTT), speaking at the Fourth World Congress of Anaesthesiologists in 1968, traced the ancestry of his profession back to the "handlers" and "beadles" who restrained surgical patients in pre-anaesthetic days;[280] be that as it may, there were undoubtedly male Operating Theatre Attendants or Porters in civilian hospitals between the First and the Second World Wars. They were doubtless still needed to restrain the patient during the induction of anaesthesia, especially before the intravenous barbiturates were introduced, but their main function was to fetch patients from the wards and to lift them on to the table in the operating theatre. They often learned to adjust the operating light to the satisfaction of the surgeon and looked after the larger unsterile items of equipment in the operating theatre such as the lithotomy poles, the diathermy machine, and the then simple anaesthetic machine which was still amenable to the use of the screwdriver. They also, to a greater or lesser extent, assisted the anaesthetist with his relatively simple techniques. The professional nursing staff of the prewar operating theatre, which looked after the aseptic and the antiseptic needs of the surgeon, would be almost entirely female, being composed of the familiar grades of Theatre Sister, Staff Nurses and Student Nurses. There would also probably be a "maid" to brew tea and scrub and polish between operating lists.[280]

There was however a very different staffing structure in the military hospital operating theatre during the Second World War, in which many of those who became postwar civilian consultants in the NHS began their specialist careers (Chapter 5). There were no pupil or noncommissioned female personnel in the Armed Services in those days. The only lady member of the team would be the commissioned Theatre Sister, and her staff would consist of a hierarchy of male other ranks. The latter, in addition to supporting the work of the surgeon, were responsible for the Medical Officer anaesthetist's equipment and became his assistant in his increasingly complex tasks which included transfusion, resuscitation and endotracheal intubation.

The new breed of postwar professional physician anaesthetists in the District General Hospitals, equally with those in Teaching Hospitals, were consequently used to, and needed, a male assistant to assist them and look after their apparatus. The older theatre attendants extended their role and were joined by a considerable number of demobilised other rank exservicemen looking for careers in the NHS similar to those in which they had felt fulfilled in wartime. The former Operating Theatre "Orderly", or "Attendant" or "Porter" thus became the "Operating Theatre Technician" (OTT); however, the Department of Health failed, or chose not, to recognise that the OTT in the NHS had much enhanced status and increased responsibilities in comparison with his predecessor the Operating Theatre "Attendant" or "Porter", and declined to pay him what he was worth, or put him on a satisfactory incremental scale reflecting career experience. Anaesthetists and the Association of Anaesthetists were deeply concerned about the plight of their valuable technical colleagues; however, despite frequent memoranda, committees, and conferences with health officials, the establishment of a qualification, and a change of name to Operating Department Assistant (ODA), little progress in improving status or remuneration resulted throughout the sixties, seventies and eighties in the face of the obstinate bureaucracy at the Department of Health.[281] It has only been in the early nineteen nineties that the pecuniary lot of their successors (now having their name changed once again to "Operating Department Practitioner", ODP) has been improved to a level comparable to that of the nurses but, at the time of writing in 1998 they still await the accolade of professional registration.[276,282]

(Sir) Ivan Magill[283] was one of the first to recognise the importance of the OTT. This was not surprising, as he was engaged in thoracic anaesthesia which was a pioneer subspecialty involving complicated technical manoeuvres such as endobronchial intubation for which trained assistance was essential. Magill was instrumental in persuading a group of OTTs in London to form the Association of Operating Theatre Technicians (AOTT) in 1945.[280]

The Association of Anaesthetists drew the attention of the Ministry of Health to the poor pay and conditions of these essential members of the operating theatre team in 1950 (Annual Report 1950). The 1953 Annual Report notes that "Council has been glad to learn that the Association of Operating Theatre Technicians has now been accepted by the Board of Registration of Medical Auxiliaries"; but this was a hollow victory. It did not mean professional registration for the OTTs which would enable them to claim higher pay within the NHS.

Shackleton[3] informed the 1964 Annual General Meeting[155] that a meeting with the OTTs was about to take place at the request of the AOTT to discuss the possibility of establishing a Diploma. Peter Dinnick (Honorary Secretary) reported to Council that, Shackleton[3] (Vice President), T Cecil Gray (the Dean of the Faculty) and Dinnick himself had met Messrs Faulkner, Higgs and Vince of the AOTT (Council Minutes 8.1.1965).[155] A Memorandum was presented asking the Association of Anaesthetists to support the AOTT in forming an academic body to prepare a syllabus for a diploma, with a view to seeking recognition by the Ministry of Health. Some members of the Council of the Association of Anaesthetists expressed doubts about the desirability of OTTs gaining professional status at all (it may even have been that the spectre of a grade of technician anaesthetist once again raised its ugly head!). Great sympathy was felt for the plight of the OTTs however, and it was decided to approach the Chief Medical Officer at the Ministry of Health (Council Minutes 8.1.1965).[155] This decision was, however, reversed at the next Council Meeting on 5 March 1965 (Council Minutes 5.3.1965), and it was decided to set up a Subcommittee under Shackleton[3] instead to consider the educational requirements and future role of the OTTs.

The Ministry of Health was, however, also giving some consideration to the position of the OTTs and later in 1965 issued a circular on the matter (Training and Duties of Operating Theatre Attendants HM (65) 76). The Subcommittee made a report to Council on Circular HM (65) 76 on 3 December 1965.[155] They noted that the document "at least recognised that the Operating Theatre Attendants [sic] were a distinct group of men and that they needed special training". A six months period of training was proposed (the Association of Anaesthetists' Subcommittee thought that this was too short) and a Trainee Grade below OTT and a Higher Grade above OTT was suggested. The Honorary Secretary was asked to write to the Department of Health "for clarification and to enquire about the proposed salary scales" (Council Minutes 3.12.1965).[155]

The 1966 Annual Report was hopeful but the 1967 Report and intervening Council Minutes report "little progress" despite interviews with the Chief Medical Officer and considerable correspondence with the Ministry. The authorities were obviously determined to procrastinate (Council Minutes 7.7.1967).[155]

Another Memorandum was sent to the Ministry of Health for the attention of the Zuckerman Committee on Hospital Scientific and Technical Services in 1968 (Annual Report 1968), but in its report that Committee specifically excluded OTTs from their consideration (Annual Report 1969).

The decade ended with the depressing acknowledgment that "The deadlock over the pay and career structure [of OTTs] still exists" (Annual Report 1969), but the Association of Anaesthetists nonetheless hopefully gave evidence to "The Joint Subcommittee of the Standing Medical Advisory Committee and the Standing Nursing Advisory Committee of the Ministry of Health on the Organisation and Staffing of Operating Departments" (the Lewin Committee) which was destined to report in 1970 (Annual Report 1969), but, in the event, the ambitious recommendations of the Lewin Report resulted in only minimal improvement in the lot of OTTs (Chapters 9 and 10).[284]

The Annual Meetings of the Association 1960-1969

All the Annual Meetings of the Association of Anaesthetists in the nineteen sixties were held in October or the first half of November. The successful practice of combining an Annual General Meeting with an increasingly sophisticated scientific programme, which had been established in the late fifties, continued, and a pattern of holding meetings in alternate years in London and elsewhere in the British Isles developed. The 1961 Annual Meeting took place outside the United Kingdom for the first time. It was held in Dublin, the capital of the Republic of Ireland, the other constituency of the Association of Anaesthetists; in 1965 the Annual Meeting was in Edinburgh, the Scottish capital, and, in 1967 in Belfast, the capital of the United Kingdom Province of Northern Ireland.[285-300] The Association was host to the Fourth World Congress of Anaesthesiologists in September 1968 and, consequently only an Annual General (business) meeting was held.

Annual Meetings of the Association of Anaesthetists of Great Britain and Ireland 1960-1969

Year	Location	Members Attending
1960	Royal College of Surgeons of England, London	c.200
1961	Dublin, Republic of Ireland	310
1962	Royal College of Surgeons of England, London	275
1963	Harrogate, England	270
1964	Royal College of Surgeons of England, London	290
1965	Edinburgh, Scotland	330
1966	Russell Hotel, London	(not recorded)
1967	Belfast	230
1968	Business Meeting only, Royal Society of Medicine, London	49
1969	Manchester, England	248

The 1961 Annual Meeting in Dublin was an outstanding success both scientifically[285] and socially.[286] The present writer remembers only a somewhat kaleidoscopic medley of brilliant receptions at the Royal Colleges in Ireland, a presentation of a peculiarly Irish play at the Abbey Theatre, a convivial luncheon at the Guinness Brewery and an Annual Dinner attended by over 500 members and guests (Annual Report 1962).[286] The profits of the meeting were £205.0s.10d (1996: £2,500) and were donated to the funds of the Faculty of Anaesthetists of the Royal College of Surgeons in Ireland which had been founded in 1959 (Council Minutes 8.1.1960[151] and Annual Report 1962).[287]

The 1963 Annual Meeting at Harrogate was notable for the construction of a mock-up of an anaesthetic induction room by the British Oxygen Company and equipped in association with other commercial companies at a cost of £3,000 (1996: £33,000) (Council Minutes 7.12.1962 and 5.7.1963).[151,155] This project was largely the brainchild of R E Loder of Peterborough, a member of Council and a member of a Subcommittee set up to advise members on planning new departments of anaesthesia and operating theatres (Annual Report 1964 and Council Minutes 2.6.1961).[151] Registrants at the Harrogate meeting were asked to fill in a questionnaire and make suggestions and Robert Loder published a consensus view in *Anaesthesia* in 1964.[288] The initiative created great interest but sadly the Ministry of Health issued its Hospital Building Note 22 on Operating Department design without consulting the Association of Anaesthetists (Council Minutes 7.2.1964).[155] A protest was made! The demonstration Anaesthetic Room was exhibited again by the King Edward VII Hospital Fund for London in 1965 and Members of Council took part in an associated symposium (Council Minutes 13.11.1964: Annual Report 1965).[155]

The 1965 Meeting in Edinburgh was also a most enjoyable occasion in that beautiful city. The Association of Anaesthetists was honoured both by the delivery of the first Sir James Young Simpson Memorial Lecture entitled "James Y Simpson. *Victor dolore*", appropriately delivered by the great man's successor R J Kellar, Professor of Obstetrics at Edinburgh, and by the John Snow Lecture on the "Evaluation of drugs" by Sir Derrick Dunlop (Annual Report 1966).[289] The scientific business included, a symposium on recovery rooms (by no means universal in British hospitals at that time), and a prototype recovery room exhibit in the technical exhibition, which was once again provided by the British Oxygen Company (Council Minutes 9.10.1964).[155,290]

The 1967 Meeting in Belfast featured a very successful scientific programme (as one might expect under the guidance of Professor John Dundee)[291] and a pleasant social programme in a city not then torn apart by sectarian violence.[299]

Trade exhibitions at the Annual Meetings

There was a small trade exhibition organised by that doyen of anaesthetic apparatus manufacturers Charles King[292] at the 1960 Annual Meeting at the Royal College of Surgeons of England (Council Minutes 4.3.1960).[151] The first major trade exhibition of any size was that organised by the Irish anaesthetists for the Dublin[286] meeting in 1961 which brought in exhibitors' fees of £655 (1996: £7,925). Another small exhibition was held at the meeting at the Royal College of Surgeons of England in 1962. This was organised by Jarman,[1,293] the reigning President (Council Minutes 1.12.1961).[1,151,293,294]

"Two large corridors" were available for a trade exhibition in the Royal Hall at the very successful Annual Meeting in Harrogate in 1963 (Council Minutes 7.12.1962).[151] This exhibition was very satisfactorily organised by T G H Wiley Ltd, a firm of exhibition contractors (O P Dinnick personal communication)[295] but, despite the trade exhibitors' fees there was a deficit of £23 (1996: £250) on the meeting as a whole (Annual Report 1964). The trade exhibitors were very pleased with the amount of space provided at Harrogate but, despite this and the expression of some misgiving about the venue (Council Minutes 1.11.1963),[155] the 1964 Annual Meeting was held at the Royal College of Surgeons of England in London and T G H Wiley Ltd were again engaged to organise the exhibition. The space available was certainly restricted and the administrative authorities at the surgeons' College were not expecting the noise and disruption occasioned by the erection of exhibition stands; moreover, these had to be set up in limited time with additional labour due to another function being held in the College the previous evening. Relations with the administrators of the Royal College of Surgeons were consequently considerably strained (O P Dinnick personal communication). This technical exhibition was run at a loss although there was apparently a profit of £202 (1996: £2,120) on the meeting as a whole (Council Minutes 9.10.1964[155] & Annual Report 1965).[296] The Edinburgh

Annual Meeting in 1965 also included a trade exhibition. An overall surplus on the meeting of £57 (1996: £590) was recorded (Annual Report 1966).[297]

More ambitious plans for an exhibition were made for the 1966 Annual Meeting in London. The Russell Hotel was chosen as the venue and T G H Wylie Ltd were once again engaged as exhibition organisers. There were 27 stands but T G H Wylie Ltd had planned for five more which they failed to sell. This was possibly partly due to a concurrent American Exhibition of Medical Equipment in London (Council Minutes 10.11.1966).[155] The exhibition should nevertheless have made a surplus of £1,314 (1996: £11,800); unfortunately T G H Wylie Ltd became insolvent and went bankrupt owing this sum to the Association of Anaesthetists. This could not be recovered and, on solicitor's advice, it was written off as a bad debt in the 1968 accounts (Council Minutes 1.12.1967, Annual Reports 1967 & 1968, and personal communication).[155]

The Trade Exhibition had, however, become an established and financially important element at the Annual Meetings, (even at the last Annual Meeting held at the Royal College of Surgeons of England in 1970 despite the 1964 contretemps described above).[298] There were 29 stands in Belfast in 1967,[299] and in 1969 in Manchester 25 stands,[300] (there being no Association Annual Scientific Meeting in 1968 because of the World Congress).

The Association and Europe

The European Economic Community (EEC) came into being on 1 January 1958 under the terms of the Treaty of Rome; in 1961 the United Kingdom began negotiations with a view to joining. John Beard attended "a long and complicated meeting conducted in France, of representatives of the original EEC countries as an observer in 1962 (Council Minutes 7.12.1962).[151] The purpose of the meeting was to determine the position of anaesthesia in the EEC; but, after the British bid to join was rejected early in 1963, the Association of Anaesthetists disbanded the Subcommittee which had been formed to consider EEC matters (Council Minutes 6.12.1963);[155] subsequently however, despite the rejection, the Association continued to be asked to send observers to the meetings of the EEC "Union Européenne des Médecine Spécialistes" to keep a watching brief. Patrick Shackleton[3] and Douglas Howat were appointed as representatives in 1966 (Annual Report 1966). They subsequently reported having attended a meeting at which considerable differences emerged about the length of training required for specialist anaesthetists (Council Minutes 1.4.1966). United Kingdom entry into the EEC again began to be a possibility in the second half of the decade (Council Minutes 7.10.1966) and in 1968, Shackleton,[3] Howat and Organe[155] attended a meeting called by the Royal College of Physicians of London to examine the implications of possible EEC Membership (Annual Report 1968). The United Kingdom finally joined the EEC on 1 January 1973 and thereafter the Association of Anaesthetists of Great Britain and Ireland has played a leading part in shaping the development of the specialty in Europe.[301]

The Association was also active in the affairs of the European Region Section of the WFSA. Douglas Howat was the Association of Anaesthetists' representative on the Standing Professional Committee of that body (Annual Report 1967).

International and National Congresses 1960-1969

The Minute Books,[151,155] Annual Reports, and the News items in *Anaesthesia* (1960-1969) indicate that the Association of Anaesthetists was officially represented at most international and foreign national meetings during the period.

These included three World and two European Congresses under the auspices of the burgeoning WFSA.

World Congresses of Anaesthesiologists

2nd - 1960 Toronto, Canada
1,700 delegates and associates from 23 countries[302]

3rd - 1964 Sao Paulo, Brazil
"Over 1,500" delegates from 42 countries[303]

4th - 1968 London, England
2,437 anaesthesiologists, "over 350" trainees and 923 family members from 66 countries[155]

European Congresses of Anaesthesiology

1st - 1962 Vienna, Austria
"Nearly 2,000 delegates" from all over the world[304]

2nd - 1966 Copenhagen, Denmark
"181 papers". "17 symposia"[305]

The Second World Congress in Toronto in 1960[302] was notable as the occasion when the United States joined the WFSA.

The Third World Congress in Sao Paulo in 1964[303] saw the election of (Sir) Geoffrey Organe as President of the WFSA after nine gruelling years as the first Secretary-Treasurer.

The First European Congress in Vienna in 1962[304] started out as a venture initiated by the European Societies themselves (Annual General Meeting 1957 & Council Minutes 3.10.1958)[151] but was later taken under the wing of the Executive Committee of the WFSA as the First Regional European Congress of Anaesthesiology (Council Minutes 7.10.1961).[151] The Congress was an outstanding success and reflected great credit on the organisers led by Professor Otto Mayrhofer.[304] It laid the foundation for the important series of European Congresses which have taken place every four years and have attracted delegates from all the WFSA Regions at the halfway mark between World Congresses of Anaesthesiology, which are also spaced at four year intervals.

The Fourth World Congress of Anaesthesiology 1968

The Association of Anaesthetists issued its invitation to the WFSA to hold the Fourth World Congress of Anaesthesiology in London in July 1964 (Council Minutes 24.7.1964)[155] and its delegates returned from the Third World Congress in Sao Paulo with a verbal acceptance of the proposal (Council Minutes 9.10.1964).[306]

A provisional booking of the entire Festival Hall complex for 9-12 September 1968 had already been made by the Officers of the Association by the Council Meeting on 9 October 1964. Peter Dinnick, the Honorary Secretary, recalled his "trepidation on being dispatched to book the Festival Hall Complex and to pledge a sum almost equal to the Association's total resources" (O P Dinnick personal communication).

The Organising Committee of the Congress was appointed as a Subcommittee of Council in January 1965 after written confirmation had been received of the acceptance of the invitation of the Association of Anaesthetists (Council Minutes 8.1.1965:[155] Annual Report 1965). All members of the Committee were present or past Members of Council with the exception of the Chairman George Ellis (1909-1998) of St Bartholomew's Hospital, and they in turn, as Chairmen of Subcommittees, gathered their own teams around them.[155] Patrick Shackleton,[3] who had represented the Association on the WFSA Council was chosen to be President of the Congress (Council Minutes 2.7.1965: Annual Report 1965). H H (Tony) Pinkerton,[2] had taken over as President of the Association at the Annual General Meeting in October 1965 but, with the courtesy which reflected his personal modesty despite his considerable public achievements, he intimated his intention of not seeking re-election at the end of 1967. This enabled Pat Shackleton to be both President of the Association of Anaesthetists of Great Britain and Ireland and President of the Congress during 1968. This gesture, in fact, ended the previous tradition of three year Presidential terms of Office; with the single exception of Philip Helliwell, (Chapter 8)[7] all subsequent Presidents have had two-year terms.

The choice of George Harold Ellis as Chairman of the Congress Organising Committee from outside the immediate circle of past and present Council Members, was inspired. George had a reputation for an uncomplicated and relaxed approach as an anaesthetist. He was noted for his outward sang-froid at times of stress, and for kindness, loyalty and very generous hospitality to his contemporaries and his juniors alike. He needed all these qualities as head of a virtually independent organisation which, starting from nothing, ultimately had a budget of nearly £100,000 (1996: £925,000),[155] and a responsibility to at least break even. His unruffled approach to problems, his ability to make rapid decisions (sometimes not without an element of risk!), his careful selection of his coworkers, and his capacity to delegate to them and to trust them, promoted harmony amongst the Members of the Organising Committee and thereby contributed greatly to the success of the Congress.

The Secretariat and the general administrative organisation of the Congress was placed in the hands of Miss P R Cridland, a professional Congress Organiser (Council Minutes 2.5.1969).[155] Her confident and accurate predictions of the ultimate attendance figure as early registrations were received was a considerable reassurance to the Members of the Organising

Committee (Annual Report 1968).

The Congress received Royal recognition when Her Majesty the Queen was graciously pleased to grant her patronage (Annual General Meeting 1969).[155]

The 1968 Fourth World Congress Organising Committee

(Past, contemporary or later office in the Association Council in brackets).

President of the WFSA	Sir Geoffey Organe[156] (President 1953-56)
Congress President	R P W Shackleton[3] (President 1967-69)
Chairman	G H Ellis (Vice President 1969-71)
Vice Chairman	C B Lewis[307] (Council 1965-68)
Senior Committee Member	R Jarman (Council 1958-65, President 1959-62)
Committee Hon Treasurer	F G Wood-Smith[308] (Council 1957-60)
Association Hon Treasurer	A J W Beard[4] (Council 1960-1963, President 1969-1971)
Committee Hon Secretary	D D C Howat (Council 1964-67 and 1978-81, Honorary Treasurer 1969-74)
Association Hon Secretaries	O P Dinnick (1963-66) (Council 1961-63 and 1966-68) P J Helliwell (1966-68)[7] (Council 1963-66, President 1973-76)
Scientific Programme	C F Scurr (Council 1956-65, President 1976-78)
Site Arrangements	R B Wright (Council 1965-68)
Scientific Exhibition	I R Verner (Pask Award 1992)
Technical Exhibition	G E H Enderby (Council 1966-68)
Social Programme	S A Mason (Council 1969-72, Honorary Treasurer 1974-78, President 1978-80)

Ladies Committee	Mrs O P Dinnick (Wife of the Honorary Secretary 1963-66)
Publications and Proceedings	T B Boulton (Assistant Editor *Anaesthesia* 1964-73, Editor *Anaesthesia* 1973-82, President 1984-86)
Public Relations	H C Churchill-Davidson (Westminster Hospital)
Secretariat	Miss P R Cridland, Congress Organiser

The funding of the Congress was started with an interest free loan of £1,000 (1996: £9,250) from the Association (Council Minutes 5.3.1965).[155] George Ellis imposed a strict financial discipline on Organising Committee Members. All were asked to pay a full Registration Fee of £25 (1996: £230) and to act as personal guarantors against the Congress making a loss to the tune of £200 (1996: £1,850) apiece (Council Minutes 6.5.1966 & Annual Report 1967). The writer remembers that the latter seemed to be a considerable sum for a young wholetime Consultant with a growing family to put at risk but, fortunately "money on the table" was not required! Wood-Smith[308] (the Honorary Treasurer of the Congress), Enderby, Jarman[1] and others, armed with the information that Committee Members themselves were prepared to personally underwrite the Congress, went forth to secure major guarantors. This they did very successfully (Council Minutes 6.5.1966 & Annual Report 1967).[155] Guarantors included £10,000 (1996: £92,500) each by the British Oxygen Company Committee, and Imperial Chemical Industries, £5,000 (1996: £46,250) each by May and Baker Ltd and Vickers Ltd, and, by Arthur Guinness Ltd, £2,500 (1996: £23,125) (Annual Report 1967). Considerable sums were also raised from the trade and others in the form of donations (Annual Report 1967). A request to the Council for International Organisations of Medical Sciences (a United Nations body) for a loan was refused (Council Minutes 5.3.1965 and 23.9.1965).[155] The Dean of the Faculty informed the Committee that the President of the Royal College of Surgeons of England raised no objection to the College being named as cosponsors of the Congress, but there was no financial commitment (Council Minutes 6.5.1966)![155] The Association of Anaesthetists itself made a further loan of £4,000 (1996:

£37,000) to the Organising Committee from the Research and Education Trust Fund in January 1967 pending the receipt of registration fees (Council Minutes 10.11.1966 and 6.1.1967).[155] The Association also lent £800 (1996: £7,400) to the Congress Committee to enable eight of its members to attend the Second European Congress in Copenhagen in 1966 to publicise the Congress and to gain further insight into the methods of organising a large Congress (Council Minutes 1.5. 1966).[155]

The Registration Fees for the Congress were set at £25 (1996: £230) with an additional late registration fee of £5 (1996: £46).[154] The writer recalls that these were considered to be excessive by a number of British anaesthetists and some consumer resistance resulted. It may be observed, however, that experience with the organisation of subsequent international congresses has revealed a reluctance on the part of some individuals in host countries to pay appropriate fees compared in absolute terms with the registration fees asked for one or two day national meetings; however, the same individuals seem to happily pay the same level of fees to congresses which they attend in other countries without undue protest! A suggestion made by Cyril Scurr, (Chairman of the Scientific Programme Committee) that there could be a special day registration rate of £2.50 (1996: £23) for Senior Registrars and Registrars sponsored by Members of the Association was accepted (Council Minutes 7.7.1967).[155] A corps of Senior Registrar Stewards was also recruited on a basis of one day's service for one day's free registration at the Congress. These stewards gave invaluable service under firm but kindly Naval discipline imposed by Surgeon Lieutenant Commander A L Revell (now, in 1998, Vice Admiral).

The registration fees raised over £90,000 (1996: £800,000) from 2,437 full Congress participants, 389 day Members and 923 accompanying family members, and this sum, together with donations and dues from 73 trade exhibitors from 12 countries, enabled the Congress to make a surplus of £4,715 (1996: £43,700) after all loans had been repaid. One thousand pounds (1996: £9,250) of this sum was donated to the WFSA to be used as a loan for future World Congress organisers, a further £1,000 was made over to the WFSA earmarked for educational purposes, and £2,715 (1996: £25,000) was retained in the Research and Education Trust Fund of the Association of Anaesthetists "for a research and educational project, not necessarily in this country [the

United Kingdom]" (Annual Report 1968: Annual General Meeting 1968: Council Minutes 5.2.1971).[155]

The Scientific Programme in the five halls of the Royal Festival Hall Complex was organised with great precision by Cyril Scurr. There were seventeen symposia and thirteen Free Paper sessions as well as a continuous programme of medical films. The subjects covered the growth points of the specialty of anaesthesia and intensive care in 1968, and included computer applications, circulatory and ventilatory physiology, pharmokinetics, communication, training, monitoring, the development of apparatus, toxicity of anaesthetics, intensive care, pain therapy and paediatric and neurological anaesthesia. A comprehensive proceedings volume was published in the International Congress Series of the Excerpta Medica Foundation of Amsterdam on a 'no profit, no loss' basis. It included the full text of over 95% of all the papers presented at the Congress.[155,309]

The Fourth World Congress of Anaesthesiology was indeed an important milestone for the specialty both in the United Kingdom and worldwide. It took place against a background of great political disturbance (the tanks of the USSR had entered Prague, the capital of Czechoslovakia on 20 August 1968) and at a time of uncertainty in the British NHS, but despite this it was an enormously successful scientific and social event. R B Wright, of St Thomas' Hospital, London, a Member of the Organising Committee in his Congress Retrospect in *Anaesthesia*[309] admirably captured the wonderful spirit of comradeship and common purpose that prevailed amongst physician anaesthetists whatever their nationality, creed or colour. The Fourth World Congress in London was undoubtedly the largest, and most important and spectacular meeting of anaesthetists that had been held up to that date, and it set a standard for the future; once again the Association of Anaesthetists of Great Britain and Ireland had blazed a trail. The knighthood for Geoffrey Organe[156] and the honour bestowed on Patrick Shackleton[3] (Commander of the Order of the British Empire) were fitting accompaniments (Annual Report 1968). The only note of sadness was that the Queen's cousin, Her Royal Highness Princess Alexandra who had been elected an Honorary Fellow of the Faculty of Anaesthetists in 1967,[310] was unable to open the Congress due to the death of her mother, the much loved and respected Princess Marina, Duchess of Kent.[306,309]

Messrs Hempsons, Solicitors to the Congress and the Association of Anaesthetists

An important by-product of the Congress was the adoption of Messrs Hempsons, first as legal advisers to the Congress and thereafter to the Association of Anaesthetists (Council Minutes 6.5.1966);[155] thus began a long and important professional association which has continued to the present time. Hempsons gave much advice to the Organising Committee during the years of preparation for the Congress. This was specifically directed to the question of financial liability in the case of failure to achieve a remunerative level of attendance. The legal fact that all Members of the Association of Anaesthetists were liable in case of failure was overcome by the generosity of guarantors. The possibility of failure was anticipated in 1980 when the Association organised the Sixth European Congress by the formation of a limited liability Company and, in 1985 it was considered wise to incorporate the Association of Anaesthetists itself and the Education and Research Fund as Limited Companies.

The Association of Anaesthetists and the manufacturers of anaesthetic equipment

Richard Bodman (Hillingdon and St Peter's and St Paul's Hospitals, London) drew attention to the poor showing of British manufacturers at foreign congresses in September 1963 (Council Minutes 6.9.1963) and, in December (Council Minutes 6.12.1963).[155] He reported that the Board of Trade was willing to assist, but only if the Association of Anaesthetists or some other body would sign a contract to supervise the exhibits. Council deferred its decision for further information but, in February 1964, Bodman stated that the replies of 23 firms which he had approached about the possibility of forming a Trade Association sponsored by the Association of Anaesthetists had not been enthusiastic. Council therefore decided that the only action they could take was to offer to act as a source of information about foreign congresses (Council Minutes 7.2 .1964).[155]

G E Hale Enderby, one of the very successful fund raising and organisers of the technical exhibition at the Fourth World Congress, again raised the question of the formation of a "joint working party with the trade" in a Memorandum to Council at the end of 1968 (Council Minutes 1.11.1968).[150]

A Subcommittee to consider the matter was formed. The Council Minutes show that there was a considerable difference of opinion in Council over the question of the Association of Anaesthetists, as a professional body being directly involved in a trade organisation (Council Minutes 10.12.1968 and 17.2.1969) but, after the deliberations of a Joint Working Party formed with the manufacturers, Council agreed in May 1969 "that the Association should take the initiative in setting up the proposed Group [of manufacturers of anaesthetic equipment]" (Council Minutes 2.5.1969).[155] Draft Articles of Association were drawn up by the Joint Working Party for an Association initially composed of 12 invited manufacturers with the Association of Anaesthetists as a subscribing member (Council Minute 4.7.1969). The proposal was referred to the Association of Anaesthetists Advisory Committee whose main function at that time was to advise on constitutional matters. The Minutes of the next meeting of Council in October 1969 imply that the decision of the Advisory Committee was against the Association of Anaesthetists participating directly as a member of the new organisation. It is simply recorded, without preamble, that Council "agreed to accept the Advisory Committee's recommendation that Council should consider favourably the possibility of cooperating with industry in the establishment of a British Pavilion at the Third European Congress in Prague [Czechoslovakia] in 1970". The prime object of this project was to centralise the British exhibits and contributions (Council Minutes 2.10.1969). John Zorab (Bristol) played an important part in advising on the "British Pavilion" on behalf of the Association (Council Minutes 6.2.1970 and 3.7.1970).[155] This was organised with the cooperation of the Government's British Hospitals Export Council and was very successful.[311]

Council was still concerned about possible misunderstanding about the relationship of the profession with the trade however. The Minutes record that Council found it necessary to caution "that it is most undesirable that anaesthetists be involved in staffing or organising the exhibit [in Prague]" (Council Minutes 3.7.1970).[155] There is no doubt, however, that the initiative shown by the Association of Anaesthetists in bringing together various British manufacturers resulted in the foundation of the independent organisation now known as the "British Anaesthetic and Respiratory Equipment Manufacturers Association (BAREMA)" in 1976 (personal communication B R Sugg). The relationship between the Association of Anaesthetists and BAREMA remains close and cordial in 1998. The Council of the Association of Anaesthetists sends representatives to the BAREMA Council, and BAREMA is represented on the Association's Safety Committee and on the Working Party on the limited life of anaesthetic equipment and both are represented on the British and International Standards Commitees.[282] This happy relationship has many mutual benefits and it provides a united front when dealing with the Department of Health and other governmental bodies. The Association of Anaesthetists has reason to be grateful for the support, financial and otherwise, which it has received from the manufacturing houses, including willing participation in the trade exhibitions at its meetings, and in a number of other ways.

Death Certification and Coroners

One of the earliest concerns of the Association in prewar days was the matter of distinguishing between "deaths due to anaesthesia", and "deaths associated with surgical procedures", and considerable progress was made after evidence had been given to the Committee on Coroners which published its report in 1935 (Chapter 4).

The Brodrick Committee on Death Certification and Coroners was appointed by the Government in 1965. The Council of the Association of Anaesthetists appointed a Subcommittee to make recommendations, and evidence was submitted based on a memorandum drawn up by G B Lucas (University College Hospital, London) (Council Minutes 2.7.1965, 6.5.1966, 3.6.1966).[155]

H V Morton[6] (at that time Vice President) and O P Dinnick gave verbal evidence to the Brodrick Committee in 1968 (Annual Report 1968). An important feature of the evidence was the submission of a draft form for reporting deaths under anaesthesia (Council Minutes 1.12.1967 and 5.4.1968).[155] It was gratifying to find that, when the Brodrick Report was finally published in 1971,[312] this form was included unaltered as the basis of a standard form for general use (Annual Report 1971). Versions of this document have since been adopted by many coroners.

Miscellaneous matters in the sixties

The relentless business of advising individual members on such matters as staffing, fees, contracts, etc, went on continuously as it does today in 1998; in the early sixties such problems were often considered by Council itself, but nowadays they are dealt with by the Honorary Secretary and other Officers in personal letters except when principle is involved.

Advice to Government and other bodies. A newsletter to Members published in September 1970[313] gives an impressive list of evidence and memoranda presented to various Government Committees and organisations. Many of these have already been considered in this Chapter and others will be mentioned below. The list of Government Committees included the Platt Committee on Medical Staffing Structure, the Accident Services Review Committee, the Working Party on Ambulance Training and Equipment, the Committee on the Standardisation of Medical Records, the Brodrick Committee on Death Certification, the Bonham Carter Committee on the Function of District General Hospitals, the Zuckerman Committee on Scientific and Technical Services, the Royal Commission on Medical Education (Todd Report 1968), the Working Party on the Organisation of Medical Work ("Cogwheel" Report 1969), the Working Party on the responsibilities of the Consultant Grade and the (Lewin) Working Party on the Staffing of Operating Departments. Other important committees to which verbal or written evidence was given, included the General Medical Council Committee on Basic Education and the BMA Porritt Committee.

Distinction Awards. The relatively low position of anaesthetists in the table of the distribution of NHS Distinction Awards was raised by members of the Association of Anaesthetists several times in the sixties. The Association made representations. There was some improvement towards the end of the decade; in 1965 only 12.7% of anaesthetists in England and Wales had awards whereas by 1969 the percentage had risen to 18.8%.[313] The latest figures available at the time of writing are 28.7% for anaesthetists compared with the overall percentage for all consultants of 34.3% ranging from 20.7% in

Accident and Emergency to 63.8% in immunopathology.[314]

A meeting of "Regional Advisers" was convened by the Association on the suggestion of (Professor) Andrew Hunter[178] of Manchester (Council Minutes 24.7.1964 & 7.5.1965).[155] "Regional Adviser" was not an official position either for the Association or the Faculty of Anaesthetists at the time and the representatives were apparently hand-picked (Council Minutes 24.7.1964).[155] The meeting was held on 1 July 1965 at the Royal College of Surgeons of England and attended by the Officers of the Association of Anaesthetists and (Sir) Geoffrey Organe,[156] the Adviser to the Chief Medical Officer (Council Minutes 2.7.1965).[155] The meeting took place against the background of an acute shortage of both Consultant posts and Junior medical staff. The Annual Report for 1965 records that "a valuable interchange of information took place on a wide range of subjects". One gets the impression from the minutes that this was certainly the case (Council Minutes 2.7.1965).[155] The meeting was unofficial and had no executive power but, as a result of it, the leaders of the specialty were undoubtedly better informed and more appreciative of the problems faced by the rank and file of provincial anaesthetists than perhaps they had been previously, and those at the centre were able to indicate to what extent measures had been initiated already to alleviate some of the difficulties their colleagues were facing. It was agreed that more Consultants were needed if the degree of supervision which was by then being demanded by the Faculty, was to be achieved, the Association position on the Medical Assistant grade was explained and accepted, more uniform provision for study leave for juniors was required, and it was stressed that there was already provision for an increase in the number of Senior Registrars and encouragement was given for appointments which included rotation between Regional and District Hospitals (Council Minutes 2.7.1965).[155]

Medical women anaesthetists. Reform in the immediate postwar period had opened up the previously male dominated medical schools to women, and by the mid sixties Council was aware that a considerable number of ladies were taking up anaesthesia (Annual Report 1967) and their potential as members of the anaesthetic work force, particularly in a time of shortage, was of great importance (Annual Report 1967). The very distinguished

Katherine Lloyd-Williams, CBE,[165] Dean of the Royal Free Hospital Medical School, had served on Council from 1947 to 1950 and had played an important part in the early meetings which led to the establishment of the WFSA (Chapter 6) but, although the Association had to wait until the sixties, the next three ladies were, or subsequently became, equally well known. Margaret Hawksley,[315] of the Hospital for Sick Children, Great Ormond Street, London, one of the earliest specialist paediatric anaesthetists and anaesthetist to the Royal children (appointed Member of the Victorian Order (MVO) in 1969), Aileen Adams of Cambridge (appointed Commander of the Order of the British Empire (CBE) in 1988), and Sheila Kenny, later Vice Dean of the Faculty of Anaesthetists of the Royal College of Surgeons in Ireland). Aileen Adams was the first lady to be elected as an Officer of the Association in 1967 when she became Assistant and then Honorary Secretary in 1968.

The 1969 Annual Report noted that the taxation laws in force "strongly discourages women from remaining in employment", and there were (and to some extent still are) "difficulties experienced by married women in obtaining Consultant posts with less than fulltime or maximum part-time commitment. The Association responded by lobbying both the Chancellor of the Exchequer (Annual Report 1969) and the Postgraduate Deans.[313]

Basic medical education and the relationship of the Association of Anaesthetists with medical students was another area with which Council was deeply concerned. The Association joined the Faculty of Anaesthetists in emphasising the need for the inclusion of anaesthesia in the undergraduate medical curriculum. This they did by lobbying the Royal (Todd) Commission on Medical Education through the General Medical Council (Annual Report 1967).[313] The aim was not to produce a practitioner capable of giving an anaesthetic on qualification, as would have been the case in the past, but to interest suitable students in the work of the specialty so that they might consider it when choosing their future careers. It is interesting in this regard that as late as September 1965 (Council Minutes 1965)[155] a Member of the Association asked what the attitude of Council was to the drawing up of rotas for "Gynaecological Housemen, Medical Housemen and others" to give anaesthetics in Casualty Departments. It was stated (presumably by Organe,[156] the Adviser to the Chief Medical Officer) "that the official Ministry view is that every doctor is entitled to give an anaesthetic but he is also entitled to refuse to give one". The Council also "deplored" anaesthetics being administered by someone insufficiently trained (Council Minutes 3.9.1965).[155]

A guest lecture scheme for student medical societies provided lectures sponsored and paid for by the Association of Anaesthetists was introduced in 1969 (Annual Report 1969) with the same objective of recruitment in view: this initiative met with some success (Annual Report 1970).

Anaesthetic Equipment. The painstaking work of the British and International Standards Organisations (Chapter 6) continued. This was an important area in which O P Dinnick continued to represent effectively the views of the Association of Anaesthetists for several years after he finished his term on Council (Council Minutes 2.10.1969).[155]

The Association of Anaesthetists also advised the Ministry and other bodies on matters of safety related to anaesthetic apparatus. These included assessment of the Bosun and other oxygen failure devices (Council Minutes 7.5.1965: Annual Report 1965), memoranda on anomalies of the colour coding of carbon dioxide fire extinguisher devices (Council Minutes 2.7.1965: Annual Report 1965) and the interchangeability of the connections of larger medical gas cylinders (Annual Report 1961).[151,155]

A proposal to increase the fee charged by the British Oxygen Company for rental of medical gas cylinders caused some sabre rattling (Council Minutes 1.2.1963 and 5.7.1963).[151,155] Council and the Ministry of Health investigated, but, as the scheme resulted in the return of 20,000 cylinders and consequently held out the olive branch of a possible reduction in the price of medical gases, Council decided that "no further action" was required (Annual Report 1963)!

Anaesthetic Records

The Ministry of Health requested the Association of Anaesthetists to design a suitable record form for inclusion in hospital records (Council Minutes 15.10.1965).[155] A Subcommittee was appointed under Professor Mushin. Lengthy deliberations took place and, in the end, a very simple form was submitted to the Ministry. The attitude of the time to record keeping is interesting: - "In order to allow maximum flexibility of usage the form is deliberately non-specific and care has been taken to ensure that failure to fill in a detail will not expose the doctor to any medicolegal criticism" (Annual Report 1966).

Chiropodists and local anaesthesia. It was reported in December 1968 that the chiropodists were seeking to be trained in the use of local anaesthesia; predictably Council did not approve of training being given to chiropodists in the use of local anaesthesia (Council Minutes 10.12.1968).[155] Some years later the limited use of local anaesthesia by chiropodists was sanctioned and agreement was reached concerning training by anaesthetists.

Tobacco shares. A protest by Langton Hewer[8] in 1967 resulted, in the Association disposing of its tobacco shares (Council Minutes 7.7.1967 and 8.12.1967).[155]

The grave of William Russ Pugh. The Association of Anaesthetists contributed 25 guineas (1996: £275) towards the restoration of the grave in Brighton cemetery, England, of the pioneer anaesthetist William Russ Pugh who administered the first recorded anaesthetic in Australia in Launceston, Tasmania in 1847 (Annual Report 1967).

The Association Tie

The suggestion that the Association of Anaesthetists should have its own tie, that ultimate mark of corporate identity, came from Richard Bodman in 1961 (Council Minutes 1.12.1961).[151] The execution of the proposal had a lengthy gestation, chiefly owing to hesitation about the number which the manufacturer decreed as a minimum (Council Minutes 2.2.1962).[151] Finally 10 dozen ties made in a rayon mixture were ordered at eleven shillings and sixpence (56p) each (Council Minutes 1.2.1963)[151] and sold on to members at fifteen shillings (1996: £6.70) (Annual Report 1963).

The tie was blue and had a gold all-over device depicting an opium poppy plant with seed capsule and leaves and an Aesculapian snake entwined around it (Annual Report 1963).[316]

It is a matter of record that, some years later, when a repeat order was made, the manufacturers substituted an owl for the poppy seed box. These erroneous ties are now collectors pieces! The Officers had the courage to authorise their sale without any comment - few members noticed !

The nineteen sixties in retrospect and the seventies in prospect

Nineteen sixty nine marked the end of an era. The administrative structure of the NHS had remained virtually unaltered during the first twenty years of its existence, and the funds available to it, though not excessive, had at least been adequate, although the way in which they were allocated had left something to be desired. The Association of Anaesthetists and the specialty of anaesthesia had learned to work within the boundaries of this stable environment and, in fact, to considerably enhance the status and influence of the specialty. The basic techniques of modern anaesthesia had been established and, with their aid, surgery had conquered the challenges offered by operations on the heart and the brain. The British specialty of anaesthesia had also extended its influence outside the operating theatre specifically into the fields of postoperative and intensive care and pain therapy. British anaesthetists were highly regarded the world over and the Fourth World Congress of 1968 had further enhanced their reputation. The Association of Anaesthetists and the Faculty of Anaesthetists had cooperated well, each in its own defined territory, and the older established and independent Association had been able to give both moral and financial support to the Faculty within the surgeons' College as and when they were needed.

The seventies were to be different. The Government and its civil servants were already becoming concerned about the cost of the NHS in the second half of the sixties. The writing was on the wall. Several reports aimed at reorganising the Service had already appeared by nineteen seventy, and the Government of the day was insistent on introducing a series of politically inspired "reforms". These were overtly designed to make the Service more cost effective but covertly intended to lessen the influence of hospital Consultants. The turmoil thus created was not to be helped by the political instability of the seventies with several changes of Government in a climate of runaway inflation. The two main political parties as they came in and out of office had perforce to inherit the problems and half developed solutions of the previous administration despite having different political philosophies. Medical education, too, was about to undergo a change from unstructured apprenticeship to a defined and controlled academic system.

The most important domestic issue facing anaesthetists in the seventies was, however, to be "the College question". Would academic anaesthesia be best served by remaining as a dependent Faculty within the surgeons' College, or would it be better if it was established as an independent, but perhaps less influential, institution? The issue was destined for some years to polarise opinion within the specialty and to bring about a marked difference of opinion between the majority of the Council of the Association of Anaesthetists of Great Britain and Ireland and a majority of Members of the Board of the Faculty of Anaesthetists of the Royal College of Surgeons of England (Chapter 8).

8

Turbulent Years
1 January 1970 to 31 December 1982

"Double, double toil and trouble;
Fire burn and cauldron bubble".

William Shakespeare (1564-1616); *Macbeth III:iii*

Executive Officers:

Presidents:- A J W Beard (1969-1971)[1]
J A Lee (1971-1973)[2]
P J Helliwell (1973-1976)[3]
C F Scurr (1976-1978)
S A Mason (1978-1980)
W D Wylie (1980-1982)
M D A Vickers (1982-1984)

Honorary Treasurers:- D D C Howat (1969-1974)
S A Mason (1974-1978)
M Rosen (1978-1983)

Honorary Secretaries:- Aileen K Adams (1968-1970)
M P Coplans (1970-1972)
J S M Zorab (1972-1974)
M D A Vickers (1974-1976)
M Rosen (1976-1978)
P J F Baskett (1978-1980)
Jean M Horton (1980-1982)
W R MacRae (1982-1984)

Editors:- R Bryce-Smith (1966-1973)
T B Boulton (1973-1982)
J N Lunn (1982-1990)

Chairmen Junior Anaesthetists' Group:-

J C Simpson (1969), F R Ellis (1970/71), P A D Williams (1972/73), G Smith (1974), J C Sugden (1975), M E Rimmer (1976), R L Hughes (1977/78), C J Barham (1979), D White (1980/81), A Chambers (1982).

Problems at home and abroad

The period (1970-1982) which is covered by this chapter was one of the most unstable in recent world and British national history. The "cold war" was at its height but Britain, now shorn of its imperial responsibilities, could only play a minor part in the confrontation between the two superpowers, the USA and USSR, as they faced each other with ever increasing stockpiles of horrific armaments.[4]

The recently independent countries of the British Commonwealth were no longer the direct responsibility of the United Kingdom, but many of them were convulsed with internal dissension and subject to dictatorial rule (often with the assistance of communist Russia or China), instead of the democratic systems with which they had been endowed at independence. Some of them, for example India and Pakistan in 1971, engaged in fighting one another; but the British Government was powerless to intervene in such conflicts. Rhodesia, a remaining independently governed crown colony, made its unilateral declaration of independence (UDI) in 1970, and the issue of majority rule remained in dispute until it accepted the inevitable in 1980 and became the independent state of Zimbabwe.[4]

Britain and Iceland confronted each over fishing limits in the so called "Cod War" in 1973, which was fortunately a skirmish of manoeuvre without gunfire or casualties; but in 1982 the United Kingdom was compelled to defend successfully the remote but British Falkland Islands and meanwhile the running sore of confrontation between the communities in the Province of Northern Ireland deepened and became more violent.[4]

The United Kingdom, dependent as it was, and is, on earning a living by supplying international services and exporting, was faced with the decline of many of its traditional British Commonwealth markets. It subsequently turned its back on the remainder (notably Australia and New Zealand) and threw in its lot with Western Europe in the shape of the European Economic Community, (EEC, now the European Union, EU) of which it became a fully participating member on 1 January 1974.[4]

The financial problems of the United Kingdom due to the loss of its traditional markets and its uncompetitive and outmoded industrial base, were greatly aggravated in 1973 by the decision of the oil producing Arab States to restrict the worldwide supply of oil and raise prices. The price of imported oil to Britain increased almost threefold. Inflation reached over 25% in the mid-seventies, and the position did not begin to be alleviated until the output of North Sea oil, which came on stream in 1975, reached reasonable levels by the end of the decade. Britain was forced to negotiate an enormous loan from the International Monetary Fund (IMF) and governments from alternating right and left wing parties strove to control inflation with price freezes and price limitations. The control of wages in the face of accelerating inflation led in turn to industrial unrest, not least in the National Health Service.

Medicine and Surgery 1970-1982

The basic research which had been a feature of the sixties began to bear fruit in the nineteen seventies.

Transplantation. The introduction of the immunosuppressive agent cyclosporin enabled renal transplantation to become a routine and successful procedure during the seventies and early eighties and gradual progress was made in heart and liver transplantation.[5,6]

Cardiology and cardiac surgery. The pharmacological control of angina and cardiac irregularities was greatly enhanced during the seventies by the increasing use, first of the adrenergic beta blocking agents (practolol, propranalol, etc)[7,8] and later of the calcium channel blockers (verapamil, nifedipine, etc).[9]

Coronary artery bypass grafting (CABG) was also gaining in importance and, by the late seventies had become the commonest cardiac operation.[10] Right at the end of the seventies the alternative of nonoperative transluminal coronary angioplasty was being developed.[11]

Fibroscopic endoscopy. Flexible instruments for the exploration and the performance of therapeutic procedures in the respiratory tree, the gastrointestial tract, the urinary bladder and the peritoneal cavity were developed in the late sixties and early seventies and gradually came into use in the later seventies and early eighties. These techniques considerably improved the facility of diagnosis and treatment of a number of conditions.[5,12,13]

Computerised Axial Tomography (CT scan) brought about a revolution in imaging internal organs during this period.[14] The improvement was particularly felt in the management of head injuries and in the diagnosis of intracranial lesions of all kinds. It took time for District Hospitals in the NHS to be equipped with this facility; however; on the one hand, prognosis of many head injury cases could have been improved and, on the other, escorting anaesthetists could have been spared many unnecessary and anxious ambulance journeys to centres of tertiary referral if the admittedly expensive funding for this technology had been available earlier!

Ultrasound and Nuclear Magnetic Resonance (NMR) techniques were also on the horizon by the early eighties.[14]

Gastroenterology. The introduction of the H_2-receptor antagonist cimetidine in the mid seventies had a profound effect on the successful medical treatment of peptic ulcers and dramatically reduced the number of cases presenting for emergency and elective gastric surgery.[15,16]

Obstetrics. The seventies brought increasing use of amniocentesis to diagnose genetic and congenital abnormalities in utero (including Down's syndrome and spina bifida),[17] and on 25 July 1978 as a result of research and development in Oldham, Lancashire, the world's first "test tube" baby was born following extracorporeal in vitro fertilisation (IVF).[18] These developments have resulted in undoubted benefits in succeeding decades, but they have also occasioned many moral and ethical dilemmas for both patients and the medical profession, as well as "complications" such as multiple pregnancies. There has also been much political debate as to whether IVF should or should not be available free of charge in the financially stressed NHS which is not yet resolved in 1998.

Day-case surgery began to come to the fore during the seventies. It had developed in the United States earlier for obvious economic reasons. It was unfortunate that some surgeons saw the considerable advantages of handling a number of cases without having to occupy inpatient beds, but did not fully appreciate the potential dangers inherent in undertaking "unsuitable operations on unsuitable patients at unsuitable times".[19] Administrators, on the other hand eagerly considered the apparent economic advantages without providing for the necessary expense of developing suitable units and procedures, and the very special nursing and anaesthetic skills which would be required. Anaesthetists played a major part in organising such units and ensuring that patients were safely and compassionately managed.[19-22]

Clinical anaesthesia 1970-1982

Important anaesthetic agents and drugs were introduced into clinical practice in the nineteen seventies and there were also considerable developments in special techniques.

Volatile agents. The hepatic and renal toxic complications consequent upon the metabolic breakdown of inhaled halothane (up to 25%) and methoxyflurane (45%) led to a search for agents which were exhaled after minimal biotransformation.[23] The result was the introduction of first enflurane (released for general use in the United Kingdom in 1978[24] with 2.4% breakdown)[23] and later isoflurane (0.2% degradation).[23] The latter agent was released for general use in North America in 1980,[25] but not in the United Kingdom until 1984.[26]

Ketamine was introduced into the USA in 1965 and into the United Kingdom in 1970.[27] It was unfortunate that emphasis was placed on its use as a single injection anaesthetic. Its propensity to cause emergence hallucinations if used without pharmacological supplementation with benzodiazepines or general anaesthesia consequently made it unpopular. Its undoubted value as an intensely analgesic and cardiovascularly stable induction agent was, therefore, not generally recognised until well into the eighties.[28]

Short acting intravenous agents. The gradually increasing use of day-case surgery stimulated an interest in agents which would promote a more rapid recovery to normality than thiopentone, which still led the field for inpatient anaesthesia.[29] Methohexitone, which had been in use since the nineteen fifties continued to be popular but is to some extent cumulative. Propanidid (Epontol) and Althesin (a mixture of the steroids alphaxalone and alphadalone) were first used clinically in the United Kingdom in 1964 and 1971 respectively.[30,31] Both were presented as oily emulsions because of low water solubility;[29] though popular with many anaesthetists both agents were voluntarily withdrawn by the manufacturers in 1984. This was because of what was considered to be an unacceptably high incidence of allergic reactions which engendered a fear of legal consequences.[32,33]

Etomidate (Hypnomidate) was introduced into clinical practice in the United Kingdom in 1976 and remains in use as an occasional induction agent in the nineties. This is chiefly because, alone amongst the intravenous agents except for ketamine, its administration is less likely to cause hypotension, although it is not otherwise a very satisfactory agent; it is painful to inject and liable to produce muscular twitching and spasm.[29,34,35] The short action of etomidate at first made it popular as an infused agent to maintain sedation in intensive care units, but its use for this purpose was discontinued in 1983 because of its propensity for causing adrenocortical suppression.[35]

Propofol (di-isopropyl phenol) dissolved in the surfactant Cremophor EL (the same solvent as used for Althesin) made an appearance as a trial drug in the seventies.[36] It was withdrawn because of the pain which it caused on injection and a possible association of Cremophor EL with anaphylactic reactions. Propofol, reformulated as an oil and water emulsion, was destined to make a considerable impact in the mid eighties (Chapter 9).[37]

Sodium nitroprusside. This hypotensive agent came into general use in the nineteen seventies, after the pharmaceutical problems were solved and the freeze-dried commercial preparation Nipride (Roche) became available. It became the agent of choice for hypotension in a number of situations including specialist neurosurgery, the management of phaeochromocytoma and of patients undergoing surgery for aortic aneurysm. Difficulties were encountered initially due to the catastrophic effects of cyanide poisoning due to overdosage.[38]

Extradural[39] **and intradural**[40] **narcotic administration** techniques were introduced in the nineteen seventies and rapidly became popular both for the relief of chronic and of acute pain (particularly postoperative pain).[41,42]

Monitoring in anaesthesia and intensive care made considerable progress. Balloon tipped flow directed flotation catheters were introduced. They enabled right sided cardiac pressures to be measured and blood samples to be withdrawn, and provided a means of estimating indirectly the pressure in the left atrium. Blood gas measurement, transducers and the monitors themselves had also improved dramatically as the science of electronics developed, and computers were beginning to be used in the operating theatres.[43]

Acupuncture attracted a great deal of interest in the seventies. The particular aspect which caught popular attention at the time was the apparent success of its use in revolutionary China instead of conventional anaesthesia for surgical operations.[44] There is little doubt that the ancient use of acupuncture does relieve pain, but the mechanism of action is in doubt. It may be to a degree the result of suggestion, the placebo effect, counter irritation, the gate theory principle but also, as seems to be proven, by the release of endogenous opiates.[44,45] The use of acupuncture for surgery is of more recent origin; despite the impression created by earlier reports, closer examination of the facts suggests that the technique is used in China for only about 2% of operative procedures for a limited number of selected patients, and that considerable supplementation with opiates and local anaesthetics is often required.[44,46] Photographs of patients undergoing surgery under acupuncture in China bear a remarkable resemblance to those of major surgery under hypnosis in the United Kingdom in the fifties![44,47]

The pollution issue (the danger to anaesthetists of chronic exposure to gaseous and volatile anaesthetics) gave rise to considerable concern in the early seventies. This was initially as a result of studies that apparently indicated that, amongst female anaesthetists and other women working in operating rooms, "spontaneous abortion" was, either more frequent than might have been expected, or greater than occurred in control groups. Other studies seemed to indicate a greater incidence of infertility, fetal abnormalities and cancer, and there was also the question of depression of the bone marrow (vitamin B12 deficiency) possibly due to nitrous oxide. "The dissemination of such reports, and the consternation to which they gave rise, were mainly the result of abstraction by various elements of the media who chose to sensationalise the implications rather than look objectively to the quality of the studies."[48] Many of the studies were indeed found to be statistically flawed.[49] The Association of Anaesthetists did much to initiate measures to investigate the problem to allay anxiety amongst its members, and to collaborate with the Department of Health (DH) in preparing guidelines.[50,51] These advised health authorities that reasonable measures should be taken to reduce the levels of contamination including the introduction of scavenging devices for waste gases, and that operating theatre nurses who planned to become pregnant should be given the opportunity to work in another area of the hospital. No official guidance was provided by the DH for lady doctors however![51]

Spence, Wall and Nunn,[48] research workers who have been intimately concerned with the evaluation of the risk presented by contamination of the atmosphere of operating rooms with volatile and gaseous anaesthetics, concluded in 1989 that there is "reasonably convincing evidence of a moderate increase in the risk of spontaneous abortion amongst exposed females, although it is possible that even this result is attributable to reporting bias. There is no convincing evidence of any other hazard." [48] Spence and his colleagues go on to say that, in the light of the results of an ongoing prospective enquiry, it is possible that even the finding of the moderate increase in spontaneous abortion may be challenged and that it is not definitely possible to dismiss the probability that "earlier environmental hazards (known or unknown) have diminished in the last decade",[48] possibly in part to the measures that have been taken to reduce atmospheric pollution. It must be acknowledged that many anaesthetists have at least a subjective feeling that they are less tired since scavenging has been introduced, and that they are less tolerant to the odour of volatile agents in the atmosphere of an operating theatre than in the past (personal experience).

The pollution problem again became an issue in 1994 when the Governments' Advisory Committee on Toxic Substances proposed to bring in unrealistic, Occupational Exposure Standards for anaesthetic gases and vapours under the Control of Substances Hazardous to Health Regulations (Council Minutes 4.2.94) despite the lack of evidence of dangers to personnel. Representation at the highest level with the Department of Health and the Health and Safety Executive have led to more realistic proposals (Annual Reports 1994 and 1995; *Anaesthesia*; **50**: 272-82 and *Anaesthesia*; **51**: 295-306).

Reorganisation and disorganisation within the NHS in the seventies

The optimism of the comparatively affluent early nineteen sixties gave rise to a situation in which thoughtful planning for changes in the efficiency with which many institutions were organised was possible, because of an atmosphere in which fear of inflation did not play too large a part. The NHS was no exception[52-58] but, by the end of the decade and during the seventies increasing, and then rampant, inflation (up to 27%), partly caused by the world oil crisis, led to desperate measures to try to search for putative efficiency as a way of cutting costs in the face of an increasingly difficult financial situation; from the early seventies onwards the NHS has been a prey to the theories of nonmedical politicians, management consultants, economists and pontificating pundits.

The Cogwheel report of a working party chaired by Sir George Godber, the Government Chief Medical Officer, was published in 1967.[52] It was so called because of the enmeshed cogwheels on its cover which some critics said were inextricably jammed. This was unfair however. This report put forward reasonably sensible proposals for the organisation of consultant medical staff within the unified District General Hospitals which had resulted from Enoch Powell's 1962 Hospital Plan for England and Wales (Chapter 7). The Report recommended the formation of Clinical Divisions of related specialities. Each Division would have an elected Chairman and they in turn, under an elected Chairman of the Medical Staff, would form a powerful Advisory Committee. This Committee would liaise with the hospital administration over such matters as the allocation of the budget provided for new equipment, manpower, and bed and space provision. Most hospitals adopted this system by the early seventies and it put an end to the massive and ineffective staff committees of 100 or more individual Consultants, although some of these continued to exist separately as talking shops.[52-55]

The Divisional system of organisation persisted reasonably successfully through the 1974, 1982 and 1984 reorganisations of the NHS until the 1991 reorganisation occurred (Chapter 9). This last reorganisation has resulted in the appointment of medically qualified Clinical Directors by lay General Managers, often, but unfortunately not always, after nomination by their colleagues. Departments of anaesthesia who succeeded in forming independent Cogwheel "Divisions of Anaesthesia and Intensive Care" fared well, but those which were incorporated into larger Divisions of Surgery had many problems, particularly as the money allocated for equipment became less and less adequate for the needs of the speciality of anaesthesia whose techniques were developing rapidly.

The Salmon Report on Senior Nurse Staffing Structure was the work of a Committee chaired by Brian Salmon, Director of the Joe Lyons catering company.[53-56] The Report was published in 1966 and its recommendations were implemented in most NHS hospitals by the early seventies. The evidence which the Association of Anaesthetists presented to the Royal Commission on the National Health Service in 1977 describes its effects as "catastrophic" and continues:-

> *"More and more experienced nurses have been removed from practical nursing into administrative posts for which many of them had neither the inclination nor the ability. Clinical areas have been downgraded in importance and put in charge of younger and less experienced nurses who have lacked the authority and incentive to regard their work as a vocation."*[57]

Those redoubtable ladies, the greatly experienced Senior Ward Sisters who dedicated their whole career to looking after patients in the wards, and who, together with the medical Consultant staff, formed the backbone of the British hospital system, were destined to disappear. The only way to promotion in the nursing service was henceforth to be up an extended and graded administrative ladder which many dedicated nurses were reluctant to ascend. The honoured post of Hospital Matron, responsible for all aspects of nursing within the hospital unit, who was a frequent visitor to the wards and familiar to medical and nursing staff at all levels, was replaced by a desk bound District Nursing Officer separated from bedside nursing by a hierarchy of clip-board carrying nurse-managers. Consultants used to solving problems by direct access to the Matron found themselves confronted by assertive "grade seven" nursing officers, who sometimes lacked the authority to take decisions and were loathe to refer matters to higher authority for fear of being labelled as "indecisive".

The Salmon system created a progressively remunerative career structure for the nursing profession and enabled them to ascend the administrative ladder, but how much better it might have been for patients if senior nurses could have remained as valued clinical colleagues in the wards, with gradually increasing salaries as their careers progressed, alongside Consultant medical staff who have fortunately remained in direct contact with patients. The principles which govern the hierarchy of an industrial firm are not necessarily those which are best applied to a national health service! The NHS has been fortunate in being able to call upon part-time married nurses who, not being too interested in promotion, have given dedicated service at the bedside.

The 1974 Reorganisation of the NHS was conceived in the sixties because of a desire to achieve unification of the service and, at the same time, to attempt to enable local authority and health authority boundaries to coincide ("become coterminous"). This, it was thought, would make the NHS more administratively efficient and more responsible to the aspirations of local communities. Early on in the planning the need to make the service more cost efficient was less important but, later in the seventies, when the economic crisis began to bite, the need to economise became the principal driving factor and, indeed, was itself partly responsible for the 1974 reorganisation becoming discredited and ultimately abandoned in 1982.[53-55]

The NHS structure which had emerged after the compromises which led to the setting up of the NHS in 1948 had resulted in a "tripartite" system - the hospital services, run through the Regional Hospital Boards and Hospital Management Committees, Family Practitioner Services, and the Local Authority Services (public health, school and child welfare, clinical domiciliary maternity, ambulance services, home helps etc.).[53-55] This system seemed to be somewhat fragmented and uncoordinated and was administratively untidy, but, in practice, it must be said, functioned reasonably well.

The concept of unification of the health services of the United Kingdom was not new. It dated back to Aneurin Bevan's original proposals for the NHS in 1946. The Porritt Committee of the BMA had also advocated unification under Area Health Boards, as did the Labour Health Minister Kenneth Robinson's "Green Paper" in 1968 (without a Regional Tier). The idea was endorsed by Richard Crossman, by then the Minister responsible for a combined Department of Health and Social Security (DHSS), in February 1970 (this time with a Regional planning tier). Edward Heath's Conservative government came into power in June 1970 and the DHSS, headed by Keith Joseph, continued and accelerated the march towards reorganisation.

McKinsey and Company Incorporated, a firm of American Management Consultants, was called in, as was the Health Services Organisational Research Unit of Brunel University, and the "Grey Book" (*Management Arrangements for the Reorganised NHS*) was finally published in 1972. It became law as the National Health Service Re-organisation Act in July 1973, just 25 years after the NHS had come into existence.[53-55]

It was left to the incoming Labour administration to bring the reorganisation scheme into operation in 1974 virtually unchanged, with medically qualified David Owen as Minister of Health under a DHSS dominated by the veteran politician Barbara Castle.[53-55]

> *"The aims of the 1974 reorganisation attempted to reconcile conflicting policies; to promote managerial efficiency but also to satisfy the professions, to create an effective administrative structure for establishing national policy but also to give delegated scope to those running the services at the far reaches of the NHS. Consequently, while the organisational outcome had the potential to unify the delivery system, it contained the seed bed of further trouble."*[54]

The principle objective of the 1974 reorganisation was the very difficult one of "maximum delegation downward, maximum accountability upwards".[54]

The 90 new Area Health Authorities (AHA) were intended to be the key to the success of the new systems. Their boundaries were generally "coterminous" with the local authority areas, and one third of their members were appointed by the local authorities. There were also representatives of the executive tier above the Area (the Regional Health Authority), and medical staff, including both hospital doctors and general practitioners, nursing and non-medical staff nominees. The General Practitioners themselves had, however, negotiated their own separate Family Practitioner Committees financed directly by the DHSS. University Teaching Hospitals lost their direct link with the DHSS and joined "Teaching Districts".

The Area Health Authorities had a management team responsible to the AHA consisting of Administrator, Treasurer, Community Physician, Consultant, General Practitioner and Nurse.[53-55]

The Districts controlled by the AHA were managed directly by a District Management Team (DMT) with a composition echoing that of the AHA, but there was no equivalent to the old Hospital Management Committee (HMC) at District level. "Units" (individual hospitals) were run by a Unit Management Team (UMT) consisting of administrator, nurse and consultant. Sometimes, between Unit and District, there was a Sector administrator attempting to coordinate two or more hospital units.

Community Health Councils (CHC) were appointed at District level to represent the public and monitor hospital performance. These often included many of the kind of people who would previously have been members of the HMCs such as local councillors. Their role was converted from being one of support for those who actually cared for patients when they were involved in management, to one of constant criticism of the service from the sidelines.[53-55]

The administrative structure of the NHS was greatly extended by these changes, 16,700 extra administrative staff had been taken on by 1977.[53] Many experienced Unit Administrators were promoted to the upper and more remunerative tiers, many with reluctance, leaving youthful juniors to try to supply the needs of hospitals at unit level. The various management teams were directed to take their decisions by "consensus". This was a lengthy process and resulted in endless meetings and discussions. The process of consensus was moreover fundamentally flawed. It was weighted against the clinical medical component because, while the administrators, community physicians and nurses on the various teams had only administrative functions, the consultants were active clinicians with many other commitments, not least the responsibility of treating patients. There were too many tiers and the teams in the higher levels interfered in the simple day to day decisions with those below them and controlled the detailed distribution of diminishing financial resources. Unit and even District administrators were often almost powerless. This was especially the case as many services such as supply of equipment, laundry, personnel recruitment etc. were managed by Area rather than District.[55]

The 1974 reorganisation resulted in a ceaselessly active but ineffective and expensive bureaucracy about which the medical profession became increasingly frustrated and angry. This was not all however. The whole creaking edifice was bedevilled by changes in political ideology as opposing parties alternatively took over the government.[53-55,59]

Industrial unrest in the NHS 1972-1979

Incomes did not keep pace with rampant inflation throughout the nineteen seventies. Both wage earners and salaried professionals in the public sector, including nurses and doctors, became increasingly militant. Trade Union membership and activity increased dramatically, both generally and within the NHS, and strikes became frequent.

The ancillary workers strikes in 1972 and 1973 involving the admittedly lowly paid catering, cleaning, maintenance, telephone and portering staffs were precipitated by a pay freeze under the Conservative government of Edward Heath. These disputes breached the emotional barrier against strike action in hospitals which had its roots in the idea of service to the sick inherent in the old voluntary system. It is estimated that 59,000 staff were engaged in strike action in 1973 with a loss of 298,000 working days.[55] Widespread action in many hospitals continued intermittently throughout the nineteen seventies particularly in major cities like London and Liverpool.[55,60-62] The other ancillary workers were joined by ambulance staff after 1974, when transfer from the local authorities to the NHS revealed regional discrepancies in pay rates.

The situation was compounded by the weakness of administrators at hospital level and their lack of experience of dealing with industrial disputes. They often continued to pay ancillary workers even when they were on strike, and even paid them overtime for coping with the extra work occasioned by the strikes![61,62] Trades Union militancy seriously disrupted the work of the hospital services. Admissions were limited to emergencies at many hospitals; at some even emergency admissions were prevented or delayed by arguments between doctors and union officials. Strikes by catering, laundry and other workers in support services affected patient care. It must be acknowledged, however, that nation-wide the response to the call for strike action was patchy, some hospitals escaped almost unscathed where relationships between the ancillary workers and the medical and nursing staff were traditionally good, but the uncertainty of the situation added to the chaos.

Trades Union militancy in general reached its peak in the "winter of discontent" at the end of 1978. The situation had been aggravated by politically inspired legislation on labour relations which was favourable to the Unions. Public disquiet about the power of the trade unions ultimately was one important factor which led to the election of Mrs Thatcher's Conservative government in May 1979 and the passage of legislation designed to regulate the conditions for strike action.

The dispute by nurses over pay in the face of increasing inflation came to a head in 1974. A Ward Sister at the time had a take home pay of 60 pence (1996: £2.50) per hour for a 40 hour week excluding meal breaks.[55] The militant Confederation of Health Service Employees (COHSE) staged demonstrations and marches[55] which brought some formidable nursing characters to the barricades! It must be said, however, that on the whole nurses honoured their professional commitment not to impair the care of patients. The *cause célèbre* of the Normansfield psychiatric hospital, which provoked a lengthy and very expensive enquiry in 1976, was an exception; in this case nurses struck and "exposed their patients to needless and serious danger" in the face of "the failure of the authorities [over a long period] to demonstrate that they were treating the nurses' complaints seriously and urgently".[55]

The members of the Royal College of Nursing maintained their traditional policy of refusing to strike, a position favoured by the majority of dedicated nurses; however their President did threaten at one stage to withdraw her members from the NHS and offer them back to the service for hire. The confrontation was diffused by the Inquiry into Nurses Pay under Lord Halsbury which recommended a 30% average pay rise for both nurses and the "professions supplementary to medicine" (including physiotherapists and radiographers).[55]

Industrial action by senior hospital doctors lasted for two relatively brief periods (from December 1974 to April 1975 and again from October 1975 to February 1976). The consultants' actions did not amount to full blown strikes however but an imposition of sanctions; in the first of the two periods the BMA recommended a "work to rule" in which the Consultants were asked to withdraw from any voluntary actions (such as attendance at committees) which were strictly outside the terms of their professional contracts. The sanctions which were to be imposed in the second period were more severe. These officially involved the limitation of consultant activity to emergency work alone and coincided with similar action taken by the junior doctors over their own dispute over pay and conditions (see below).[59] Anaesthetists, as members of a speciality of tertiary referral, were not generally concerned with initiating the sanctions and, with a few exceptions, dealt with the patients presented to them in the operating theatre or the intensive care units. Surgeons were not averse in practice in ceasing to attend committees, especially those involving hospital administration, or to reduce the number of patients seen as outpatients, but they were less prepared to limit what they liked doing best - cutting surgery - and, by hook or by crook, continued to operate! It is significant that although there is a passing reference to the "political decision to proceed with the phasing out of private beds in the NHS" there is no direct reference to the senior or junior doctors' disputes in the 1975-1976 Annual Report of the Council of the Association of Anaesthetists.

The dispute with the Consultants was not primarily about NHS pay even though the real value of money fell dramatically during the seventies due to inflation.[53] The Review Body machinery functioned shakily, but sufficiently effectively during the decade, to encourage doctors and their BMA negotiators to behave with considerable restraint over remuneration. There were, however, many hard fought arguments with Barbara Castle, Secretary for Health and Social Security, over the implementation of the various awards. This was especially the case in 1974 after the government breached their own guidelines in granting the miners a disproportionate increase. There was, however an award of 30% in medical pay in 1975, and 30.4% staged over 3 years in 1978.

The reasons for the dispute with the Consultants were, in fact threefold; first the apparently increasingly inadequate financial provision for the NHS and the inefficiency of the cumbersome administrative structure created by the 1974 reorganisation, which was failing to deal with the disruption caused by the industrial action of ancillary workers; second was the matter of the prolonged negotiation over a new contract for hospital Consultants and its pricing; and thirdly, and most important, the doctrinaire attempts of Mrs Castle and the Labour government to eliminate pay-beds from NHS hospitals. This stemmed from an almost fanatical determination to abolish private practice within the NHS as well as, at the same time placating the trade unions, who, at various times withdrew their labour from providing catering, cleaning and other services from pay-bed facilities to the discomfort of the patients.[55,59]

It was unfortunate that the proposed abolition of the pay-beds was linked to the introduction of the new contract for consultants. This was because a working party was established under (Lord) David Owen charged with implementing both policies.

The new contract for consultants was first proposed by the BMA in 1972 to replace the contract which had been in existence since the beginning of the NHS. The latter was considered to be out of tune with the working conditions of the nineteen seventies. The reason for this was that it was based on five and a half day (11 sessions) NHS working week, with an undefined and unlimited work load which was exploited by the government in pay negotiations. The aim was to replace it with a defined contract for a five day (10 session) NHS working week with Consultants having the right to engage additionally in non-contractual work, including extra NHS sessions, as well as private practice.[55,59]

Negotiations over the new contract dragged on for 7 years, latterly partly because they were inextricably linked in the terms of reference given to the Owen working party concerning the elimination of private pay beds in the NHS, and partly because the Review Body (for once) priced the putative contract proposals unfavourably in 1979. The new contract was finally implemented in a modified form by the incoming Conservative administration in 1980. This unexpectedly included the provision for "whole-time" (now to be 10 instead of 11 sessions) consultants to earn up to an additional 10% of their salary in private fees in addition to the provision for extra sessions to the basic contract to be worked for additional remuneration when the service required it. The 10% provision was particularly welcome to whole-time consultant anaesthetists in relation to the anaesthetising of private patients of their part-time surgical colleagues on NHS lists. A long-standing anomaly (Council Minutes 6.6.1972) was consequently eliminated.[55,59]

Pay-beds in the NHS. The details of the prolonged confrontation between the BMA representing the medical profession and the Labour government over pay-beds can not be considered in detail here. They are well described in the official history of the BMA.[59] The Prime Minister (Harold Wilson) attempted to cool the passions aroused by the dispute by announcing the establishment of a Royal Commission on the NHS in October 1975, but he only succeeded in inflaming the situation by refusing to delay legislation on the abolition of pay-beds.[59] The eminent lawyer Lord Arnold Goodman was called in to mediate between the government and the profession. His proposals were for a gradual phasing out of pay-beds in NHS hospitals by an independent board over a lengthy period of time when, in each locality, there was adequate provision of beds in private hospitals. These proposals were accepted by the Consultants (Council Minutes 2.1.1976) who called off their sanctions; they were embodied in law by an Act in 1976. The acceptance of the proposals by the medical profession may seen rather surprising, but the BMA negotiators probably recognised the value of procrastination in the face of the possible change in the political colour of the Government after a general election. This in fact came to pass in May 1979 when the policy of phasing out pay-beds in the NHS was reversed by the incoming Conservative Administration under Mrs Thatcher.[59]

The industrial action by the junior hospital medical staff at the end of 1975 amounted to restricting work to emergencies, and it coincided with the second period of sanctions imposed by the Consultants. The action was immediately triggered by a dispute concerning the interpretation of the pricing of a new contract which has been negotiated for Junior Staff,[63,64] but the real causes went deeper.[65] This was undoubtedly a time of low morale and conflict in the NHS, and the juniors felt that their very considerable contribution to the work of the service was not valued by their employers, the Department of Health and Social Security or their agents (the administrators). Trainees in the hospital service, as before the introduction of the NHS, had "worked long hours for low pay spurred on by a crock of gold at the end of the tunnel - consultant status" but this prospect had "now collapsed into a heap of dust", Consultants pay had fallen behind, the wards were "understaffed (and the old-style ward sister was now yet another legend of the golden age)". There was also a shortage of basic equipment, and there was an atmosphere of discontent in the service.[65]

The new contract had its origins in the proposals of the then newly formed autonomous Hospital Junior Staffs Group Council of the BMA.[66-68] The implementation of the contract had subsequently been negotiated step by weary step with a reluctant Department of Health and was ready for implementation in 1975. It is amazing that, prior to the New Contract, junior doctors were theoretically committed to a working week of 168 hours (7 days of 24 hours)! Any off duty or other conditions such as compulsory residence were at the whim of the employer.[63] The juniors' new contract was a compromise between the traditional professional concept of the medical practitioner's open-ended responsibility for his patient, which had undoubtedly been exploited by the NHS administration both centrally and locally, and the need to regularise the hours of junior doctors. The concept of Units of Medical Time (UMTs) was introduced. There was to be a basic working week of 40 hours (10 UMTs) for which a basic salary was to be paid, and two tier salary supplements for duties above 44 hours paid at a lesser rate. These rates were to be 30% of the equivalent basic salary rate for actual extra working time in the hospital (class "A") and 10% for available on call (class "B"). The number of additional UMTs applicable to each post on average was to be negotiated with local employers and paid as a regular salary.[63,64]

The pricing of the contract[64] precipitated the industrial action by the juniors following a ballot in October 1975.[65] This was because the Department of Health had apparently refused to fully endorse a promised "no detriment" provision, and it was feared that some juniors (a minority who had previously managed to negotiate local extra duty payments) would lose financially. The juniors were in a frustrated and militant mood and, consequently voted for industrial action.[69] Industrial action by juniors, which involved a commitment to treat emergencies only, had already started in a number of hospitals before it was made official by the BMA on 27 November 1975 at the same time as similar sanctions were imposed by the consultants.[70,71] The official action by the junior doctors was short lived. Further discussions with (Lord) David Owen, Minister of Health, resulted in some concessions and the allocation of additional funds, and the industrial action was suspended on 16 December 1975.[72,73] The Consultants' sanction involving declining to treat patients other than emergencies lasted until 12 February 1976.[73] The involvement of junior anaesthetists in the industrial action was minimal; as was the case with the Consultants they continued to deal with the work presented to them in the operating theatre and intensive care units by colleagues in the bed-owning specialties.

The significance of the industrial action by senior and junior medical staff and of the new contracts has been described by Brian Edwards, in his book *"The National Health Service; a Manager's Tale (1993)"* as a "watershed" in the history of the NHS.[55] This is undoubtedly the case. Short though the industrial actions of the senior and junior medical staff were, and even though they did not result in the neglect of patients suffering from emergency or life threatening conditions, they nevertheless caused an estimated additional 100,000 people with elective conditions being added to waiting lists, "not to mention the suffering caused to individual patients by delays in diagnosis and treatment".[53] The medical profession has not taken industrial action again but its actions in 1975 and 1976 leaves administrators and those nurses who were and are members of the Royal College of Nursing, as the only groups of NHS workers who have never been "prepared to risk the well-being of patients by disrupting or withdrawing services".[55,74] The provocation was undoubtedly great, but it must be said that doctors compromised their status as members of a caring and learned profession, and to some extent their credibility as the leading group amongst the workers of the NHS, by their actions in 1975 and 1976.

Edwards is, however, not correct in saying that the dispute "finally removed any lingering deep rooted ethical objections [on the part of the medical profession] to industrial action". The Presidents and Deans of the Medical Royal Colleges and Faculties, while recognising the provocation and the deplorable record of the government of the day (which "could no longer claim to fulfil" a role "as spokesmen for the interests of the community"); would not "associate themselves with the profession's proposals to limit their services to the treatment of emergencies,"[75] and the correspondence columns of the *British Medical Journal* of the period (1975 Volume 4 and 1976 Volume 1) indicate that many ordinary hospital practitioners, both senior and junior, were appalled at the decision of the Council of the British Medical Association to call for industrial action,[55,59,76] and many would no doubt oppose industrial action if it was proposed in the nineties.

The new junior hospital doctor contract also broke new ground. An attempt had been made to preserve the tradition of open-ended professional care by medical practitioners by fixing a relatively low level of the pricing for "Units of Medical Time" for on call commitments over the basic 40 hours; but the concept of "overtime payments" had been irrevocably introduced into medical remuneration in the NHS for the first time. There is no doubt however that the idea of supplementary payments was a matter of expediency to obtain more money.[65] Many juniors, especially the more senior trainees would have preferred an adequate professional salaried structure without overtime payments, coupled with a more reasonable attitude to a reduction in the "excessive hours" worked by many of them which they regarded as a separate issue. Twenty junior doctors wrote a letter to the *British Medical Journal* which included this passage:-

> *"A preoccupation with remuneration for hours worked will lead to a lowering of professional standards in medicine.... It will limit the freedom of individual clinicians and will introduce restraint on patient care. ...... the many situations when doctors do not have time off duty is to be deplored; a solution to this problem must be achieved urgently, but it cannot be circumvented by an overtime system when the real need is adequate staffing."*[77]

It may also be observed that, although the new Consultants' contract agreed with the incoming Conservative government in 1979 preserved the concept of continuous responsibility for patient care with its nominally paid ten session ("maximum part-time") and nominally paid eleven session ("whole-time") contracts, it also offered a contract paid for nine sessions "for those consultants preferring a more defined NHS commitment;" in the latter case "a Consultant's obligation to give substantially the whole of his time to the NHS and to give it priority at all times [does] not apply".[78] This was certainly a new departure for the NHS: some Consultant Anaesthetists found it attractive.

The General Medical Council

The Merrison Committee into the Regulation of the Medical Profession was established in 1972 under the Chairmanship of the eminent physicist (Sir) Alec Merrison, Vice Chancellor Bristol University, under a Conservative government. This followed an acrimonious dispute with the BMA over the institution of fees for retention on the medical register.[59,79,80] The Committee was widely representative and its report under the Labour government in 1975 was generally welcomed by the medical profession. It proposed a more representative General Medical Council (GMC), with a majority of elected members. It recommended continued self regulation of the profession and renewed emphasis on specialist training, but its suggestion for a specialist register was not implemented by the Medical Act which followed in 1978. It also courageously expressed concern about the standard of some overseas immigrant doctors (a matter of considerable concern at the time), but paid tribute to the immense contribution they had made to keeping the NHS going over the recent difficult years. The Merrison Committee said in its report "We do not accept that doctors in the British Isles are trained to an unnecessarily high standard, and we doubt whether the assertion of the contrary by the Health Department would be accepted to be a disinterested comment."[79,80]

The Association of Anaesthetists set up a special working party to prepare evidence for submission to the Merrison Committee. The submission was published as Appendix B to the 1972-1973 Annual Report. The document proposes a "Regulatory Body" to replace the GMC. This was presumably because the remit of the GMC as it then existed was considered to be too narrow to be effectively reorganised; however, in general the proposals of the Association of Anaesthetists were not very dissimilar to those which were subsequently contained in the Merrison Report for a reorganised GMC with wider membership and powers.

Particular emphasis was placed in the submission for the need of the Association of Anaesthetists for statutory representation on the GMC of the Faculty of Anaesthetists of the Royal College of Surgeons of England. This was supported by the surgeons' College. There was apparently some opposition to this proposal, including hesitation on the part of the GMC itself, and the Council of Association of Anaesthetists joined in pressing the authorities for its implementation (Council Minutes 11.3.1977).[81] Considerable satisfaction was therefore felt when, in due course, after the 1978 Medical Act had been passed, John Edmund Riding (Dean of the Faculty 1976-1979) took his seat on the GMC and continued to represent the Faculty as Past Dean and Member of the Board of Faculty for several years thereafter.[82]

The Royal Commission on the National Health Service and its consequences

The Royal Commission on the National Health Service was announced in 1975 by the Labour Prime Minister Harold Wilson at the height of the confrontation between the government and the medical profession over private practice in the NHS and the new contracts for junior doctors. It was almost certainly a delaying tactic.[83] Sir Alec Merrison, who had just completed the report of his Committee on "The Regulation of the Medical Profession" [79,80] was appointed Chairman in 1976, but the membership of the Commission was not made public until the following May, when the announcement caused considerable dismay to the BMA and the medical profession.[84,85] (Lord) David Owen has stated that the "membership (of the Commission) had been carefully chosen,"[53] but with what objective, or whether or not he was serious, is open to doubt. The total medical input amongst the members was to be provided by a Professor of Psychiatry and two politically orientated General Practitioners; NHS hospital doctors, senior or junior, were not represented, but a dental professor and a senior nurse were included. Representations to the Secretary of Health and Social Security failed to induce him to widen the membership.[83]

The Honorary Secretaries of the Association of Anaesthetists (Michael Vickers and Michael Rosen) produced an exceptionally comprehensive and well reasoned document of evidence for the consideration of the Royal Commission.[85] Many of the problems of managing and funding the NHS are covered as well as the particular problems of anaesthetists. A dedicated insurance based service divorced from general taxation was recommended, as was an end to the short term annual allocation of funds which had made long term planning difficult throughout the history of the NHS. Stress was also laid on the need for undergraduate exposure to anaesthesia to aid recruitment, structured postgraduate and continuing education, the need for flexible working patterns to cover activities outside the operating theatre; and the special needs of women in medicine.[85] The paper makes fascinating reading even today for all who are interested in the history and future development of the NHS and its funding of anaesthetic services. Council approved the content of the document after wide consultation and discussion through the Linkman organisation which had been established in 1974 (see below), and it was distributed to all members of the Association of Anaesthetists (Council Minutes 12.11.1976, 7.1.1977 and 11.3.1977).[81,85]

The Report of the Royal Commission was published in July 1979, three months after a Conservative government had replaced the Labour administration which had initiated it.[86-88] The leading article in the *British Medical Journal* described it as "pragmatic and generally low key" and states that "so well phrased and logically presented is the report that the reader is in danger at times in mistaking elegant prose for rigorous argument".[88] Merrison and his colleagues recognised that the NHS had "achieved a great deal and embodied aspirations and ideals of great value" and they believed that it was "not suffering from a mortal disease susceptible only to major surgery." They were, however, rather too complacent about the morale of the service. They did not recommend a great increase in provision from general taxation (which pleased the politicians and administrators but not the BMA and the medical profession)[53,55,83] but, on the other hand, they were not "satisfied with the nation's present level of expenditure on health"; however they did not suggest how funding could possibly be increased (for example by an insurance system).[83] They differed from the BMA on manpower planning and raised the question of the subconsultant grade once again but, on the positive side, they introduced the concept of peer review and audit, and recommended a slimming down of the administration and peripheral delegation of responsibility for the day to day affairs of hospital management.[53,55,83-88]

Patients First, published in December 1979, embodied the response of the Department of Health to the administrative proposals of the Royal Commission.[89] This envisaged the abolition of the Area tiers and the establishment of District Health Authorities with the responsibility for the day to day management of the services, and staff delegated to the hospital level as far as possible. Medical input to administration was to be much more on an advisory basis with a strengthened executive role for the Hospital Administrator. These proposals were embodied in the Health Services Act of 1980 and led to the second reorganisation of the NHS in 1982.[53-55] It is interesting in the light of future developments in the organisation of the NHS that the document stated:

> "It is the doctors dentists and nurses and .... other health professions who provide the care and cure of patients and promote the health of the people. It is the purpose of management to support them in giving that service."[89]

The 1982 Reorganisation abolished the Area Health Authority, and this resulted in much uncertainty for the administrative staff of the NHS. Once again they had to reapply for what were in effect their own posts, but this time, unlike the 1974 reorganisation, there was contraction and not enough jobs to go round; in the end there were 2,830 early retirements and redundancies at a cost of £54 million (1996: £97 million).[55] The old system of "top-sliced" cash-limited budgets was continued. There should theoretically have been a devolution of the taking of decisions to District and Units, which should have resulted in flexibility to arrange their own staff structure and manage their own budgets. They should also have gained authority to practice the much talked about "virement" (a new word for the NHS meaning the use of savings from one budgetary commitment for another purpose); in practice the powers of Unit Administrators were very limited, and there was continued pressure from the centre to cut costs within the limits of the cost capping system which had been introduced by the Labour government in 1976.

The period from 1982 to the next reorganisation in 1984 was a time when actual clinical services were not greatly curtailed but support services deteriorated. This particularly applied to the catering facilities and the maintenance of the physical conditions in which patients were cared for and in which staff worked. The imposition in 1976 of the RAWP (Resource Allocation Working Party) formula (an attempt to divide inadequate funding more equally amongst Regional Health Authorities) improved provision in some Regions but caused severe problems in others, notably in London.[53,54]

The 1982 Health Workers pay dispute involved almost all unionised workers in the NHS led by the Trade Union Congress Health Services Committee. The industrial action mainly took the form of intermittent withdrawal of labour by targeted groups. Patient care was disrupted, some hospitals were reduced to providing accident and emergency services only, and police sometimes had to provide emergency ambulance services. Medical staff were not involved but suffered great frustration, while waiting lists of non-urgent patients increased. The Royal College of Nursing stuck to its no-strike policy and gained considerable press sympathy. Other unions, not directly concerned with running the NHS, took supporting action. Sixty thousand people were protesting on the streets of London on 22 September 1982, and pits, ports and daily newspapers were closed. This dispute lasted to December 1982 while the Conservative government rode out the strike. The unions settled in the end for much less than the 12.5% rise "across the board" which they demanded originally. The patients and staff suffered a great deal in terms of reduced patient comfort and the lowering of morale. The only really positive gain was the introduction of the Review Body system for nurses. This provision stood the nurses and the NHS in good stead as it did in the case of the medical staff, but this happy state of affairs for both groups has been threatened by the latest (1991) "internal market" re-organisation (Chapter 9).[55]

The period chosen for the coverage of this chapter (January 1970 to December 1982) was indeed stormy for the NHS. This, as has been noted above, was largely occasioned by the alternating policies of left and right wing political parties with contrasting ideologies attempting to control expenditure in the face of mounting inflation. The administrative structure which remained after all the political manoeuvring was weak and ineffective. Further reorganisation was inevitable.

The business of the Association 1970-1982

The years between the first day of 1970 and the last of 1982 (the Golden Jubilee year of the Association of Anaesthetists) were a period of considerable developmental activity for the specialty of anaesthesia both nationally and internationally, and this was reflected in the conduct of the affairs of the Association.

The membership of the Association almost doubled during the period, from 2,229 to 4,434 and the active United Kingdom membership (Ordinary and Junior) from 1,830 to 4,326. The most dramatic rise was in the membership of the Junior Anaesthetists' Group (from 276 to 1,092) (Annual Reports 1969 and 1982).

These figures reflect transition from a shortage specialty with relatively poor recruitment to one which was attractive to young postgraduates, particularly towards the end of the period.[90-93] It will be noted however that, although Junior Membership had increased fourfold, Ordinary Membership (mostly Consultants) had only increased by 30% (1,554 to 2,033). This reflects a persistent resistance on the part of the Department of Health to create new Senior Registrar and Consultant posts.[94] Trainee anaesthetists were undertaking a disproportionate amount of the anaesthesia in the NHS hospitals and there was a bottleneck at Registrar to Senior Registrar level. There was consequently a considerable loss of well qualified Registrars during the early nineteen seventies in emigration to the United States and the major British

Commonwealth countries, but this became progressively less towards the end of the decade when immigration into the United States and other older Commonwealth Dominions began to be restricted, national qualifying examinations were introduced in various countries including the USA, and anaesthesia became an increasingly attractive option in the United Kingdom.

A programme for the seventies. Philip Helliwell on becoming President announced the formation of four working parties (Council Minutes 2.11.1973[81] and Annual Report 1974). These were initiated to study:-

Working party 1: The pattern of representation on and the method of election to the Council of the Association of Anaesthetists. This working party was chaired by John S Inkster of Newcastle upon Tyne.

Working party 2: The financial implications of the establishment of a College of Anaesthetists; chaired by the Honorary Treasurer S A Mason of King's College Hospital, London.

Working party 3: The options available to meet the service and educational demands made upon the specialty; chaired by E Brian Lewis of Ashford Kent (then and for many subsequent years a prominent member of the Council of the BMA).

Working party 4: The implementation of the Lewin report on the organisation and staffing of operating theatres; chaired by Peter J Horsey of Southampton.

The remits of the first two working parties are indicative of two of the central issues on which the Council of the Association of Anaesthetists were to have lengthy deliberations during Helliwell's Presidency . The other two working parties collected a considerable amount of important data which was of great value in negotiations with the Department of Health over the manpower problems of the medical profession itself and the working conditions of Operating Department Assistants.

National and International commitments

The status of the Association of Anaesthetists as an essential contributor to the work of governmental and other national organisations was established and greatly enhanced during the seventies. The Annual Reports 1970-1982 record that *inter alia* the Association gave evidence or advice to the Zuckerman Committee on Scientific Services in the NHS, the British Pharmacopoeia Commission, the Committee on Safety of Medicines, the Lane Committee on the working of the 1967 Abortion Act, the Lewin report on the staffing of operating theatres, the Advisory Committee on Ancillary Staff training, the City and Guilds Examination Board, the Central Manpower Committee, the Brodrick Report on Certification of Death and Coroners, the International Standards Organisation, the Merrison Committee of Enquiry into the Regulation of the Medical Profession (General Medical Council), the Central Distinction Awards Committee, the Medical Defence Union and, of course the Department of Health and Social Security on many topics. The latter included, pollution of operating theatres, obstetric analgesia, the use of Entonox (50% oxygen and nitrous oxide mixture) by ambulance crews, the use of local anaesthesia by chiropodists, the testing of newly installed pipelines, women in medicine, complaints procedures, acupuncture, hospital administration and design ("Community" and "Nucleus" hospitals), fees for family planning procedures and the perennial question of remuneration for anaesthetics in dental surgeries.

The Association was also represented on international organisations, specifically the Union of European Medical Specialists (UEMS) and the Regional and Central Committees of the World Federation of Societies of Anaesthesiologists (WFSA), directly or either through their Officers.[95]

Accommodation for the Association

The conduct of the administrative and secretarial functions of the Association of Anaesthetists in the prevailing circumstances of the Joint Secretariat in the surgeons' Royal College in Lincoln's Inn Fields had its lighter moments, but conditions there became intolerable in 1971, especially for an Administrative Secretary of the calibre of Miss Joyce Baxter (Chapter 7) A move to a small suite of offices in the British Medical Association complex in Tavistock Square was organised very rapidly, chiefly through the resourcefulness and initiative of the Honorary Secretary Michael Coplans (1922-1997), who reported to Council on 4 June 1971[96] the impending move on 24 June 1971 to Room 126, Tavistock House North (Annual Report 1971). The small office only provided secretarial space, but the Council began to meet in the larger accommodation of other organisations in BMA House, notably that of the Medical Defence Union (Council Minutes 3.12.1972).[96]

There was an attempt by the Officers of the surgeon's College to lure the Association of Anaesthetists back into a proposed expanded and reorganised Joint Secretariat accommodation during 1972 (Annual Report 1972: Council Minutes 1.9.1972),[96] but fortunately the Ladies Guild of the Royal Medical Benevolent Fund vacated a 1180 square feet (110 square metres) suite of offices in the BMA complex (Rooms 475-8 in Tavistock House South), and the Association moved in the 15 May 1973.

The accommodation included an adequate room for Council meetings which was re-equipped "to an appropriate standard", as well as smaller rooms for secretarial offices (Council Minutes 2.3.1972 and 4.5.1973:[96] Annual Report 1973). The Association of Anaesthetists remained in this suite of offices until it moved to 9 Bedford Square in November 1985.

A resolution was passed at the 1977 Annual General Meeting during Cyril Scurr's Presidency authorising the Officers to investigate the possibility of purchasing separate premises for the Association and, if necessary, to raise a "mortgage or loan not exceeding £200,000 (1996: £1,000,000)" (Council Minutes 30.10.1981).[97,98]

The next real move in the search for a purchase of property was a proposition put to Council by President W D Wylie on 30 October 1981; this was that the Officers should actively look for suitable premises, and this was agreed. The reasons for proposing the purchase of a suitable property were exclusively for the benefit of the Association of Anaesthetists. This was firstly, because it would be an investment, secondly because the Association of Anaesthetists would no longer have to pay the £10,000 (1996: £20,400) annual rental to the BMA, and thirdly because it would be a more suitable headquarters for the rapidly developing Association of Anaesthetists (Council Minutes 30.10.1981);[97] despite the suspicions of some who expressed opposition at a time when the College controversy was at its height (personal communications J Alfred Lee and others), it should be appreciated that there was no intention of obtaining a premises for a unilaterally declared College of Anaesthetists. A factor which was initially perceived as an additional spur to the search was that the lease of the suite in Tavistock House South was due to expire at the end of the year. This was not important in the end however as the lease was actually twice extended by mutual agreement with the BMA until the end of 1985, by which time the Association of Anaesthetists had moved into 9 Bedford Square (Chapter 9 and W D Wylie, personal communication).

The estate agents Hillier and Parker were engaged to assist with the search (Council Minutes 5.3.1982).[97] Two properties in Wimpole Street were considered during 1982 but rejected because of failure to obtain planning permission for the necessary modifications to listed buildings (Council Minutes 3.12.1982 and 4.2.1983).[97] Derek Wylie, who completed his term of office as President at the Annual General Meeting in October 1982, was invited by Michael Vickers, the incoming President, to personally continue the search for a suitable property (Council Minutes 3.12.1982).[97]

The Secretariat of the Association 1970-1982

Miss Joyce Baxter (Chapter 7) had first Mrs Karen Davis and then Mrs C L Somers as her Secretarial Assistant, and Mrs M Campion kept the accounts "on a part-time basis" (Annual Report 1977).

Miss Baxter retired at the end of 1973 and was dined out by the Officers and Council with honour and regret at the Royal Automobile Club (Annual Report 1974).[99] She was succeeded by the charming Miss Ann Muir who was destined to superintend the administrative affairs of the Association through ten presidencies until the Diamond Jubilee Year of the Association of Anaesthetists in 1992 (Chapter 9)!

The reconstruction of the Council of the Association

Elections to Council and its composition. The system of Council itself nominating suitable candidates to fill vacancies carried on into the nineteen seventies; in 1970, for the first time since 1959, two additional nominations were received (Council Minutes 6.11.1970).[96] A postal ballot was held; in the event the five Council nominees were elected to the five vacancies. The rules relating to Council membership were redrafted in 1970 to make certain that there was a reasonable representation from outside London. There were to be 12 elected Members of Council, at least five of whom were to be elected from Ordinary Members who neither "resided nor practised within the area of the Metropolitan Police District". Such a system could only be guaranteed to produce the desired balance in Council by Council itself nominating a list of candidates. There were three vacancies in 1971 and one of the Council's nominees was not elected, and, in 1973, there were originally six Council nominations (Council Minutes 7.4.1972)[96] and one very important later addition, M D Vickers, for four vacancies (Council Minutes 3.11.72 and 8.11.1972).[96] There was obviously increasing interest in election to the Council of the Association of Anaesthetists. Council resolved that they would retain the right to nominate but in future would only nominate the exact number of additional candidates to fill the vacancies (Council Minutes 7.4.1972):[96] in the event Vickers and three of the other Council nominations were elected.

Aileen Adams (Honorary Secretary (1968-1970) and later Dean of the Faculty) originally suggested that the Single Transferable Vote system should be adopted for election to Council (Council Minutes 16.6.1972),[96] and this change was made from 1973 onwards (Annual Reports 1972 and 1973). It was actually used for the first time in 1973 to select council nominees for five vacancies; it was however resolved to accept the first four names voted in at the election, and that of the Scottish candidate who had obtained the most votes (Council Minutes 2.3.1973 and 4.5.1973).[96] A sixth vacancy was created by the election of Michael Vickers to the post of Assistant Honorary Secretary. There were two additional nominations and there was a postal vote using the single transferable vote, which in fact made no difference to the result (personal recollection). The vote resulted in the election of four of the Council nominees (including the Scotsman) and the two counter nominees (Council Minutes 26.9.1973).[81] The procedure was obviously becoming complicated and untidy and the President (Helliwell) referred the problem to the working party which he had set up under John Inkster. This Working Party reported to the Council on 5 April 1974;[81] as a result it was agreed that:

1. Council should continue to make nominations, but that first nominations should be invited from the electorate, and only subsequently should Council make their nominations "if they saw fit". The identity of the nominators should not appear on the

voting papers so that there would be no apparent distinction between Council and other nominees.

2. No special voting arrangements or cooptions would be made to ensure Scottish, Welsh or Irish representation but that the Dean of the Irish Faculty should continue to be coopted to Council.

3. A map showing the residential location of Officers and current Council Members should be provided with the voting papers.

4. Each candidate should be permitted to provide brief curriculum vitae.

Council did not finally relinquish the practice of making its own Council nominations until the Annual General Meeting of 1979 when the bye-laws were altered to provide solely for nomination in writing by two Ordinary members and, at the same time, all geographical limitations on candidates were removed (Council Minutes 2.3.1979)[97]

The rules were revised again at the 1982 Annual General Meeting (Council Minutes 8.1.1982);[97] from 1983 onwards three candidates have been elected each year for four year terms with no provision for casual vacancies which might arise (for example, by election of an Ordinary Member as Assistant Honorary Secretary).

The increased general awareness of the purpose and influence of the Association of Anaesthetists in recent years has ensured that highly motivated and competent candidates have come forward to offer themselves for election, and groups and societies have seen to it that geographical and specialist professional interests have been well looked after. The Chairman and Secretary of the Group of Anaesthetists in Training (formerly the Junior Anaesthetists Group) are elected by the Trainee (Junior) Members and have had full voting rights within Council since 1970 (Council Minutes 3.7.70).[94,96]

The policy of cooption to the Council of those anaesthetists who hold high Office in other major organisations ensures that the Association of Anaesthetists has available expertise and advice at the highest and widest possible level. The 1998 list of cooptions included the President of the Royal College of Anaesthetists, the Dean of the Faculty of Anaesthetists of the Royal

College of Surgeons in Ireland, the Adviser in Anaesthesia to the Chief Medical Officer, the President of the WFSA (who is currently from the United Kingdom), the Chairman of the Advisers in Anaesthetics of the Armed Forces, the Convenor of the Irish Standing Committee and the Editor of *Anaesthesia News* (Chapter 9). The Editor of *Anaesthesia* is, of course, an Executive Officer of the Association.

Association Officers were, and are, nominally elected annually and, although the constitution provides for counter-nominations, the list proposed by the existing Officers and endorsed by Council was, and subsequently always has been, elected at the Annual General Meeting without dissent (a system which probably owes its origin to the foundation of the Association by Officers of the Section of Anaesthetics of the Royal Society of Medicine) (Chapters 2 and 3). Presidents and Vice Presidents are usually elected and re-elected for two year terms but, in fact can be re-elected annually thereafter. The lengths of normal tenure of the Officers of Honorary Treasurer and the Editor of *Anaesthesia* were not specified, as was the case of the terms of the Honorary Secretaries (four years in total), until the nineteen seventies when maximum periods of five and ten years were agreed (Council Minutes 2.3.1973),[96,100] The limitation on the period of office of officers in any organisation is a wise precaution and saves embarrassment both from the point of view of the organisation and the holder of the office! The pattern of the individual serving one year as Assistant Honorary Secretary, two years as Honorary Secretary and a further year as Immediate Past Honorary Secretary was also instituted in the nineteen seventies and ensured continuity (Annual General Meeting 1974).

The reorganisation of the Advisory Committee. The Annual Report for 1972 during J Alfred Lee's Presidency records that "almost the entire business of Council has been initially discussed by the Advisory Committee". This is a very different function from that of the Advisory Committee of the sixties where only personal problems of Members and particularly important specific administrative matters, often concerning the Constitution, were referred to it (Chapter 7).

The composition of the Advisory Committee, which was previously appointed by name, was reconstituted to be by appointment by office during 1972. It was to consist of the President, the President Elect, the Honorary

Treasurer, the two Honorary Secretaries, the Chairman of the Junior Anaesthetists' Group, the Dean of the Faculty and the Chairman of the BMA CCHMS Subcommittee, plus one other member of Council. The Minutes imply that the ordinary elected members of Council were not very happy with this proposal, particularly the statutory appointment (rather than cooption) of the Dean of the Faculty and the Chairman of the CCHMS Subcommittee of the BMA (Council Minutes 2.3.1973).[96] The inclusion of the Editor of *Anaesthesia* was unsuccessfully challenged at the Council Meeting of 26.9.1973.[81] The composition was however finally allowed to stand provisionally, with the addition of a second member of Council for one year, and the change was reported to the 1973 Annual General Meeting at which Helliwell succeeded to the Presidency.

Helliwell defined the future functions of the Advisory Committee at his first Council meeting as President on 2nd November 1973[81] as:-

1. having *"executive authority to dispose of matters that need not worry Council."*

2. charged with giving *"careful consideration to the Agenda for Council, presenting matters for discussion in a form that would ensure full consideration of the alternatives available".*

The composition of the Advisory Committee was modified again at the Council Meeting on 6 December 1974[81] when it was agreed that, in addition to those appointed *ex officio*, there should be three Ordinary Members elected by ballot each year from amongst the Ordinary Members sitting on Council; a proper balance between the powers of the Advisory Committee and of the Council as a whole was thus maintained. The reorganisation of the Advisory Committee meant that fewer meetings of the full Council were required. The custom of the Executive Officers meeting before each Advisory and Council to discuss the agenda developed, and was formalised during Michael Rosen's Presidency (1986-1988). The system developed out of necessity because of the increasing volume of business to be transacted, but it none the less works well.

Changes in the Rules and Bye-laws. All these changes in the middle of the seventies, particularly during the Helliwell Presidency (1973-1976), and catalysed by the hard work and inspiration of the Honorary Secretaries of the period (John Zorab, 1972-1974 and Michael Vickers, 1974-1976), greatly enhanced the professionalism of the Association of Anaesthetists and prepared it for its ever expanding role in the nineteen eighties. The administrative revolution was not achieved without considerable changes in the constitutional rules and bye-laws. These provided a series of field days for the more pedantic and legally minded Members! Many new measures were "sent back" for rewording before they were finally ratified. Philip Helliwell confided that he dreaded introducing a new constitutional measure because of the fear of "having to withdraw it with a red face" (personal communication)!

The legal status of the Association was discussed with the Association's solicitors (Messrs. Hempsons) during 1973 (Annual Report 1973). The possible change was that of incorporating the Association of Anaesthetists as a Limited Liability Company so that its financial liabilities fell on a corporate body rather than on individual members. It was however concluded at that time that "there would be few, if any, advantages to be gained by such a move and Council agreed to take no further action in the matter" (Annual Report 1974). This decision was not entirely propitious. The failure to incorporate at this stage might have resulted in a problem when it came to the purchase of the lease of 9 Bedford Square in 1983; however the difficulty was overcome by the courage and initiative of Derek Wylie and Michael Vickers who were by then the Trustees of the Association. The General Fund of the Association and the Education and Research Trust were incorporated as separate companies in 1985 (Chapter 9).[100]

An economic miracle 1974-1982

Philip Helliwell[3] was the last holder of the prestigious Office of Medical Superintendent of Guy's Hospital, London before the convulsive reorganisations of the NHS in the late seventies and eighties abolished the post. The Treasurer and Chief Accountant and Controller of the Investments and Endowment Fund of the Guy's Group of Hospital during that period was Ernest Warburton. Warburton was greatly respected by the senior medical staff of Guy's Hospital for the support which he gave them and his willingness to give them timely advice about pensions and investments (Helliwell personal communication). Philip Helliwell introduced Ernest Warburton to Council of the Association of Anaesthetists in 1974 and he was then invited to become the Honorary Financial Advisor to the Association (Council Minutes 4.10.1974).[81]

The financial affairs of the Association were transformed between 1974 and 1982 as a result of the advice given by Ernest Warburton, and the work of two very able Honorary Treasurers (Stanley A Mason and Michael Rosen).

The original key to the reorganisation, in addition to careful management of the investments of the Association of Anaesthetists, was the separation of the accounts of the General Fund from those of the Research and Education Fund (later the Education and Research Trust), and the transfer by variable covenant of the annual surplus form the General Fund to the Research and Education Fund which was registered as a Charity (Council Minutes 7.2.1975).[81] This transaction achieves very considerable tax advantages for the Association.

The accounts of the Association of Anaesthetists show that, in 1975, the General Fund had an income from the interest on investments of £2,205 (1996: £9,800) and that the total income (including members' subscriptions and profit from the journal *Anaesthesia* was £25,208 (1996: £112,400) with capital gains on investment of £5,431 (1996: £24,200); while by 1982 the investment income was £29,612 (1996: £55,700) and the total income was £191,990 (1996: £361,000).

The Research and Education Fund received a payment from the variable Deed of Covenant from the General Fund in 1975 of £8,649 (1996: £38,600) and interest income from investments of £4,880 (1996: £21,800) with capital gains of £530 (1996: £2,400); whereas in 1982 the variable covenant amounted to £57,664 (1996: £108,400), the interest income was £20,579 (1996:£34,700) and capital gains in that year were £3,103 (1996: £5,800).

The assets of the Association of Anaesthetists and its income continue to rise steadily in the nineteen nineties. This has enabled the Association to increase its work and its contribution to the well being of the specialty of anaesthesia. Its activities have included the acquisition of a prestigious headquarters in Bedford Square, and the contributing of donations and loans to the Royal College of Anaesthetists (Chapter 9). Truly there has been an economic miracle. The Association of Anaesthetists expressed its gratitude by electing Ernest Warburton to Honorary Membership in 1981. Ernest was the first Honorary Member to be elected who was not medically qualified, since 1962 and only one of 6 such out of the 105 Honorary Members who have been so honoured in the whole 64 year history of the Association. He continued to advise the Association until its Diamond Jubilee year (1992) when the accountant Francis Wirgman took over.[101]

Subscriptions to the Association have risen in real terms since 1974. Ernest Warburton convinced the Finance Committee early on that the Association of Anaesthetists was undersubscribed for a professional organisation![101]

The annual Ordinary Members rates including receipt of the Journal *Anaesthesia* have been:- 1974:£12 (1996: £60), 1982:£40 (1996: £75), and 1996: £120. It must be remembered also that the 1974 rate was fixed when the journal *Anaesthesia*, the cost of which is included in the subscription, had only just increased its publication rate from four to six times each year while, by 1982 it was being published monthly.

The debate concerning the need for a College of Anaesthetists

The result of increasing specialisation in the United Kingdom in the mid twentieth century was a desire of members of the emergent medical disciplines to aspire to founding independent academic bodies, separate form the traditional general Colleges of physicians and surgeons, to provide for their own educational, training, examination and registration requirements.[102]

The "British" College of Obstetricians and Gynaecologists separated fairly amicably in 1929 from the Royal College of Surgeons of England, and became "Royal" in 1939; the Faculty of Radiology, always independent although for a time resident in the surgeons' College in Lincoln's Inn Fields, was formed in 1939 and became the Royal College of Radiologists in 1974; the College of General Practitioners was founded in 1953 ("Royal" in 1967); and the College of Pathologists ("Royal" in 1970), and the Royal College of Psychiatrists in 1963 and 1971 respectively.

The pattern could have been different; a multidisciplinary College or Academy might have been formed on the lines of the Royal College of Physicians of Canada; but an attempt to found an Academy of Medicine in

1945, immediately after the Second World War, foundered because of the traditional insistence on their own independence of surgeons and physicians. The existence of separate colleges does not mean that they can not, and do not, act in unison when occasion demands, and this had become increasingly apparent since the formal Conference (now the Academy) of the Royal Medical Colleges and their Faculties was established in the mid nineteen seventies.[102]

The functions of the Royal Medical Colleges in the United Kingdom were defined by Sir Rodney Smith (President of the Royal College of Surgeons of England 1973-1977) as being that of maintaining the standards of the services offered by their Fellows and Members to the public.[102] "This responsibility included the supervision of training, the determination of standards for qualification [which always includes specialist qualification, but may include basic qualifications entitling the holder to practice medicine or dental surgery as well], and efforts to improve further education and research". In recent times these functions, besides the conduct of examinations leading to diplomas of Fellowship and/or Membership, have involved the holding of meetings and lecture courses to facilitate postgraduate and continuing education, inspection and approval of hospitals engaged in the training of specialists, and advice to the government on the recruitment and deployment of manpower.[103] No College should as a body take up cudgels purely on behalf of the self-interests of its Fellows or Members;[102,103] indeed they can not do so as they are not permitted under the provisions of their charitable charters to negotiate terms and conditions of service with employers and, in particular, with a near monopoly state employer such as exists in the National Health Service. It could be said that the Medical Royal Colleges look after the interests of patients but other bodies must look after the interests of the practitioner! This is only a half truth however. Rodney Smith emphasises that the limitations should not prevent the Colleges drawing attention to the dangers if the conditions under which the Fellows and Members are forced to work effect the standard of care which can be given to patients; and indeed they have frequently done so. Smith acknowledges that there is "a narrow line of distinction between areas which should be of legitimate concern to Colleges, and areas where Colleges would be well advised to keep out of".[102] There have certainly been times since the introduction of the NHS, when to an outsider, the older Colleges and their Presidents have seemed to come near to political confrontation with the Government.[102,104] Conversely the Council of the Association of Anaesthetists of Great Britain and Ireland, while not concerning itself with the details of the conduct of academic anaesthesia since it promoted the formation of the Faculty in 1948, has not hesitated to campaign for remedial action when it was felt that the arrangements made for organising academic anaesthesia were inadequate.

The position of the Faculty of Anaesthetists of the Royal College of Surgeons of England in 1970. Anaesthetists were, and still are, grateful to the surgeons' College for taking them under their wing at the time of the inauguration of the National Health Service in 1948, and thereby giving them the academic status which enabled those suitably qualified to become Consultants in the NHS (Chapter 5). The specialty of anaesthesia had developed in size and importance by 1970, however, to such an extent that it had become the largest single specialty in the NHS, and Fellows of the Faculty of Anaesthetists accounted for over 25% of practitioners with Fellowship status in the Royal College of Surgeons of England. Their position within the surgeons' College was, however, anomalous despite their numerical strength. The anaesthetists were represented by a Faculty which neither controlled its own funds nor awarded its own diplomas. All the decisions of the Board of Faculty, on which three surgeons (the President and two Vice Presidents of the College) sat *ex-officio* as voting members with 20 anaesthetists, were, moreover, subject to ratification by the Council of the College which was comprised of 29 surgeons, one dental surgeon, and one anaesthetist. There was, consequently a growing feeling amongst anaesthetists by 1970 that this position was unsatisfactory. It was known that the Council of the College were seeking a new Charter. Many anaesthetists hoped (and indeed expected) that this would include what came to be known as the "three Faculty" or "tripartite" solution. This would have involved the creation of a structure of three virtually independent Faculties (surgery, anaesthetics and dental surgery) managing their own affairs and equally, or at least proportionately, represented on a common Royal College Council.[103,105-107]

There is little doubt that the failure to achieve this "three Faculty" objective was a big factor amongst those which led ultimately, and probably fortunately, to the establishment of an independent Royal College of Anaesthetists. It is significant that, when the independent College of Anaesthetists finally received its Royal Charter in 1992, it was difficult to find any anaesthetist who objected; and yet there had, at one time, been very considerable and powerful opposition both amongst the leaders of the specialty and the rank and file.[108]

It is to the credit of successive Officers and elected Council Members of the Association of Anaesthetists in the seventies and eighties that their single minded perception and refusal to accept second best, led finally to the establishment of the independent Royal College of Anaesthetists. They had first to persuade the majority of anaesthetists practising in the United Kingdom, many of whom were initially doubtful, and then the Board of Faculty itself, that the foundation of the independent Royal College of Anaesthetists was both viable and necessary.

The question of unification or integration. The first mention in the Council Minutes of the consideration of "the relationship between the Association and other bodies concerned with anaesthesia" was by Philip Helliwell[3] who was at that time Chairman of the Advisory Committee. Helliwell reported that, at a meeting of the Advisory Committee held that morning (6.2.1970) "discussions had taken place as to whether existing arrangements [for co-operation between the Association of Anaesthetists, the Faculty, and the BMA] were in the best interests of the specialty."[96] The following September (1970) John Beard,[1] the reigning President of the Association, in a newsletter addressed to all Members of the Association,[109] stated:-

> *"The cross representation and close friendship of the Council of the Association and the Board of Faculty enable mother and daughter [!] to work amicably together. Nevertheless, other people, including the Department of Health and even many anaesthetists, find the differentiation of the more academic functions of the Faculty from the wider interests of the Association confusing."*
>
> *"To complete the picture, but not I am afraid to simplify it, the Association asked the BMA in 1946 to set up an Anaesthetists' Group in order that there might be specialist anaesthetic opinion on the Central Consultants Committee of the Hospital Medical Services."*
>
> *"The relationship between these bodies, or even their unification,*

are much in our minds, but the issues are involved and will need much consideration."[109]

It is difficult to understand the use of the word "unification" by an anaesthetist of Beard's seniority and medicopolitical status as both President of the Association and a member of the Board of Faculty. He must have known that the charitable charter of any future Royal College would inevitably prevent it being involved directly with those interests of anaesthetists which concerned their terms and conditions of service. It may be that he had in mind "integration" rather than "unification" between the Association of Anaesthetists and a putative College with a joint secretariat.[110] Beard was obviously also concerned about the relationship of the Council of the Association of Anaesthetists with the Anaesthetists Group of the British Medical Association, (The BMA being the only recognised national negotiating agency between the medical profession and the administrators of the NHS). The Association Council and the Committee of the BMA Anaesthetists' Group conducted their affairs more or less independently at that time although they did have cross representation.[59] The BMA Group of Anaesthetists was, however, disbanded in 1973 and replaced by the Anaesthetists Subcommittee of the Central Committee for Hospital Medical Services (CCHMS), which later became the Central Consultants and Specialists Committee (CCSC). This reorganisation resulted in the direct representation of the Council of the Association of Anaesthetists, and consequently, its influence was increased to a very satisfactory level (Annual Reports of Council 1972 and 1973), and there was no longer any cause for anxiety that the voice of the Association of Anaesthetists was not being adequately represented through the BMA.

There should not have been any confusion between the roles of the Association of Anaesthetists and the Faculty of Anaesthetists as, as mentioned above, the functions of the Faculty were limited to academic matters by the charitable nature of the Charter of the Royal College of Surgeons. Such matters as the conduct of the Fellowship examination and the organisation of training and the certification of hospitals for training purposes were clearly the sole responsibility of the College as they had been since the foundation of the Faculty. There are however areas where it was and is legitimate for both the Association of Anaesthetists and the Faculty of Anaesthetists to have a view.

These included such matters as the use of manpower and the presentation of evidence to government and other enquiries, albeit at times from different standpoints. Both bodies could also rightly participate in providing postgraduate and continuing education by holding meetings and conferences. Confusion may have arisen however because the original Royal Colleges of Physicians and Surgeons tended to be the predominant voice for all issues other than a remuneration for their specialties and had at times adopted a quasi-political role. The Faculty of Anaesthetists, on the other hand, from its position within the surgeons' College tended to confine itself more narrowly to academic matters and leave other issues to the independent and historically powerful Association of Anaesthetists.

The concept and presumed value of "unification" was very much in the minds of anaesthetists early in the seventies[111], but by the end of the decade, the distinction between academic functions (Faculty or College) and functions related to terms and conditions of service (Association of Anaesthetists) was more fully understood.

The 1971 resolution. Informal meetings on the "possible integration of the Association with other bodies concerned with anaesthesia" took place between the Officers of the Association and the Dean of the Faculty (Cyril Scurr, 1970-73, later President of the Association of Anaesthetists, 1976-78) and others during 1971 (Annual Report 1971); however; the event which really stimulated progress was a motion submitted by Peter J Tomlin of the Birmingham University Department to the Annual General Meeting of the Association of Anaesthetists which took place at Birmingham on 24 September 1971 (Annual Report 1972).[112] The motion was passed, as amended by W Derek Wylie. It resolved:-

> *"That the Council take steps to determine the views of all anaesthetists after all the relevant information had been made available, concerning a unified organisation for all anaesthetists; and to report back as soon as possible to the membership of the Association, if necessary to an Extraordinary General Meeting, the conditions of an acceptable arrangement."*[112]

The only real difference between the resolution as passed and the original was the significant substitution for "all anaesthetists" for "other bodies concerned". The words "unified organisation" featured in the resolution, and no mention was made of a possible "College".

The 1972 Document of Information and Referendum, and the 1973 Special General Meeting and Resolutions. J Alfred Lee (1906-1989)[2] took over as President at the Annual General Meeting in November 1971. He was not at that time, nor subsequently, an advocate of a College of Anaesthetists.[108] He believed that the future of anaesthesia lay within the surgeons' College (personal communication); like a number of other senior anaesthetists he remembered with gratitude the assistance which the Royal College of Surgeons of England gave to the aspirations of anaesthetists in 1948 at the inauguration of the NHS. It is to Lee's great credit that he presided with absolute impartiality over a difficult period when the opinions of the Council of the Association were crystallising into a stance which firmly favoured seeking to persuade the Faculty to progress towards independent collegiate status.

In order to activate the resolution passed at the 1971 Annual General Meeting Council resolved that a Document of Information should be prepared and a referendum should be conducted by questionnaire by an *ad hoc* Committee under the chairmanship of Philip Helliwell[3] who was at that time Chairman of the Advisory Committee. The Committee included Michael Vickers, W D Wylie, George H Ellis and F Richard Ellis (Chairman JAG).

The Document of Information was masterly and exhaustive and extraordinary measures were taken to ensure that it was not biased. Professor W Holland of the Department of Clinical Epidemiology, St Thomas' Hospital London and Dr M E Abrams, Senior Lecturer in Medicine at Guy's Hospital London, gave their approval of its impartiality (Council Minutes 16.6.1972).[96]

The Charter Committee of the Royal College of Surgeons of England had been meeting meanwhile to draw up proposals for the new Charter for the College. The circulation of the Document of Information was delayed until these proposals were known. The Charter Committee of the surgeons' College had been chaired by the reigning Dean of the Faculty of Anaesthetists Cyril F Scurr, but his initial proposal for the Three Faculty College was rejected by the surgeons from the outset (personal communication). One can have sympathy with this point of view for, after all, their College was, and always had been, a college of surgeons. The proposed changes of the Charter Committee were approved by the Faculty of Anaesthetists on 17 May 1972 (Council Minutes 16.6.1972).[96] They can be summarised as follows:-

1. A declaration in the preamble to the effect that the Fellows of the Faculty were equal in status to surgical Fellows of the College. (The meaning of this was difficult to understand in the face of the rejection of the three Faculty College concept with a proportionately representative Council).[105,110]

2. There was to be an increase of the representation of anaesthetists on the Council of the surgeons' college from one to three.

3. There was to be an opportunity for anaesthetists to become President or Vice President of the Surgeons' College (if elected by the Council consisting of 24 surgeons, three dental surgeons and three anaesthetists).

4. Authority to appoint examiners and award diplomas was to be delegated to the Faculty.

5. There was to be an opportunity for an anaesthetist to be awarded the College Gold Medal.[105,108,113]

The President and two Vice Presidents of the Surgeons' College were to remain voting members of the Board of Faculty, and the finances of the Faculty were not to be separately identified, but were to remain under the control of the College Finance Committee.

A copy of these proposals was circulated with the Document of Information to approximately 6000 anaesthetists with a questionnaire, but the Council of the Association of Anaesthetists expressed "neither approval nor disapproval".

The content of the responses to the questionnaire were carefully reviewed by Vickers. They were equivocal and again demonstrated that the obstacles to the "unification" of the various bodies of anaesthetists were not fully understood.[110] Council therefore decided to hold a Special General Meeting

The debate concerning the need for a College of Anaesthetists 323

at the house of the Royal Society of Medicine on 2 June 1973 and to put two resolutions to those present (Annual Report 1973):-

> 1. *"The meeting proposes that the Council of the Association, having regard to the views expressed in the Referendum, should urge the Board of Faculty to explore the possibilities of further reorganisation within the Royal College of Surgeons. The meeting believes that such reorganisation should clearly indicate that the academic and relevant professional affairs of each of the three specialties, surgery, dental surgery and anaesthesia, are under the independent control of its own academic body; in addition, the policy and managerial affairs of the College should be placed in the hands of a governing authority on which the Fellows in these three specialties are appropriately represented."*

This resolution was carried by 71-1 votes (Annual Report 1973).

> 2. *"The meeting is of the opinion that, should the objectives set out in the previous resolution prove to be unattainable, an independent College of Anaesthetists would be to the ultimate benefit of the specialty, providing it is introduced at an appropriate time and under appropriate conditions. Pending the outcome of such further negotiations, the meeting instructs Council to undertake a detailed examination of the options available and hopes that the Board of Faculty of Anaesthetists will join in discussions with Council at a suitable time".*

This resolution was also carried, but only by 37-35 votes (Annual Report 1973).

The present writer believes that these results were thoroughly representative of the views of anaesthetists as a whole in 1973. They were not satisfied with what the proposed new Charter for the Royal College of Surgeons of England was offering but were hesitant about supporting a move to total independence. One important factor was the fear of the economic cost of purchasing suitable premises and the consequent size of the subscription which would be required to sustain and support the purchase; to quote Lady Macbeth there was a prevailing atmosphere of "letting I dare not wait upon I would"[114] at that time. There were, in addition, a considerable body of anaesthetists who were indifferent and, as has already been mentioned, a number of the senior members of the specialty who felt a strong sense of loyalty to the Royal College of Surgeons of England for historical reasons.[105,108]

Further discussion 1973-1975. Alfred Lee[2] handed over the Presidency to Philip Helliwell[3] at the Annual General Meeting in Bristol in September 1973; before doing so, however, he announced that Council had appointed a group consisting of P J Helliwell,[3] D D C Howat, Michael Rosen and J S M Zorab (Hon Secretary), to give effect to the hope expressed in the resolution of the Special General Meeting of June 1973 that meaningful discussions on the College question should take place with the Board of Faculty (Minutes of the 1973 Annual General Meeting).

It is no secret that Philip Helliwell,[3] the new President, shared the opinion that the proposed College Charter did not go far enough to satisfy the needs of the speciality of anaesthesia. He was supported in this view by the executive officers (S A Mason, who became the Hon Treasurer in 1974, the Hon Secretaries (J S M Zorab and M D Vickers) and the Editor of *Anaesthesia*, (T B Boulton). They, and the majority of the elected members of the Council, were of the opinion that further negotiations were necessary. They believed that the aim should be to extend the provisions of the College Charter to gain greater autonomy for the Faculty within the College of Surgeons or, if this was not possible, to seek a separate Charter for the foundation of the independent College of Anaesthetists. It was, however, necessary to first convince the majority of anaesthetists that the latter action was desirable and practicable.

One of Helliwell's first actions as President was to set up the Working Party to determine the financial implications of founding and maintaining a College of Anaesthetists under the Chairmanship of Stanley Mason. It was hoped that the Faculty would nominate representatives to join this Working Party (Council Minutes 1.2.1974)[81] but it declined to do so (Council Minutes 5.4.1974).[81] The Working Party concluded that the project would be viable at an annual subscription of £30 (1996: £150), although this figure was contested as an underestimate at the 1974 Annual General Meeting by the then Dean of the Faculty (Professor (Sir) Gordon Robson). Helliwell had also had correspondence with the President of the Royal College of Surgeons Sir Rodney Smith. The latter was adamant that the provisions of the new proposed Charter of the surgeons' College would represent a satisfactory position for the Faculty of Anaesthetists.[105]

At the 1974 Annual General Meeting Helliwell[3] stated that the opinion of Council was that "not only does the revised Charter of the [surgeons'] College fail to satisfy their interpretation of the first Resolution at the Special General meeting in June 1973, but it does not represent a long-term arrangement". A resolution was then presented and passed with 63 votes in favour and only 7 against. This resolved that:-

"This meeting believes that Council should take all necessary steps to determine the strength of support for the formation of a College of Anaesthetists."

Professor Sir Geoffrey Organe's enquiry was instituted in response to the resolution at the 1974 Annual General Meeting. Sir Geoffrey was asked, as an elder statesman, to assess the strength of academic support for the independent College. This he did by postal ballot and personal consultation. The definition of "academic" was fairly widely drawn. It included Consultants of all teaching hospitals and University Departments, Members of the Boards of Faculty of the English and Irish Colleges, Examiners, and Members of the Council of the Association of Anaesthetists. Few of these, except for some Members of the Association Council, were Consultants in District General Hospitals who did not have teaching appointments; however, it was agreed that "Sir Geoffrey, at his discretion might canvass the opinion from others." (Council Meeting 7.2.1975)[81]

Sir Geoffrey presented his report to Council on 5 September 1975[81] and its content was conveyed to the membership in the 1975 Annual Report. Sir Geoffrey's opinion was:-

"That, though there was strong support for the concept of independent status for anaesthetists, this was subject to reservations. The major reservation concerned the ability to raise funds for a respectable independent College outside the College of Surgeons. Whilst the majority would support such a venture they did not relish the prospect

of leading such a move or trying to raise funds. There was, however, strong support for the independence if it could be obtained in close relationship within the College of Surgeons." (Council Minutes 5.9.1975)[81]

Further discussion in 1975 and 1976. Sir Geoffrey Organe's conclusions were rather disappointing for the Council of the Association of Anaesthetists; however, Council resisted a suggestion by the retiring Dean of the Faculty (Gordon Robson) and the immediate past Dean (Cyril Scurr) to the effect that "public acknowledgment that a move to total independence was no longer contemplated", should be made "because this would enable further advances to be made for anaesthetists within the College of Surgeons". This proposal was rejected because a clear idea had not been obtained of what such advances might consist (Council Minutes 5.9.1975).[81] This was wise; the official grant of the new Charter for the surgeons' College was still three years into the future!

More frank discussions ensued between the President (Helliwell) and the Hon Secretaries Vickers (also a member of the Board of Faculty) and Zorab, on behalf of the Association, and the President of the surgeons' College (Sir Rodney Smith), the Dean of the Faculty (Gordon Robson) and the Secretary of the College (R Johnson-Gilbert). The position of the officers of the surgeons' College remained the same, either the proposed new Charter provision must be accepted as a satisfactory position, or the anaesthetists would have to form an independent College and move out of the premises of the Royal College of Surgeons of England; even the possibility of simply changing the name of the Faculty of Anaesthetists to the College of Anaesthetists was considered by the President of the surgeons' College to be unacceptable to the Privy Council (Council Minutes 5.3.1976).[81] The latter surmise was, of course, subsequently proved to be incorrect (Chapter 9).

The concept of "Unilateral Declaration of Independence" (UDI) was much in the public mind at the time (1975-76) because of the apparent success of the UDI proclaimed by the Government of Rhodesia. Some anaesthetists canvassed the possibility of UDI in the form of a College of Anaesthetists outside the College of Surgeons and independent of the Faculty, but this was not seriously considered by Council until 1978. The perceived obstacles were the question of control of the specialist Fellowship Diploma, which the Faculty of Anaesthetists and the College of Surgeons would certainly not surrender, and the absence of suitable premises. The theoretical possibility of the College of Anaesthetists with a separate Charter retaining accommodation within the Royal College of Surgeons building was discussed with the officers of the surgeons' College in 1976, but rejected by them out of hand.[105]

The official attitude of the Board of the Faculty of Anaesthetists in 1976 was supportive of the view that the proposed terms offered in the new Charter of the Surgeons' College were satisfactory. In order to facilitate the application for the Charter by the College, the following resolution was introduced on 17 March 1976 by (Sir) Gordon Robson, just prior to handling over the office of Dean to J E Riding of Liverpool:-

"The Board of the Faculty of Anaesthetists firmly requests Council to press forward with all possible speed to implement the Consolidated Charter, secure in the knowledge that the Faculty sees its future to be within these walls in close association with our surgical and dental colleagues as described in the Charter and in common endeavour to maintain the College."[105]

An attempt was made to amend the resolution by deleting everything in it after the words "Consolidated Charter" but a vote was not taken for procedural reasons.[105]

The inauguration of the anaesthetists' Academic Foundation. Helliwell[3] was re-elected as President for a third year at the Annual General Meeting in Cardiff in September 1975 (Council Minutes 7.6.1974).[81] The Presidency had customarily been held for only two year since 1967 (Chapter 7) but, in view of Helliwell's commitment and extensive knowledge of the intricacies of the independent College issue, and the conversations with the Officers of the surgeons' College which were then taking place, it was considered that it was desirable to maintain continuity. There was some degree of optimism that a solution would be found at the end of 1975 but, as has already been noted, by the middle of 1976 it was clear that, for the time being, no further progress could be made.

The Officers and Council of the Association reviewed the options and determined to maintain a flexible position, but, meanwhile to initiate a charitable trust to accumulate funds which could ultimately be transferred to a truly independent academic body responsible for the specialty of anaesthesia (Council Minutes 21.5.1976).[81]

Members of the Association of Anaesthetists were circulated with a letter from Council signed by the President in September 1976.[105] This document announced the intention of setting up the Trust and outlined the possible options for establishing a College of Anaesthetists and reviewed the negotiations which had already taken place. The decision to initiate the Anaesthetists' Academic Foundation and to fund raise for it, was reported and endorsed by the 1976 Annual General Meeting in London.

The Trust Deed was signed on 22 March 1977 by W D Wylie, P J Helliwell, and D D C Howat who were the Trustees of the Association of Anaesthetists.[116] The last named (a Member of the Board) was deemed to be "the person acceptable to the Board of Faculty" under the terms of the Trust Deed (Council Minutes 7.1.1977).[81,117] Douglas Howat resigned as a Trustee of the Foundation in 1978 and Aileen K Adams (later Dean of the Faculty) replaced him. She resigned in 1985 on becoming Dean and was replace by another member of the Board of Faculty, P J F Baskett.

The intention of the President and Officers of the Association of Anaesthetists and the overwhelming majority of the elected members of its Council was "to facilitate the evolution of a truly independent status for the academic body responsible for the specialty of anaesthesia".[115] The objects defined in the Trust Deed of the anaesthetists Academic Foundation were drawn up very widely however:-

1. *To advance the art, science and teaching of anaesthesia.*

2. *To advance education in anaesthesia and for that purpose to organise courses of instruction.*

3. *To promote research in all aspects of anaesthesia and arrange for the publication of the useful results thereof.*

4. *In the event of another charity being formed which has such objects including all those set out above to transfer its assets (if the Trustees so decide) to such other charity.*[116]

The word "independent" was not mentioned, nor the word "College"; under these terms any money collected could actually have been immediately handed over to the Royal College of Surgeons for the use of the Faculty of Anaesthetists! Whatever the legal niceties, the present writer (then Editor of *Anaesthesia*) believed then, and still believes, that this ambiguity was a pity. The apparent reluctance of the Council of the Association of Anaesthetists to nail its colours to the mast caused confusion and some irritation amongst those who wished to subscribe money aimed at establishing an independent College of Anaesthetists.[103,118] It can indeed be argued that the fund would have obtained more donations if the intention to work for the formation of a College of Anaesthetists inside or outside the surgeons' College had been made explicit.

It must be emphasised that, once inaugurated, the Anaesthetists' Academic Foundation was entirely independent and its disposal was solely in the hands of its Trustees.[116,117] The Trustees kept faith with the intentions with which it was founded. The donations were invested, but the Fund received relatively little publicity after the initial appeal because events began to indicate that the Faculty was moving towards administrative and financial independence, and the Association of Anaesthetists began to raise funds for its own premises; but, despite this, just over £172,000 (1996: £246,000) was handed over to the College of Anaesthetists in 1988 when an amendment to the Charter of the Royal College of Surgeons of England enabled the Faculty to be granted collegiate status within the surgeons' College.[119] The Anaesthetists' Academic Foundation continues as the main fund raising organ for the present Royal College of Anaesthetists. Its trustees are now appointed by office. They are the President of the Royal College of Anaesthetists, the President of the Association of Anaesthetists of Great Britain and Ireland and the Chairman of the Finance Committee of the Royal College of Anaesthetists. This is surely a further happy example of the collaboration between the two organisations which now exists.

A Coordinating College? This solution was originally suggested in 1976 by R Johnson-Gilbert, Secretary of the Surgeons' College (Council Minutes 5.3.1976). Such a College, it was proposed, might issue joint diplomas in anaesthesia in the names of the Royal College of Surgeons of England and the Royal College of Surgeons in Ireland. The idea was discussed further but not encouraged by the then President of the Association in his newsletter.[105] It was not really a practical proposition.

A College of Anaesthetists temporarily separate from the Faculty? This form of UDI was discussed in a paper tabled by Cyril Scurr early in 1978 (Council Minutes 6.1.1978).[81] It was proposed that a College should be founded, which would be complementary rather than competing with the Faculty with the ultimate aim that the two would coalesce. It was suggested that the new College might take over the educational activities of the Association of Anaesthetists and develop an examining body to issue diplomas in intensive care and dental anaesthesia. It was thought that the Irish Faculty might be interested. A working party was set up and did a considerable amount of work on the project; as the status of the Faculty gradually improved over the next decade however, the project gradually merged into support for conversion of the Faculty into a College within the surgeons' College.

Fund raising for the Anaesthetist' Academic Foundation and the furore over "the Unity of the College". The beginning of active fund raising for the Anaesthetists' Academic Foundation was supported by an Editorial in *Anaesthesia* in the January 1978 issue.[115] It suggested that "in preparing their new Charter[113] (which was due to be enacted on 18 March 1978) the Royal College of Surgeons of England have given an indication that they would respect anaesthetists for seeking their independence." This was because the idea of a "three Faculty" or "tripartite" College had been rejected. The view of the elected members of the Council of the Association of Anaesthetists that they were "unequivocally" in favour of the foundation of the independent College of Anaesthetists was reiterated and, in accordance with the then current thinking of Council, it was suggested that an independent College should be formed with which it was hoped the Faculty would ultimately coalesce. The Editorial also called upon "Anaesthetists who believe in the foundation of an independent College .... to ensure that those whom they elect to the Board of Faculty will not only be individuals of the highest academic and administrative ability, but will also reflect their views and facilitate a smooth transition to independence".[115]

In the event, the publication of the 1978 Editorial in *Anaesthesia* coincided with the issue of a joint newsletter from the President of the Royal College of Surgeons of England, (Sir) Reginald Murley, and the Deans of the Faculties of Dental Surgery and Anaesthetists. The newsletter, entitled "The Unity of the Royal College of Surgeons", called for unity within the surgeons' College, and proposed a "moratorium" of 10 years on moves towards the foundation of a separate College of Anaesthetists during which the practical effect of the Charter could be assessed.[106,108,117,120,121]

The letter from the President and Deans of the Royal College of Surgeons of England stated incontrovertibly that "There is nothing ignoble in such sentiments [the desire for the development of an independent College of Anaesthetists], nor do we regard those who hold them as being in any way disloyal to the College (of Surgeons of England)".[120] This civilised assertion was greatly appreciated especially by those who were members of the Board of Faculty.[120,121,122] Others chose to take a contrary view.[108,117] A letter in the *British Medical Journal* signed by ten senior anaesthetists, prominent in the affairs of the specialty, objected strongly to the contents of the Editorial in *Anaesthesia* and suggested that it was disloyal to encourage the election to the Board of Faculty of those who supported the concept of the independent College. It was even suggested that the plan was to "disrupt" the Faculty.[108] The letter resulted in considerable correspondence in the *British Medical Journal* from members of the specialty. This was almost exclusively in favour of an independent College.[123,124] The single exception was a letter which suggested that his colleagues in Scotland would prefer that "no change in the present arrangements" was preferable to an "independent College of Anaesthetists in London," or, rather surprisingly, "to an independent College of Anaesthetists in Scotland".[125] Vernon Hall (President of the Association and a former Vice Dean of the Faculty) expressed himself as being strongly in favour in the correspondence pages of *Anaesthesia*,[126] and Professor Andrew Hunter of Manchester (another former Vice Dean of the Faculty) was equally strongly against.[127] Denis (W D A) Smith from Leeds considered the pros and cons of the problem in a very learned dissertation[128] to which the Immediate Past Secretary of the Association (M D A Vickers) replied with wit and wisdom.[129] *The British Journal of Anaesthesia*, broke its usual silence on political matters and contributed a wise and balanced Editorial over the signature of its Editor, Professor Alastair Spence (later President of the Royal College of Anaesthetists 1991-1994) and its Editor of Postgraduate Education numbers (Professor John Norman of Southampton).[103] They concluded that fresh negotiations were desirable to further improve the status of anaesthetists within the surgeons' College to give parity to anaesthetists.[103]

Stanley Mason of King's College Hospital, London succeeded to the Presidency (1978-80) at the Annual Meeting in Wembley on 1 December 1978 after a very successful four years as Honorary Treasurer. Official relations with the President, Dean of the Faculty of Anaesthetists and the Officers of the surgeons' College continued to be strained, and private discussions were not without rancour (S A Mason personal communication).

One can sympathise with the optimism of the Officers of the Faculty in 1979. The Faculty was certainly beginning to enjoy the limited benefits of the new College Charter (three representatives on the College Council, control of the Fellowship examination, independent representation on national bodies, and the election of an anaesthetist, ((Sir) Gordon Robson) as Vice President of the surgeons' College (1977-79) under the new ordinances). The outgoing Dean of the Faculty expressed the opinion at the Annual General Meeting of the Faculty in March 1979[130] that the Association and its Officers had no business to continue to argue in favour on an independent College and he called in question the veracity of some of their statements. He also asserted that the only discussions "of real importance (were) those within the College and Faculty". It is not easy to accept this view; after all the overwhelming majority of members of the Association of Anaesthetists (let alone of its Council) were also Fellows of the Faculty, and surely, therefore, they had a right to be heard! There was, however a ray of hope from the point of view of the Council of the Association of Anaesthetists; the Dean stated that "in the months ahead" it was planned "to look constructively and in detail at the whole position of the Board of Faculty. The Dean believed that:-

> "We [the Board of Faculty] shall approach our problems in a mature and adult manner and shall look at the facts and realities rather than hopes and assertions, and that our attention shall be concentrated... on what should be our sole concern, namely the unity and effective future development of our specialty in a stable environment".[130]

Progress towards reconciliation. John F Nunn took over the Office of Dean of the Faculty in June 1979. He considered that it was "an over simplification to believe that the only option open to us [the Faculty of Anaesthetists] was to stay as we are or to move and establish a totally independent College", and he set up working parties to consider various aspects of the problem.[131]

The membership of the Board of Faculty had begun to change towards support for the foundation of a College of Anaesthetists following retirements and subsequent elections in favour of further constitutional change, and, on 8 May 1980 the Dean (John Nunn) presented a series of resolutions to the Council of the Royal College of Surgeons of England which had been passed by the Board of the Faculty of Anaesthetists in Committee in April 1980. These crucial resolutions recognised:-

1. that a "substantial number" of Fellows believed that the specialty of anaesthesia had developed to the stage at which they should be represented by an autonomous College.
2. that the close relation of the academic bodies of anaesthesia and surgery should be preserved.
3. that the Board would like to explore the possibility of autonomous Collegiate status under the aegis of an" Academy of Surgical and related Science" (an idea which had been suggested in the discussion paper by the Secretary of the surgeons' College).
4. that in addition to discussions with the Council of the College of Surgeons the matter should be discussed with the Regional Educational Advisers of the College, the Association of Anaesthetists of Great Britain and Ireland, the Association of Professors of Anaesthesia, the Trustees of the Anaesthetists' Academic Foundation and the Fellows of the Faculty in general.

A new working party of the Faculty was appointed to discuss the future constitutional position with the Council of the surgeons' College.[132,133] It seemed at last that some progress would be made and this was even more the case when Sir Alan Parks[134] became President of the Royal College of

Surgeons of England in mid-1980. Sir Alan, though comparatively young for the office (59), was a man of wide experience as surgeon, research worker and administrator. He showed great sympathy for the aspirations of anaesthetists, and he persuaded his Council to inaugurate the vital process of the complete separation of the budget of the Faculty from that of the surgeons' College. It was a sad loss, both to the College and the Faculty when Sir Alan died suddenly and unexpectedly in November 1982.[134]

The discussions between the Faculty and College moved slowly despite the heroic efforts of the Dean, (John Nunn). Conversations between the considerably experienced and greatly respected Derek Wylie, who had taken over as President of the Association in September 1980,[135] and the Secretary of the College (R Johnson-Gilbert) were not fruitful either, while the Faculty-College discussions were *sub-judice*.[136]

Derek Wylie had been involved in very early discussions concerning a separate College of Anaesthetists when he was Vice Dean and subsequently Dean of the Faculty; he "never believed that [the Faculty] could succeed in getting a final resting place as a College within the College of Surgeons building." He believed also that the surgeons "missed a wonderful opportunity to bring together on one site a body of medical and dental practitioners, but to be a success it would have to become a College of Surgeons, Anaesthetists and Dental Practitioners with a proper representation on Council for all three groups running three Faculties, not two!" (W D Wylie personal communication).

John Nunn was succeeded by Professor Donald Campbell of Glasgow as Dean of the Faculty in June 1982. Nunn's time as Dean has been extremely fruitful in many ways (it had included *inter alia* the restructuring of the Fellowship examination and the start of an interdisciplinary effort to regularise training in intensive care), but he expressed regret at the March 1982 Annual Meeting that progress in the matter of "the constitutional future of the Faculty" had been slow and the issue remained unresolved.[137] Nunn believed however that "solutions involving the curtailment of the sovereignty of the College are unlikely to be acceptable to surgical Fellows, but real progress is being made on the further evolution within the College which might be made if the Board resolves to remain within the College".[137] These changes were to include the extension of the premises allocated to the Faculty within the surgeons' College[106] and the appointment of Stanley Alan, LLB as Secretary to the Faculty. Stanley Alan had already served the Faculty for 10 years as Assistant Secretary while the Secretary of the College of Surgeons (R Johnson-Gilbert) had also been Secretary to the Faculty.[138]

Professor Michael Vickers (Cardiff) succeeded Derek Wylie as President of the Association on 22 October 1982 at the Annual Meeting during the Golden Jubilee celebrations of the Association (Annual Report of Council 1982-83).[107,139] Vickers reviewed the twists and turns of the seemingly interminable discussions over the College question 'both with and within' the surgeons' College throughout the previous decade, in an Editorial in the November 1982 issue of *Anaesthesia*.[107] He listed the changes in the status of the Faculty which had already taken place which marked "a significant degree of practical independence, albeit unacknowledged in its title or legal status". He believed that these changes were as far as the surgeons were prepared to go. The three Faculty (tripartite) College solution, which would have satisfied many anaesthetists, had been rejected, and it was his "impression that, in the College, it is the surgeons who now seem more certain that anaesthetists are inevitably going to separate than even the most independently inclined anaesthetists, and surgeons who seem most sure that they are representing grass-roots opinion, both surgical and anaesthetic." It appeared to Vickers and many others that "the most stable endpoint was a College of Anaesthetists quite separate from the College of Surgeons."[107] Amazingly it took another ten years for this objective to be achieved!

Association Honours 1970-1982

John Snow Silver Medals were awarded to three former Presidents of the Association of Anaesthetists whose names have figured prominently in previous chapters during this period (R P W (Pat) Shackleton,[140] Sir Geoffrey Organe[141] and T Cecil Gray) and to William W Mushin,[142] former Vice President and Dean of the Faculty and Dean and first holder of the Chair of Anaesthetics at the Welsh National School of Medicine.

The Pask Certificate of Honour was initiated in 1975 and first awarded in 1977. The institution of the award resulted from dissatisfaction expressed in Council at the absence of official recognition of the contribution of anaesthetists from St Bartholomew's Hospital, London who acted with considerable gallantry in the rescue operation which followed the Moorgate Underground Railway disaster on 28 February 1975 (Council Minutes 4.4.1975, 5.9.1975).[81,143] It was recalled that, although the first three John Snow Medals were awarded in 1946 to anaesthetists who had been decorated for gallantry in the Second World War (Chapter 5), by subsequent usage the John Snow Medal had become the highest award for services to the British and Irish specially of anaesthesia in general and to the Association of Anaesthetists in particular. It was therefore decided to institute a new award named after the holder of the first John Snow Medallist Professor E A Pask, OBE who had served with such conspicuous gallantry (Council Minutes 3.9.1976 and 12.11.1976).[144] The Certificate of Honour would however also be awarded for other categories of service besides those of gallantry.[145] The award was to be made:-

"On the direction of the President and Council of Association of Anaesthetists of Great Britain and Ireland to honour those who have rendered distinguished service, either with gallantry in the performance of their clinical duties, to the specialty of anaesthesia as a whole or to the Association itself, either in a single meritorious act, or consistently and faithfully over a long period".[145]

The first awards were presented by the President Cyril Scurr at the Annual General Meeting in Dublin on Friday 30 September 1977. The Certificate was designed by (Professor) Peter Cull, Medical Artist to St Bartholomew's Hospital, London who was himself awarded a Pask Certificate in 1986 for the advice and support which he had given to the Association of Anaesthetists.

The names and deeds of the first recipients illustrate the type of service for which the award has continued to be made. The first award was made to Mrs Pask "in recognition of the outstanding services to anaesthesia of her husband". The second acknowledged the gallant devotion to duty at the Moorgate disaster of P M Finch a Registrar at St Bartholomew's Hospital. The other awards were to O P (Peter) Dinnick, past Honorary Secretary and Vice President and long serving representative of the Association on the British International Standards Committee, Roger Bryce-Smith, past Editor of *Anaesthesia* and Chairman of the Editorial Board, Professor W W Mapleson, the physicist in the Department of Anaesthesia of the University of Wales, and Erik Jacobsen, the President of the Danish Society at the highly successful joint meeting held the previous year.[145] The complete list of Pask Award holders appears in Appendix C together with brief notes giving the reason for each award.

Honorary Membership was bestowed on nine eminent senior British anaesthetists between 1971 and 1975. Four of these were former Presidents and two distinguished Vice Presidents whose names have figured prominently in this volume. The other three were T Philip Ayre the leading paediatric anaesthetist and inventor of his eponymous T-piece of Newcastle upon Tyne,[146] C J Massey Dawkins of University College Hospital, London,[148] pioneer of extradural analgesia in the United Kingdom, and Major General Keith Stephens, Commandant of the Royal Army Medical College, the first anaesthetist to reach that rank.

It had been decided not to make any further appointments to the category of Corresponding Membership ("distinguished anaesthetists practising outside Great Britain and Ireland") after 1976. Three eminent Americans and the pioneer Swedish anaesthetist Professor Torsten Gordh, who were previously Corresponding Members, were elected to Honorary Membership at the Annual General Meeting that year (the first foreign anaesthetists to be so honoured since 1960, and before that since 1955). J Alfred Lee[2] and Professor T J Gilmartin of Dublin[149] were also elected to Honorary Membership in 1976. There followed a period of six years (1977-1982) when, in addition to two former Presidents (T Cecil Gray, and P J Helliwell) and five other senior United Kingdom anaesthetists, an unprecedented seven foreign anaesthetists (three from the United States, and one each from France, Germany, India and the Philippines) were elected. Professor Sir William Paton, the Oxford pharmacologist, who besides researching many drugs related to the practice of anaesthesia, had been an invaluable adviser to the Editorial Board of *Anaesthesia*, was also honoured in 1980 and as, as has already been mentioned, was Ernest Warburton, Financial Adviser to the Association in 1981.

Postgraduate training following the (Todd) Report of the Royal Commission on Medical Education

The Royal Commission on Medical Education under the eminent scientist Lord Alexander Todd, FRS, Master of Christ's College, Cambridge, reported in 1968.[59,150,151] This report initiated a structured and programmed approach to postgraduate training organised and supervised by the medical Royal Colleges (including the Royal College of General Practitioners). This was to replace the previously haphazard service-based apprenticeship training. The House Officer (preregistration year) was to be followed by three years "General Professional Training" with specialist elements, culminating in certification by the appropriate Royal College; in the case of the anaesthetists this would be by the passing of the examination for the diploma of Fellowship of the Faculty of Anaesthetists (FFARCS). There was to follow a further three year period of "Higher Professional Training" at Senior Registrar level leading to accreditation and eligibility for Consultant Status in the NHS.[94,152] This is the system which defined and controlled postgraduate training from the mid seventies until the Calman Report of May 1993 proposed concentrating and shortening postgraduate specialist training to conform with regulations introduced by the European Union (EU).[153-155] It is of interest that in 1973 the Junior Anaesthetists' Group suggested a shorter integrated General Professional and Higher Professional Course of four years.[94] The Minutes of the 1973 Annual General meeting of the Association of Anaesthetists indicate that Allan C D Brown[156] (a British Senior Registrar anaesthetist and a prominent leader of the BMA Hospital Junior Staff Group Council at a critical time for the BMA and its negotiations with the Government) pointed out that the six year training period might put British anaesthetists at a disadvantage compared with EU anaesthetists if they sought to work in other EEC countries. This was because the period of training before the continental Europeans were recognised as specialists was only three or four years. This dilemma was resolved by the granting by the Faculty of Anaesthetists of a European specialist certificate after passing the FFARCS plus one year of further training (a total of four years). It was this procedure which led ultimately to the challenge in the nineteen nineties about specialist recognition designed to bring the United Kingdom into line with her European partners.[153-155] Allan Brown[156] also suggested at the 1973 Annual General Meeting that periodical specialist recertification might be the logical outcome of the structured training programme proposed by the Todd Committee.[59,150,151] This has also become a medicopolitical issue of the nineties!

The Joint Committee on the Higher Training of Anaesthetists (JCHTA) was established in 1971 and its successor is the Training Committee of the Royal College of Anaesthetists (TCRCA). The institution of this

Committee brought together representatives of the Faculty, the Association of Anaesthetists of Great Britain and Ireland, the Association of Professors of Anaesthesia, the postgraduate Deans and the Department of Health, for the strategic planning of Higher Professional Training and the accreditation of Senior Registrars prior to their application for Consultant appointments. The Association of Anaesthetists thus gained, and still retains, an important voice in the provision of Higher Professional Training, an area which might reasonably be considered to be the preserve of the Royal College of Anaesthetists alone. The Junior Anaesthetists' Group were invited to send a representative to attend the JCHTA from 1976 onwards. This was an important and far sighted development which was initiated by (Sir) Gordon Robson (then Dean of the Faculty and Chairman of the JCHTA). The proposal was accepted by Council despite some rather unnecessary concern about confidentiality on 5 May 1976.[81] The Junior Anaesthetists' Group (now Group of Anaesthetists in Training) is in a unique position to nominate for committees such as the TCRCA as there is as yet no equivalent organisation within the collegiate structure. The Royal College of Anaesthetists changed its ordinances in 1993 in order to be able to invite a member of the Group to attend its Council as an observer.

The Linkman organisation

The President (Philip Helliwell)[3] reported to the 1974 Annual General Meeting that it was proposed to institute a nationwide network of "link-men" (the hyphen was soon dropped). The scheme had been initiated by the then Honorary Secretary, Michael Vickers.[157] The objective was, and is, to "provide Council with a means of transmitting information to and from Members". The Faculty Regional Education Advisers were asked to nominate one anaesthetist from each District General Hospital who could be relied upon to act as a linkman (Annual Report 1974).

The 1975 Annual Report of Council records that the Linkman organisation had been used six times during the year to obtain grass roots opinion and disseminate Council opinions on various topics; these included (inevitably) efforts to improve dental fees and the number of salary increments that could be awarded if more experienced anaesthetists were appointed to Consultant posts, and opinions on the revision of the Abortion Act. The 1976 Annual Report of Council paid tribute to the conscientiousness of Linkmen whose advice had been sought on many topics, including the adoption of the international Système International units by the United Kingdom, family planning fees, consultant job descriptions and evidence to the Royal Commission on the National Health Service.

The First Conference for Linkmen was held on Wednesday 17 November 1976 on the day before the Annual General Meeting[157] and Linkmen Conferences have been held, usually before the Annual General and Scientific meeting, in every succeeding year. These conferences provide an invaluable occasion for the Honorary Officers and Council to exchange opinions with Ordinary Members. They have undoubtedly contributed to the success with which the Association of Anaesthetists has been able to make its voice heard and to achieve effective action in the medicopolitical arena.

The complimentary organisation of an annual meeting of Faculty (now Royal College) of Anaesthetists' Tutors from District General Hospitals was started in 1979 and carries out a similar role in exchanging views with the College Council concerning training in anaesthesia and the conduct of the Fellowship examination.

The journal *Anaesthesia* 1970-1982

Roger Bryce-Smith of Oxford retired at the end of 1972 from the Editorship which he had held with distinction since the retirement of Langton Hewer in 1966. The Editor from 1973 to the end of 1982 was Thomas B Boulton (when appointed of St Bartholomew's Hospital, London but, later of Reading and Oxford), who had previously been Senior Assistant Editor. Bryce-Smith became Chairman of the Editorial Board and served in that capacity until 1975 (Annual Report 1975), when the then President (Philip Helliwell)[3] took over and continued as Chairman until 1987. John N Lunn (Cardiff) joined Tom Boulton as Joint Editor in 1982 and continued as Editor until 1990.

Stuart Warne, the senior partner of H E Warne Ltd of St Austell, retired unexpectedly because of ill health in 1972. Warne's were a relatively small firm who had printed and distributed the journal since 1962 and the success of the arrangement had been Stuart Warne's personal interest (Annual Report 1972). The severance of this personal link and the impending change of Editorship provided a suitable opportunity to unify and reorganise the mechanics of the publication of *Anaesthesia*; consequently, and chiefly as a result of negotiations conducted by Roger Bryce-Smith, Blackwell Scientific Publications (BSP) of Oxford took over the management of publication from the beginning of the 28th volume in January 1973. This was the end of the "cottage industry" phase in the history of *Anaesthesia*. The freelance Technical Adviser (A W Mycroft) and the freelance Advertising Manager (Mrs Dorothy Mitchell), both of whom had served the journal well for a number years, amicably stood down. Their functions were taken over by BSP, and printing was undertaken by their near neighbour Alden Press of Oxford (Annual Reports 1972 and 1973). The relationship of *Anaesthesia* with BSP was a relaxed and happy one during a period in which the journal developed considerably both in size and quality. It was based on mutual respect and flexibility both on the part of the Chairman of the firm (Per Saugman) and especially also of the late Keith Bowker, the Director who managed the difficult interface between the professional publishing house and the part-time amateur Editor with great tolerance and good humour.

The connection with BSP lasted until it was terminated with mutual expressions of regret at the end of 1981, when BSP was outbid in a purely commercial competition for the award of the contract for the publication of *Anaesthesia* by Academic Press Ltd of London and New York.[158,159] Commercial competition once again dictated that BSP (now called Blackwell Science) took over publication of *Anaesthesia* from January 1997 onwards (Annual Report 1996).

The quantity and quality of material submitted to *Anaesthesia* increased steadily throughout the seventies; in 1976 the Editor estimated that one quarter of the articles received were unsuitable, five per cent were irresistible and deserved priority, and the remainder contained solid and important material which deserved publication.[160]

Delays concerning the publication of individual articles caused some anxiety (Annual Report 1975);[160] consequently the frequency of publication was increased from four to six per year and the size to standard A5 when BSP and the new Editor took over in 1973, to nine issues in 1976 (Vol 31),[160] to ten in 1977, and *Anaesthesia* finally became a monthly journal in 1980 (volume 35). The modern double column style was adopted in 1977 to enable slightly more words to be printed to the page. The number of pages in Volume 25

(1970) was 598 and, by contrast, the total in Volume 37 (1982) was 1266.

The Système Internationale. A consequence of the entry of the United Kingdom into the European Economic Community (EEC) was felt in 1975 when an early EEC directive was hastily passed on by the Department of Health. This decreed conversion to the Système Internationale (SI) units of measurement, and *Anaesthesia,* in agreement with the *British Journal of Anaesthesia* began to use the system at the beginning of 1976.[161,162] Out went the mEq/litre and mmHg for blood gas tensions and in came the mmol/litre and the kiloPascal (kPa); fortunately as the result of howls of protest by many organisations (including the Association of Anaesthetists Council) millimetres of mercury (mmHg) was retained for blood pressure (Council Minutes 14.11.1975 and 2.1.1976).[81] The change to SI units was achieved remarkably easily in the United Kingdom despite some grumbling (Council Minutes 14.11.1975).[81] This was probably partly because of the apparent advantages of the change, but also because of the *de facto* unity of health care under the NHS. It was not however, to be the last time that the British Government were ahead of other member states of the Europe in their enthusiasm to comply with an edict from the EEC! The discrepancy which was created between the usage of nomenclature in British journals and those of their cousins and North America is regrettable.[163,164]

The Vancouver Convention. A more harmonious move towards the standardisation of medical scientific journalism was achieved by the publication of a set uniform requirements for manuscripts. This was promulgated by an informal meeting in Vancouver in 1978 of medical editors from the United States, Canada and Britain of which Stephen Lock of the *British Medical Journal* was a prominent participant.[165,166] *Anaesthesia* has conformed with the Vancouver Convention from volume 35 (1980) onwards. The change in the style of listing references was not as great as that required by those journals which had employed the alphabetical "Harvard System" because *Anaesthesia* had always used a form of referencing involving sequential numbering. The *British Journal of Anaesthesia* did not change from the Harvard system until 1988.

Editorial Policy 1973-1982. The Editor of the day was cognisant that the journal was, not only an international scientific journal, and had a readership ranging from the novice to those in retirement, but that it was also the house journal of the Association of Anaesthetists; as such, he believed that it was right that it should carry news and views and information about the British specialty of anaesthesia as well as up to date clinical scientific material. The policy at that time was to produce "a scientifically and socially informative, readable and, at times, amusing journal for members of the Association which it serves and all others who care to peruse its pages" (Annual Report 1975);[160,167,168] nor did its editorials hesitate to express views on medicopolitical matters when it believed this to be desirable![106,107,110,115,168]

A useful survey conducted by a questionnaire in 1978 suggested that, for the seventies, *Anaesthesia* "was generally on the right course" but that the Editors would be well advised "to trim their sails a little and give a touch on the tiller in response to fashion and the slightly veering wind of readers' opinions".[167]

Personnel. The journal was served by a distinguished team of loyal Assistant Editors between 1970 and 1982:- M K (Sir Keith) Sykes (later Nuffield Professor at Oxford), M D A Vickers (Professor at Cardiff), R S Atkinson (Southend and later Vice Dean of the Faculty), J N Lunn (Cardiff, Editor from 1982), J S Inkster (Newcastle upon Tyne), A P Adams (Professor, Guy's Hospital, London), P J Horsey (Southampton), M Morgan (Royal Postgraduate Medical School; appointed editor from 1991), I Corall (King's College Hospital, London) and C E Blogg (Oxford).

Others who contributed to the success of *Anaesthesia* by compiling specialist sections were: Leon Kaufman (University College Hospital) who for twenty five years coordinated the Anaesthetic Literature section until it was discontinued at the end of 1990 (having been superseded by electronic retrieval systems) when he received a Pask award; Kaufman was assisted during this lengthy period by Edward Sumner of the Hospital for Sick Children, Great Ormond Street and Professor A R Hunter of Manchester; D V Bateman of Epping and St Mark's Hospital who was Honorary Proof Reader from the mid seventies to 1982, who also received a Pask award; R H Ellis (St Bartholomew's Hospital, London) who subedited the Correspondence Section; E O Parbrook (Glasgow) Audiovisual Section; and Adrian Padfield (Sheffield), Calendar of National and Local events. One trusted "guide philosopher and friend" of the Editors was Miss Dorothy Atkins[169] who, despite considerable respiratory incapacity, served *Anaesthesia* from her home for many years as Reference Librarian and Indexer with great good humour and forbearance.

The expanding business of the journal also necessitated properly financed and defined secretarial assistance for the Editor at his place of work. Mrs Una J Spanner, former Librarian of the Royal Berkshire Hospital, Reading was the Personal Assistant, organiser and prompting conscience of Tom Boulton at the Royal Berkshire Hospital, Reading from 1978 to 1982, and Mrs Susan Campbell was Personal Assistant to John Lunn at Cardiff from 1982, when he became Joint Editor before taking over as sole Editor at the beginning of 1983 (Annual Reports 1982 and 1983).[170]

A Cumulative Index for the first 30 years of publication of *Anaesthesia* (1946-1975) was compiled by the leading Indexer Doreen Blake in 1982 and has since proved to be invaluable.[171]

The cover of *Anaesthesia* was redesigned on white card in 1973 with the version of the Association Coat of Arms drawn by (Professor) Peter Cull of St Bartholomew's Hospital for the World Congress in 1968. The cover was made water repellent in 1978.[167] Special covers were produced for the Silver Jubilee of the first publication of *Anaesthesia* in 1971, the Silver Jubilee of the accession of Her Majesty Queen Elizabeth II in 1977, the Golden Jubilee of the foundation of the Association in 1982 and the 6th European Congress of Anaesthesiology also in 1982.

The financial affairs of *Anaesthesia* were conducted on a somewhat notional basis up until the arrival of Ernest Warburton as Financial Adviser in 1974. Blackwell Scientific Publications (BSP) published the journal for the Association of Anaesthetists and collected nonmember subscriptions and the advertising revenue and the Association contributed a *pro rata* sum for Members' copies; BSP then deducted the expenses of publication and printing and paid over any profit to the Association. Whether or not a normal profit showed in the annual accounts of the Association depended upon the precise timing of the various payments and the way the accounts were presented; on occasion an apparent loss gave rise to unfair adverse comment from the floor at Annual General Meetings. Ernest Warburton's first action in 1974 was to recommend the incorporation of the A*naesthesia* account within the General Account of the Association and then, in 1981, with the expiry of the current contract with BSP, the privilege of publishing *Anaesthesia*, collecting subscriptions and the advertising income and supplying and mailing members copies free of charge, in return for the payment to the Association of a contractual sum (indexed related to inflation), was put out to tender. The principal bids were made by BSP and the international publishing house of Academic Press (AP) and, in the event, the AP bid of £30,000 (1996: £61,000) per annum for three years was accepted for publication to begin with the January 1982 issue (Annual Report 1981); from then on the only direct expenses incurred on the debit side of the balance sheet of *Anaesthesia* have been for editorial and secretarial expenses and allowances for in house office and accommodation expenditure. The contract with AP was renewed at intervals; in 1992 it provided for an annual payment of £90,000 to the Association (indexed linked). The surplus derived by the Association from the publication of *Anaesthesia* in 1983 at the end of the first year of operation of the AP contract was £18,305 (1996: £34,400) and by 1991 it was over £50,000 (1996: £57,000). The figures demonstrate the increasing importance of *Anaesthesia* as an international scientific journal.

The change of publisher occurred in the last year of the ten year editorial stint of the present writer in a year (1982) in which he and John Lunn were Joint Editors prior to the latter succeeding to the Chair as sole Editor. The change represented another milestone in the life of *Anaesthesia*. The separation from BSP was taken with regret but for sound financial reasons, but the contrast between visits to the relaxed atmosphere of BSP building, on its green field site within easy walking distance of the dreaming spires of Oxford,[159] and the more competitive efficiency of the AP offices and their urban surroundings in Camden Town took some time to get used to. There was moreover the new experience of having to deal within the first year with three successive youthful, and upwardly mobile technical subeditors, to whose responsibility the affairs of *Anaesthesia* seemed to have been delegated, rather than communicating directly with the friendly BSP senior executives who were always prepared to accommodate an amateur Editor over a few extra pages or a copy date missed by a few days! There is no doubt however that the efficient and disciplined business acumen of Academic Press (later, due to amalgamation, W B Saunders Company Ltd) subsequently served *Anaesthesia* well and assisted John Lunn to raise its status as an international scientific journal to a very high level of excellence during the eighties; even so, John had to "train" a further five technical subeditors during that time (J N Lunn personal communication).

The Junior Anaesthetists' Group 1970-1982

The Junior Anaesthetists' Group (JAG) (since 1991 the Group of Anaesthetists in Training (GAT)) was founded in 1967 (Chapter 7). It is a unique organisation for a medical specialist society. The numerical size of JAG continued to grow apace in the seventies. There were only 320 members in 1970, but by the end of 1982 there were 1293. These figures represented 16% and 37% of the overall United Kingdom voting membership of the Association of Anaesthetists respectively.

The influence of the JAG also increased enormously; by 1982 its nominated representatives were members within the Association of Anaesthetists of its Council, the Advisory Committee, the Linkman Conference and the Editorial Board as well as most Association Standing committees and Working Parties; and outside the Association on, the BMA Anaesthetists Subcommittee and its Hospital Junior Staffs Council, on the Joint Committee for the Higher Training of Anaesthetists, the Education Committee of the Faculty of Anaesthetists, and the Council of the Section of Anaesthetists of the Royal Society of Medicine (Annual Report 1981).

Representation on the JAG Committee was initially on a regional basis, but this was abandoned in 1975 after a change in the constitution to allow cooption to ensure a balanced representation. A representative nominated by the Hospital Junior Staff Group of the BMA was also coopted after 1975. The JAG (now GAT) is the only organised body representing anaesthetists in training; consequently, whenever trainee representation is needed in bodies other than the Association of Anaesthetists, it is to the Group which they turn for advice and nominations. The range of topics discussed by the Committee of the JAG is sometimes even broader than those considered by the Council of the Association itself, because it includes matters concerning training and examinations, which Council would normally regard as being in the remit of the Faculty or College. The JAG Committee has occasionally made direct representations to the Faculty and College on its own behalf. The essential business of the JAG Committee at Annual Meetings from its origins in the sixties to 1992 is considered in Elizabeth Spencer's monograph.[94]

Topics discussed (some of which were researched by questionnaire), and representations made, included General and Higher Professional Training during its evolution, recruitment to the specialty, study leave, fatigue (many junior anaesthetists were compelled to work 100 hours per week in 1971 but considered they were only safe for 80 hours), the revised examination structure, examination fees, the refusal of some Hospital Administrators to honour their commitment to "study leave with pay", the provision of regular study days (40% of Senior Registrars did not have any such provision in 1979), overtime payments, part-time training for "doctors with domestic commitments" (the Department of Health were painfully slow in implementing their own policies), the block at the Registrar to Senior Registrar interface, housing problems of rotating Senior Registrars, and the "Sick Doctor" scheme (see below).[94]

Support for the formation of a separate College of Anaesthetists was strong from the beginning amongst trainee anaesthetists and increased steadily between 1970 and 1982; at the Annual Meeting of the JAG in 1972 at Liverpool there were 45 in favour, 26 against and 17 of those present abstained, at the 1978 Annual Meeting at Exeter there were 80 in favour, none against, and only three were undecided. There was also unanimous approval for specifically earmarking the profits from that meeting to the Anaesthetics Academic Foundation.[94,172,173]

Junior Linkmen. Communication between the JAG Committee and rank and file junior anaesthetists was not easy early in the decade. The senior Linkmen were asked to distribute information and the difficulty was alleviated by a steadily increasing amount of space to affairs of the JAG in *Anaesthesia*,[172,173] but the position was still further improved by the institution of a Junior Linkman scheme in 1985.

The production of career guides has been a special responsibility of the JAG Committee. *Anaesthesia in the Seventies*, with its attractive line drawings as illustrations, was produced in 1972 during the Chairmanship of F Richard Ellis (later Professor of Anaesthesia at Leeds). The booklet was aimed at senior medical students and provisionally registered house officers, with the intention of stimulating recruitment to the then shortage specialty and was funded by the Association of Anaesthetists for between £500 and £600 (1996: £3,400-£4,000), (Council Minutes 7.4.1972: Annual Report 1972).[94,96] The emphasis had changed by the time *Anaesthesia: A Career Guide* was produced in 1981 with the support of BOC Medishield; this publication was largely the work of John Evans (Oxford) and provided a detailed account of the work of a well established and recruited specialty and guidance on the posts and examinations which formed the rungs of the career ladder (Council Minutes 30.10.1981: Annual Report 1981).[97] The Career Guide was again revised by Philip Bickford Smith with up to date photographic illustrations in 1985 to take account of the changes in the Diploma of Anaesthetics and Fellowship examination structure. Publication was achieved with the support of Ohmeda, the successors to BOC Medishield, (Annual Report 1985). The career guides were widely distributed to Linkmen, Deans of Medical Schools, Postgraduate Deans, Heads of Academic Departments and at Career Fairs (Council Minutes 30.10.1981).[94,96]

Career Fairs for hospital specialties at medical schools began to be popular in the nineteen seventies. A transportable exhibit was prepared by the JAG Committee under the guidance of Michael Rosen in 1974 with the cooperation of the Medical Illustration Department of the Welsh National School of Medicine. This exhibit was replaced by an up to date version based on the career guide in 1985.[94]

Annual Scientific Meetings for Registrars began in the nineteen sixties and continued into the seventies. The meetings in 1970 and 1971 were in Glasgow (140 registrants) and at Westminster Hospital, London (180 registrants), respectively. The 1972 meeting at Liverpool was renamed as "the Annual Scientific Meeting for Junior Anaesthetists" and attracted 270 participants. The series continued with increasing sophistication (Sheffield 1973, Brighton 1974, Birmingham 1975, Newcastle upon Tyne 1976, Cambridge 1977, Exeter 1978, Oxford 1979, Leicester 1980, Guildford 1981 and Southampton in 1982 with 370 registrants).

The guest and Pinkerton lectures. The series of guest lectures at the JAG Annual Scientific Meeting was inaugurated by J Alfred Lee, the reigning President, at Sheffield in 1973,[94,174] and became the eponymous Pinkerton Lecture in 1982 in recognition of H H Pinkerton[175] the President at the time of the foundation of the JAG in 1967.

A bronze medal similar to that awarded to the John Snow Lecturer is awarded to the Pinkerton lecturer in addition to the financial honorarium (£300 in 1994). The first Pinkerton lecture was delivered by Chris (C J) Hull, Professor of Anaesthesia, Newcastle upon Tyne.[94]

The Registrars Prize for ten minute presentations was inaugurated at the Brighton meeting of the JAG in 1974. The first prize winner was Paul Griffiths. Subsequent prize winners are listed in Appendix C. Since 1985 the President's Medal has accompanied the monetary award.[94]

Social events at the JAG and GAT meetings have often been robust occasions! The appreciable proportion of ladies in JAG and GAT (even by 1981 26% of Senior Registrar anaesthetists, were female) possibly accounts for the "lack of enthusiasm" for an accompanying persons' programme, the possible provision of which, so far as can be recalled has not been discussed since 1973![94]

The study of mortality associated anaesthesia 1979-1980

The Association of Anaesthetists of Great Britain and Ireland had had a long and enviable record of being concerned to elucidate the reasons for deaths during the administration of anaesthesia as has been noted in previous chapters, and had, in fact, begun its first formal investigation into "deaths associated with anaesthesia" in 1949 (Chapter 6). The 1979-1980 investigation was instigated by the reigning President Cyril Scurr at the Council Meeting on 7 January 1977.[81] He believed that "at a time when the Health Service was under attack, it was important to have some index of a fall in anaesthetic mortality". He pointed to the record of the Association in this context in the past, and emphasised that "now that deaths associated with anaesthesia were probably less than a hundred cases a year" an enquiry would be administratively containable. (Sir) Gordon Robson, at that time a coopted Member of Council as Adviser in Anaesthetics to the Chief Medical Officer, supported the idea of an enquiry and drew attention to the forthcoming editorial in the *British Journal of Anaesthesia* by D Bruce Scott of Edinburgh (Council Minutes 7.1.1977)[81] (Robson must have had an advanced copy as the Editorial was published a month later). Scott,[176] in his editorial, drew attention to the fact that cases of deaths during anaesthesia had to be reported to the authorities when anaesthesia was clearly not a contributory factor "regardless of the enormous advances in anaesthesia ..... and the decline in mortality attributable directly to anaesthesia". He stressed on the other hand, that it was important that all deaths associated with anaesthesia should be scrutinised by "a body which is competent to judge them". Scott went on to recommend a confidential and peer reviewed enquiry such as that conducted by the Department of Health into maternal deaths in obstetrics.[176,177] Some Members of Council were concerned about the legal implications but, upon being reassured that the investigation could be absolutely confidential and anonymous, a working party was set up to look at the problem consisting of Robson, Scott, John S Robinson (then Professor of Anaesthesia in Birmingham) and the Officers of the Association (Council Minutes 7.1.1977).[81]

The initial intention had been to study both mortality and morbidity but, in the event, because of the inherent difficulties in defining and obtaining data about morbidity, it was decided to study only the definite end point of mortality (Council Minutes 7.1.1977, 4.5.1977).[81]

W W Mushin[142] (Emeritus Professor of Anaesthesia of the University of Wales) was recruited to the Committee (Council Minutes 11.3.1977)[81] and was shortly afterwards elected to its Chairmanship. The Nuffield Provincial Hospitals Trust were approached and provided generous funding for three years.

The study which resulted was "most carefully planned"[179] and was "modelled on the triennial enquiry into maternal deaths of the Royal College of Obstetricians and Gynaecologists",[177-180] as Scott had suggested.[176] The organisation which was set up consisted of a broadly based Central Committee, chaired by Professor Mushin with D B Scott as Secretary, on which sat the President, Honorary Treasurer and Honorary Secretary of the Association of Anaesthetists of Great Britain and Ireland, the Dean of the Faculty of Anaesthetists (J F Nunn), Professor Harold Ellis (Royal College of Surgeons of England), and representatives of the Faculty of Community Medicine of the Royal College of Physicians of London, The Department of Health and Social Security (two representatives), the Office of Population and Census Studies, and J N Lunn (Cardiff) as Chairman of the Regional Assessors' Subcommittee;[180] and it was upon John Lunn that the success of the enterprise ultimately depended.

It was accepted, on the advice of Professor A L Cochrane (the representative of the Faculty of Community Medicine), that the initial study should be limited to "about one third of the hospitals (in England, Wales and Scotland) represented by five regions (three in England, and Wales and the whole of Scotland)".[180] The English Regions were North Western, West Midlands and Trent. The Scottish Home and Health Department funded the study in Scotland separately. The study was also limited to patients who died within six days of surgery for several acceptable reasons.[178]

The Central Committee appointed one or two Assessors in each of the Regions, and the Assessors appointed respected local Correspondents in individual hospitals in collaboration with the staffs of the local Departments of Anaesthesia. The local Correspondents identified patients in their hospitals who had died within six days of surgery and sent separate letters and questionnaires to the anaesthetist and surgeon concerned. The surgeon and anaesthetist were asked to return the questionnaire directly to the Regional Assessor. The Regional Assessor, in collaboration with a second Regional Assessor, would then determine whether the conduct of the anaesthetic was wholly or partly responsible for the death, or not implicated at all.[180] It was unfortunate that various surgical organisations were initially suspicious and, in the end, surgical cooperation was only "conditional on the exclusion of, or comment on, possible surgical factors"; thus the study had perforce to limit its aims to the identification and quantification of those features within the whole practice of anaesthesia in the hospital environment of the which may influence the incidence of death" and "sophisticated treatment of the data" had "on the whole [to be] avoided".[180]

The report of the mortality study (112 pages and 44 tables) was published early in August 1982 by the Nuffield Provincial Hospital Trust.[180] A summary of its conclusions by Lunn and Mushin was also published in *Anaesthesia*,[181] and this was accompanied by an expertly composed analytical Editorial by John Nunn, who had just retired as Dean of the Faculty of Anaesthetists.[179] The report was based on 6060 patients who had died in hospital within six days of surgery out of 1,147,362 operations embraced by the study.[179-181]

Lunn and Mushin concluded that:-

"The overwhelming message of this report is that the process of anaesthesia is remarkably safe. Although one in 166 (0.6%) patients die within six days of an operation, only one in 10,000 dies totally as

a result of anaesthesia. Thus the number of deaths totally attributable to anaesthesia is in the region of 280 per year in the United Kingdom and the majority of these are probably avoidable. In a much larger number 1800 deaths (one in 1700 or 0.06%) anaesthesia may have played some part and these too could, in large measure be avoided. The events which cause the deaths have not changed over 30 years."[181]

Lunn and Mushin go on to list a number of deficiencies in administrative practice. They included; trainee anaesthetists were "too often left unsupported by Consultants for supervision and by other staff for assistance; the inadequate provision and use of essential monitoring; insufficient consultation between surgeons and anaesthetists; inadequate pre-operative preparation of the patient; disregard by the surgeons of the implications of intercurrent disease for the anaesthetist, and th\e absence of recovery rooms in 17.5% of deaths".[179-181]

It was unfortunate that the Association of Anaesthetists was not consulted by the Nuffield Provincial Hospital Trust about the precise mechanism for the release of the report.[182] The lay press, including regrettably the quality papers, chose to ignore the enviable safety record of anaesthesia and to sensationalise its contents with headlines such as "Anaesthesia could cost 900 lives each year".[183] Editorials in the *British Medical Journal*[184] and the *Lancet*[185] were supportive, however. A considerable correspondence followed in the *British Medical Journal* (1982 volume 285). The acknowledged deficiency concerning the lack of data on surgical causes for operative and postoperative deaths was stressed, and there was considerable support for the assertion of Lunn and Mushin themselves that "the difficulty of assigning causative factors in postoperative deaths to anaesthesia or to surgery make it important that future epidemiological studies should be combined ones between anaesthetist and surgeon".[180,181,186-189] This pioneer audit stimulated interest in audit amongst surgeons and led directly to the cooperation of the Association of Anaesthetists of Great Britain and Ireland with the Association of Surgeons of Great Britain and Ireland in the Confidential Enquiry into Perioperative Deaths (CEPOD), which reported in 1987. This collaborative investigation was supported by the Nuffield Provincial Hospitals Trusts and the King Edward's Hospitals Fund for London.[190] CEPOD has been succeeded by the National Confidential Enquiry into Perioperative Deaths (NCEPOD), an independent body supported by the Associations of Anaesthetists and Surgeons and the Royal Colleges and their Faculties.[191,192]

Anaesthetists voiced concern about the comparative lack of recovery rooms and intensive care units in the United Kingdom;[184,193,194] some attributed this to a deficiency of funding by the National Health Service,[184] but others stressed the reluctance of surgeons and others to have their patients cared for in locations other than their own wards.[193] It seems almost incredible that in 1994 John Lunn, who was still prominent on the NCEPOD Steering Group, should find it necessary to draw attention to the fact that there are still a few hospitals undertaking surgery in the NHS and the independent sector, which do not have recovery rooms or do not staff them adequately.[195]

It is also interesting, in view of the emphasis which was destined to be put on the importance of monitoring in the mid-eighties, that a group of anaesthetists in 1982[196] criticised the modest opinion of Lunn and Mushin[180] that the minimum acceptable standard of monitoring should be a blood pressure cuff and an electrocardiograph for every patient, with a volume meter for those who were artificially ventilated. Those who disagreed were concerned both about the utility of such instruments in all circumstances and the legal implications which might result in a claim for negligence if these devices, having been defined in the report, were not used on particular occasions; fortunately others strongly supported the provision of proper monitoring![197]

A lone surgeon in the correspondence pages of the *Lancet* acknowledged that the safety of anaesthesia had increased, but he believed that this was only a reflection of the improvement in medical practice in general and was not the result of formal training and academic standards in anaesthesia ("the academic game"). He also believed that the report "would be used to support demands for further diversion of limited resources to this already large and powerful specialty, but that the money could be better spent in other areas![198]

The original mortality study was continued for a further year. One hundred and ninety seven detailed reports were received during 1981. Analysis of these confirmed the earlier results.[199]

Help for the Sick Doctor

The Merrison "Report of the Committee of inquiry into the Regulation of the Medical Profession", which had reported in 1975[79] had *inter alia* critically appraised the arrangements, within the NHS and by the GMC, for action for the protection of patients when a previously competent and adequately qualified medical practitioner became clinically incompetent through illness or addiction to drugs or alcohol.[79,200] The options available in 1975 were indeed limited and inappropriate for the management of medical practitioners who might be potentially curable. The NHS "Three Wise Men" semi-official procedure in which three senior Hospital Consultants acceptable to the local hospital medical staff, first considered an allegation of incompetence from patients or NHS staff, and then made recommendations to the employing authority as to whether or not the individual's services to the NHS should be "curtailed or discontinued with consequent effects upon his livelihood".[200]

It was not surprising that this official mechanism was only invoked by medical colleagues in the case of a fellow practitioner in extreme circumstances. A Committee of Enquiry into Competence to Practise was set up by the BMA in 1973[200] in anticipation of the publication of the Merrison Report on the Regulation of the Medical Profession in 1975.[79] The BMA committee continued its deliberations and took into account the recommendations of the Merrison Report before it reported itself in 1976. This BMA committee acknowledged that there had been many instances in which administrators and administrative officers had pursued complaints about the possibility that the health of a practitioner was adversely affecting his competence with "tact and diplomacy", and had been able to solve many problems informally by "consent and co-operation of the doctors concerned", but it was felt that a structured but less formalised early warning mechanism was required.[200] The GMC, at the time of the publication of the Merrison Report in 1975, could only act if the incompetence resulted in a disciplinary offence with all the penalties that implied, which included public exposure and supervision or erasure from the Medical Register. The GMC subsequently established a Health Committee in 1980. The procedure and sanctions of the Health Committee were more sympathetic to the sick but potentially dangerous practitioner but, even as late as 1981, a practitioner suspended by the Health Committee on the grounds of ill health was not eligible for sick pay from the NHS.[201] It should be emphasised that the BMA Committee[200] considered competence to practise in its totality, including the basic requirement of initial medical education and specialist training which were necessary to produce a competent practitioner, linguistic ability, continuing medical education, the benefits and dangers of medical audit, legal and complaints procedures, as well as loss of competence due to ill health including addition to drugs and alcohol.

The composition of the BMA Committee was broadly based and, in addition, took written evidence from many organisations, including the Association of Anaesthetists, and verbal evidence from a number of individuals, including Kenneth Rawnsley,[202] Professor of Psychological Medicine at the Welsh National School of Medicine. Cyril Scurr was one of the five representatives of the "Specialists Royal Colleges and Faculties in England" on the BMA Committee.[200]

The Association of Anaesthetists Help for the Sick Doctor Scheme. The BMA Committee had "studied in detail" the non-coercive approach to the problem of the sick doctor instituted by a Committee of the Medical Society of New York drawn from "doctors skilled in dealing with alcoholism, drug addition and mental illness, the principal areas in which the sick doctor lacks insight into his need for help." The procedures of this scheme ensured confidential separation between the practitioners who confronted the sick doctor to ask if he needed help, and those who supplied the information. Many other States in the USA also had similar informal schemes in operation.[201]

Cyril Scurr (by then President of the Association of Anaesthetists) drew the attention of its Council to the New York scheme in 1977 (Council Minutes 7.1.1977 and 11.3.1977.[81] It was a happy coincidence that Michael Rosen was a colleague of Kenneth Rawnsley,[202] (later President of the Royal College of Psychiatrists and Honorary Member of the Association of Anaesthetists) on the staff of the University of Wales in Cardiff. Rosen and Rawnsley together were largely responsible for cementing a partnership between the Association of Anaesthetists and the Royal College of Psychiatrists. This resulted in the initiation of the "Help for the Sick Doctor" scheme of the Association of Anaesthetists which pioneered the concept in the United Kingdom.[203] This scheme predated the subsequent establishment of the GMC Health Committee in 1980[204] and was the stimulus for the establishment of the National Counselling and Welfare Service for Sick Doctors in 1986.[205]

The scheme was initially given the title of the "Competence to Practise Scheme", but because, unlike the comprehensive BMA report of 1976,[200] its function was limited to loss of competence to practise through illness or addiction, it was renamed the "Help the Sick Doctor scheme" (Council Minutes 4.5.1979).[81]

The scheme was introduced by Michael Rosen at the Linkman Conference in November 1978,[206] and explanatory notices were placed in *Anaesthesia,* the *British Journal of Anaesthesia* and the *British Medical Journal* in 1979.[207,208]

The Help for the Sick Doctor Scheme of the Association of Anaesthetists was succinctly described in complimentary terms in the *British Medical Journal* in January 1981, in a leading article.[201] This also acknowledged its uniqueness (details of the operation of the scheme had been supplied to the leader writer by the Association of Anaesthetists through the Anaesthetic Sub-committee of the Central Committee for Hospital Medical Services of the BMA, so far as confidentiality permitted - Council Minutes 9.1.1981).[97] The leading article states:-

> *"In this scheme a doctor worried about an anaesthetist telephones the Association and without having to disclose his identity, is given the name and telephone number of a referee whom he can contact. The referees are all retired, distinguished anaesthetists; because they are retired they cannot influence the sick doctor's future career, and their distinction should allow them to be known to and trusted by the sick doctor. The referee will satisfy himself that a problem exists by talking to the reporting doctor and another doctor if possible. The*

referee will then contact a psychiatrist from another region, who will get in touch with the sick doctor. The Royal College of Psychiatrists cooperates in the scheme by providing a list of recommended psychiatrists. If the sick doctor accepts treatment then the referee destroys all records of phone numbers and names and trusts the treating psychiatrist. If after a month the sick doctor has not accepted treatment then the referee is told, and he in turn informs the original reporting doctor. There is no formal link with the GMC health committee, but the referee will make it clear to the reporting doctor that he has an ethical duty to take the matter further."

"Because the scheme is highly confidential and keeps no records it is hard to know how well it is working, nevertheless, in two years of operation one referee (who has done most of the work) has dealt with 11 cases, and in none of them did the sick doctor refuse to accept treatment".[201]

If the sick doctor had declined treatment the reporting practitioner would have the option of initiating the "Three Wise Man" procedure or, more likely after 1981, of informing the Health Committee of the GMC.[204,205]

The original list of "retired, distinguished anaesthetists"[206] was A J W Beard,[1] P J Helliwell,[3] J Alfred Lee,[2] W W Mushin,[142] A C Forrester, Sir Robert Macintosh[209] and Sir Geoffrey Organe;[56] S A Mason became a referee in 1981 when Sir Robert Macintosh and Sir Geoffrey Organe retired (Council Minutes 1.5.1981).[97] It is apparent, however, that, from the start, Philip Helliwell dealt with the majority of the cases,[201,203] and continued to do so until Maurice Burrows took over as Chairman of the Referees in 1992.

The Medical Defence Union contributed £1000 (1996: £3,200) towards the initial running costs of the scheme (Council Minutes 2.3.1979),[81] but the Department of Health did not contribute any funds. The first answerphone was originally installed at the offices of the Association of Anaesthetists so that initial requests by informants to be put in touch with a referee could be received at any time (Annual Report 1979).[210]

Philip Helliwell[3] reported in 1982 that the scheme had been helpful on "some twenty occasions".[203] The confidential nature of the scheme prevents assessment of the outcome in individual instances, but it is known that assistance is rarely if ever declined by the sick anaesthetist.[201] It is also established that, though it is possible for a doctor who has been treated for alcoholism to resume his career in anaesthesia, it is unwise for an anaesthetist who has once become addicted to other drugs and agents to continue to be permitted to practice as an anaesthetist, even if he has apparently been cured, although a career change within medicine is often possible (P J Helliwell, personal communication).

The advantages of the scheme are acknowledged to be its flexibility, and informality as an early warning system before serious problems develop or culpable offences involving patients occur.[203] Health Authorities, knowing that a careful watch is being kept by responsible colleagues, have usually been sympathetic and cooperative in regarding the individual as a sick employee, and in tolerating prolonged absences for treatment or in arranging reasonable financial terms for early retirement.

Great interest was generated by the "Help for the Sick Doctor Scheme" of the Association of Anaesthetists.[201] A seminar organised jointly by the Association of Anaesthetists and the Royal College of Psychiatrists took place at the premises of the Royal College of Psychiatrists on 8 March 1982. There were 50 participants representing 28 organisations. W D Wylie (President of the Association 1980-1982) chaired the morning session during which both Rosen and Helliwell spoke. The General Medical Council held an informal meeting to discuss the need for counselling and the welfare of such doctors on 16 June 1982 at which Stanley Mason represented the Association of Anaesthetists.[211] The General National Counselling and Welfare Service for Sick Doctors, the procedures of which owe much to the original scheme of the Association of Anaesthetists, was initiated by the GMC and the BMA in consultation with the Royal Colleges and their Faculties in 1986 with Professor Rawnsley[202] as its Chairman and Helliwell as a member of the management committee.[205] The special dangers to anaesthetists due to their ready access to anaesthetic agents and other drugs is recognised, and the Association of Anaesthetists own scheme for help for the sick doctor has been kept in existence alongside the national scheme.

The Association and the European Union (formerly the European Economic Community)

The United Kingdom became a member of the European Economic Community (EEC), now the European Union (EU), on 1 January 1974. The EU Directives relating to the free movement of doctors within the EEC were implemented in the United Kingdom on 16 June 1977, after some hesitation over the omission of a safeguard which would make it necessary for a doctor who wished to practise in another country to show linguistic competence in the language of the host country. The position in the EU is that any doctor who received his or her basic medical qualification in one of the other EU member states (Germany, France, Belgium, Luxembourg, the Netherlands, Denmark, Italy, Spain, Greece, Portugal, Austria, Finland, Sweden and the Republic of Ireland) can be temporarily registered in any of the other states without a test of linguistic competence, and can obtain full registration after being employed for a year or on demonstration of a nominal linguistic standard. United Kingdom doctors, of course, have reciprocal privileges in other EU states.[212-214]

The problem of specialist training and qualifications presented a real difficulty. Most EU states other than the United Kingdom have a very different system in which recognition as a specialist depends on a statutory period of training, usually involving clinical responsibility under supervision, in a single programme in a single hospital. Training in these countries culminates in the individual receiving a certificate of satisfactory completion of training and registration as a specialist. Specialist registration is necessary because in most countries the practitioners are in independent practice. The health services in these states are financed by insurance based systems under which patients reclaim the practitioners' fees from the government to a greater or lesser extent. It is therefore necessary for specialists to be identified and registered.[214] The minimum period of training in anaesthesia decreed by the EEC (now the EU) at the time of entry of the United Kingdom in 1974 was three years, though, even at that time, several countries already required a longer period.[215]

The position in the United Kingdom and Ireland was, very different; already by 1974 a system of postgraduate training had been set up by the

Royal Medical Colleges which involved a period of General Professional Training (GPT) of three years, usually completed by passing the appropriate examination for a Fellowship or Membership diploma. A further period of at least three years of Higher Professional Training (HPT) as a Senior Registrar followed. Satisfactory completion of a total of six years specialist training after the year of provisional registration implied that the individual was ready for the responsibility of a Consultant post in the British National Health Service, or in the Irish Republic, even though this requirement was not and subsequently never had been officially mandatory. The question of specialist registration did not arise because independent private specialist practice in the United Kingdom or Ireland was almost exclusively dependent on promotion to Consultant rank. The entry of the United Kingdom into the EEC (EU) coincided with the completion of the period during which the Medical Royal Colleges were formalising their training schemes, and it was believed at that time that the General Medical Council might introduce a Specialist Register in conformity with the other EU states.[216] It was therefore decided to issue a "Certificate of Accreditation". This entitled specialists trained in the United Kingdom to practise in other countries in the EU. It very soon became obvious, however, especially when GMC did not in fact institute a specialist register, that confining the right of United Kingdom trained specialists to practise in other EU countries to those who were accredited in the United Kingdom after six years training, put them at a disadvantage, compared with those from the EU states who received their certificates after only three years. The General Medical Council, who are the "competent authority" for EU purposes, therefore agreed to issue EU certificates of equivalent specialist qualification to specialists who wished to work in other member states after they had completed three years of GPT, passed the appropriate Fellowship or Membership examination (in case of anaesthetists the FFARCS), and had undertaken a further year of HPT, and were approved by the appropriate Higher Training Committee serviced by the Medical Royal Colleges. The award of an EU certificate was not considered to entitle the holder to be regarded as an independent specialist in the British NHS and, perhaps more importantly, the British health insurance companies and provident associations by and large only paid fees to practitioners who were accredited or who held Consultant posts[217] (a privilege which has only been won by hard bargaining by anaesthetists).[210] Specialists in these categories, but not those with an EU certificate, were entitled to request that the letter "T" is printed beside their listing in the British Medical Register since 1 January 1991[218] but, in fact, perusal of the Register indicated that remarkably few established Consultants chose to have this accolade added to their entries!

John Zorab in his review in 1977 of the position of anaesthetists in the EEC sagely remarked that this two tier system of registration "may present a major problem for resolution in the future."[212] How right he was; although, in fact, it was well over a decade before the position was seriously challenged in the Courts in 1991 when, after a series of legal battles, the anomalous position emerged that apparently "the holder of a European specialist qualification (certificate) issued in another member state was entitled to appear as such in the British Medical Register, but not the holder of the equivalent (EU) certificate issued in Britain."[219,220] Underlying dissatisfaction with the whole edifice of postgraduate training in the United Kingdom and accreditation became apparent after this well publicised legal confrontation especially amongst trainees.[219,220] This was not only because of the two tier specialist registration issue, but also because of the lengthy specialist training system in the United Kingdom with its major element of service commitment to the NHS.[221-224]

The publicity in the United Kingdom apparently drew the attention of the European Commission in Brussels to the problem and they raised the subject with the Department of Health in 1992. A working group was set up under the Chief Medical Officer of England, Kenneth Calman.[218] The Calman working group reported in 1993 with medical proposals for the reorganisation of shortened, "seamless", structural specialist training.[153,225-227]

The implementation of the recommendations of the Calman report envisaged a major reduction in the service element contributed by trainees. This in turn implies a marked expansion of the Consultant grade, or the creation of a new intermediate specialist grade with full responsibility for the clinical care of patients, and yet, apparently, the Minister for Health implied that there would be no additional funding. The Officers of the Association of Anaesthetists have been deeply involved with this problem (Chapter 10).[227]

The Association and the European Union (formerly the European Economic Community)

The Section Monospécialisèe d'Anesthésiologie et de Réanimation is the official Subcommittee through which the views of the anaesthetists of member states are conveyed to the Union Européenne des Médicins Spécialistes (UEMS) and thence to the EU Commission.[212,215] The Association of Anaesthetists had originally sent observers during the abortive bid which the United Kingdom made to join the EEC in the early nineteen sixties and were invited to continue to attend as observers despite the failure of the initiative. Interest by the Association revived in 1972 as the renewed negotiations for the entry of the United Kingdom into the EEC (EU) seemed likely to succeed. A request for two fresh nominations to the anaesthetists' European subcommittee was made through the British Medical Association to the Faculty of Anaesthetists in 1972, and it was agreed that the Faculty and the Association should each send one representative. Sir Geoffrey Organe was nominated to represent the Association of Anaesthetists and Douglas Howat the Faculty (Council Minutes 1.9.1972).[96,215] The initial meeting of the anaesthetists' subcommittee in 1972 defined the scope of the specialty as including:- the administration of anaesthetics, the care of the patient before, during and after surgery including monitoring and therapeutic intervention, the management of respiratory failure, oxygen and inhalation therapy, blood transfusion and parenteral nutrition, the treatment of pain and the management of extra corporeal circulation and renal dialysis. A meeting in 1974 recommended a minimum period of training for anaesthesia of four years, compared with the three years current in some member states, but this proposal was blocked by the UEMS itself.[212,215]

John Zorab replaced Sir Geoffrey Organe as the representative of the Association of Anaesthetists in 1976. The Association originally set up its International Affairs committee in 1976, primarily in an attempt to deal with the discrepancies between United Kingdom practice and that of the other EU countries and to press for the reactivation of the EU subcommittee which had not met since 1974. (Council Minutes 21.5.1976 and 2.7.1976: Annual Report 1976).[81,212] The EU subcommittee has met regularly since that time and the British contribution has been considerable. Douglas Howat became Chairman in 1984 and Peter Baskett, who took over as Association representative from John Zorab in 1982, succeeded him in 1986. W R MacRae served as Association Representative from 1987. Perusal of successive Association

Annual Reports (Annual Reports 1982-1996) reveals many problems which have been encountered by anaesthetists in the other EU countries. Few of these have been directly relevant to British practice, but guidelines and recommendations have been promulgated, and a great deal of moral support has been given to anaesthetists of our EU continental partners, who have gradually experienced an improvement in their medicopolitical status; as has already been described however the contrast with the United Kingdom has resulted in discrepancies in the way in which completion of specialist training is recognised. The standard of 5 years of training in anaesthesia was finally accepted by the UEMS in 1988 but has not been made mandatory by the promulgation of an EU directive.[224] The mechanisms by which our standards are monitored in the United Kingdom and Ireland are foreign to other EU countries (inspection of training hospitals and compulsory assessment by examination for example), but there is growing evidence that some of these practices may ultimately be adopted.[227] There is little doubt that the continued input of the Association of Anaesthetists of Great Britain and Ireland, has played a not inconsiderable part in changing opinion with regard to the possible acceptance of such concepts. A European Board in Anaesthesiology Reanimation and Intensive Care (EBAR) was set up by the Committee in 1993 on the recommendation of the UEMS. This body is charged with "harmonising educational standards for the specialty in the European Community and will advise on training, on mutual recognition of qualifications, and on the possibility of recommending the introduction of examinations."[227] This is a tall order since, in addition to the present twelve countries of the old European Economic Community, the European Medical Boards and Committees of its successor the European Union (now comprised of fifteen nations (Belgium, France, Germany, Italy, Luxembourg, the Netherlands, Denmark, Ireland and the United Kingdom, Greece, Portugal, Spain, Austria, Sweden and Finland) now has representation from the other European trade organisation EFTA (the European Free Trade Area Association which includes Norway and Switzerland), and is shortly likely to admit observers from Poland and Hungary. William MacRae (President 1992-1994) has aptly remarked, "It was difficult enough to find some common ground with the original (twelve) EU members but this rapid expansion has compounded the problem."[227]

The European Academy of Anaesthesiology

The idea of a European Academy had its origins in informal discussions at the 6th World Congress of Anaesthesiologists in Mexico City in 1976.[228,229] The 1976 Annual Report of the Association of Anaesthetists, which covers the last year of the Presidency of Philip Helliwell,[3] records that "unofficial soundings" had been taken in various countries with regard to the possible formation of an "Academy of Anaesthetists of Europe". This was conceived as an organisation which would have comparable functions in Europe as a whole to the Royal Medical Colleges in the United Kingdom in maintaining academic standards.

The Council Minutes of 7 January 1977,[81] reporting a meeting of its new International Relations Committee on 17 September 1976, recorded that the new President of the Association of Anaesthetists (Cyril Scurr) and the new Dean of the Faculty of Anaesthetists (J E. Riding) had written to the doyen of French anaesthesia, Professor Jean Lassner, suggesting a meeting to "discuss the foundation of an "Academy of Anaesthesia" for Europe". The involvement of the Faculty at this early stage is interesting. It is the present writer's recollection, as a member of both the Council of the Association of Anaesthetists and the Board of the Faculty, that some of those who favoured the establishment of an independent College in the United Kingdom, but were frustrated by the lack of progress in that direction at the time, saw a European Academy as a body that could possibly become more important throughout Europe than the Faculty; on the other hand there is no doubt that, later on, when the Academy was about to be an established fact, some members of the Board of Faculty who did not believe that an independent College would be viable, were distinctly cool about the foundation of the Academy. They may indeed have seen it as a potential possible challenge to the Faculty; in the event the Academy has proved to have much greater influence in continental Europe than in the United Kingdom, though the contribution which individual British anaesthetists have made to its development has been considerable.

Professor Lassner replied to the British letter to the effect that "his French colleagues were in favour of such a meeting (to discuss the formation of an Academy) as were the Germans, Spaniards and Austrians" (Council Minutes 3.3.1977),[81] and from then on Lassner became the chief architect of the foundation of the Academy. He wrote to all the societies of anaesthetists in Europe and convened a meeting of 32 nominated delegates from 16 countries in Paris. This meeting was addressed by Madame Simone Veil, then the French Minister of Health, and a steering committee was formed.[229] The first General Assembly of 46 delegates nominated by 22 European Anaesthesia Societies was held in Paris during the 5th European Congress of Anaesthesiology in 1978.[228] Officers and a Senate were elected. Professor Lassner was elected President, W S Wren of the Republic of Ireland (a member of the Association of Anaesthetists) was elected Secretary and, of the twelve senators, two were British (Sykes and Vickers) and the United Kingdom was the only nationality to have more than one member. Michael Rosen was elected Chairman of the Finance Committee. It must be stressed however that, though of necessity national societies were asked to nominate the founder Academicians, the Academy is not composed of delegates from the national societies. Academicians are elected individually on their merits irrespective of nationality. There were just over 100 Academicians by the end of the first year and 275 by 1984. [228,229]

The First Scientific Meeting of the Academy was held in October 1979 at the Royal Postgraduate Medical School (Hammersmith, London) with Professor (Sir) Keith Sykes as organiser and host.[230]

The European Journal of Anaesthesiology came into being in 1984 with Michael Vickers and Professor E Nilsson of Sweden as Editors.[229]

The European Diploma of Anaesthesiology was also instituted in 1984. This was principally to encourage specialists from those countries which do not have their own examination to achieve an academic standard. Some states have made it a mandatory part of their own system of training. Five hundred and sixty diplomas had been awarded by 1994. All of these have been by examination as no honorary diplomas have been granted. The Diploma can be sat in a number of centres in Europe in any one of five languages chosen by the candidate. European diplomates were granted exemption from the first part of the Fellowship examinations of the Royal College of Anaesthetists and the Irish Faculty.[227,229,231]

The work of the International Relations Committee 1976-1982

The International Relations Committee was originally set up in 1976 to monitor and influence the manner in which the EEC directives of the European Economic Community were introduced (Council Minutes 21.5.1976).[81]

Aileen Adams became Chairman of the Committee in 1977 and, after making recommendations with regard to the formation of the European Academy (see below: Council Minutes 6.1.78 and 7.7.1978),[81] the Committee began to turn its attention to an old interest of its Chairman (Chapter 7), that of providing aid in the field of anaesthesia for developing countries, and liaison with others outside the EEC. The Committee defined its principle task as that of fostering cooperation between the various bodies who were endeavouring to assist the developing countries (Annual Report 1979);[232] under Aileen Adams and her successor John Zorab (later Secretary General and then President of the World Federation of Societies of Anaesthesiologists), the Committee came to be recognised as the coordinating body in the United Kingdom for anaesthesia by many organisations. These included the governmental Overseas Development Administration (ODA), the Crown Agents, the World Federation of Societies of Anaesthesiologists, (WFSA), the British Council and its Committee for International Relations (originally the Inter-University Council), the Appropriate Health Resources and Technologists Action Group, and the Bureau for Overseas Medicinal Services (Annual Report 1979 to 1981:[232-234] personal communication R J Eltringham).

J A (Tony) Bennett of Bristol was assisted by the ODA to visit Sudan in 1979 and set up a teaching project in Khartoum, which was also visited by Douglas Howat and Professor J A Thornton of Sheffield in the same year.[232]

The British Council funded a "somewhat hazardous" visit by Tony Bennett to Uganda early in 1980 in the unstable situation following the end of the Amin regime in 1979 (Council Minutes 11.4.1980),[97,233] and also visits by William MacRae to Bangladesh in February 1981 and Aileen Adams to Zambia in October of the same year, and all of them made comprehensive reports to the Association Committee. Advice was also given on recruitment for many other countries including Kenya and Malawi, and assistance was provided to Patricia Coyle (Australia) when she took up a post at Mulago Hospital, Uganda in 1981 (Annual Report 1981).[234]

The International Relations Committee thus established itself as a clearing house for information about many countries during this period, and was able "to act as a forum for the exchange of experience and ideas, with the aim of supporting the development of the practice and teaching of good safe anaesthesia, wherever it was needed" (Annual Report 1982).[235]

The Exchange with East Germany (the German Democratic Republic, GDR) came about as the result of an intergovernmental cultural agreement a decade before reunification in 1990. The Association of Anaesthetists were designated as the nominating body (Council Minutes 11.4.1980 and 6.6.1980)[97] Douglas Howat paid a visit to East Germany in April 1982 (Annual Report 1982)[235] and Professor Borchert came to the United Kingdom in October 1982 (Council Minutes 3.12.1982).[97] Clifford Franklin (Manchester), was Association Visitor to East Germany in 1984.[236]

Training in outpatient dental anaesthesia and sedation

The administration of anaesthesia for dental outpatients was the last bastion of the belief that any qualified medical or dental practitioner should be considered to be capable of safely administering a general anaesthetic by virtue of his undergraduate training alone. The position was most jealously guarded by Dental Practitioners who had no means of obtaining adequate postgraduate training in anaesthetics, and to a lesser extent by medical General Practitioners, many of whom practised dental anaesthesia for exodontia as an interesting and moderately remunerative sideline, without formal postgraduate training.[237] The number of ambulatory cases deemed to require general anaesthesia fell during the seventies.[237-239] It certainly was not possible for dental or non-specialist medical undergraduates to obtain adequate training, nor, indeed, could it be assumed that those who completed their postgraduate training in the specialty of anaesthesia from the seventies onwards were necessarily adequately trained in this branch of practice (although, of course, by reasons of their general training in anaesthesia they would naturally be better equipped for the task than the new graduate).

A considerable number of general anaesthetics were then, and in 1998 still are being administered in the United Kingdom to unintubated ambulant patients for minor dental surgery, particularly to children for both exodontia and for orthodontic indications. This outpatient technique has been a peculiarly British practice for many years; most other countries having opted for local anaesthesia, with or without sedation. Sedation techniques had an enviable safety record, whereas, in the case of general anaesthesia, there was a relatively small but significant mortality in the seventies;[240] these isolated deaths were given prominence in the public press and gave rise to considerable professional and public concern, especially bearing in mind the minor nature of the surgical procedures.[237-241]

The Wylie Report 1978. A Working Party was convened by the Deans of the Faculties of Dental Surgery and of Anaesthetists in 1976 under the Chairmanship of W Derek Wylie. The terms of reference were "to make recommendations with respect to the safety of patients under dental anaesthesia and the training which must be undergone to achieve this." The Association of Anaesthetists and the British Dental Association were invited to take part. Philip Helliwell and Michael Coplans represented the Association of Anaesthetists.[242,243]

The Wylie Report was published in April 1978;[242] significantly it noted that nothing had been done at a national level to implement the recommendations on postgraduate training in anaesthesia since the publication of the report of the Joint Sub-committee in 1967 and the Windeyer Report of 1969 (Chapter 7). The Wylie Report emphasised that postgraduate training in anaesthesia was required for both medical and dental undergraduates who wished to administer outpatient dental anaesthesia. It also clearly distinguished sedation from general anaesthesia. It defined the former as a condition "in which the use of a drug or drugs produces a state of depression of the central nervous system enabling treatment to be carried out, but during which verbal contact with the patient is maintained throughout the period of sedation." It was stressed that "the drugs and techniques used should carry a margin of safety wide enough to render unintended loss of consciousness unlikely," and the report acknowledges that such methods "may demand less comprehensive training." It also emphasised that dental undergraduates should be given training in sedation techniques. The report provided a comprehensive list of the basic "core" skills required in medical diagnosis, anaesthesia, sedation and resuscitation, and detailed the facilities and equipment which a practitioner would require to have available before undertaking the administration of general anaesthesia for dental outpatients. It also called for a "national policy for training in dental anaesthesia", and it emphasised that a "training programme should include the practice of general anaesthesia in a hospital, preferably in a resident appointment, and experience of general anaesthesia in a general dental practice, as well as the appropriate theoretical components". The question of a Diploma in Dental Anaesthesia was "left open", but the Wylie party was of the opinion that "a mechanism must be found for the establishment of a list of recognised dental anaesthetists, the gateway to it being ....an approved training programme" as proposed in the report. Such a list should be without detriment to the rights of existing practitioners. The report also suggested that "a small joint committee of the two Faculties of Dental Surgery and Anaesthetists should be responsible for national developments in this field of education and should hold a register of recognised teachers and training programmes."[242]

The Seward Report.[243,248] The two Faculties of the Royal College of Surgeons of England (Dental Surgery and Anaesthetists) set up an inter-faculty Working Party to consider the implementation of the Wylie Report with Professor Gordon Seward of the London Hospital (later Dean of the Faculty of Dental Surgery) as Chairman; neither the Association of Anaesthetists nor the BMA or the BDA were represented on the Working Party because training and standards were deemed to be the remit of the Royal College of Surgeons and its Faculties, but two out of the three Board Member representatives of the Faculty of Anaesthetists were also members of the Council of the Association (T B Boulton and Michael Vickers). The draft report was also circulated to the Association and the BMA and BDA for comment.

The draft Seward Report endorsed the core skills and facilities and equipment which should be required for the practice of dental anaesthesia as defined in the Wylie Report. It also very importantly specifically categorised the ultra-light methohexitone technique as being firmly within the Wylie Working Party definition of general anaesthesia, and thus outside the scope of the practice of the operating dentist-sedationist, whether assisted by competent nurses or dental surgery assistants or not. The report did however recognise conscious sedation techniques with nitrous oxide or the benzodiazepines, in which verbal contact with the patient was not lost, as being permissible for use by the trained operator-sedationist working with trained assistance. The draft Seward Report also envisaged a properly funded full-time course in dental anaesthesia, supervised by a special joint committee of the two Faculties, which would last seven months (one month theory and six months practice both in hospitals and general dental surgeries). The Working Party also proposed, that after safeguarding the rights of dental and medical practitioners already practising outpatient dental anaesthesia, there should be a limited list of dentally and medically qualified dental anaesthetists who would be entitled to a higher level of remuneration from NHS sources. This concept was similar to the scheme for the practice of obstetrics by General Medical Practitioners, which had been in operation for a number of years.

The Association of Anaesthetists gave qualified support to the draft report, but Council were of the opinion that training in dental anaesthesia should be for one year full time or equivalent (Council Minutes 8.4.1977).[81] The BDA, through the *British Dental Journal,* welcomed the report when it was published in 1981, but stated prophetically "Questions of financing postgraduate training and funding suitable ways of rewarding practitioners will prove extremely difficult", and called for "the BDA and the BMA to set aside sectional interests and take action which will demonstrate their commitment to the continuance of a service which commands the confidence of the public".[248]

This latter appeal fell on deaf ears so far as the General Medical Services (General Practitioner) Committee (GMSC) of the BMA were concerned![244,249,250] General Practice was undergoing a period of introspection in the early eighties which was designed to enhance the image, importance, and scope of "primary care" (vocational training for general practice became compulsory for new entrants in 1982).[249] There was great emphasis on extending the meaning of the word "general" to cover specialist procedures undertaken in general practice! The GMSC objected to the concept of a seven month course in anaesthesia, despite the no detriment proposal and the fact that the original recommendation for a whole time course had been modified to include the possibility of recognising a flexible part-time equivalent. They also rejected the idea of a list of qualified dental anaesthetists on the grounds that Consultant Anaesthetists might be automatically included while most general practitioners would not be.[244,250-254] The reports of the debates in the GMSC on this topic show a regrettable degree of self interest and misrepresentation of the aims and intentions of the Wylie and Seward Working Parties.[250-254] A suggestion was made in the Council of the Association of Anaesthetists that the Research and Education Fund might be used to fund teaching programmes in dental anaesthesia, but it was pointed out that governmental "Section 63" funds for medical and dental general practitioner postgraduate education were theoretically available (Council Minutes 5.3.1982).[81]

There was a limited attempt by the Dental Section of the Department of Health to meet the proposals for a course in anaesthesia for dental practitioners. The two Faculties were not invited to set up a joint committee to oversee the training courses as proposed by the Seward Working Party however, nor were arrangements made for an initial theoretical course. The Department of Health confined itself to offering Regional Health Authorities funding for an overall national quota of eight dental practitioner trainees to be paid as Senior House Officers for six month periods to be attached to departments of anaesthesia. The content of the course of training was not clearly defined. Almost all the trainees, selected by the Regional Health Authorities without reference to the Faculties, were recently qualified dental practitioners waiting to find suitable practices or appointments, and the majority of them were women graduates. Individual Consultant Anaesthetist trainers made considerable efforts to give these trainees a basis in anaesthesia and resuscitation, but the Seward proposal for an apprentice component in general dental practice was neither funded nor generally implemented, especially with regard to conscious sedation. A large part of the training, in fact consisted of the administration of general anaesthesia under supervision in general operating theatres (personal recollection).

The Faculties of Dental Surgery and of Anaesthetists did their best to support the scheme voluntarily. They organised joint five day courses, but "hands on" experience was not possible and the practical element was limited to observation of demonstrations. Almost all the young dental practitioners who took part in the scheme stated that they enjoyed the experience, but it was a pale shadow of what the Seward Working Party had so carefully considered and recommended. The scheme started in 1986 and was discontinued in 1988 as it was considered to be unsatisfactory both by the two Faculties and by the Department of Health (personal recollections).

The Spence Report 1981. The Chairman of this Scottish Working Party was Professor A A Spence (at that time Professor of Anaesthesia in Glasgow). It ran in parallel with the Wylie Working Party to consider the position in Scotland. It concluded that it would be possible for all general anaesthesia for dental outpatients to be practised by Consultant Anaesthetists in special units within a decade, and it suggested possible interim training schemes for medical and dental practitioners.[248]

The Nuffield Foundation Committee on Inquiry into Dental Education. This independent inquiry was appointed in 1977 and its report was published in 1980.[255] The section of the report on outpatient anaesthesia recommended postgraduate training and a special list of dental surgeons trained to administer general anaesthetics.

New guidance on the administration of outpatient anaesthesia. Two deaths in dental surgeries involving operator anaesthetists, at a time when a new Dentists Bill was under consideration by Parliament, led to public and professional pressure on the Department of Health (DH) and the General Dental Council (GDC) to attempt to ensure greater safety in the administration of dental anaesthesia in general dental practices (Council Minutes 21.5.1982:[97] Annual Report 1983[257]).[256] The Association of Anaesthetists played an important part in stimulating interest. Public relations consultants were employed (Council Minutes 6.10.1978),[81] questions were asked in Parliament

(Council Minutes 4.2.1983)[97] and the Association took part in discussions with the DH which also included representatives from the BMA, the BDA and the Faculty of Anaesthetists (Council Minutes 8.4.1988),[97] Annual Report 1983).[256,257] The Department of Health at last abolished the iniquitous NHS payment of a fee to the dental surgeon for administering his own general anaesthetic in 1983, and in the same year the GDC outlawed the practice.[256] The GDC went even further in its "Guidance". It stressed that the second medical or dental practitioner who administered an anaesthetic to dental outpatients, must be adequately trained and that proper apparatus, including resuscitation equipment, must be provided. Operator sedation with an appropriate margin of safety (benzodiazepine or "relative analgesia" (RA) nitrous oxide) was permitted but a trained assistant was required to be present, and adequate resuscitation equipment was to be provided.

The guidance concluded by stating that "A dentist who carried out treatment under general anaesthesia or sedation without fulfilling these conditions would almost certainly be considered to have acted in a manner which constitutes infamous or disgraceful conduct in a professional respect".[256] This verdict would carry with it dire penalties including erasure from the Register. The ultra-light methohexitone technique was included as unsuitable for the operating dentist by invoking the Wylie Report definition already mentioned. The GDC does not have jurisdiction over medical practitioners but the guidelines had obvious implications regarding training for those who had not specialised in anaesthesia. Many dental surgeons gave up the use of anaesthesia in their own practices as the result of these guidelines and, where general anaesthesia was deemed necessary, patients were increasingly referred to hospitals and the Community Dental Service. There was also a coincident continued fall during the nineteen eighties in the absolute number of patients requiring general anaesthesia as a dental outpatients. This was the result of better hygiene, including fluoride supplementation,[258] improved conservation techniques, and the use of inhalation and intravenous sedation. The latter gained further popularity after the introduction of the shorter acting and safer intravenous benzodiazepine midazolam.[259] The problem of a national policy for the postgraduate training of dental surgeons in anaesthesia remained unresolved however.[260] The report of the Expert Working Party chaired by Professor David Poswillo and published in 1990, was destined to attempt to tackle this problem as part of a comprehensive review of the question of the provision of outpatient anaesthesia and sedation for dental patients. This review has had important consequences (Chapter 9).[261]

Fees for the administration of anaesthetics to NHS patients in General Dental Practice

This perennial problem has occupied the attention of the Association of Anaesthetists from its foundation, and particularly since the inauguration of the National Health Service.[262] A satisfactory solution has never been found, or rather "conceded" by the Department of Health (DH). The difficulty stemmed from the system of paying for the administration of anaesthesia as a dental "item of service" from the "dental pool" as negotiated between the Government and the British Dental Association.[262] Deduction from the Dental Pool diminished the amount available for purely dental earnings. The 1970 Annual Report of the Association of Anaesthetists records:-

"Discussion with the Department of Health regarding anaesthetic fees for dental work has arrived at an impasse, since "It is a matter of law that a general anaesthetic given in connection with any item of general dental service is part of that treatment."

1970-1976. Early in the seventies, when the Association was attempting to negotiate directly with the DH for a simple increase in dental anaesthetic fees, no response was received either from the British Dental Association (because of the possible deprivation to the dental pool) or from the DH, presumably because the Association of Anaesthetists was not itself a negotiating body (Annual Reports 1970, 1971 and 1972); however, once the British Dental Association (BDA) accepted that the claim was for monies separate from the dental pool, they cooperated fully. The establishment in 1973 of the Anaesthetists Subcommittee of the Central Committee for Hospital Medical Services within the BMA organisation, with predominant Association of Anaesthetists Council membership, also provided the Association with direct access to the NHS negotiating machinery (Annual Report 1973).

Various attempts were made to suggest mechanisms to the DH which could be used to allocate funds for dental anaesthetic fees under "Category 2" payments (a system most used to reward pathologists for reports on investigations outside their usual hospital work) as proposed in 1973 (Annual Report 1973). This concept was rejected by the DH. An "attendance" fee to cover travel and other expenses to supplement the fees in individual cases (similar to a "call-out" fee for the domestic attendance of an electrician or plumber) was proposed in 1975, and, at the same time, attention was called to the reluctance of Dental Estimates Board to approve the payment of the "Special Anaesthetic Fee" which was supposed to be available when there were particular medical or dental difficulties (Annual Report 1974).[263]

The DH continued to be resistant to the idea of an attendance fee but agreed to ease the terms upon which the payment of the special fee was payable in 1975 (Annual Report 1975).[264,265]

1976-1979. The DH asked for evidence that dentists were experiencing difficulty in obtaining the services of medical anaesthetists on account of the low fees (Annual Report 1976). The evidence was obtained by the Association of Anaesthetists but rejected by the DH. The President of the Association (Cyril F Scurr) at the Council Meeting on 8 July 1977 deplored the fact "after eleven years of bad faith on the part of the DH anaesthetists were being asked to administer anaesthetics for a fee that was only a fraction of what was being paid to repair men", and he went on to ask for the authority of the Council of the Association of Anaesthetists to advise members not to administer anaesthetics in dental surgeries for NHS fees except in the cases of extreme hardship, and for children and pensioners. It was also agreed that general practitioner anaesthetists should be approached through the General Medical Services Committee of the BMA (Council Minutes 8.7.1977).[81] A comprehensive letter from the President to all Members of the Association of Anaesthetists was prepared. This explained the history of the dispute and detailed the protracted negotiations with the DH.[262] The proposal to withdraw services under the NHS conditions was endorsed by the Linkman Conference in September 1977,[264] and the full cooperation of the BMA was obtained; then, in December 1977 letters were sent to the *British Medical Journal* and the *British Dental Journal* advising that "anaesthetists (whether Consultants or General Practitioners) should discontinue giving dental anaesthetics under the NHS as from January 1978". The letters were signed by the Chairman of the BMA Council, the Chairman of the CCHMS, the Chairman of the General Medical Services (General Practice) Committee and the President of the Association of Anaesthetists.[265] The fees that were current in 1977 are listed in the letter. They range from £2 (1996: £6) for an anaesthetic for the extraction of 1-3 teeth to £4.60 (1996: £14) for "more than 20" teeth with the exceptional fee of £11.50 (1996: £34) for cases of special medical or dental difficulty. The fee of 60p (1996: £2) for the operating dentist was still available at that time and not discontinued until 1983. The aims of the anaesthetists are stated in the letter to be, (a) payment of an attendance fee, (b) payment of fees from NHS medical funds and available to part-time and wholetime Consultants alike (as well as General Practitioners) and (c) negotiation of realistic fees when the Government's "pay policy", at that time operative, permitted.[265]

It is doubtful whether the call to cease to administer anaesthesia had a marked effect in reducing the number of anaesthetics administered under the NHS terms despite the solidarity of the BMA committees with the Council of the Association of Anaesthetists. Many Consultants and General Practitioners were earning useful if modest additional incomes from the NHS fees, especially in towns in which general dental practices were conveniently located in relation to hospitals or general medical practices,[264] and some were making good use of the special fee provision, although this rather begged the question as it also came out of the dental pool (Council Minutes 5.1.1979).[81] Anxious questions were asked in Council about the effect of the "ban" in March and June 1978, but the Association Officers could not give a positive reply other than "the BDA felt the sanctions were creating pressure",[81] however, after some hesitation, the ban was lifted in October 1978 after "the Minister of State (Health) had ..... agreed to negotiations on this subject".[266] These negotiations did not result in the provision of an attendance fee, but the anaesthetic fees were increased (as before according to the number of teeth extracted) to between £4.60 (1996: £11.50) and £5.75 (1996: £14.50) for the administration of "nitrous oxide or ethyl chloride", and between £7.65 (1996: £20) and £9.55 (1996: £24) for "other general anaesthetics"! These fees from the dental pool should be compared with £10.90 to £12.30 (1992:

£27 to £31) from medical funds for each patient who received a domiciliary visit from Consultants of other disciplines, with the addition of extra payments for mileage and use of equipment.[267]

1979-1983. The election of the Conservative government in 1979 and the appointment of a psychiatrist (Gerald Vaughan) as Minister of Health gave rise to optimism and, after an interval to allow the new administration to "settle in" (Council Minutes 4.5.1979),[97] representatives of the Association of Anaesthetists, the BDA, and GMSC of the BMA met the Minister. The meeting is reported to have been "cordial" but no concessions were made (Council Minutes 5.10.1979:[97] Annual Report 1979).[232] The DH continued to procrastinate (Annual Reports 1980, 1981, 1982, 1983!)[233-235,257] The only concession obtained from the DH in this period was the abolition of the fee for anaesthesia administered by the operating dentist (Council Minutes 8.4.1983:[97] Annual Report 1983).[256,257] This, coupled with the new "guidelines" issued by the General Dental Council (GDC) on the necessity for training and proper equipment for outpatient dental anaesthesia,[256] and other factors already noted, led to a further decline in the number of general anaesthetics for outpatient dentistry which were administered. There was a still greater relative decline in the number administered in general practice dental surgeries, because of the tendency to refer those patients who were still considered to require a general anaesthetic for outpatient dental treatment to properly equipped hospital or Community Dental Service Units. The anaesthetists for these clinics were funded on a salaried or sessional basis. It is true to say that, fees for visiting anaesthetists to general dental practices, though of course still important to a limited number of individuals, ceased to be a major problem for the Association of Anaesthetists. Procrastination on the part of the DH had paid off with alterations in the way in which dentistry was practised!

Research and Education 1970-1982

Business for the Research and Education Committee began quietly in the seventies. Large funds were not available, but nonetheless the 1970 Annual Report records that applications for research grants were "disappointingly few"; however, it also warns that, "Whilst in the past full time Research Fellows have been supported increasing salaries and other costs means that this is becoming beyond the (Research and Education) Committee's resources". It goes on to say that grants of more than £1000 per year (1996: £8,250) would be exceptional. Travel grants would not be given to take up posts abroad or to attend a Congress but might be granted to extend such visits.

Joan C Scott, working with Professor E A Cooper in Newcastle upon Tyne, was awarded a "part-time research fellowship" in 1971 to investigate acid-base changes resulting from controlled ventilation under anaesthesia. This work was later extended by a Medical Research Council Grant to include several papers and an MD thesis (Annual Report 1972).

The Research and Education Committee continued to make a considerable number of grants for apparatus and technicians' salaries throughout the nineteen seventies (Annual Reports 1971-1979).[232] The amounts awarded were not large by some standards, for example the Research Grants totalled £4,328 (1996: £19,300) during 1975 and, apparently, no travel grant were made during that year (Annual Report 1975); however, these disbursements must have been very helpful to the recipients, many of whom were already, or later became, well known for important research work. They included Professor J W Dundee (Belfast), J Selwyn Crawford of Birmingham (depression of the fetus due to anaesthesia), (Professor) F R Ellis of Leeds (malignant hyperthermia), Professor M D Vickers of Cardiff (investigations into the cardiovascular effects of acrylic cement), Professor J S Robinson (Birmingham) and (Professor) T E J Healy (Nottingham) for investigations into the effect of muscle relaxants, as well as a number of investigators from non-teaching hospitals.

The Chairman of the Research and Education Committee (Alastair Spence) reported to Council on 1 December 1979 that the available research funds had not been fully used, even though ample funds were by now available (in large part due to the financial prowess of the Association Financial Advisor Ernest Warburton). Spence proposed that the limit for any one project be raised to £5,000 (1996: £12,500) to attract more ambitious applications; when inflation is taken into consideration this increase was actually a comparatively modest rise from £1,000 (1996: £8,250) limit set in 1970. An improved system of scrutiny of applications by assessors was instituted at that time.

"Under the influence". Council guaranteed £1,000 (1996: £2,300) to underwrite the collection and publication by MacMillan in book form of the classic articles from the *British Journal of Anaesthesia* by Denis (W D A) Smith on the history of nitrous oxide, under the title "Under the influence"[268] (Annual Report 1980)[233] but, in the event, this potential subsidy was not required.

The Association Research Fellowship was instituted following a proposal to Council by John Norman (Professor of Anaesthesia, University of Southampton) in January 1981 (Council Minutes 9.1.1981).[97] The salary was set at Senior Registrar level and the availability the Fellowship was widely advertised. There were eight applicants from amongst which Geraldine (E G M) O'Sullivan (then at Oxford and later Consultant at St Thomas' Hospital, London) was appointed to study the gastric secretory activity of obstetric patients employing non-invasive methods (Annual Report 1982).[235]

Fellowships and Grants financed by Industry. Several firms provided money for grants during this period. They included, the British Oxygen Company Medishield Travel Grant, the Hoechst Fellowship (which enabled a European physician anaesthetist to be attached for six months to a British University Department) and the Surgicon and Critikon Travel Fellowships (Annual Reports 1979, 1980 and 1981).[232-234]

The Fatigue Working Party. A meeting of the Section of Anaesthesia of the Royal Society of Medicine on 5 April 1974 under the Presidency of A R Hunter of Manchester (1914-1991) was entitled "The Anaesthetists' Environment"; more specifically it was concerned with the influence with external factors might have on the health and performance of working anaesthetists. W D A (Denis) Smith of Leeds (Member of the Council of the Association 1976-1980) discussed the topical concern at that time of the effect of the chronic inhalation of trace concentrations of volatile and gaseous anaesthetics in the operating theatre;[269] amongst the others speakers that evening, R T Wilkinson, of the Medical Research Council Applied Psychology Unit at Cambridge, provided information about tests which had been used experimentally to measure the influence of sleep deprivation on vigilance and the performance of routine tasks in other circumstances. He believed that such tests might be applicable to measuring the lack of sleep on the performance of anaesthetists.[270] This was a matter of concern with particular reference to the possible danger of lack of sleep on the performance of junior anaesthetists working long hours. Professor M D Vickers of Cardiff prompted Council to set up the Fatigue Working Party with Denis Smith as Convenor in May 1977 (W D A Smith personal communication). [232,233,271,272]

Four projects were envisaged:-[232,271,272]

1. A study of the role of anaesthetists by the social scientist Lisl Klein. This project was completed and the report was published in 1980.[272,273] It is considered in more detail in the next section together with a separate investigation into the personality of the anaesthetist which was not part of the Fatigue Working Party project.[274]

2. An ergonomic study of the work of anaesthetists by Paul Branston (ergonomist) and David Osborne (psychologist) of University College, Swansea. This involved the use of a time lapse video recorder to monitor the activities of anaesthetists at work at the Royal Free Hospital, London. Posture, head, eye and hand movements were noted, and pulse and eye blinks were monitored by telemetry. The investigators hoped to assess the anaesthetists vigilance; they were enthusiastic, but there were difficulties in communication between the disciplines of ergonomics and anaesthesia which, Denis Smith believed, might have been avoided if an anaesthetist had been a member of the investigating team. A paper was presented at a Congress on Research and Psychology in Medicine at Swansea in 1978, but the Fatigue Working Party and the Research and Education Committee found their conclusions unconvincing.[271,272]

3. A study of the sleep and work activity using activity logs. Thirty-five Senior Registrars and 52 anaesthetists of other grades (from

Senior House Officer to Consultant) compiled logs but the investigation was not completed.[271,272]

4. A study of reaction times using Wilkinson's Reaction Timer Mark II. A certain amount of preliminary data was collected by the Convenor, but the definitive study was not undertaken due to technical and staff changes and other difficulties.[271,272]

The investigations of the Fatigue Working Party collected a considerable amount of pilot information which would be of value to any investigator who wishes to undertake a similar study, but the project was discontinued after due consideration by the Research and Education Committee and the Council in 1981.[272] These were an ambitious series of studies undertaken at a time of great industrial stress in the British National Health Service and they were probably inadequately resourced. Denis Smith reviewed the projects in a paper at the World Congress of Anaesthesiologists in Manila in 1984.[271]

The personality and role of the anaesthetist. Two very interesting and contrasting research studies on the nature of specialisation in anaesthesia were initiated and/or supported by the Association of Anaesthetists in the early nineteen eighties. The reports of both are well worth reading.[273,274] Perusal of the then customarily anonymous contemporary background Editorial in the *Lancet*[275] suggests that it was probably written by someone in the know, possibly an Association Officer. It indicates that the two investigations were undertaken at a time when it was considered that anaesthesia was a shortage specialty which was not recruiting well and that there was a disturbingly high rate of attrition from the junior grades; however, these are points which the authors of the reports of the two studies do not overemphasise.

The first study was initiated by the Fatigue Working Party.[271,272] Lisl Klein, a social scientist of the Tavistock Institute of Human Relations, London, made an exploratory case study by interview and observation of a limited population of 6 Consultants, one Senior Registrar and 7 junior anaesthetists, two Consultant Surgeons and a Senior Nursing Officer in a District General

Hospital of 850 beds in London.[273] The quoted opinions of the subjects are interesting. They are perhaps a little outdated but compatible with the rather critical but submissive attitudes of some anaesthetists of that period. Lisl Klein's comments are perceptive for an outsider, but the degree with which they could or should be applied generally is speculative, especially as the small sample includes a high proportion of junior trainees. Klein, in fact, does not claim that her conclusions should be so applied.

The other study by Peter Reeve of the Department of Applied Psychology of the University of Wales endeavoured to arrive at a conclusion about the typical personality of anaesthetists by psychometric testing by means of a personality questionnaire (Cattells 16PF Form C).[274] Reeve's sampling was carried out in the Department of Anaesthetics in the University of Wales, and more extensively at the November 1978 Annual Scientific Meeting of the Association in London[276] and at the Junior Anaesthetists' Group Meeting at Oxford in March 1979.[94] The sample to whom the questionnaire was administered consisted of 171 male and 60 female anaesthetists (about 6.6% of anaesthetists in the United Kingdom at that time). This group consisted predominantly of established anaesthetists (Consultants and Senior Registrars) in contrast to Lisl Klein's Group. The picture that emerged was that, as a whole, anaesthetists were "more reserved, intelligent, assertive, serious, conscientious, self sufficient and tense and less socially bold and self assured" than the general population.[274] Reeve's findings were subsequently used as part of the procedure for selecting 62 Senior House Officers and Registrars out of 140 short-listed candidates for the Department of Anaesthetics of the University of Wales between 1980 and 1987, and the careers of successful applicants were monitored over the following three to eight years.[277] The results of the study "demonstrated validity of this personality questionnaire in identifying those doctors who have a high probability of being successful and satisfied in the specialty of anaesthesia as well as those who will not". Ten (16%) of the successful 62 appointed candidates left anaesthesia during the follow up; the "wastage" in the three years prior to the study in Cardiff and London teaching hospitals was estimated to 35% to 40%.[277]

Both the Klein and Reeve studies provided interesting information. There was, however, a contrast between the philosophical approach of sociology and the quantitative gathering of data by the experimental psychologist. This resulted in a brisk exchange of view between investigators in the pages of the journal *Anaesthesia*![278,279]

The Lewin Report and the Operating Department Assistants

The long awaited report on "The Organisation and Staffing of Operating Departments" by a joint Subcommittee of the Standing Medical Advisory Committee and the Standing Nursing Advisory Committee of the Department of Health, was published in 1970.[280,281] The Committee was chaired by the eminent neurosurgeon and medical politician Walpole S Lewin, of Addenbrookes Hospital, Cambridge (later Vice-President of the Royal College of Surgeons of England, Chairman of the BMA Council and a BMA Gold Medallist).[282] The Association of Anaesthetists gave evidence to the Lewin Subcommittee but was not directly represented; however, Geoffrey Spencer (Consultant Anaesthetist and Consultant-in-Charge of Intensive Care at St. Thomas' Hospital, London) was a member of the Subcommittee.

Anaesthetists and the Council of the Association of Anaesthetists hoped that the Lewin Report would at last provide a means of recognition for their loyal and valued assistants (the operating theatre technicians), with a progressive career-long ladder and an appropriate and adequate incremental salary scale. It was also recognised that once those of suitable standard were assimilated into the new career structure, proper training courses with a recognised examination or assessment before qualification would be required for new entrants.

The deliberations of the Lewin Subcommittee were not solely or primarily concerned with improving the conditions of service and pay for those who assisted anaesthetists however. Its main objective was "to consider the organisation of work in the operating theatres and the patterns of staffing required" as a totality. The proposals which emerged were revolutionary and complex and, though the recommendations of the report were accepted in principle by the Department of Health, they were never fully implemented, and resulted in only minor improvements in the lot of Operating Theatre Technicians, now to be called Operating Department Assistants (ODAs).[283-286]

It should be remembered that the Lewin Report was produced at a time (1967-1970) when there was both a shortage of rank and file nurses in general, and recruits for operating theatre nursing in particular. The senior nursing hierarchy were also determined to create an administratively structured profession in the wake of the Salmon Report, and there was a great deal of argument at the time concerning what was, and what was not, "nursing work". The nurses' leaders considered that, as they saw the situation, the passing of instruments to surgeons to enable them to perform operations on unconscious patients was not nursing work, however much skill was involved, and however much it contributed to the success of the operation. A qualified nurse could be an operating theatre supervisor but should not be employed as a scrub nurse.

Lewin had had a distinguished career as a surgeon in the Second World War and was the Commanding Officer of a Territorial Army Reserve Field Surgical Team (FST) thereafter. He seems to have had a vision of operating theatre organisation based on the wartime military model, with perhaps a commissioned female theatre sister in overall charge, but male technical assistants for the surgeon, and to a lesser extent for the anaesthetist. The Lewin Subcommittee proposed the creation of a new class of staff in the NHS, to be known as Operating Department Assistants (ODA), to both carry out the duties of the operating theatre technicians (including assisting the anaesthetist) and also trained to scrub up and assist the surgeon.[280,281,283,284] The implication was that, once the new ODA grade was established, it would have an interchange with some of the nurses' duties, and consequently an appropriately enhanced salary scale. That was all very well, but the DH, as it has done so often in the history of the NHS, having issued a decree that the Lewin report should be implemented by the peripheral Regional and District Health Authorities, sat back, ignored the problems created, and did not provide funds for training and other necessary administrative processes.[283,284]

The Council of the Association of Anaesthetists initially generally welcomed the Lewin Report (Annual Report 1971). Many anaesthetists believed that at last it would "provide a marked improvement in the terms and conditions of service of theatre attendants (technicians)". The process of assimilating experienced operating theatre technicians already in post into the new grade of ODA was achieved unevenly but relatively successfully, though the methods of assessment by which this was accomplished varied enormously. The requirement for the ODA to be able to scrub up to assist the surgeon was fortunately often ignored, as were other aspects of the strict criteria for assimilation laid down by the Lewin Report.[287] Less experienced operating theatre assistants were graded as Operating Department Orderlies (ODOs), especially in the minority of Health Authorities where the Lewin criteria for assimilation were strictly applied. Some Health Authorities opted to employ only ODOs who required only in-house training. The higher grading of Senior Operating Department Assistant (SODA) was often given to senior ODAs in a unit for organising the service of ODAs, rather than for professional prowess; thus, in a given unit, there was only one SODA, and a rank and file ODA could not aspire to the higher grade as he became more senior, unless, of course, the SODA left or retired.

The real trouble began when new Trainee Operating Department Assistants (TODAs) were recruited. Nursing recruitment for theatre work began to improve especially amongst the increasing number of married nurses who appreciated the defined hours. There was therefore less need for ODAs to be trained directly to assist the surgeon and, moreover, this possibility was strongly resented by many nurses in the theatre team and by some surgeons.[283-286] The City and Guilds of London Institute (Syllabus No 752) introduced a national examination for a diploma as the outlet examination for promotion from TODA grade to ODA in 1975, but the provision of courses leading to the diploma for TODAs was by no means universal; only 64 (51.6%) of 124 respondents to a questionnaire issued to Association of Anaesthetists Linkmen in 1982 intimated that their TODAs had access to City and Guilds courses and scrubbing up (though theoretically essential for promotion to ODA) occupied less than 5% of Trainees time overall; in other words many TODAs were often trapped in that grade.

There was little improvement in the financial position of ODAs and SODAs. There was in fact too small a difference between ODA and SODA pay scales to recognise the difference in responsibility adequately. Despite the many representations by the Association of Anaesthetists and others they remained included in the remit of the Whitley Ancillary Staff Council, the negotiating body for the lowest paid workers of the NHS. Attempts were made to recommend transferring them to the Council in 1974, and to the Professional and Technical B Council in 1981, but to no avail (Annual Report 1981).[234,286]

It is a sad reflection on the attitudes within the Department of Health that, despite all the investigations, reports, and the representations of the Association[283,284,286] (Annual reports 1975, and 1981)[234] the lot of the ODA was only marginally improved between 1970 and 1982. An Editorial in *Anaesthesia* in 1970 stated, "It is now 25 years since the Institute of Operating Theatre Technicians came into being and it is sad that they have passed their majority without achieving a reasonable salary scale and without even the most primitive element of a career structure",[285] and in 1982 an Association working party reported "Anaesthetists feel strongly that ODAs have not received the recognition they should".[286] The confused and unsatisfactory position was summarised in an excellent Editorial in *Anaesthesia* by Professor Andrew Hunter of Manchester in 1978.[287]

Assistance for the Anaesthetist

The concern with the terms and conditions of service of ODAs on the part of anaesthetists and the Association of Anaesthetists was primarily the result of a desire to see that the lot of this loyal group of colleagues were fairly remunerated and given the recognition they deserved.[280-287] There was a deeper issue however. That was the problem of providing adequate assistance for anaesthetists at all times and in all locations where anaesthesia was administered.[285,288]

The Lewin Report (1970)[280] stated:-

"In our view, ... except for very minor procedures, the minimum non-medical membership of a basic team within the operating theatre should be three people; one should be a scrubbed assistant in charge of the instrument table; the second a qualified operating department assistant who would be primarily assisting the anaesthetist and attending to the necessary equipment; and the third a circulating assistant."[280]

An investigation by the 1974 Association Working Party on the implementation of the Lewin Report based on 179 replies (a 95% response) by Association Linkmen concluded:-

"ODAs might provide night and weekend cover in four [NHS hospital] groups for every one in which they did not. Unless nurses

are trained when most emergency surgery is done an anaesthetist will have to take on this work under conditions which do not comply with the recommendations of Lewin. .... It seems doubtful from the information supplied by Linkmen if any hospital is able to supply such cover [Lewin's minimum three non-medical members of the basic operating theatre team] round the clock for emergency operating."[283]

The Department of Health (DH) accepted the Lewin Report and directed that action should be taken by the Regional Boards and in the hospitals to implement it but, despite this, the official attitude of the DH in 1975 to providing assistance for the anaesthetist was:-

"there are likely to be occasions, particularly outside working hours, where it will not be possible to achieve.......[constant assistance for the anaesthetist]......The role of the ODA is developing and it is hoped that doctors can continue to provide a good service to their patients with the facilities now available and that they will not find that the patient's safety is endangered."[283]

The report of the 1975 Working Party of the Association of Anaesthetists reacted to this statement:-

"Council can only deplore this attitude. ......Anaesthetists may well find themselves under pressure to forego their assistance and their attitude to this should be considered now. This is a matter on which the anaesthetist's need and the patient's welfare go hand in hand."[284]

It was extraordinary that the DH and local administrators continued to deny anaesthetists assistance at the most vulnerable times - emergencies out of hours and, in particular, in obstetric units, and, most unfortunately, during the conduct of anaesthesia for Caesarean section. It is not surprising, however, because of the pittance that was payable for standby duty, that, when there was a deficiency in ODA staffing levels, the first element of their services to be discontinued or not implemented was the out of hours commitment.

The Joint Board of Clinical Nursing Studies (JBCNS) at last acknowledged that some nurses found satisfaction assisting anaesthetists and instituted the

JBCNS Course ENB182 in 1982 to provide formal training for State Registered Nurses (SRN). The 1982 Working Party of the Association of Anaesthetists identified only four JBCNS courses and only 28 nurses so trained in post in the whole of the United Kingdom. Some local courses for SRNs or the more practical State Enrolled Nurse grade were also identified.[286] Those hospitals which adopted properly organised nurse assistants found them very satisfactory especially as they were totally dedicated to assisting anaesthetists and had no other duties in the operating theatre. The JBCNS Course ENB182 anaesthetic nurses were also trained to institute intravenous infusions and prepare the patient for surgery in other ways.[286]

The 1982 Association Working Party on Assistance for Anaesthetists[286] summarised the situation as follows:-

"....in most areas anaesthetists were happy with the standards of such helpers that they had, but many were very unhappy with the number of assistants available to them. Deficiencies undoubtedly occurred, even in routine lists, but these deficiencies were accelerated with emergency situations, and glaring shortages were identified in maternity units, being particularly poor in labour wards. Other areas of specific weakness identified were X-ray Departments, Accident and Emergency Departments, Cardiology Departments, small hospitals and out of hours emergency situations."[286]

The 1982 Working Party Recommendations emphasised that "The anaesthetist requires the help of a trained assistant wherever anaesthesia is administered" and that "the level of cover must be adjusted so as to ensure the presence of adequate assistance throughout the 24 hours."[286]

The 1982 report of the inquiry into mortality associated with anaesthesia also pointed out the need for trained assistance for anaesthetists at all times.[180]

The Board of Faculty of Anaesthetists insisted from the early eighties onwards that to be recognised for the training of anaesthetists "It is expected that all locations where anaesthetics are administered will be properly equipped and staffed at all times."[289]

Many hospitals achieved a satisfactory service by the mid eighties but it often needed dogged and obstinate persistence with local administrators. The writer had the duty of writing a number of strong letters in support of colleagues who were insisting that their Health Authorities should provide adequate assistance for anaesthetists when he was Chairman of the Faculty's Hospital Recognition Committee from 1982-1984 (confidential correspondence). It was unfortunate that some anaesthetists were prepared to accept second best for the sake of local peace and quiet. It was also a source of regret that many of their senior surgical colleagues were not forthcoming in giving their support. The writer himself recalls, with some embarrassment, that, at one of his hospitals, the very lengthy argument with the authorities, including the Medical Advisory Committee, was finally settled, not by the insistence of the Consultant Anaesthetists, but by the Senior Nursing Officer in charge of the operating theatres putting her foot down by making and enforcing a rule which decreed that no procedure would start in the operating theatre unless the full Lewin operating team, including an assistant for the anaesthetist, was present. This was an interesting reflection on the shifting balance of power within the hospitals of the National Health Service!

The campaign for universal provision of assistance for the anaesthetists at all times, and in particular in obstetric units had to be maintained throughout the eighties however. An investigation conducted by the Obstetric Anaesthetists Association in 1992 reported that of "around 200 obstetric units many did not have anaesthetic nurses to assist the anaesthetist."[290] This does not mean to say, of course, that anaesthetists were not assisted by midwives or other nurses with varying degrees of expertise during the induction of anaesthesia, but personal experience suggests that conditions under such circumstances are rarely entirely satisfactory! Problems relating to the recruitment status, remuneration and training of ODAs persisted through the eighties and into the nineties. These difficulties are given further consideration in Chapter 9.

The Consultant Workload and the Consultant Contract

The Memorandum on the Workload of Anaesthetists published in January 1976 (Annual report 1976) was one of the earliest, and has subsequently proved to be one of the most important, guideline documents issued by the

Association of Anaesthetists. It, and its successive revisions, in 1983, 1984, 1990, 1991 and 1997, have had an important impact in ensuring that successive NHS contracts for consultant anaesthetists have been reasonably phrased and interpreted by the employer. The 1990, 1991 and 1997 Working Parties have been Joint Working Parties with the Royal College of Anaesthetists.[291]

The original Working Party was set up in 1974 under the Chairmanship of Stanley Mason with the title "Working Party on present terms and conditions of service and the way in which they might be varied" (Annual Report 1974). This was at a time of unrest when "working to contract" was proposed. It was therefore clearly necessary to define more closely what the then existing contract really involved for anaesthetists, bearing in mind the professional commitment of the Consultant grade to continuing care of patients.

The document as it emerged in 1976 after the danger of further industrial action had abated to some extent, owed much to work (including careful analysis of Ministerial utterances concerning the interpretation of the NHS Terms and Conditions of Service) by Brian Lewis, Michael Coplans and John Zorab; in the words of the 1976 Annual Report:-

> *"The document draws the crucial distinction between a notional half day ($3\frac{1}{2}$ hours) and a theatre session (which might last for many hours longer) in contractual terms and presents several sample work programmes which appear to be within the terms of the contract. ..... The principle use of the document lies in the hands of divisions [of anaesthesia] in preparing job descriptions for new appointments and adjusting the workload of Consultants where it considerably exceeds reasonable bounds."*

The specimen programmes in the document included provision for ward work, emergencies and administration; in general it was proposed that wholetime anaesthetists should not undertake more than seven of their eleven sessions in the operating theatre. The document and its revisions, brought to the attention of Health Authorities by Divisions of Anaesthesia, and later by the Regional Education Advisors of the Faculty and Royal College of Anaesthetists, has done much to demonstrate to the employers that anaesthetists have duties outside the operating theatre, such as preoperative visiting, and has generally been accepted by them. Previously it was not unknown for a new consultant to be presented with a contract involving nine or ten operating theatre sessions (some of them lasting far longer than the "notional $3^{1}/_{2}$ hours"), as well as an emergency commitment.

The Association of Anaesthetists document was "enthusiastically received by the CCHMS Committee of the BMA when presented to it by the Anaesthetists' Subcommittee, and other specialty groups were requested to produce similar documents" (Annual Report 1976).

Distinction awards

The relatively small number of anaesthetists receiving distinction awards continued to cause concern in the seventies as it had in the sixties. The primary bed-owning specialties which had been in existence when the scheme was set up at the inception of the NHS in 1948, had received the lion's share of the awards and this was perpetuated. There were also difficulties at a local hospital level in getting anaesthetists nominated for "C" awards due to the variations in the way in which District representatives on the "C" award Committee (of whatever specialty) consulted their colleagues![292,293] Most members of "A" and "B" Higher Award Committees must have had the frustrating experience of not being able to recommend an outstanding individual for a "B" award because he did not have a "C". The composition of Regional Distinction Award Committees gave rise to some anxiety; although many anaesthetists sat on these committees, it was, in fact, not until 1982 that Sir Stanley Clayton (then Chairman of the Central Advisory Committee on Distinction Awards) ruled that anaesthesia should be one of the specialties that were always represented (Council Minutes 21.5.1982).[97]

The Association of Anaesthetists made a big effort to overcome some of the secrecy surrounding the awards, and to improve both the quantity and quality of advice presented to the Regional and Central Advisory Committees. Machinery was set up by the Association which was unique amongst the specialties. A senior award holder in each NHS Region (hopefully an "A" award holder, and ideally one who sat on the Regional Higher Awards Committee) was invited by the President of the Association (P J Helliwell)[3] to convene an *ad hoc* Committee of award holders. They were asked to convey the views of the award holding anaesthetists of each Region to the Regional

Committees and to the Committee of the Faculty of Anaesthetists, as well as to Cyril Scurr who had a seat on the Central Awards Committee (Annual report 1975). The names of the members of all members of the Regional "C" Awards and Higher Awards Committees were also published in *Anaesthesia*.[294,295]

These measures did much to make certain that the speciality spoke with a single voice, and generally ensured that anaesthetists who were regarded by their peers as meritorious, received awards. They have probably been less successful in promoting an increase in the percentage of anaesthetists holding awards. The percentage of anaesthetists with Distinction Awards in England and Wales rose from 25.9% in 1976 to 29.2% in 1988, but fell again to 28.7% by the end of 1992 which is the latest figure available. The percentage for all consultants in the NHS is 34.3%, with, for example, accident and emergency consultants 20.7%, general surgeons 44.7%, general physicians 49.3%, and neurosurgeons 53.1% (31 December 1992 figures).[296,297]

Another change in the nineteen seventies after the 1975 reorganisation of the NHS was the amalgamation of the former Regional and Teaching Hospital "C" Award Committees.[293] The advantages or disadvantages of this change depend on the point of view of the individual consultant and to which side of the fence he or she was appointed!

Private (Independent) Practice

The first Linkman Conference on 17 November 1976 requested Council to press for the linkage between anaesthetists' and surgeons' fees as paid by the Provident Societies (the "global" system) to be broken, to prepare a guide of fees set out in relative but not monetary terms, and to prepare a booklet which explained to the patient the basis of the fees.[157] Council responded by appointing a Committee (Council Minutes 7.1.1977).[81]

Leon Kaufman (University College Hospital, London) presented a report on the work of the Committee to the Second Linkman Conference in 1977 (3.11.1977).[298] Discussions had taken place with the Provident Societies who had agreed that anaesthetists were underpaid. The global system of the combined allocation for the fees of surgeons and anaesthetists caused problems. The Provident Societies paid out the full amount asked for by whoever presented his bill first, and the remainder of the global sum to the second applicant whatever amount was billed; the second applicant was then left to apply to the patient for any deficiency. There had been occasions when surgeons had claimed the whole fee from the global sum! Kaufman advised anaesthetists to submit their bills promptly! The Provident Societies disclaimed responsibility because the contract was legally between the patient and the practitioners.[298]

Another difference of opinion had also arisen. The Provident Societies claimed that they only allowed their patients to be treated by specialists, but disagreed between themselves on the definition of specialist. The Private Patients Plan (PPP) would only accept a Consultant in the NHS, whereas the British United Provident Association (BUPA) were equivocal about the term "specialist", especially where anaesthetists were concerned, and would in practise remunerate any practitioner who the surgeon chose, who might be unqualified and/or untrained as an anaesthetist. It is sad, that when asked in 1979, the Royal College of Surgeons of England and their Faculty of Anaesthetists declined to comment on this issue which so obviously affected the standard of anaesthetic service.[299,300]

The Association also produced a document entitled "Your Anaesthetic" which described the anaesthetic procedures, the responsibilities of the anaesthetist and the basis upon which fees were calculated, for the patients and the public at large to peruse. A unitary scheme of "relative values" for assessing fees was also described in another pamphlet (so much for pre-operative assessment - graded according to physical condition and length of operation - so much for monitoring, so much for administering drugs, etc).[300] Some linkmen in 1978 thought this system too complicated and proposed that operations and anaesthetics should be grouped and graded into three or four categories. Two intrepid linkmen were moved to quote their own fee scales - for minor procedures (£20: 1996: £60), for intermediate (£30-£40: 1996: £90-£120), and for major (£50-£60: 1996: £150-£180); neither of these two anaesthetists took account of any special medical difficulties as they accepted the "swings and roundabouts" principle.[299]

Discussions continued with the Provident Societies. Those positive advances which resulted in this period owe much to the tenacity of Peter

Baskett and Maurice Burrows; by 1979 the term "independent practice" was being commonly used and the Provident Societies had conceded in principle that only anaesthetists of NHS Consultant rank, or those accredited by the Faculty of Anaesthetists, would be recognised, but "without detriment to existing practitioners" who were not specialists but who were engaged in independent practice;[232] however, the Association of Anaesthetists found it necessary to refer to this matter again in 1990. Negotiations with the Provident Societies continued. The Association suggested in 1979 that the sum to be paid to the anaesthetist should be one third of the global sum allocated for the particular operation. This was on the basis that the anaesthetist spent about half the time overall with the patient as did the surgeon. The "swings and roundabout" concept was to be adhered to with regard to special difficulties except in the most extreme cases.[232] Initial reaction to this proposal was described as "not unreasonable",[232] nevertheless BUPA in 1980 responded by proposing that anaesthetists should limit their fees to a five point scale in return for direct payment.[233] Protracted discussions followed in which it transpired that the Provident Societies led by BUPA wished to fix the Anaesthetists share of the global sum to 20%. This was unacceptable to Council of the Association of Anaesthetists, which then drew up its own recommended fees for operations grouped in bands ("minor", "intermediate", "major", "major plus" and "complex major") with a figure for each.[234,235,301,302] These guidelines were updated according to nationally agreed principles every two years and, it must be said, during the next decade the Provident Societies paid out benefits in accordance with them in the majority of cases, until the investigations of the Monopolies and Mergers Commission which were started in 1992 (Chapter 9).

Fees for family planning

The institution of a free family planning service in the NHS is often associated with the incoming Labour administration after the General Election in February 1974 and the appointment of (Baroness) Barbara Castle and (Lord) David Owen to the Department of Health and Social Security. This is not the case; the concept was part of the 1974 reorganisation which the outgoing Conservative Government had already set in motion. A contract for additional fees for various family planning procedures in general practice had already been negotiated before the General Election and sent to the Review Body for pricing. Female sterilisation for medical indications had always been undertaken in the hospital service on ordinary routine operating lists, but now it was envisaged that a very large additional element of elective female sterilisations should be added to gynaecological surgeons' work load and routine vasectomies to that of the general surgeon;[303] it should also be remembered that this was at a time when the movement for day surgery was in its infancy.

The best solution, especially as ethical and religious attitudes were involved, would have been to institute extra separately funded sessions outside the normal consultant contract, in which surgeons, anaesthetists, and other staff could take part, if they so desired, for additional remuneration. This would also have been the better solution when the Abortion Act of 1967 came in to force, but the Department of Health, under pressure, took the anomalous decision to pay surgeons and anaesthetists fees to operate on family planning cases (whether for medical or social reasons) during routine operating lists,[304,305] as indeed was already the case with private NHS patients. This seems to have been a rather extraordinary decision from a government dedicated to the abolition of private practice within NHS hospitals. It was, however, stipulated rather nebulously, that the fee was to be for the operation only, consultation being part of the surgeon's NHS contractual duty, the usual amount of NHS work "should not be affected", and that surgeons must come to an arrangement with the Health Authorities with regard to the amount of time and resources which should be devoted to other NHS work.[304]

Various procedures were covered by the scheme including reversal of male and female sterilisation and the insertion of intrauterine contraceptive devices; as examples, the surgeon's fee for a female sterilisation as a separate procedure was £22 (1996: £98), and the anaesthetist's fee £10.75 (1996: £48) Many medical practitioners (including surgeons) were affronted by the ethical and practical implications of these payments. They regarded them as an illogical use of funds to further "one of the Government's pet schemes" in an impoverished health service and wrong in principle.[305,306] The overall cost of the new comprehensive Family Planning Scheme in general and hospital practice was estimated at forty million pounds (1996: £180 million) in a full financial year November 1975.[307]

Many anaesthetists felt that, since the fee was stated to be for the operation only, in this instance the anaesthetist's fee should be equal to the surgeon's.[308] This view was represented strongly to the Department of Health through the Anaesthetists Subcommittee of the (BMA) CCHMS Committee, but without avail (Annual Reports 1975 and 1976). Some Health Authorities even refused to pay anaesthetists at all until the Association of Anaesthetists and the BMA took legal advice and made representations (Annual Report 1979).[232]

Miscellaneous matters 1970-1982

Safety and Standards. The interlinked business of the Council of the Association and its Safety Committee (established 1974) and the British Standards Institution (BSI) and the International Standards Organisation (ISO) continued and increased.[309] The long service O P Dinnick (Middlesex Hospital, London) (Chapter 9) and Peter W Thompson (Cardiff) in representing the Association of Anaesthetists in the exacting work of the BSI and ISO will be particularly remembered.

The Safety Committee itself considered many matters; amongst these were the pollution of operating theatres and scavenging of anaesthetic gases (Chapter 7), the installation and maintenance of medical gas pipe-line systems, oxygen supply pressure failure devices,[310] electrical safety, safety valves in breathing systems, and disconnection and misconnection of anaesthetic equipment. The Safety Committee also discharged a very important duty in advising members on safety questions, and supporting them when necessary when they had problems with their local Health Authorities in obtaining funds for safer equipment (Annual Reports 1970-1982).[232-235]

The Safety Committee influenced two strictly clinical decisions. The members of the Committee were "alarmed" to learn that one Defence Society believed that it would not be possible to defend an anaesthetist if his patient suffered thrombosis after an elective operation if she was receiving the contraceptive pill. The question of the responsibility of the anaesthetist to be aware of such medication arose. The Committee discussed the problem with "two surgical associations" and the Defence Society, and asked the Editor of the *British Medical Journal* (BMJ) to publish an Editorial on the subject (anonymous as was customary in the *BMJ* of the time). This made special reference to the low oestrogen preparations and stated *inter alia* "Withdrawal of oral contraceptives for four to six weeks before surgery is of doubtful

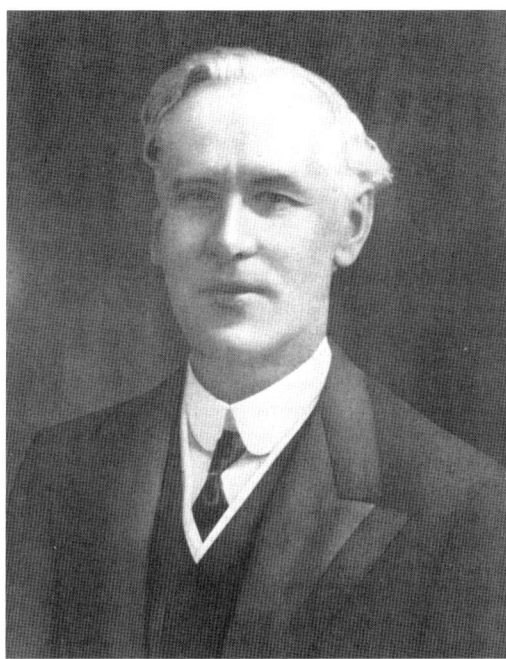

Figure 1

J.Frederick Silk
(1848 - 1943)

The Founder of the first Society of Anaesthetists in 1893 which became the Anaesthetic Section of the Royal Society of Medicine in 1909.

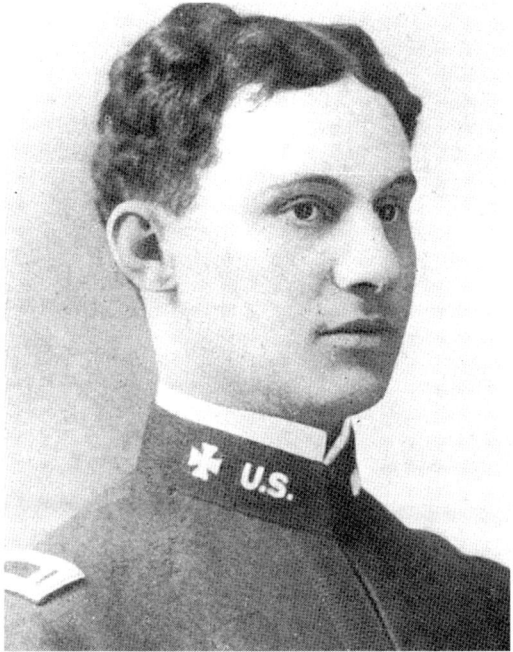

Figure 2

Hyman Morris Cohen
(1875 - 1929)

Founder Editor of the *British Journal of Anaesthesia*. The main mouthpiece of the physician anaesthetists in the United Kingdom and Ireland from 1923 until the foundation of the Association of Anaesthetists in 1932 and thereafter of the Association of Anaesthetists of Great Britain and Ireland until the start of publication of the Association journal *Anaesthesia* in 1946.

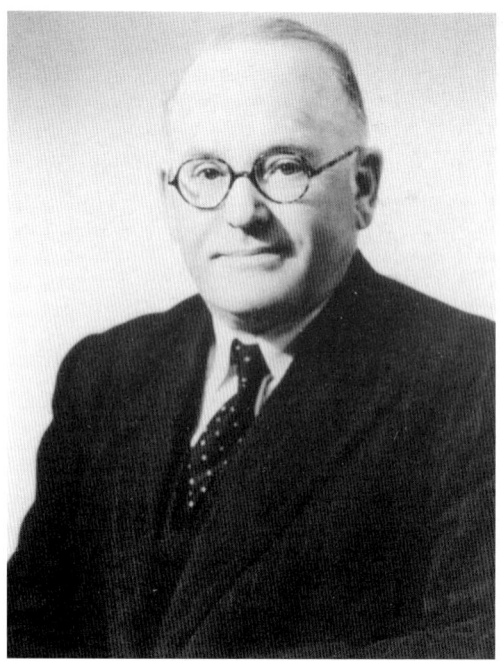

Figure 3

Henry Walter Featherstone, OBE (1894 - 1967)

Founder of the Association of Anaethetists of Great Britain and Ireland in 1932.

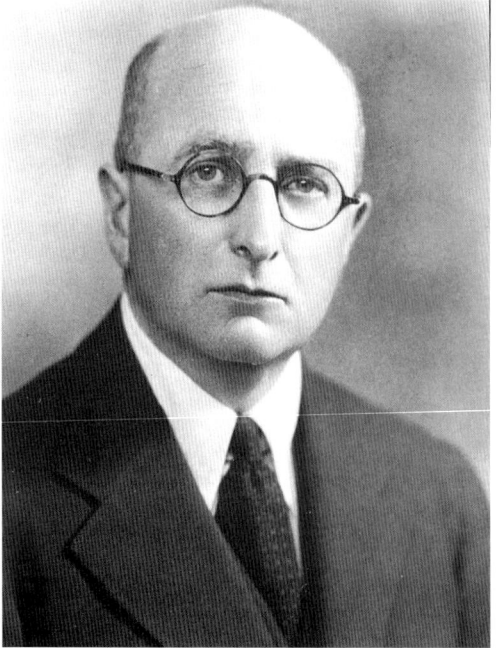

Figure 4

W Howard Jones (1895 - 1935)

The first Honorary Secretary of the Association of Anaesthetists. His untimely death was partly attributed to depression brought on by the poor conditions in which university hospital anaesthetists worked in the nineteen thirties.

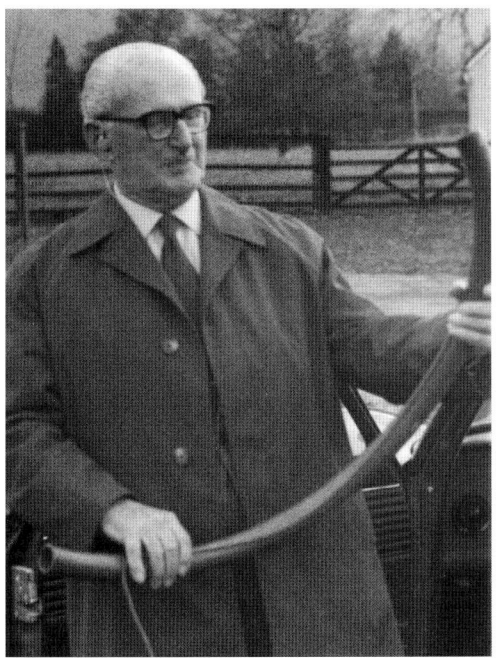

Figure 5

Sir Ivan Whiteside Magill. KCVO
(1888-1986)

Doyen of British physician anaethetists and initiator in 1935 of the Diploma of Anaesthetics (DA) of the Conjoint Board in England of the Royal College of Physicians of London and the Royal College of Surgeons of England. This was the first examination for a diploma in anaesthesia in the world.
Photograph J.S.M. Zorab

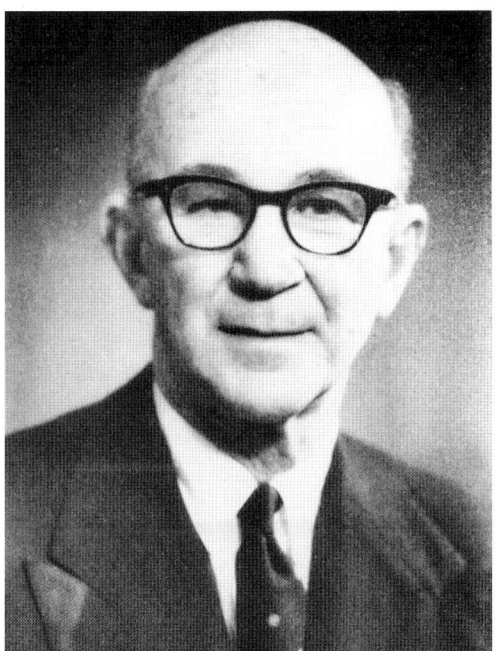

Figure 6

Professor Sir Robert Reynolds Macintosh
(1897-1989)

Nuffield Professor of Anaesthesia at the University of Oxford (1937-1965) and the first anaesthetist to be appointed to an independent university chair in anaesthetics.

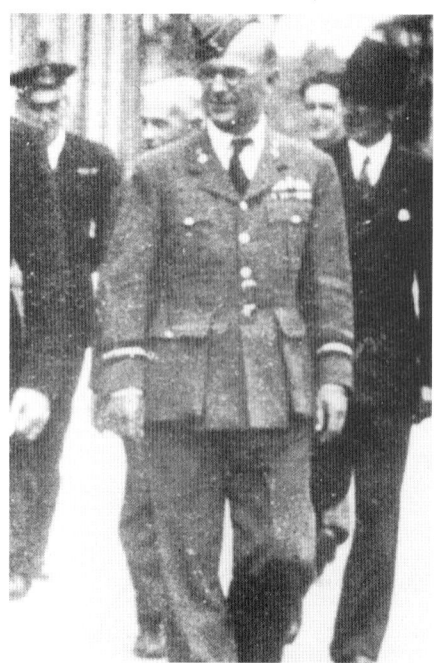

Figure 7

Air Commodore R R Macintosh, RAF (1941-1945)

Professor Robert Macintosh in his Second World War role as Adviser in Anaesthesia to the British Armed Forces.

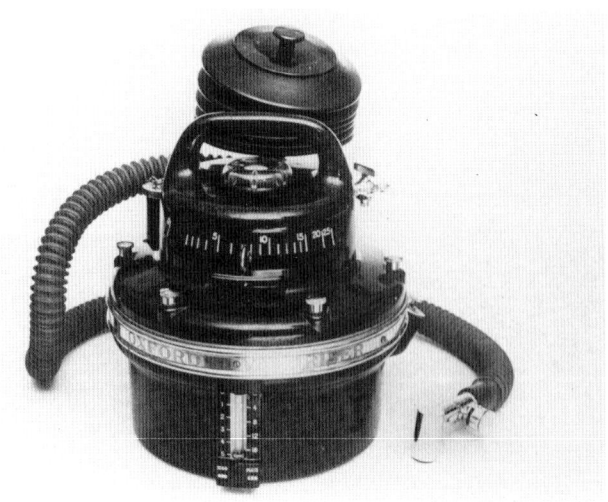

Figure 8

The Oxford Vaporiser (1942) was designed by the Nuffield Department of Anaesthesia at Oxford, headed by Professor Macintosh, for the accurate administration of ether in air by the British Armed Forces; it was manufactured by Lord Nuffield at the Morris Motor Works at Oxford.

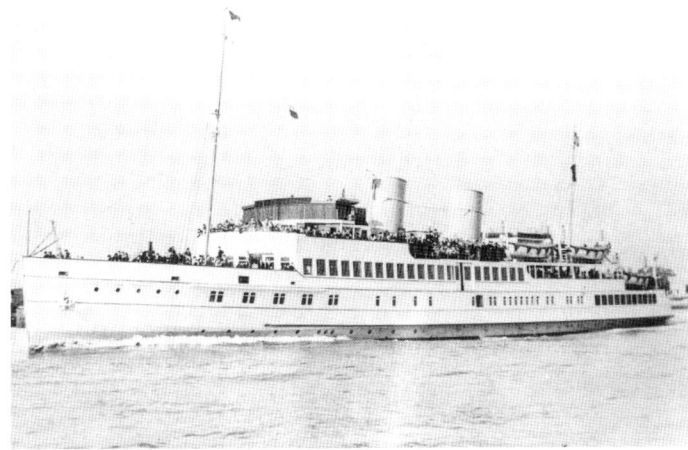

Figure 9

SS Queen of the Channel. The London to Southend Ferry in which Major H W Featherstone, the Founder President of the Association of Anaesthetists, escaped from Boulogne when the British Expeditionary Force was evacuated from France in 1940.
Photograph with the permission of the National Maritime Museum

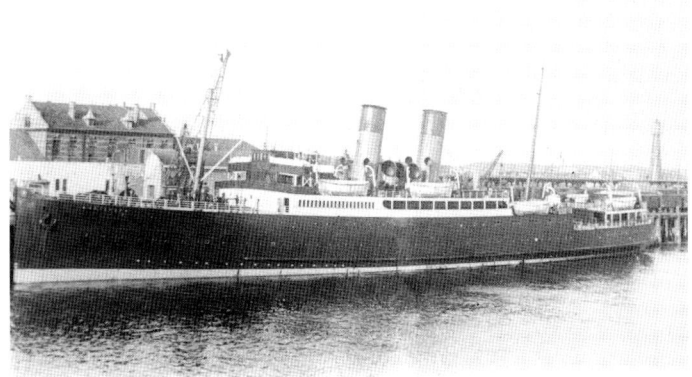

Figure 10

SS Amsterdam (Hospital Carrier 64). Lieutenant Colonel Featherstone was medical officer in charge of Hospital Carrier 64 during the D-Day landings in Normandy in 1944 when she was sunk; as a result of the impeccable training which the unit had received under Featherstone many lives were saved and 200 patients transferred to a naval cruiser. Featherstone was appointed OBE in recognition of this exploit.
Photograph with the permission of the National Maritime Museum

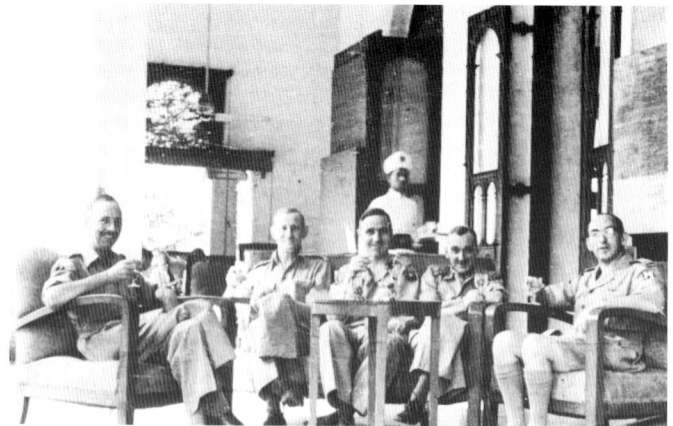

Figure 11

RAMC Regional Advisors in Anaesthesia in India (c. 1943). Left to right: W S McConnell (Guy's Hospital, London), V F Hall (King's College Hospital, London), K Ashworth (of Manchester and later of Charing Cross Hospital, London), T A B Harris (Guy's Hospital, London) and V Goldman (Eastman Dental Clinic, London).

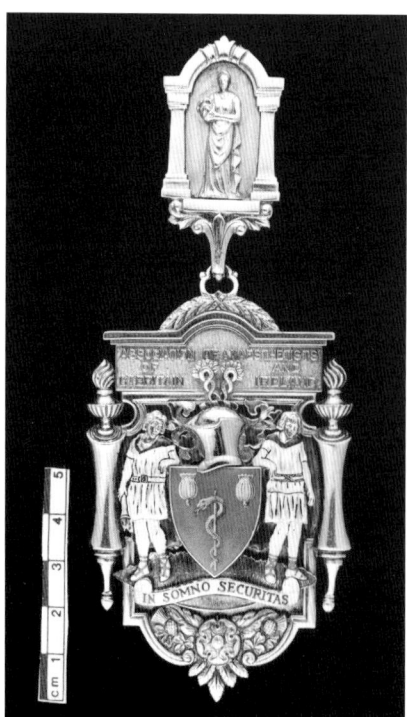

Figure 12:

The badge of the President of the Association of Anaesthetists of Great Britain and Ireland. Presented by the membership 1946.

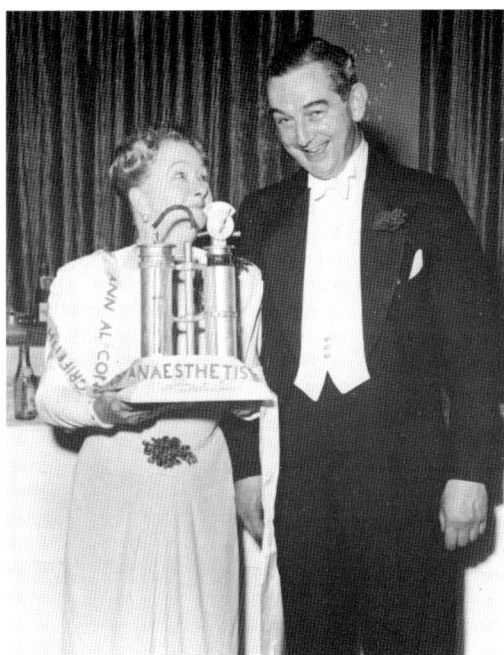

Figure 13

Ronald Jarman. DSC (1898 - 1972).

President of the Association of Anaethetists 1959 - 1963, on the occasion of the 26th Congress of Anaesthetists of the (North American) Anaesthesia Research Society in London in 1951.

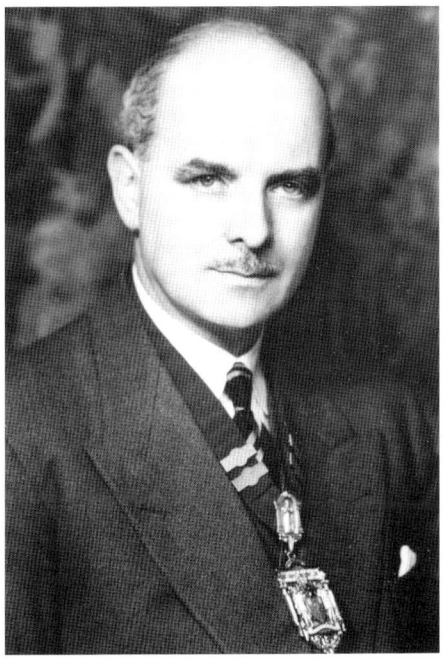

Figure 14

Professor T Cecil Gray. CBE when President of the Association of Anaesthetists (1956 - 1959).

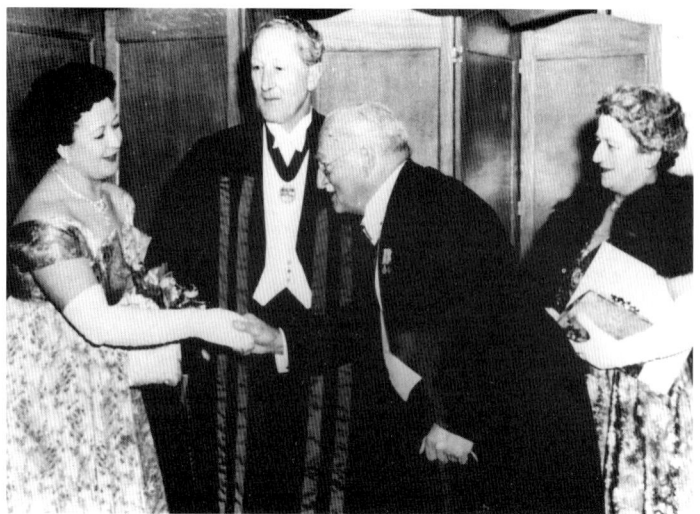

Figure 15

(Sir) Geoffrey and (Lady) Organe welcoming Mr Martin Clover (grandson of the pioneer physician anaesthetist Joseph T Clover. 1825 - 1882) and his daughter during the celebrations of the 10th anniversary of the foundation of the Faculty of Anaesthetists of the Royal College of Surgeons of England in 1958.

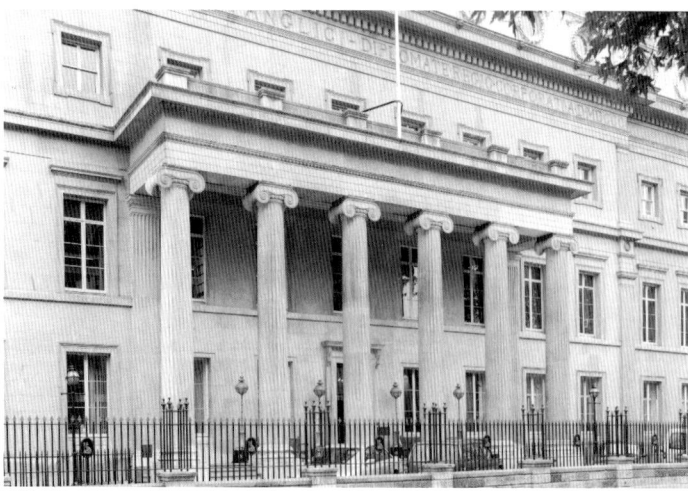

Figure 16

The Royal College of Surgeons of England. Home of the Joint Secretariat. This included that of the Association of Anaesthetists from 1944 to 1971.
Phil McCarthy Photography, London

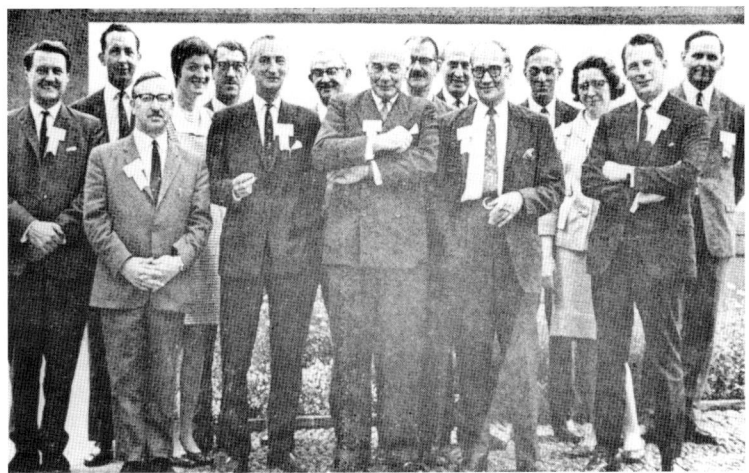

Figure 17

The Organising Committee of the 4th World Congress of Anaesthesiologists, London, 1968. Left to right; front row: D D C Howat, S A Mason, C B Lewis, R P W Shackleton, G H Ellis, I R Verner; back row: C F Scurr, Miss P R Cridland, R B Wright, R Jarman, F G Wood-Smith, O P Dinnick, A J Beard, Mrs O P Dinnick, T B Boulton. *(see also page 264)*

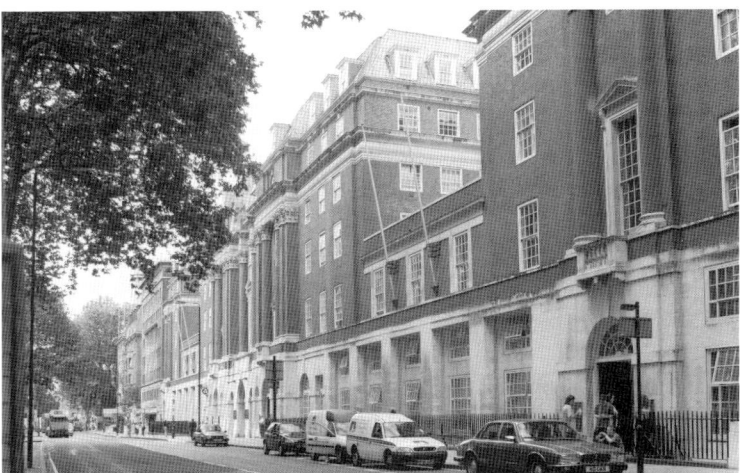

Figure 18

British Medical Association House, Tavistock Square, London, in which the Council of the Association of the Anaesthetists occupied a suite of offices from 1971-1985.

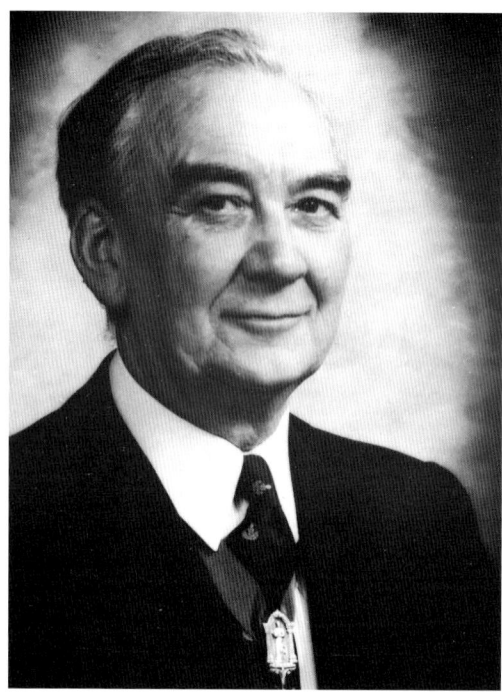

Figure 19
Phillip J Helliwell
(1915 - 1994) when President of the
Association (1973-1976).

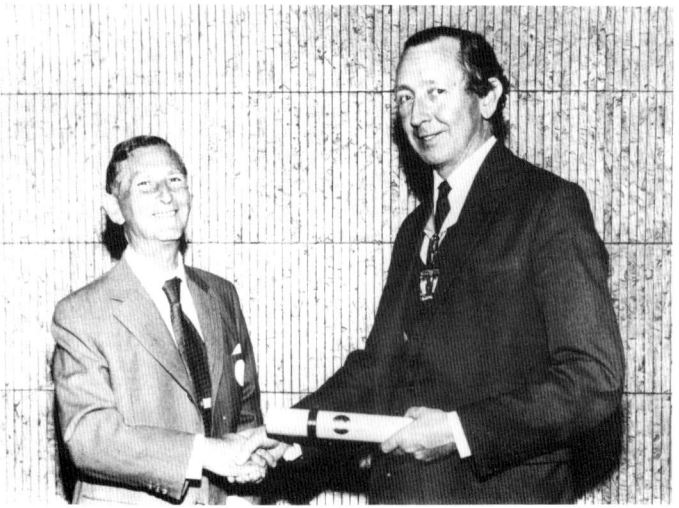

Figure 20
Z Lett (Hong Kong) and C F Scurr, CBE (President) on the occasion of the presentation of a Pask Award of Honour to Z Lett at the Annual Meeting of the Association of Anaethetists in 1978.

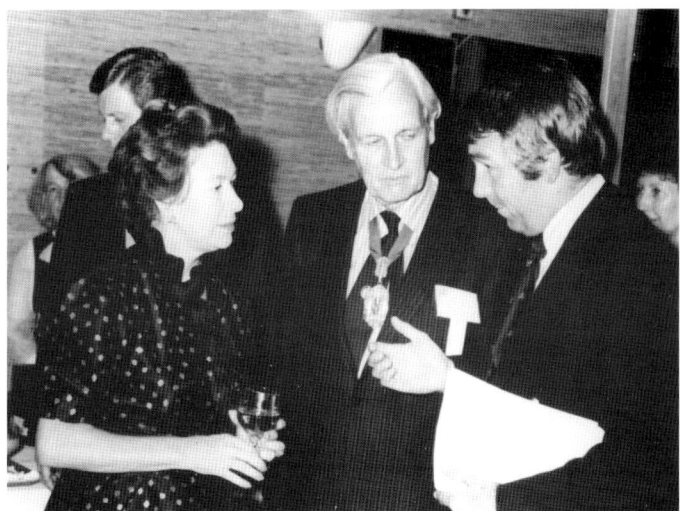

Figure 21

HRH The Princess Margaret, Countess of Snowdon (Patron), W D Wylie (President of the Association of Anaesthetists) and a representative from the extensive Trade Exhibition at the 6th European Congress of Anaesthesiology in London in 1982.

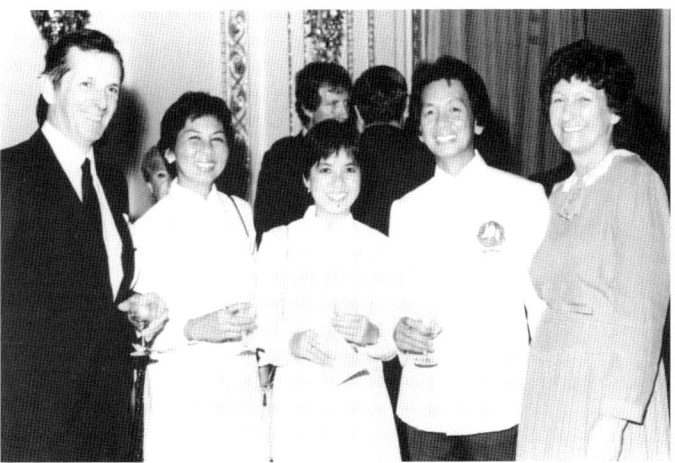

Figure 22

J S M Zorab (Secretary General of the WSFA and of the 6th European Congress of Anaesthesiology) and Mrs Zorab and Filipino delegates during the Congress in London in 1982.

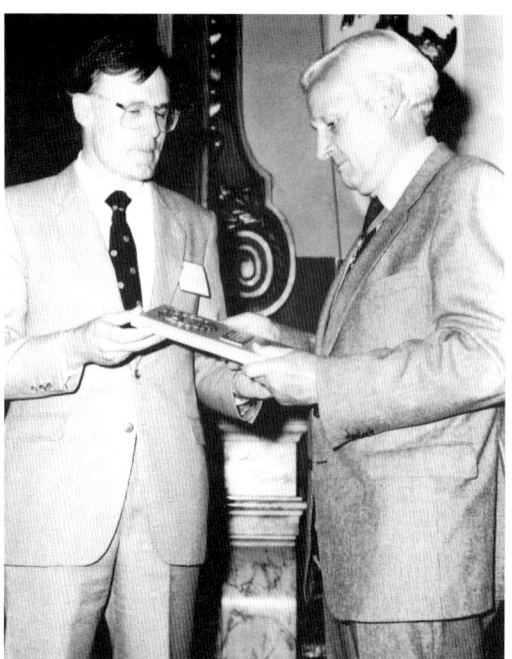

Figure 23

Robert Hare (President of the Australian Society of Anaesthetists and W D Wylie (President of the Association of Anaesthetists of Great Britain and Ireland) on the occasion of the presentation of a plaque from the Australian Society during the Golden Jubliee Celebrations of the Association of Anaethetists in 1982.

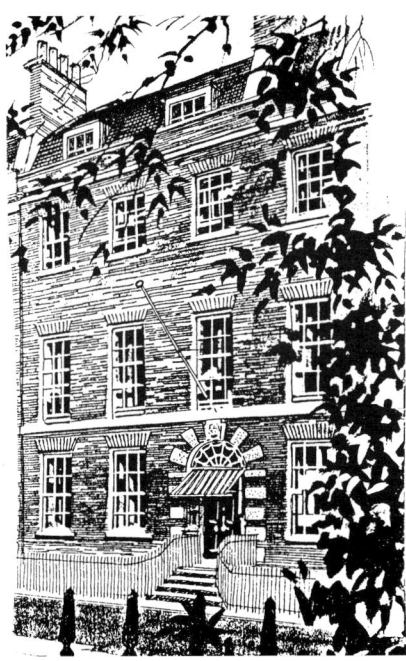

Figure 24
9 Bedford Square, London.

Headquarters of the Association of Anaesthetists of Great Britain and Ireland since 1985.
Drawing reproduced with the permission of Glaxo Wellcome PLC

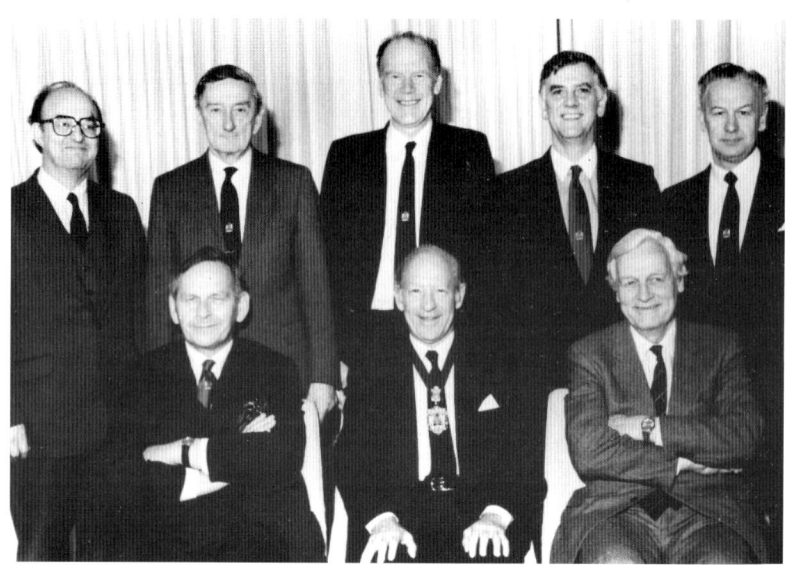

Figure 25

Officers of the Association of Anaesthetists of Great Britain and Ireland at the time of the official opening of 9 Bedford Square in 1987. Left to right; front row: T B Boulton (President 1984-1986), M Rosen (President 1986-1988), W D Wylie (President 1980-1982) and Trustee of the Association); back row: J N Lunn (Editor of Anaesthesia), M M Burrows (Honarary Treasurer and President elect), M J Inman and P Morris (Honarary Secretaries) and W R MacRae (Honorary Treasurer elect).
Phil McCarthy Photography, London

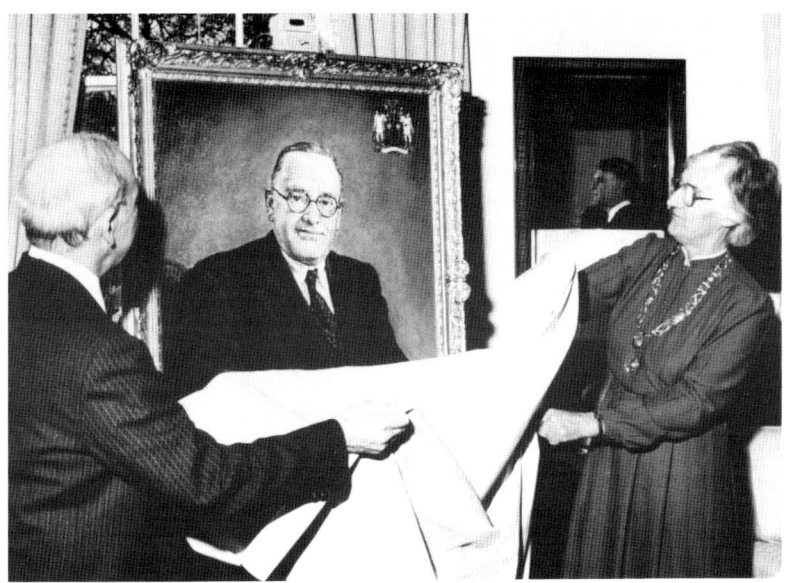

Figure 26

Presentation to the Association of Anaesthetists of the portrait of H W Featherstone (Founder President) by the Dean of the Faculty of Anaesthetists (Aileen K Adams, CBE) in 1988.
Phil McCarthy Photography, London

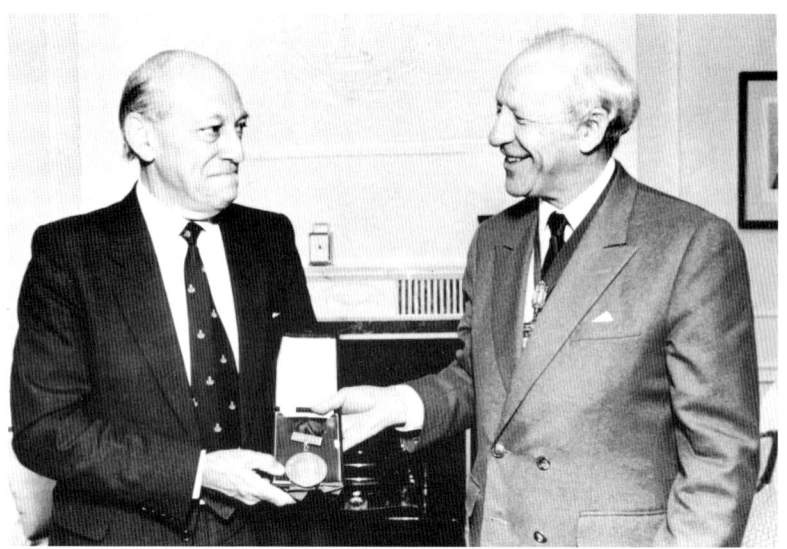

Figure 27
The first and second recipients of the Sir Ivan Magill Gold Medal for Innovation. J F Nunn (1988) and Michael Rosen, CBE (1993).

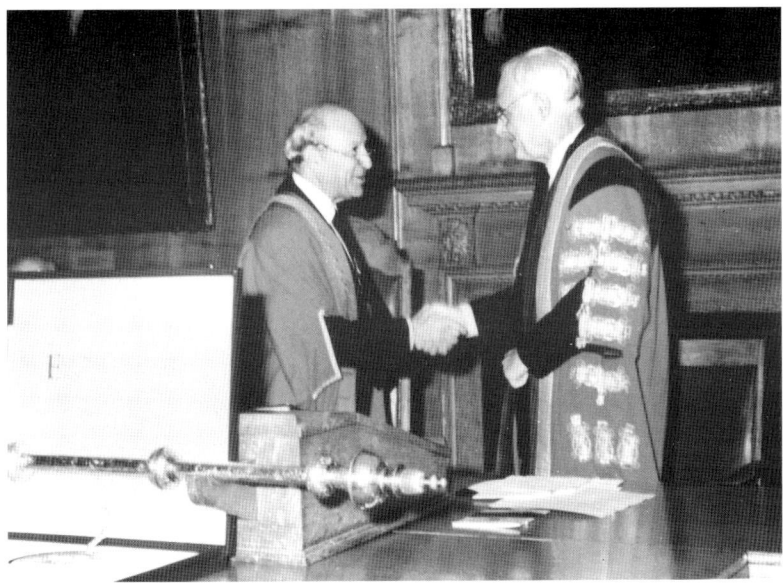

Figure 28
Michael Rosen, CBE (President of the College of Anaesthetists) and Sir Ian Todd, KBE (President of the Royal College of Surgeons of England) at the inauguration of the College of Anaesthetists in 1988.
Jalmar Photographers, London

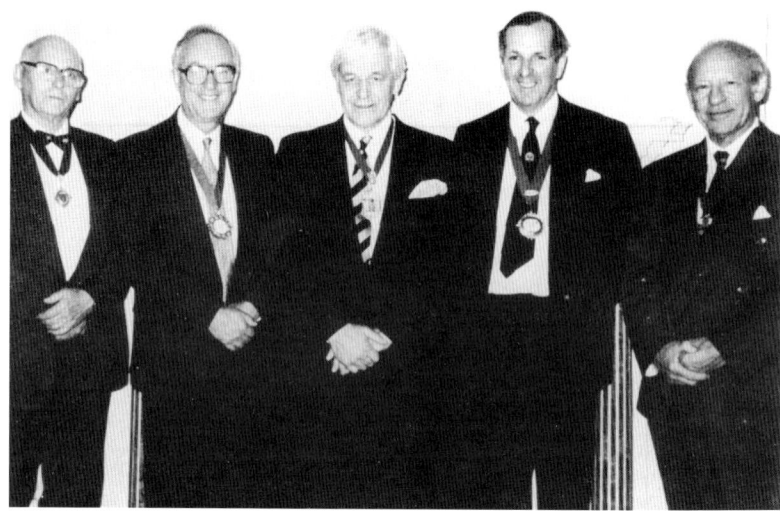

Figure 29

The five members of the Association of Anaesthetists of Great Britain and Ireland who, in 1991, were concurrently Presidents of (left to right) the Anaesthetic Section of the Royal Society of Medicine (P W Thompson), the European Academy (M D A Vickers), the Association of Anaesthetists of Great Britain and Ireland (P J F Baskett), the World Federation of Societies of Anaesthesiologists (J S M Zorab), and the (Royal) College of Anaesthetists (M Rosen).
Phil McCarthy Photography, London

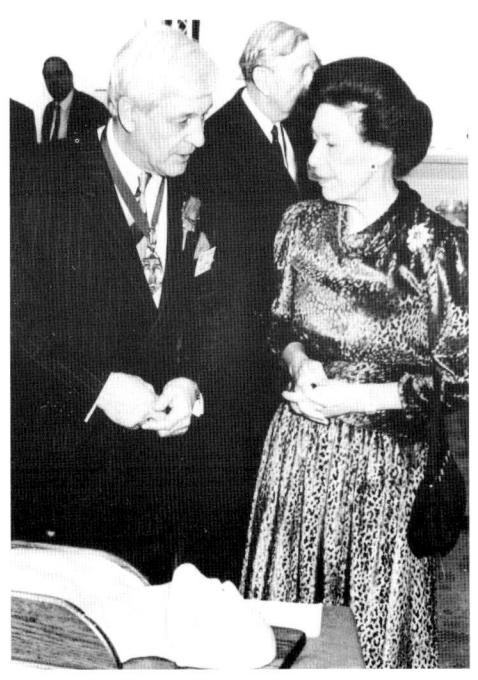

Figure 30

HRH The Princess Margaret, Countess of Snowdon (Patron) and Peter Baskett (President) during the Diamond Jubilee celebrations of the Association of Anaesthetists of Great Britain and Ireland in 1992.
Phil McCarthy Photography, London

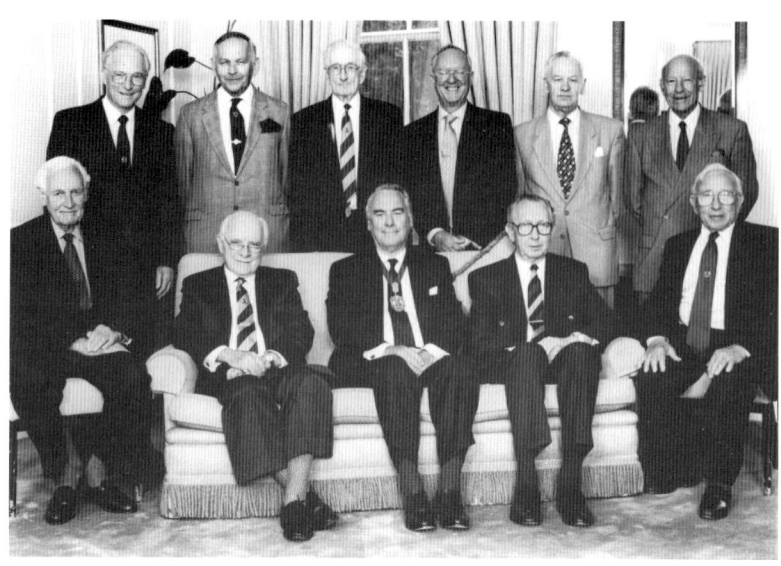

Figure 31

The reigning President with Past Presidents of the Association of Anaesthetists at the Past Presidents' luncheon, 1997. Seated left to right: W D Wylie (1980 -1982), T C Gray (1956-1959), W L Baird (1996-1998), C F Scurr (1976-1978), S.A. Mason (1978-1980), standing (left to right): S M Lyons (1994-1996), T B Boulton (1984-1986), M M Burrows (1988 -1990), M D A Vickers (1982-1984), W R MacRae (1992-1994), M Rosen (1986-1998).

Phil McCarthy Photography, London

rationale".[311] The Committee also succeeded in getting some changes made in the regulations concerning ampoule labelling in 1976; specifically the printing of the "approved name in prominent letters" (Annual Report 1976).

The neurological complications of spinal and epidural anaesthesia. A small *ad hoc* Committee consisting of R Len Hargrove (Westminster Hospital, London), Andrew G Doughty (Kingston-on-Thames) and Richard S Atkinson (Southend-on-Sea) was formed in 1972 to study the complications of spinal and epidural anaesthesia (Council Minutes 4.2.1972: Annual report 1972). An interim report was presented as an Editorial in *Anaesthesia* in 1974,[312] and Len Hargrove presented a further report in 1981 to the Obstetric Anaesthetists Association after "over 120" cases had been collected. Hargrove writes in his abstract, "The majority of complications are both mild and transient but there is a significant incidence of serious complications resulting in permanent disablement or death. In most of the latter it is possible to trace an avoidable factor which has directly contributed to the accident".[313]

The Joint Working Party on consultant posts remaining unfilled after repeated advertisements was a useful example of cooperation between the Association of Anaesthetists and the Faculty of Anaesthetists. The Chairman was Douglas Howat. Representatives of the two bodies visited the hospitals concerned at the invitation of the Consultant Anaesthetists and the Area Medical officer. It was found that "The major factors in failing to fill posts [was] the unattractive reputation or names of some of the areas concerned and the unimaginative advertisements and job descriptions" (Annual Reports 1980-1982).[233-235]

Doctors with Domestic Commitments. Another Joint Working Party with the Faculty considered this problem at length, which of course, mainly concerned married women despite its politically correct title. Considerable advance had been made since the nineteen sixties but much remained to be done. The working party was chaired by the President Stanley Mason and benefited from the expertise of Dr R H McNeilly (Acting Regional Medical Officer of the Oxford Region, where a great deal had been done to accommodate married lady anaesthetists). An important and helpful report was published in *Anaesthesia*.[314]

Trichloroethylene. The Association was successful in persuading the manufacturers (Imperial Chemical Industries Ltd) to continue to produce the volatile agent trichloroethylene, much beloved of British anaesthetists,[315] for a further four years in 1980. ICI stated that its continued manufacture thereafter would depend upon the amount used (Annual Report 1980);[234] alas the whole point about trichloroethylene was that each anaesthetic used so little and that it was so inexpensive! The agent was finally withdrawn in 1984.

Intravenous Regional Analgesia (IVRA). Council became concerned about several deaths which had resulted when IVRA was being used. The Department of Health issued a hazard warning about the technique in 1982. Margaret Heath of Lewisham (Member of Council 1979-1983: Vice President 1992-1993) drew attention to the hazards in an editorial in the *British Medical Journal*[316] and spoke about the technique at the Linkman Conference in October 1982.[317] The initial concern was chiefly about the possibility of leaks beneath the arterial cuff used in the procedure, but it became apparent that there were particularly dangers from the cardiotoxicity of bupivacaine (Annual Report 1983).[257] The Committee on Safety of Medicines were informed and the manufacturers of bupivacaine subsequently modified their data sheet.[318]

Suicide and the anaesthetist. Philip Bickford Smith (Honorary Secretary of the Junior Anaesthetists Group - JAG) at the 1982 Linkman Conference expressed the concern of the Group about four junior anaesthetists who had recently committed suicide, and the possible relationship with the stress of their appointments; all four had recently taken up duty in new posts.[319] A confidential inquiry by the Council of the Association "could not identify any common factors directly related to their work as anaesthetists" (Annual Report 1983).[235]

Scientific, General and Special Meetings 1970-1982

Year	Month	Location	Attendance
1970	November	Royal College of Surgeons of England	350
1971	September	University of Birmingham	360
1972	November	Bloomsbury Conference Centre, London	410

Year	Month	Location	Attendance
1973	September	University of Bristol	425
1974	November	Tara Hotel, London. Joint Meeting with the Danish Society	c.450
1975	September	University of Cardiff	c.450
1976	November	Tara Hotel, London	"a record"
1977	September	Royal College of Surgeons in Ireland, Dublin, Joint Meeting with the French Society	c.600
1978	November	Wembley Conference Centre, London, Joint Meeting with the German Society	801
1979	September	University of Stirling	550
1980	September	Royal Festival Hall, London Anglo-American Meeting	c.800
1981	September	Queens Medical Centre, University of Nottingham	c.500
(1982	September	6th European Congress of Anaesthesiology, Royal Festival Hall, London	c.2000)
1982	October	Royal College of Surgeons of England, London	c.450

1970-1979. The pattern, which had been developed in the nineteen sixties, of holding combined Annual General and Scientific Meetings alternately in London and elsewhere in the United Kingdom continued throughout the seventies, except that the September 1977 Annual Meeting was for the second time held in Dublin, the capital of the Republic of Ireland. The custom was also instituted of holding the Linkman Conference on the day before the main meeting at the same venue from 1976 onwards, after that organisation came into being. The only exception was in 1977 when the Linkman Conference was held at the Royal Society of Medicine in the November following the September Dublin Meeting. University campus complexes for the meetings, and University Halls of Residence for accommodation, catered adequately for the increasing numbers of registrants attending and the enlarging technical exhibitions outside London, but there was beginning to be difficulty in finding suitable conference facilities in London (Council Minutes 5.1.1979).[97] London meetings were usually held in November and provincial meetings in September before the start of University terms.

A new feature in the seventies was the holding of reciprocal meetings with various European societies. The Danish Society (Dansk Anaesthesiologisk Selshab), headed by their President (B Haxholdt), visited London in November for a very successful joint meeting in 1974[320] and returned the compliment in Copenhagen in June 1976.[321] The French Société Francaise d'Anesthésie, d'Analgésie et de Réanimation under their veteran President Jean Lassner invited the Association to a joint meeting in Paris in June 1975, and joined the Association at its Annual Scientific Meeting in Dublin in September 1977; both meetings were memorable occasions (Annual Report 1975).[322-324] The German Society Deutsche Gesellschaft für Anasthesiologie und Intensive Medicin were the guests of the Association at the Wembley Conference Centre in November 1978. This occasion attracted 801 delegates of which some 150 were Germans. The Wembley Centre is not in the most attractive part of London and is somewhat separated from the main hotels, and the lecture theatre had some unusual architectural features, but convivial social events in the City of London, and a well organised coach service, made up for these difficulties.[325] The German Society subsequently hosted a very successful joint meeting with the Association in Bonn in May 1985, including a first class scientific and social programme and a pleasant excursion on the Rhine (Annual report 1985).[326]

The Canadian Society of Anaesthetists issued a special invitation to the Association of Anaesthetists to attend their meeting in Kingston, Ontario in 1975.[327] Special travel arrangements were made, and a very valuable scientific and pleasant social meeting resulted.[328]

1980-1982. The Annual Meeting in 1981 was held in the University of Nottingham (Annual Report 1982).[235,329] It followed the established format (an excellent and well organised scientific programme, and the Annual General Meeting, Civic Reception and Annual Dinner); however, the Annual Meetings in 1980 and 1982 (the Golden Jubilee year of the Association) were exceptional

(Annual Reports 1981, 1982 and 1983).[234,235,257]

An Anglo-American Meeting was held at the Royal Festival Hall, London in September 1980.[330] This was not an official joint meeting with the American Society of Anesthesiologists (ASA) because the ASA have a policy of not holding meeting outside the USA, but close cooperation between Jack Moyers (Iowa City) and John Zorab (Vice President of the Association) ensured a satisfactory attendance by members of the ASA. The (British) Neurosurgical Anaesthetists Travelling Club and the American Society of Neurological Anaesthesia and Neurologic Supportive Care also held a concurrent meeting at the Festival Hall (Annual Report 1981)[234,330] The meeting was memorable for the outstanding John Snow Memorial lecture delivered by (Sir) Cecil Clothier QC (Parliamentary Commissioner for Administration and Health Service Commissioner ("Ombudsman") for England, Wales and Scotland, the text of which was subsequently published in full in *Anaesthesia*.[331] Sir Cecil has continued to take a great interest in the affairs of the Association and was elected to Honorary Membership in 1987. The Organising Committee of the Sixth European Congress regarded this meeting as a useful trial run for the Congress at which the Association of Anaesthetists would be hosts in 1982.

A meeting in honour of the ninetieth birthday of Sir Ivan Magill, KCVO[332] on 9 June 1978 was organised by the Section of the Royal Society of Medicine and supported by both the Association and the Faculty of Anaesthetists with Andrew Doughty (Kingston-on-Thames) in the Presidential Chair of the Section. A reception and buffet supper and cake-cutting ceremony followed the meeting, and many past Presidents of the Section and Association were present; they included three anaesthetist Knights (Sir Ivan Magill, KCVO[332] himself, Sir Geoffrey Organe[141] and Sir Robert Macintosh[209]).[333] *Anaesthesia* published a special issue in honour of Sir Ivan with an Editorial by Cyril Scurr (the President of the Association) and a reproduction of Magill's classic paper on endotracheal anaesthesia.[334]

A joint Meeting of the Association with the Society of Anaesthetic Laboratory Technicians was held in Cambridge on 28 March 1980. Professor Cedric Prys-Roberts (Bristol) delivered the eponymous Richard Salt lecture.

There was a number of interesting papers and a convivial dinner (Annual report 1980).[233]

The Golden Jubilee of the Association of Anaesthetists of Great Britain and Ireland

The fiftieth Anniversary of the foundation of the Association in 1982 was celebrated by three specific functions apart from the hosting of the Sixth European Congress of Anaesthesiology.

Joint Commemorative Dinner. The Councils of the Association of Anaesthetists and the Section of Anaesthetics of the Royal Society of Medicine, whose Officers founded the Association of Anaesthetists in 1932, held a joint dinner to celebrate the Golden Jubilee at the house of the Royal Society of Medicine on 5 March 1982 (Annual Report 1982).[235] The joint hosts were the reigning Presidents of the Association and the Section (Derek (W D) Wylie and Gordon Jackson Rees of Liverpool). The guests included five anaesthetists who had been Presidents of both bodies, and Sir Ivan Magill[332] and Francis Waddy (Northampton) who were Founder members of the Association (Annual Report 1982).[235]

The Golden Jubilee Annual Meeting of the Association took place at the Royal College of Surgeons of England, Lincoln's Inn Fields on 22 October 1982, a few weeks after the Association had successfully hosted the Sixth European Congress of Anaesthesiology (Annual Report 1983).[257] The one day programme included the Linkman Conference, a symposium on "Difficult Intubation" (Chaired by Professor T Cecil Gray), the Annual General Meeting, and the John Snow Memorial lecture, delivered by the incoming President of the Association, Professor Michael Vickers of Cardiff. Professor Quintin Gomez of the Philippines (former President of the World Federation of Anaesthesiologists) and George Edwards (St George's Hospital, London), another Founder Member of the Association of Anaesthetists, the first John Snow Lecturer in 1958 and the initiator of the original investigation of the Association into deaths associated with anaesthesia, were elected to Honorary Membership. Pask awards were presented to Donald Bateman (Epping), retiring Honorary Proof Reader of *Anaesthesia* after long service, and Francis Waddy (Northampton), who besides being a Founder member of the Association, was a pioneer in intensive care.[235]

The Golden Jubilee Dinner of the Association was a magnificent affair held at the Guildhall in the City of London on the evening of the Annual General Meeting on 22 October 1982. The new President, Professor Michael Vickers, was in the Chair, Sir Cecil Montacute Clothier, QC proposed the toast of the Association, and the President proposed "The Guests", to which Professor T C Gray replied. The guests included nine former Presidents of the Association and the Presidents of almost all the Royal Colleges (Annual Report 1983)[236,335]

The Association and the World Federation of Societies of Anaesthesiologists and its World and European Congresses 1970-1982

World Congresses of Anaesthesiologists and European Congresses of Anaesthesiology 1970-1982.

3rd European 1970	Prague Czechoslovakia
5th World 1972	Kyoto, Japan
4th European 1974	Madrid, Spain
6th World 1976	Mexico City, Mexico
5th European 1978	Paris, France
7th World 1980	Hamburg, West Germany
6th European 1982	London, England

The practice of holding the World and European Congresses alternately every two years has effectively enhanced the European Congresses almost to World status. They attract a considerable number of delegates from North and South America and Australasia in addition to Europeans (in 1982 from both sides of the Iron Curtain). This was a welcome development so far as registrants were concerned, but there were some reservations when it came to a choice of speakers. Many felt that a European Congress should have a European atmosphere and that there was plenty of talent in Europe to choose from. An alliance of British, Belgium and Dutch anaesthetists was moved to protest in a letter to *Anaesthesia* when the provisional programme of the 1978 Fifth European Congress in Paris was announced. They wrote "The preponderance of non-European and non-anaesthetist speakers is a cause for great concern"; some alterations were subsequently made to the final programme.[336] Speakers from the United Kingdom were prominent at all the World and European Congresses.

The Third European Congress of Anaesthesiology in Prague, Czechoslovakia was the only one in the World or European series to be held behind the Iron Curtain during the Cold War.[4] The medical hosts were most welcoming and did well to organise an international congress only two years after the "Prague Spring" and its brutal suppression by Soviet tanks.[4] Some of the officials who administered the conference were however grim of visage and hidebound and bureaucratic in their actions! The atmosphere was that of an occupied country, as well it might be with Russian troops encamped on the periphery of the City. The people were sad and resigned on the surface, but full of fun and fire underneath. There was, however, an atmosphere of suspicion and one felt that some generous individual hospitality was given at personal risk to the host for consorting with westerners. It was sad to see the beautiful buildings of Prague so badly neglected. Twenty years later, during the 8th European Congress in Warsaw in 1990, it was fascinating to compare the atmosphere in a country recently liberated from Soviet domination; the feeling of release was palpable, but the Poles were not entirely used to freedom or democracy (personal recollections)!

The Association of Anaesthetists of Great Britain and Ireland and the WFSA. The Officers and the former Officers of the Association continued to play a leading part in the medicopolitical committees and assemblies of the World Federation and its European Section (Annual Reports 1970-1982).[232-235] John Beard[1] was a member of the WFSA Executive Committee; Douglas Howat was successively Chairman of the European Section, Trustee of the WFSA Educational Anaesthesia Foundation of the WFSA, Chairman of the Executive Committee of the WFSA and finally its Vice President. John Zorab was Secretary of the European Regional Board, elected Secretary General in 1980 and President in 1984. Michael Vickers became Chairman of the WFSA Statutes and Byelaws Committee in 1980, Secretary General in 1988 and President in 1994. Peter Baskett became Chairman of the Cardiopulmonary Resuscitation Committee in the same year.

The Association being a large society of physician anaesthetists has five delegates at the various assemblies; this is second only to the USA.

Sixth European Congress of Anaesthesiology
London, 8-15 September 1982

Patron
Her Majesty the Queen

President of the Congress
W D Wylie (President of the Association 1980-1982)

Organising Committee

Chairman P J Helliwell,[3] *Deputy* S A Mason, *Secretary General* J S M. Zorab, *Deputy* P J F Baskett, *Treasurer* M Rosen, *Deputy* J N Horton, *Honorary Secretary of the Association* Jean M Horton, *Assistant* W R MacRae, *Financial Adviser* Ernest Warburton

Scientific Programme:	*Chairman* A A Spence,
	Deputy C M Conway,
	Members J Norman, C Prys-Roberts,
	C J Hull, G Smith
Social Programme:	*Chairman* Richard II Ellis
Technical Exhibition:	*Chairman* M D Vickers,
	Deputy R S Vaughan
Editorial:	*Chairman* T B Boulton,
	Deputy R S Atkinson
	Members J N Lunn, A P Adams, P J Horsey, C E Blogg, A L Revell, D B Welch
Communications:	*Chairman* D H Short
	Public Relations I R Verner
	Stewards J Mathias
	Projection C A B McLaren
	Television A W Makepiece
	Adviser P Hansell
Conference Organiser:	Caroline Roney

The Council had resolved in 1974 that an offer should be made to the WFSA European Regional Committee for the Association of Anaesthetists of Great Britain and Ireland to host the Sixth European Congress of Anaesthesiology in London in 1982, coincident with the Golden Jubilee of the

Foundation of the Association (Council Minutes 5.4.1974).[81] The offer was accepted at the meeting of the European Regional Assembly of the WFSA held at the 6th World Congress in Mexico City in April 1976[337] (Annual report 1976: Council Minutes 21.5.1976)[81]

The President Philip Helliwell[3] (1973-1976) assumed the Chairmanship of the 1982 Steering Committee (Council Minutes 12.11.1976), and continued as Chairman of the Congress Committee when Cyril Scurr took over as President in November 1976. The initial planning of the scientific programme was in the capable hands of John F Nunn (Director of the Medical Research Council, Clinical Research Unit at Northwick Park Hospital) but, when he was elected Dean of the Faculty of Anaesthetists in 1979, Professor Alastair Spence (then of Glasgow but later of Edinburgh) took over the Chairmanship of the Scientific Programme Committee.[337-339]

Choice of venue. Two venues were considered initially. These were the Wembley Conference Centre and the Royal Festival Hall (Council Minutes 12.11.1976). The Royal Festival Hall was chosen after the experience of the 1978 Annual General Meeting at Wembley.

The financial management of the Sixth European Congress. The members of the Organising Committee of the Sixth European Congress in 1982 approached their task in a less relaxed but more professional manner than did the organisers of the 4th World Congress in 1968 (Chapter 7). Commercial considerations as advocated by Mrs Thatcher's administration were much more to the fore in the eighties! (personal experience of both Congresses).

It is of interest to compare the two Congresses which were fourteen years apart with a period of escalating inflation between them. Both were held at the Royal Festival Hall which, amongst other negative factors, has only limited space for the all important (and fee paying) technical exhibition; however, better use was made of the space that was available in 1982; every odd corner on every level was utilised!

The organisers in 1982 were not asked to give a personal guarantee against the possible failure of the Congress as they were in 1968, nor were commercial guarantors sought; in 1982 a limited liability company was formed at a cost of £500 (1996: £950) to guard against possible loss, and the enterprise was regarded as a charitable function under the terms of the Education and Research Fund (Council Minutes 5.10.1979).[97]

Both Congresses took place at a time of considerable financial stringency, and both followed political crises earlier in the year (the Czechoslovakian rising in 1968 and the Falklands War of 1982); because of the international and political situation there was anxiety that there would be sufficient numbers of registrants to make the respective Congresses financially viable. There are two possible strategies when running meetings in such circumstances; one is to make the registration fee higher, thus providing a low break-even point in terms of attendance, the other is to fix a low registration fee and hope for a high attendance. The latter course of action causes a great deal more anxiety for the organisers, but it can be argued, from a purely philosophical point of view, that a low registration fee attracts more registrants and, after all, that is what the purpose of a scientific meeting is all about! The registration fee for the 1968 World Congress was £25 (1996: £230), and that for the European Congress in 1982, which again was sharply criticised by some United Kingdom anaesthetists, was £120 (1996: £225)! The attendance in 1968 was just under 2,500 full registrants at the World Congress with just over 900 accompanying persons; in 1982 at the European Congress there were just over 2,000 registrants and some 500 accompanying persons. The Surplus from the 1968 meeting was £4,715 (1996: £43,700), and from the 1982 Congress £219,242 (1996: £412,000), when the net proceeds were paid into the Association Education and Research Fund in 1986 after the affairs of the Congress Company had been wound up. The 1982 European Congress figure includes a refund on Value Added Tax (VAT) which was negotiated as a result of the charitable status of the Congress Company by the Honorary Treasurer (Michael Rosen,) and the Financial Adviser Ernest Warburton. VAT was introduced in the United Kingdom in 1973, and therefore was not a factor in 1968!

The Scientific and Social programmes of the Sixth European Congress were very successful; to gain an impression it is hardly possible to improve on quoting almost verbatim the concise report in *Anaesthesia* written by R S Atkinson (at that time Senior Assistant Editor of *Anaesthesia* and later Vice Dean of the Faculty of Anaesthetists):-[338]

The Opening Ceremony. Her Royal Highness Princess Margaret graciously opened the Congress on 8 September in a Ceremony at which Dr Derek Wylie, the President of the Congress, Professor Jean Lassner, Chairman of the European Regional Section of the World Federation of Societies of Anaesthesiology, and Kenneth Clarke, QC, MP (the Minister of Health) also spoke. HRH Princess Margaret presented the Presidents of each European Society with a commemorative certificate and, at the conclusion of the ceremony, P J Helliwell,[3] Chairman of the Organising Committee, presented a crystal glass bowl engraved with the arms of the Association of Anaesthetists of Great Britain and Ireland to Princess Margaret. The Princess then toured the exhibition area and met many of the Congress participants during an informal reception.

The Scientific Programme began on 9 September, almost 1000 papers being presented in up to seven auditoria between then and the final session on 15 September. The Scientific Committee under the chairmanship of Professor Alastair Spence, arranged 18 symposia with a number of distinguished invited speakers, the subjects being: Intravenous Anaesthesia, Obstetric Anaesthesia; Pharmacokinetics; Cellular Effects of Anaesthetics; Breathing Systems and Apparatus; Immunology; Acute Pain; The Neuromuscular Junction; Local Anaesthesia; Paediatric Anaesthesia; Infection in the Intensive Therapy Unit; Anaesthesia Toxicity; Pain Therapy; Cardiovascular Aspects of Anaesthesia; Neuroanaesthesia; Quality Control in Anaesthesia; Pulmonary Problems in Intensive Care.

There were also sessions of free papers, mostly grouped so that related topic could be considered in the same session, film presentations and posters. The total number of scientific sessions was 104. Simultaneous interpretation into English, German, French and Spanish was available in the main auditoria.

The Technical Exhibition which was organised at various sites in the Festival Hall and also in the Hayward Gallery involved over 800 companies from Great Britain and Europe and displayed information on a wide range of drugs and apparatus.

The Association of Anaesthetists of Great Britain and Ireland organised a souvenir shop, there were also stands promoting *Anaesthesia*, the *British Journal of Anaesthesia*, and the World Congress in Manilla in January 1984.

Publications. The volume of Summaries published in the form of a Supplement to Anaesthesia was the only official record of the scientific programme.[339] No proceedings volume was published. The Editors of

Anaesthesia produced a daily Congress News as a daily bulletin of information.

Social programme. On the evening of 9 September there was a concert given by the English Chamber Orchestra conducted by Michael Tilson Thomas at which the soloist in the Mozart Piano Concerto K.488 in A major was Christina Ortiz. This was followed by Open Air entertainment; a musical display by the Band of the Royal Marines and later spectacular fireworks. On Saturday 11 September, there was a Gala Evening in the Covent Garden Market area, which included street entertainment, late night shopping, dinner and dancing. On 13 September a Buffet Reception took place in the Guildhall and Glaziers' Hall in the City of London.

The Closing Ceremony was held in the Queen Elizabeth Hall. Speeches were made by Professor K. Steinbereithner (Treasurer of the European Regional Section), and Derek Wylie (President of the Congress). Scottish music and dancing by the Caledonian Highlanders and Argyll dancers then entertained the audience, and the Pipe Major 'quaifed' with the President.

The Sixth European Congress in London was an undoubted success. More than 2000 registrants enjoyed the scientific programme, while they and around 500 accompanying guests enjoyed day tours and receptions. The weather was exemplary, cloudless skies and warm sunshine throughout adding to the enjoyment. On the final day central London enjoyed its warmest September day in nine years, 27.6 C (81.7 F).

Other events in London occurring in association with the Congress included the conferring of Honorary Fellowships in the Faculty of Anaesthetists of the Royal College of Surgeons of England on Professor J J Bonica (USA), Professor T Gordh (Sweden), Professor F F Foldes (USA), and the Fellowship by Election to Professor J Lassner (France), J R McCarthy (Ireland), Professor E N Ayim (Kenya) and Professor O Norlander (Norway). M Sando (Australia), was prevented by illness from receiving a Fellowship by Election, and was conferred on him in October. The eponymous W W Mushin Lecture of the University of Wales was delivered by J F Nunn, Immediate Past Dean of the Faculty, in the Royal College of Surgeons on 10 September. It is a pleasure to record that C Langton Hewer was presented at his home with an autographed leather bound edition of *Recent Advances in*

Anaesthesia and Analgesia, Volume 14 by Churchill Livingstone to mark 50 years of personal unbroken service as author and editor of the series.

The Postgraduate Course

The Association of Anaesthetists organised a Postgraduate Course at the Royal Festival Hall on the day before the Sixth European Congress, but independent of it in that participants were not required to register for the Congress.[340] The format was based on that of the courses which precede the Annual Scientific Meetings of the American Society of Anesthesiologists each year. Several groups of lectures are held simultaneously and participants choose to attend one lecture from each group. Over 800 registrants attended the course. This event initiated by the Association (now known as the Continuing Medical Education Day) has been held annually ever since as a joint venture of the Association of Anaesthetists and the Faculty (now Royal College) of Anaesthetists (Council Minutes 3.12.1982).[97]

The turbulent and productive years 1970-1982

The twelve years 1970-1982 were certainly turbulent years, for the world, for the United Kingdom, for the National Health Service (which underwent two reorganisations and several industrial disputes), for the specialty of Anaesthesia, and for the Association of Anaesthetists itself, but they were also challenging and productive. The Association was fortunate during this period of challenge to be served by exceptional gifted teams of Presidents, Treasurers and Honorary Secretaries; together they turned the challenges into very considerable achievements.

Michael Vickers composed an erudite Editorial in 1983 towards the end of his first year in office as President.[139] He defined the activities of a professional association as belonging to three categories. These were "self preservation" (measures directed towards the organisation and smooth running of the Association itself), "rituals" (the decorous but imaginative conduct of its public administrative, professional and social business, and of such matters as the award of honours and commendations for exceptional professional merit) and, above all, "member service" (and beyond that service to the profession and community at large).

The move to a self-contained suite of offices in BMA House, the extensive reorganisation of the conduct of the business of Council, and the methods of election to it, in the Helliwell years, the establishment of the Linkman organisation, and the continued enhancement of the responsibilities and status of the Junior Anaesthetists' Group, resulted in an efficient administrative machine by 1982, and the improved access to the corridors of power through the British Medical Association Anaesthetists' Subcommittee greatly increased the effectiveness and status of the Association.

All this was achieved while the essential day to day business of advising on, and negotiating improvements, in the individual and corporate well-being of the members of the Association of Anaesthetists went on.

The Officers and Council, moreover, helped to bring about by persuasion a change of attitude and self esteem in anaesthetists, which set the specialty inexorably on a course which was to lead to the establishment of an independent Royal College and Anaesthetists at the end of the next decade.

The Association of Anaesthetists also pioneered medical audit (the mortality in anaesthesia investigations), and it had become a significant and innovative educational organisation in the field of national and postgraduate medical education. It had also been able to finance research including establishing a Research Fellowship, and its journal *Anaesthesia* had become a monthly publication and improved in contents and international status.

Some problems, notably those connected with assistance for the anaesthetist, outpatient dental anaesthesia, and independent practice, remained to be solved, and many others lay ahead, particularly those concerned with manpower and the provision and organisation of training.

The innovative "Help for the Sick Doctor Scheme" originated by the Association of Anaesthetists in collaboration with the Royal College of Psychiatrists was a model of its kind which was used to develop a national scheme for all members of the United Kingdom medical profession.

The financial status of the Association had improved out of all recognition during the twelve years 1970 to 1982, thanks to the efforts of the Financial

Adviser (Ernest Warburton) and the Honorary Treasurers. The Association of Anaesthetists of Great Britain and Ireland had celebrated its Golden Jubilee in style and successfully hosted the Sixth European Congress of Anaesthesiology in 1982. The national economic situation was improving and the prospects for the years 1983-1992, the sixth decade in the life of the Association, looked good both for the United Kingdom and the Association itself. How far this optimism was justified remains to be recounted in Chapter 9.

9

The Sixth Decade

1 January 1983 to 31 December 1992

"Congratulations and Jubilations"

Bill Martin and Phil Coulter.   Popular Song 1968.

Executive Officers.

    Presidents:-   M D A Vickers (1982-1984)
                             T B Boulton (1984-1986)
                             M Rosen (1986-1988)
                             M M Burrows (1988-1990)
                             P J F Baskett (1990-1992)
                             W R MacRae (1992-1994)

    Honorary Treasurers:- M Rosen (1978-1983)
                             M M Burrows (1983-1988)
                             W R MacRae (1988-1992)
                             W L M Baird (1992 et seq)

    Honarary Secretaries:- W R MacRae (1982-1984)
                             M T Inman (1984-1986)
                             P Morris (1986-1988)
                             W L M Baird (1988-1990)
                             J E Charlton (1990-1992)
                             R S Vaughan (1992-1994)

    Editors:-   J N Lunn (1982-1990)
                             M Morgan (1990 et seq)

Chairmen of the Junior Anaesthetists' Group (JAG): *

P J Bickford Smith (1983), Wendy Scott (1984-1985), W Hamlin (1986-1987), D L Paul (1988-1989), P J Heath (1990), Elizabeth M Spencer (1990-1993).

* From 1991 onward "The Group of Anaesthesia in Training"(GAT)

Ups and downs in world and national politics (1983-1992)

It seems paradoxical that a decade which saw steady progress in the affairs and aspirations of the Association of Anaesthetists of Great Britain and Ireland culminating in its Diamond Jubilee in 1992, should witness such dramatic fluctuations in international politics[1] and major changes in the way in which the British National Health Service was administered.[2-7]

Few foresaw, for example, the amazing consequences for the world which were to stem from the appointment of Mikhail Gorbachev as General Secretary of the Communist Party of the Soviet Union in 1985; by the time he succeeded to the Presidency in 1988 his courageous policies of glasnost (openness in government and a degree of political and economic freedom for the individual) and perestroika (restructuring and liberation of the machinery of government) were beginning to have an effect. His statemanship led not only to the end of the Cold War and agreements on nuclear weapons with the USA, but also to nationalist restlessness and liberal revolution in the Soviet satellite countries, the breaching of the Berlin Wall, and the reunification of Germany in November 1989. Less propitiously Gorbachev's reforms precipitated demands for the independence and armed unrest in the constituent republics of the USSR, to economic chaos and lawlessness in Russia, to the abortive coup by the old style communists, and ultimately to the replacement of Gorbachev himself by his arch rival Boris Yeltsin in 1992.[1]

The United Kingdom began the period under review in a somewhat euphoric atmosphere after the successful defence of its own sovereign territory of the Falkland Islands in 1982 and, apart from the ever present thorn in the flesh of terrorist activity in both Northern Ireland and mainland Britain itself, there was peace until 1991 in which year the United Kingdom found itself shoulder to shoulder with the USA in the mercifully brief, televised, and strangely technologically clinical Gulf War against Iraq, in the defence of the former British protectorate of Kuwait.[1]

The rise and fall of Mrs Thatcher who became the longest serving United Kingdom Prime Minister in the twentieth century was also both dramatic and revolutionary. When she took office in May 1979, monolithic old style trade unionism and outdated industrial management practices hampered by penal taxation were between them strangling the economy, inflation was rampant, personal taxation was punitive, and the United Kingdom was deeply in debt to the International Monetary Fund (IMF) partly due to profligate centrally controlled government spending on doctrinaire projects. The ruthlessness of the Thatcher Government was destined to solve many of these problems, but the rigid policies of the early years, involving shutting down inefficient industries, caused a steep rise in unemployment which resulted in considerable social unrest. There were riots in Brixton, Liverpool and several other cities, and industrial action in the National Health Service in 1982. Public opinion was changing by 1983, however, an optimistic feeling was abroad that the individuals and not the State were once more in control of personal destinies and there was a sense of general revival and well being. The policy of resistance to the growing attempts at bureaucratic interference by the European Economic Commission so far as it went, was also popular, as had been the courageous and successful decision to defend the Falklands. The political opposition was also weak and divided, and the elections in 1983 and 1987 were won on the strength of a booming enterprise economy.

Privatisation relieved the government of the financial burdens of various utilities and brought once and for all gains to the Exchequer ("selling the family silver" as the ageing former Prime Minister Harold Macmillan (1894-1986), once a keen supporter of Mrs Thatcher, put it), and Mrs Thatcher's undoubted stature as a world leader gained considerable respect.[1]

The writing was on the wall by 1988 however. Tax cuts, popular as they were with the middle and higher income groups, led to profligate consumer spending, inflation, and a widening trade gap once again. Changes in social security benefits also hit low earners, and once again there was industrial unrest which included a six month dispute with the ambulancemen. *The coup de grace* for Mrs Thatcher was the Community Charge or "Poll Tax". The principle, that everyone should pay something towards the cost of social services rather than the whole burden falling on the property owner, was a sound one; too often local Councillors with nothing to lose had voted for extravagant expenditure on politically motivated schemes. The concept that everyone should pay the same flat rate irrespective of means was, however, both unfair and ill-advised; a local income tax or a local sales tax would have been preferable. Resistance and violent rioting ensued. Mrs Thatcher's long rule ended and John Major, the ordinary man in the street, came into office on 28th November 1990 to face a rejuvenated opposition under Neil Kinnock, who, *inter alia,* was gunning for the Government over the reorganisation of the NHS due to take place on 1st April 1991.[1-4]

Mr Major's style as Prime Minister was conciliatory, and ostensibly promoted an avowed policy of putting the ordinary citizen and consumer into the picture. The "Citizen's Charter"[1] of July 1991 and its subsidiary the "Patients' Charter"[5-7] of the following October were typical of this approach. They re-emphasised certain fairly obvious existing consumers "rights" and set some administrative "targets" for the public services; however the public, apart from using the charters as a text for making complaints, were less easily won over and, while they had criticised Mrs Thatcher for being dictatorial, they now castigated her successor as a ditherer; nonetheless aided by a spirit of patriotism engendered by the successful prosecution of the Gulf War similar to that experienced after the Falklands Campaign, and a fear of the increases in personal taxation that the "tax and spend" programmes of the Labour party might precipitate, the Conservatives were returned with a narrow but workable majority in April 1992.[1]

One government strategy which was continued relentlessly throughout the period was the attempt to contain the cost of the NHS, and, consequently, the Service was subjected to two further politically motivated reorganisations in 1984 and 1991.[3-4] The latter, the most controversial in the whole forty-three year history of the NHS, was planned without consultation with the medical profession, and it was executed in haste apparently in order to have the reorganisation in place before the 1992 General Election in which the government of the day feared they might be defeated.[3] The resultant administrative system virtually excludes the medical profession in an advisory role except at hospital level, and includes it only at a peripheral level in executive management.[2-4] This situation has a distinct resemblance to that described in George Orwell's *Animal Farm*![4-8]

The nineteen eighties have also seen the development of the growth industries of, regulatory legislation (much of it emanating from the European Commission in Brussels), compensation seeking, "political correctness", with its supporting "thought police" and expensive consultancy lecture courses,[9] and armies of inspectors, "quango" members, and "do-gooders" seeking to impose their own pet solutions to problems in the belief that they, and they alone, are right; at the same time the broadcasters and other journalists have been granted increasing licence to invade privacy to target and persecute both private and public individuals with all the ferocity and self-righteousness of mediaeval witch hunts, whether or not the victims are right or wrong over a particular issue.

It is unfortunate that the once self-reliant and charitable British people now frequently seek someone to blame and victimise, and monetary compensation for every minor vicissitude in life. The parrot cry that they "are-not-interested-in-the-money-and only-wish-to-ensure-that-it-never-happens-again" does not ring true at times!

We entered the age of PCs ("personal computers" and "political correctness") in the eighties. Political correctness is now carried to extraordinary lengths.[9] It would be funny, if it was not so sad, that some people object to being described as "Chairman", in favour of the inanimate "Chair" or asexual "Chairperson". This is on the grounds that "Chairman" is sexually discriminatory, when the dictionary defines "man" as "human being" as its first meaning and goes on to give "person" as a synonym![10] The present writer certainly did not object to being alluded to as a "round eye" by Oriental people when he worked in the Far East, and it is a source of satisfaction that, now retired, he retains the title "Old Age Pensioner" (OAP), the erasure of which has defied all the efforts of the thought police! Society is certainly less light hearted and takes itself much more seriously than before the advent of "Political Correctness". The era of jargon and acronyms is also upon us and is to be deplored.

Medicine and Surgery 1983-1992

Acquired immune deficiency syndrome (AIDS) poses one of the major medical challenges of the twentieth century. It was first described in 1981 as an outbreak of opportunistic lung infections due to pneumocystis carinii and/or cases of Kaposi's Sarcoma in homosexual men, particularly in California and New York.[11-15] The earliest cases probably occurred, in developed countries at least, in 1979.[14] The first British report of "primary cytomegalovirus carinii and cytomegalovirus infections" in a practising homosexual appeared in the *Lancet* in December 1981; one of the authors was a physician anaesthetist practising in intensive care.[15] The causative virus was described in 1983. It was originally designated the "lymphadenopathic associated virus", then as "human T lymphotrophic virus type III" (HTLV III), and finally as "human immunodeficiency virus" (HIV).[16-20]

The potential significance of a fatal new incurable infectious disease, which could not be prevented by immunisation, which had a long latent period during which the patient was symptomless but capable of transmitting the infection, and which could be spread by homosexual and heterosexual intercourse in semen, by parenteral injection, the donation of blood, or by transplanted organs, and to infants through the placenta and by breast feeding, was not at first generally appreciated; in fact it seemed to many to be almost unbelievable at the end of the half century which had seen the conquest of pneumonia, smallpox, tuberculosis, poliomyelitis, malaria, syphilis and gonorrhoea and many other infections.

Up until 1985 AIDS was a little known quantity in the United Kingdom being limited to less than two hundred cases, though in Africa (where the disease may indeed have originated),[21] in the United States and in Australia it was well established in proportion to the populations, and in western continental Europe beginning to be so.[14,22] Articles on what was regarded as the "Gay (homosexual) plague" had however appeared in the popular press[23] and the epidemiologists had recognised the signs of a possible pandemic and its serious dangers.[22-24] The British Medical Association, "prompted by the number of enquiries" issued a statement in April 1985. This noted that the disease was transmitted "largely by sexual contact, especially homosexual, and by blood to blood inoculation", including the sharing of needles and syringes among drug abusers. It also indicated that there was a possible danger of infection from pooled blood products, and stated that the risk from single unit transfusions was small. The use of a "plastic airway" for "mouth-to-mouth" resuscitation was recommended.[25] Considerable public apprehension, sometimes almost amounting to hysteria, developed in the mid eighties and regrettably some members of the medical and nursing professions in the United Kingdom were not immune to overreaction.[26] Letters reached the Association of Anaesthetists asking whether an anaesthetist was justified and/or would avoid disciplinary action, if he or she refused to anaesthetise an AIDS case (personal recollection). This, of course, would have been unacceptable conduct both ethically and in the eyes of the General Medical Council. The Council of the Association of Anaesthetists first discussed the immunisation as the serum was largely derived from the pooled plasma of homosexual men and there was concern that it might contain the AIDS virus. This reservation was described as "absurd" by Zuckerman and other experts in 1984 because of precautions taken in preparation;[46] nonetheless the Council of the Association initially sought further guidance from the Chief Medical Officer before advocating that all anaesthetists should be immunised "provided proper precautions were taken" (Council Minutes 1.2.1985).[27] A vaccine prepared by a method which guaranteed freedom from the possibility of spreading AIDS was developed in the late eighties; thereafter the Association of Anaesthetists recommended immunisation for all anaesthetists.[28] Some Health Authorities refused to implement this policy because of the cost, but fortunately General Practitioners were more co-operative (personal recollection). The Department of Health (DH) originally confined its advice to stipulating that nurses and hospital doctors working in renal dialysis units should be immunised. It was not until 1993 that the DH decided to make it absolutely mandatory for all health workers who perform invasive procedures and, in addition, for general practitioners, dentists, midwives and their students. The cost of screening, immunisation and follow up for seroconversion was to be met by Health Authorities out of existing funds, and the DH invited the authorities to set the expenditure "against the possible legal costs if a patient is infected by a health care worker"![49]

Minimal invasive surgery had, of course, been practised as an extension of diagnostic endoscopy of the urological and gastrointestinal tracts for several decades before the nineteen eighties. It had, for example, largely transferred access for the surgery of the bladder and prostate from the incision of the lower abdominal wall to the urethra, thereby bringing benefits to patients, particularly to the elderly, by reducing the traumatic consequences of surgery and encouraging the beneficial use of regional anaesthesia.[50]

Laparoscopy was first practised in 1910[51,52] and subsequently used as a diagnostic procedure by a small minority of general surgeons (personal recollection of J P Hosford, St Bartholomew's Hospital, London 1949), and it came into its own for surgical female sterilisation in the sixties when that operation became generally ethically acceptable.[52,53]

The development of endoscopic techniques for the removal of renal and ureteric stones and the developments of second generation extracorporeal shockwave lithotripsy and other electronic, ultrasonic, and laser techniques have made it possible to treat the majority of stones in the urinary tract without anaesthesia and with minimal morbidity for the patient.[54,55] Lithotripsy and endoscopic procedures have been developed for the treatment of stones in the gall bladder and biliary tract[56] and minimally invasive techniques for arthroscopic surgery have been available since the seventies.[57] Continued progress in the use of nonoperative transluminal angioplastic coronary artery surgery, as practised by cardiologists and radiologists, has also reduced the need for open-heart surgery.[54]

The most dramatic development in minimal invasive surgery in recent years has, however, been in general abdominal surgery. This has occurred since 1990, when the French surgeons Dubois and his colleagues described the results of their first 36 laparoscopic cholecystectomies.[58] Dubois and his team had undertaken their first laparoscopic cholecystectomy in 1988[58] but the procedure was actually first reported by Mouret of Lyons in 1987[56] and laparoscopic appendicectomy had been described in 1983.[59] It was, however, the report of Dubois and colleagues in a prestigious American journal[58] which triggered enthusiasm amongst surgeons for minimally invasive abdominal surgery;[60] since then, in addition to the gall bladder, almost every abdominal organ, oesophagus, stomach, duodenum, small and large bowel, liver, spleen, kidney, ureters and pancreas have all been resected or repaired.[61]

Monson[61] has stressed that "minimal access surgery" would be a more appropriate term than "minimal invasive surgery" so far as the abdomen is concerned:-

"although the scar may be smaller and the level of postoperative discomfort may be less, the operation otherwise remains essentially unchanged with the same list of potential complications - and a few new ones thrown in for good measure."[61]

The same care in selection and preoperative preparation of the patient is required and a general anaesthetic is essential for most major procedures. It is accepted that abdominal laparoscopic procedures often take longer than the equivalent open operation even allowing for the "learning curve". There are at times further delays when an originally planned closed procedure has to be converted to an open operation because of technical difficulties. There are, however, obvious advantages when all goes well in terms of reduction of postoperative pain and the incidence of wound infection. Questions which can only be answered by the lapse of time remain; for example "can laparoscopic colectomy be as effective as open resection?", and "will the essentially different repairs to groin hernias have a higher or lower rate of recurrence than the traditional methods?"[61,62] Health economists and academics will doubtless conduct endless debates concerning the cost benefit of the reduction of hospital stay versus increase in theatre time and the provision of expensive and constantly improving equipment, as well as the charges relevant to after care in the community.[60,63,64]

Minimal Invasive Therapy and Surgery has been cited as "one of the great innovations of health care in the twentieth century",[64] and even as possibly a principle which will change the way hospitals are organised and run with the "Director of Interventional Therapy" ("probably a physician") being at the head of a team which will include an endoscopist, an interventional radiologist, a laser specialist, an anaesthetist-intensivist, an imaging specialist, a physicist-bioengineer, a health economist, and an "open" surgeon![54,65] Most anaesthetists probably take a different view![66] Time alone will tell!

There was considerable concern also that minimal invasive surgery had been introduced with undue haste without its implications being properly assessed.[63,64,67] There have been real difficulties in the field of surgical training. Many surgeons believed initially that "the basic techniques are not difficult to acquire" but ignored the implication of the following statement that "training courses will be set up all over the Western world",[60] only to find that "operations that were straightforward open procedures may require considerable laparoscopic expertise" *(British Medical Journal 1993)*.[64] The urge to adopt the new techniques was undoubtedly due to surgical enthusiasm on the part of the British surgeons but it was attributed to patient pressure in continental Europe.[63,64] Whatever the reason surgical enthusiasm inevitably led to complications especially in relation to the common bile duct.[61,64] This caused professional and public alarm in the United Kingdom. Training centres have now been set up in London, Leeds and Dundee with the aid of £2 million grants from the DH and the Wolfson Foundation[68] and the Senate of the Royal Surgical Colleges (composed of representatives of the Royal Colleges of Surgeons of Great Britain and Ireland and related surgical organisations), has issued a guidance document on the importance of the role of training on "quality assurance" in general which includes the statement:-

> *"If a technique is considered by the profession to be sufficiently novel as to require special training and assessment before being introduced into general clinical practice, its initial use should be controlled and limited to a number of specified centres for clinical trial. The Colleges are now devising mechanisms for achieving such control."*[69]

It should also be remembered that British surgeons, in contrast to their European colleagues, are prevented by law from training on pigs and other animals.[61]

There is further concern, not least for the anaesthetist. The surgeons who undeniably practice minimal access surgery with discretion, skill and confidence at the present time were trained in the era of open surgery and are well able to employ that technique when necessary, but where minimal access surgery has been adopted, there is evidence already that trainee surgeons are getting less practical experience even in laparoscopic operating because this is being undertaken by their seniors.[70] Patients can not be expected to submit themselves for open surgery if it can be demonstrated that minimal access surgery is available and equally beneficial. Will there be sufficient cases, for which the open techniques are preferable, to train surgeons to use them when necessary, or equally important, when the highly technical equipment is not available, as in developing countries?

Immediate prehospital care for cardiac and traumatic emergencies has been improved considerably in developed countries in the last two decades. It is a movement in which British doctors, cardiologists, anaesthetists, accident and emergency specialists and general practitioners have had a considerable influence, and yet in the nineties our own provision for prehospital trauma care in the United Kingdom is still far from perfect.[71-73]

Effective treatment for cardiac arrest became a practical possibility from 1960 onwards with the introduction of positive pressure ventilation, external cardiac compression and external defibrillation (Chapter 7); soon thereafter cardiac arrest protocols and teams became an integral part of in house hospital practice. The next step was the introduction of schemes designed to train ambulance crews and the general public in basic cardiopulmonary resuscitation without apparatus, or with minimal mechanical aids for ventilation, so that an oxygenated circulation could be maintained until medical assistance became available. Rex Binning[74,75] (Association Council Member 1963-1965) and many other British anaesthetists have been pioneers in this field (pages 187-188).[76]

The practice of providing specially equipped ambulances to transport a team to resuscitate a patient, and to carry out defibrillation if necessary before monitored transfer to hospital, was pioneered by the cardiologist Pantridge in Belfast in the mid nineteen sixties,[77] and a number of similar units were subsequently introduced in many parts of the world, including the United Kingdom, Continental Europe, North America, Australia and Japan.[78,79] The cardiac resuscitation teams in these ambulances were initially led by medical practitioners but, by the mid seventies, it proved to be practicable to train selected non-medical personnel to man emergency ambulances, not only to maintain the circulation but also to intubate, to diagnose ventricular fibrillation, carry out defibrillation, and to establish intravenous infusions. Douglas Chamberlain (cardiologist) and Binning and their colleagues in Brighton, and Peter Baskett have been successful in providing coronary care operated by trained ambulance crews since the seventies,[79-82] as has John Hoyle (Consultant Anaesthetist) with the Bournemouth Ambulance Service.

Previous to the sixties the primary aim of ambulance crews in densely populated counties was rapid evacuation to hospital emergency departments where medical resuscitation could begin[82] and, even up until 1970, the mandatory training of British ambulance crews amounted to little more than instruction in first aid.[83] The increasing toll of road traffic accidents led to a gradual realisation in the late sixties throughout developed countries that an appreciable number of casualties were dying of avoidable complications (primarily obstruction of the airway), either at the site of the accident or in transit.[84-89]

West Germany (the Federal German Republic as it then was) was early in the field of providing care at the site of an accident. There the first emergency ambulances with medical practitioners from Government run hospitals as members of the crew, began operating in 1957; by the nineteen seventies almost all of the country was covered by the service and, by the mid eighties a highly efficient system backed by 35 helicopter stations was operating. France has developed a rather similar system, as have Belgium and some Eastern European countries including Hungary and Czechoslovakia.[71,90]

A report of the United States National Academy of Sciences in 1966 drew attention to the deficiencies of the trauma services with the dramatic title "Accidental death and disability: the neglected disease of modern society";[85] however, systems of immediate prehospital care in the United States, for both the consequences of myocardial infarction and for trauma are not much older than the early seventies. It is pleasing to be told that the example of the work of Pantridge[77,78] in mobile coronary care in Northern Ireland had an influence;[91] but the American Emergency Medical Services were developed with the aid of Federal Funding and with the characteristic American propensity to act decisively once having seen the benefits of a particular course of action. The Vietnam conflict had demonstrated the value and success of immediate prehospital care by paramedical personnel undertaking procedures previously considered to be only the province of the medical practitioner, and many paramedics fortuitously returned to the United States at a time when there was considerable public pressure for improvement in the emergency medical and ambulance services;[91] however, like many things in so vast a country as the USA, not least in health care, the system is not yet entirely uniform nor fully developed.[90] The American pattern of paramedical prehospital care was followed in Australia and South Africa.[71]

Matters have moved more slowly in the United Kingdom![92] Britain only had prehospital care schemes of adequate standard in a relatively small number of areas of the country up until the nineties, and those that did exist had only developed as the result of individual voluntary effort. The DH did not encourage the schemes because of fears of the financial consequences, and there were trade union difficulties with the ambulance staff.[71,83]

Kenneth Easton developed a remarkable voluntary system of BASIC (British Association of Immediate Care Schemes) amongst his family practitioner colleagues from 1965 onwards, which, by 1977, had 1,200 medical practitioners participating in 73 immediate care schemes country wide using their own vehicles and equipment.[71,89,93]

The BASIC schemes were very successful in rural areas but less so in the urban situation. Several emergency teams, based on the initiative of individual hospital "Casualty" (later "Accident and Emergency") Consultants, were developed in the United Kingdom in the fifties and sixties. These enable casualty surgeons and nurses to be summoned by radio to road accidents with equipment carried in ambulances or police or private cars at the request of the ambulance or police services. They included those at Derby (since 1955),[92] Preston ("several years" before 1965),[93] and Bath (since 1966).[88,94] Gögler's mobile accident service in Heidelberg, West Germany[84] and that organised by Henning Poulsen (Professor of Anaesthesiology at Aarhus, Denmark)[95] had begun to function in 1957. All these schemes involved transporting medical and nursing personnel to the accident or emergency, but the Mobile Resuscitation Unit (MRU) organised by Peter Baskett based at Frenchay Hospital, Bristol from 1972 onwards, was manned by specially trained ambulance (paramedic) personnel.[71,74,82,83,90,96] A feature of the Frenchay Hospital Scheme was the use of 50% nitrous oxide and oxygen for the relief of pain by ambulance personnel which was developed by Baskett,[97] endorsed by the Association of Anaesthetists (Annual Report 1972), and subsequently adopted as standard equipment in British ambulances.[83]

"About a dozen" of the 64 peripherally managed ambulance services in the National Health Service which existed after the 1974 reorganisation had developed similar schemes by 1980 This was despite a Health Service circular in 1976 advising the Authorities that there were insufficient grounds for the development of such schemes,[98] which were not in fact approved by the DH until ten years later in 1986.[71]

The Association of Anaesthetists was ahead of the DH in endorsing and promoting the training of ambulance personnel to paramedical standards, encouraging members to participate as trainers, and recommending the development of a paramedical wing of the ambulance service in the seventies and early eighties.[99,100] Some reservations were expressed at the Linkman conferences but they were mainly concerned with the question of legal liability, patient consent (particularly for training intravenous infusion and intubation by ambulance staff in the anaesthetic room) and funding.[101,102] The matter of consent was again raised at the Linkman Conference in 1990 when new consent forms were introduced and various alternative procedures were discussed.[103]

The deficiencies in the trauma services in the United Kingdom came to a head after the publication in 1987 of the report of the Confidential Enquiry into Perioperative Deaths (CEPOD), an investigation which had developed out of the original study sponsored by the Association of Anaesthetists into mortality associated with anaesthesia which reported in 1982. The report showed that a significant number of trauma cases died in hospital from avoidable causes because of lack of resources in the hospitals to which they were taken, and because very often they had been managed by inexperienced staff;[71,104] moreover the trauma services of the United Kingdom, in comparison with those in parts of the United States and continental Europe, had been under severe criticism for some time from informed opinion both in the United Kingdom and abroad.[90] Trunkey, a prominent American trauma surgeon (see below) was quoted in 1991 as stating that the system in the United Kingdom was "disorganised, fragmented and producing a universally bad outcome".[71]

The Royal College of Surgeons of England (RCS) took up the challenge and appointed a Working Party on "The management of patients with major injuries", on which the then Faculty of Anaesthetists was represented by Peter Baskett. The RCS Working Party reported in November 1988.[90] A retrospective study of 1,000 consecutive trauma deaths in eleven Coroners' districts in England and Wales had been conducted. This detailed analysis was mainly concerned with the fate of 514 patients who reached hospital alive rather than the 486 who died at the accident site or during transport, but the number of casualties who died before reaching hospital varied considerably between districts. The inference was that it was likely that differing standards of prehospital care was a factor.[71,90] A prior study conducted on behalf of the Medical Commission on Accident Prevention had postulated that properly organised and delivered prehospital care had "scope for preventing something of the order of 20% of the total RTAs (road traffic accident) deaths.[105]

The RCS working party report in 1988 recommended that (except in special cases such as the trapped casualty when the assistance of a medical practitioner would be required) that:-

> *"Prehospital care should be provided by specially trained ambulancemen. In addition to a higher level of therapeutic skills they should be trained in injury severity assessment in order that patients can be conveyed to appropriate hospitals. There should be increased medical involvement in the organisation and training of the ambulance service."*[90]

There has been improvement in pre-hospital care and transport since the RCS Working Party Report in 1988.[90] An increasing number of dedicated paramedical emergency ambulances can be seen (and heard) in the towns and on the roads in the United Kingdom, and the Chief Medical Officer at the DH advised Ambulance Authorities that every front-line ambulance responding to emergencies should have a paramedic as a member of the team by the end of 1995, (the recommendation that paramedics should be trained and separate emergency front line ambulances provided was made at a Department of Health conference on the ambulance services in 1980 at which both the Association and the Faculty of Anaesthetists were represented!).[99] Training standards for all ambulance personnel and advanced training for paramedics have been improved under a National Health Service Training Authority and a minimum national curriculum has been introduced (Baskett P J F personal communication, 1994). Provision is by no means perfect yet however![72,73,106]

> *"Several [Health] Authorities now have helicopters (available to them) although cover is sporadic. Many have a combined operation with the Police.... There are few purely medically dedicated helicopters outside London*[107] *but a lot of [Health] Authorities are considering this. Clearly cost is the main deterrent. The Defence Services do respond to services inland (i.e. other than air-sea rescue)*[108] *but this is run strictly on a financial basis and the hospital has to pay for this service." (Baskett P J F personal communication, 1994)*

Such are the difficulties encountered in the peculiarly divisive "purchaser-provider" culture which has been instituted in the peripheral provision of public services in the United Kingdom in the last decade (see below)!

The care of traumatic casualties within hospitals in the United Kingdom had not been satisfactory throughout the existence of the National Health Service. The new specialty of Accident and Emergency (A & E) medicine was created after the Bruce Report of 1971.[71,90] The purpose was for the A & E Consultants to take over "Accident and Emergency" (formerly "Casualty") Departments in General Hospitals from the nominal supervision of orthopaedic surgeons, and to provide Consultant supervision for junior staff who had largely been left to their own devices.[71,90] Anaesthetists became eligible for appointments as Accident and Emergency Consultants alongside surgeons and physicians in 1978, and a four year multidisciplinary training was recognised by the Royal College of Physicians.[90,109,110]

The appointment of Consultants to A & E Departments improved the immediate resuscitation and care of patients but there were and are difficulties. First there was often (and to some extent still is) only one A & E Consultant to each A & E Department. This situation leaves juniors unsupervised out of hours particularly at night; secondly, medical politics of the interface between the A & E Departments and the bed owning specialists, the frequent need for a multidisciplinary co-operation and the difficulty of "squeezing" traumatic accident patients into routine operating lists led (and regrettably sometimes still leads) to less than optimum care for the trauma patient, and on occasion, to unnecessary death. These factors were highlighted by the report of the CEPOD investigation in 1987,[104] and led to the publication of the RCS Report on the management of patients with major injuries in 1988, to which reference has already been made.[90] The RCS Report[90] made recommendations for improved staffing and facilities for the A & E Departments in District General Hospitals. These would continue to handle the majority of patients, and multidisciplinary Trauma Centres (the RCS Report suggested 25 in the United Kingdom,[90] others believe that 8 would suffice if helicopters were used)[111] would deal specifically with the estimated 0.5% of multiple trauma patients in addition to less severely locally injured patients in an associated A & E unit.[90] Trauma centres as established in some parts of the United States were particularly advocated; they had been shown to improve the outcome of multiple injured trauma cases.[112,113] It may be noted that, even in the USA, provision of Trauma Centres was not yet fully established nationwide in 1988.[114] It is of historical interest that what was in its day a forerunner of the Trauma Centre concept was founded in the United Kingdom in 1941 by private and public subscription before the British National Health Service was inaugurated in 1948. This was the Birmingham Accident Hospital conceived to cope with major injuries in the industrial area.[71,90] This hospital became world famous and did some magnificent pioneer work in the fifties and sixties. This included the outstanding contribution of the Consultant Anaesthetist Leslie J Wolfson[115] on the management of massive haemorrhage and burns.[116] It is unfortunate that administrative failure to ally the institution closely with a major hospital as specialisation developed, and lack of funding, has led to a decline in the importance of the Birmingham Accident Hospital and an opportunity to create a major trauma centre was lost.[71,90] One experimental Trauma Centre has been funded by the NHS at the North Staffordshire Royal Infirmary since the publication of the RCS Report in 1988.[71,117]

Improvements in the management of trauma in District Hospital A and E Departments have been brought about, first, by the concentrated programme of training based on the Advanced Trauma Life Support (ATLS) course. This was initiated by the Royal College of Surgeons of England, and, by the end of 1992, over 2,000 medical practitioners had attended including many anaesthetists;[117,118] secondly by the concept of developing trauma teams to give immediate care to patients when they arrive in the A & E Department,[106] and thirdly by adopting the policy recommended by the Association of Anaesthetists of setting aside a dedicated 24 hour emergency operating theatre in many hospitals.[90,119]

The Association of Anaesthetists published a guidance booklet on "The Role of the Anaesthetist in the Emergency Service" in 1991.[120] This was well received at the Linkman conference later that year, although there was concern about manpower cover for all the responsibilities which have to be undertaken by anaesthetists in the modern hospital with the limited number of staff available.[121]

The government response to the RCS Report[90] was described as "half-hearted" in an Editorial in the *British Journal of Anaesthesia* in 1990.[122] There have been some improvements in the management of medical emergencies and training in the United Kingdom in the last few years, but much more still needs to be done in the field of prevention, as well as in improving facilities for clinical care when accidents do occur, if unnecessary deaths are to be avoided.[71,90,122]. Peter Baskett writing in 1990 described the development of the British Trauma Care as "a tale of woe".[71] He was certainly correct at that time but in 1994 he wrote more optimistically:-

> "The ATLS courses have done much to help matters and I am hopeful that the Department (of Health) will move forward in the next few years. They always do it very slowly but I think that we will get there in the end." (Baskett P J F, personal communication 1994).

Let us hope that he is right!

O'Kelly and Westaby[111] have certainly demonstrated that the provision of Trauma Centres throughout the United Kingdom could be a "relatively efficient use of resources" in the new "cost effective" NHS. Medical care for the casualties of major incidents and disasters requires careful planning in advance and specialised clinical care both at the accident site and in the hospital. British anaesthetists have been intimately concerned with all these aspects.[122] The United Kingdom had its fair share of disasters in the eighties![3,123] They included IRA (Irish Republican Army) and Protestant paramilitary terrorist incidents both in Northern Ireland and on the mainland, urban mob violence at Tottenham and elsewhere, the aircraft fire on the ground at Manchester, the Bradford City Football Club fire, the Abbeystead Pumping Station explosion, the Hungerford massacre, when a gunman ran amok, the Kings Cross underground fire, and the Lockerbie and M1 motorway air crashes.[3,124] Anaesthetists have played an important part inside and outside hospital in these incidents. Sixteen of the eighteen medical practitioners who attended on site at the Moorgate Underground disaster in 1976 were anaesthetists.[96] Three anaesthetists have been awarded Pask certificates for gallantry at the scene of disasters (Chapter 7). Hospitals in the United Kingdom have invariably responded well to a sudden influx of casualties from major accidents or disasters, but it can not be said that advance major incident plans have always functioned with effortless efficiency, improvisation has often been required; in particular communication between the incident site and the hospital has often been difficult.[124] It would seem that, with the development of trained paramedical emergency ambulance crews, on site medical and nursing teams sent out from A & E departments have often proved to be ineffective or redundant;[124] but, of course, medical expertise will still be required in certain circumstances, as when there is a trapped casualty.

Clinical Anaesthesia 1983-1992

The principle developments in this period were in the pharmacology of intravenous anaesthetics and competitive neuromuscular blocking agents, new initiatives in the control of postoperative pain, concern with the safety of the patient under anaesthesia reflected in developments in the field of monitoring, and, last but not least, the introduction of the amazing Laryngeal Mask Airway (LMA).

Short acting intravenous agents. Propofol (di-isopropl phenol), which had been withdrawn in its original formulation with cremophor EL, was reintroduced in 1983 as an aqueous emulsion. It rapidly became popular and widely accepted as an induction agent (particularly for day surgery), for continuous infusion for the maintenance of anaesthesia, for sedation in the intensive care unit, and for the control of convulsive states.[125-127]

Volatile agents. Desflurane (I-653, a fluorinated methyl ethyl ether) originally developed in the United States by Eger[128] was introduced into British practice in 1991. It has a low boiling point (23.5°C) and requires a special electrically heated vaporiser, but has not been demonstrated to have hepatic or renal effects and provides a rapid recovery because of its low solubility. The rapid recovery from its effects means that it has considerable potential, particularly in day surgery.[129,130] Sevoflurane (a fluorinated isopropyl ether) provides rapid induction and recovery and can be vaporised by standard techniques (B.P.58.5°) but it is less stable in soda lime than other agents and has a significant rate of breakdown in the body.[129]

New neuromuscular blocking agents. Atracurium and vecuronium were introduced into United Kingdom practice in 1983 and have since been widely accepted. The former was particularly welcome because of its reliable degradation by the Hofmann effect, and neither is cumulative or has major cardiovascular effects.[131,132] Later the short acting competitive blocker mivacurium and the long acting drugs doxacurium and pipecurium have been on trial.[132]

Postoperative pain is a subject which had been of concern to anaesthetists over many years,[133,134] but a cautious approach, related to concern over possible drug induced respiratory depression and supervision in general wards, and the fact that, in most circumstances, the condition was self limiting, had led to the subject being neglected.[134-136] Reports from patients in the lay and professional press,[136] the advent of new methods such as the extradural and intrathecal injection of long acting local anaesthetic agents and the introduction of the extradural and intradural injection of opioids, and patient controlled analgesia (PCA), led to renewed interest in the eighties,[134-138] A joint working party of the Royal College of Surgeons of England and the newly independent (now Royal) College of Anaesthetists, chaired by Alastair Spence (later President of the anaesthetists' college 1991-1994) issued an important report in 1990.[139] This began by stating bluntly:-

"The treatment of pain after surgery in British hospitals has been inadequate and has not advanced significantly for several years. This report describes the background to this persistent failure and makes recommendations to improve the situation."[139]

The report recognised, as others had done, that though efficacious, many of the newer methods (for example the administration of opioids by spinal techniques and PCA) had dangers or might not be used efficiently if they were not properly managed or monitored;[136,139,140] the value of "High Dependency Units" (HDU) where high risk patients could be supervised postoperatively and, *inter alia,* postoperative pain could be safely controlled by the newer methods, was recognised,[139,141] but it was emphasised that, for the majority of postoperative cases, these techniques could be adequately supervised in ordinary surgical wards provided nursing personnel were properly trained and educated, and essential monitoring equipment was provided.[139]

The establishment of properly resourced Acute Pain Services to oversee the use of techniques for the relief of pain throughout each hospital was also recommended.[139,142] The Association of Anaesthetists issued booklets on "Immediate Postanaesthetic Recovery" and "High Dependency Units - Acute Care in the Future" in 1985 (revised 1993) and 1991 respectively. The recommendations made by the various working parties of anaesthetists and surgeons have been acted upon and there has been general improvement in the management of postoperative pain in the United Kingdom, but this is by no means universal.

Monitoring during anaesthesia and afterwards in the recovery period had already attracted the attention of anaesthetists in the nineteen seventies but, with renewed interest in auditing mortality and morbidity, and the increasing cost of litigation following anaesthetic accidents, it became a prominent issue during the eighties.[143] It was fortunate that by the end of the decade the improved sophistication and reliability of the available monitors enabled the well trained and conscientious anaesthetist to improve greatly the safety of patients under anaesthesia.[143,144]

The Dutch were first in the field of establishing statutory requirements for monitoring in 1978.[143] It was, however, the publication of a report in the *Journal of the American Medical Association* by the Harvard Medical School of Boston, USA in 1986 detailing "specific, detailed mandatory standards for minimum patient monitoring during anaesthesia", which had been devised as part of their safety and risk management policies, which attracted the attention of anaesthetically developed countries.[143,146] These standards were quickly endorsed by the American Society of Anesthesiologists and have subsequently been modified to cover advances in technology. Several states in the USA have now adopted specified standard monitoring as a legal requirement. A reduction in malpractice suits against anesthesiologists in the USA and premiums for insurance for anaesthetists has followed these initiatives. Canadian anaesthetists adopted a similar policy with similar results.[143] Standard monitoring requirements have also been established in Continental Europe and Australia.[145]

The Faculty of Anaesthetists in 1987 specified a list of monitoring facilities which should be available at every location where anaesthesia was administered or where patients were recovered. This was, however, after some reluctance on the part of a minority of Board Members about the possible legal implications (personal recollection). These requirements became one of the factors taken into account before a hospital is recognised for the training of candidates for the Fellowship of the Faculty (now Royal College) of Anaesthetists (FFARCS now FRCA). The list has been updated in the light of subsequent developments;[145,147] it makes a marked contrast to the modest suggestions made in the original 1982 report on "Mortality Associated with Anaesthesia" commissioned by the Association of Anaesthetists (Chapter 8)!

The two principal monitoring techniques which became available to clinical anaesthetists in the nineteen eighties as the result of amazing progress in technical electronics, were capnography and pulse oximetry. These two techniques together with the developments of the sixties and seventies have made a very significant contribution to the safety of anaesthesia.[148]

The values at which auditory alarms sound are often set well above or below levels at which harm can come to the patient; this can be irritating to both surgeon and anaesthetist, but it generally provides a wide margin of safety for the patient and encourages a high standard of practice!

Safety in anaesthetic practice cannot be bought by the mere provision of monitors however. Monitors have to be observed and interpreted and the loop closed by necessary action. Many other factors are involved. These include careful patient assessment, appropriate selection of trainees for the specialty of anaesthesia, adequate basic and continued training, equipment checks, continuous supervision of the patient both in the operating theatre and the recovery room, audit and the detection of fatigue and decreased professional competence. The subject was reviewed in 1992 in a chapter by Professor A P (Tony) Adams of Guy's Hospital, London.[143] Monitoring the depth of anaesthesia to avoid awareness remains a problem.[149]

The laryngeal mask airway (LMA) was first described in 1983 by A I J (Archie) Brain, (then of the Royal London Hospital),[150] and, after painstaking development,[151] it was released commercially in the United Kingdom in 1989.[152] It is probably the most outstanding development in the techniques of administering inhalation anaesthesia since the introduction of wide bore tracheal anaesthesia in the nineteen twenties.[153] The LMA provides an acceptable secure airway for routine anaesthesia in adults and children without occupying the hands of the anaesthetist with a facemask, and it may also be used with controlled ventilation.[154] Its use with the potentially full stomach is controversial,[155] except perhaps, in circumstances when intubation has not proved to be possible, as may be the situation in a case of Caesarean section.[156,157] It has also been demonstrated in a multicentre trial "that the laryngeal mask airway offers advantages over other methods of airway ventilation management, such as bag-valve-mask or mouth-to-mouth methods," for use by ward nurses who have been trained in its use, for resuscitating patients with cardiac arrest.[158]

The LMA has proved to be remarkably popular amongst anaesthetists in the United Kingdom where it has been thoroughly evaluated (there were 17 citations in volume 44 of *Anaesthesia* in 1989 and 47 in volume 48 in 1993); even the usual administrative protests in the British NHS concerning "the cost" have not inhibited its widespread adoption. The LMA was welcomed and evaluated in Canada in 1990[157] The first anaesthetic with an LMA in Australia was administered (personally by the present writer) in 1989, and the device has become widely accepted in that country since its commercial release in 1991 (personal communications and *Anaesthesia and Intensive Care,* volumes 19 and 20, 1991 and 1992).[159] The LMA received Food and Drug Administration approval for use in the United States of America in August 1991.[160] A comprehensive review article in *Anesthesiology* in July 1993 concluded, "The preliminary experience gained with this device in Europe and Australia suggests that it may also transform contemporary anaesthetic practice in the United States."[161]

Archie Brain was awarded a Pask Certificate of Honour by the Association of Anaesthetists in 1992,[162] and at the 1995 Annual General Meeting he was awarded the Magill gold medal for innovation. He certainly deserves these honours.

The National Health Service 1983-1992

The NHS underwent two further reorganisations in the period 1983-1992. They finally brought to an end the old concept of a tripartite management of a hospital by a Committee of Consultants, a Hospital Secretary or House Governor, who organised domestic services, and a Matron responsible for the organisation of nursing. The 1982 reorganisation proved to be very unsatisfactory in practice (Chapter 8). Theoretically it was the expressed intention that decisions on operational matters should be devolved to Districts and Units (hospitals), but there were many disputes about responsibility for particular areas between administrators at Region, District and Unit levels, with a result that administrative chaos ensued. The consensus system and management team of unit administrator, nurse and consultant survived, as did the medical advisory machinery and the District Health Authorities with professional, trade union and local authority representation, but it became very difficult to make meaningful progress on any matter against a background of increasing financial restriction. It was a most unhappy period. The relationship between the medical profession and the administration was at best uneasy, and at worst confrontational. The administrators were charged with the absolute priority of cutting costs by various initiatives involving making "efficiency savings"; clinical activity was not greatly curtailed however except covertly by the occasional subterfuge of closing a ward for "redecoration" or the failure to commission new buildings, and delay in filling staff vacancies. The medical and nursing professions were however, painfully aware of deterioration in maintenance and in the efficiency of support services. The difficulties were aggravated by the mandatory policy of seeking cost and corner-cutting outside tenders for activities such as domestic cleaning and laundry. The consequences of all this was a further deterioration in professional morale.[2-4,163,164]

There is no doubt that a radical revision of the organisation and administration of the NHS was necessary, but the changes that have been made have been instituted without meaningful consultation with the medical profession or its leaders as a whole.[3] Those decisions have had far reaching effects which have not always, or arguably overall, been beneficial to the NHS!

The perception of Government in 1983 was that reorganisation of the administrative structure on businesslike commercial lines might result in efficiency savings which would reduce the need for ever increasing provision for an NHS which was to remain "free at the point of use". The Management Inquiry, under the Chairmanship of (Sir) E R Griffiths[165,166] was consequently commissioned in February 1983. Griffiths was at that time the Managing Director of the Sainsbury plc supermarket chain.[2,3] The sequence of events which led to two further reorganisations in the management of the NHS in 1984 and 1991 was thus begun. The consequent organisational changes have led to clinicians responding by taking on a management role at the peripheral operational interface with patient care in the form of Clinical Directorates and as individuals as Medical Directors of Hospital Trusts, but hospital medical specialists have been virtually excluded from a collective strategic, executive or advisory role in the way hospitals or the NHS are managed, or in the strategic planning of the NHS, in favour of lay managers.[2-4,163,164] This probably need not have been the case if there had been more flexibility on the part of politicians, the medical profession and lay administrators.

The Griffiths Report and the 1984 reorganisation. Roy Griffiths was assisted in his deliberations by two businessmen and a former chairman of a Regional Health Authority.[2-7] We are told that:-

"Griffiths began his task knowing little about the structure and operations of the NHS. He had relatives who worked in the service and their experience led him to start with a strong conviction that [general] management could succeed if it had not only the respect of the professions but also their active participation."[2]

The last sentence in this passage is important. Griffiths recognised that doctors should be "looked upon as the natural managers".[3,165-167] There is little doubt that Griffiths envisaged including more doctors in direct line management in the NHS at all levels than was subsequently the case after the 1984 reorganisation, based on his report, was implemented by the Government.[2-3,163-164,167,168]

Griffiths reported in October 1983 in the format of an admirably brief letter;[165-166] indeed some said "too brief" as it concentrated to a large extent only on the management of the acute hospital services. Brief though the document was the proposals contained in the document were certainly revolutionary so far as the NHS was concerned. The report was strategic rather than tactical however. It defined a general plan but did not consider the details of its implementation. It advised that the Regional, District and Unit structure should be retained but recommended the end of the consensus principle, and the appointment of General Managers with executive responsibility at all three levels. It proposed that the line of management should be continued to an NHS Management Board responsible for the leadership and control of the organisation of the NHS; this would be separate from a strategic and politically orientated Health Service Supervisory Board. Responsibility for all day-to-day decisions in the acute service was to be in the hands of the General Managers at Unit level. There were also to be delegated management budgets and performance targets and reviews. Griffiths also emphasised his belief in the importance of the closer involvement of medical clinicians in management.[2-4,163,164-168]

The idea of a General Manager who would be responsible for the whole organisation of which he was in charge was not a new one prior to or since the inauguration of the NHS. Medical Superintendents (who often had clinical responsibility as well and ran hospitals with the aid of lay Secretaries) were a feature of the administration of Local Authority hospitals before the NHS. Some Medical Superintendents continued in this role into the early days of the NHS[168] despite the general adoption of the voluntary hospital patterns of Hospital Secretary or House Governor working in conjunction with the Consultant Medical Staff Committee, with the Matron responsible for nursing. Medical Superintendents survived particularly in mental hospitals, but also in some general hospitals formerly belonging to municipal authorities such as the London County Council (LCC). The Report of the BMA Medical Services Review Committee in 1962, chaired by Sir Arthur (later Lord) Porritt also proposed a medically qualified Chief Officer at "Area" (District) level.[169] Porritt was, however, not in favour of the concept of the "hierarchical system of staffing hospitals" by the appointment of Medical Superintendents. He believed that "the influence of the Hospital Medical Committee [had] declined because it had not been given the status enjoyed before the NHS, and he favoured the traditional voluntary hospital system, albeit strengthened by an elected member of the Consultant staff to liaise with the Hospital Secretary or House Governor in conducting day to day administration.[169]

The response of the BMA Central Committee for Hospital Medical Services (CCHMS) to the Griffiths Report was positive but cautious to both the concept of general management and devolved managerial budgeting.[166] There was, however, general agreement that the period allowed for consultation was too short (25 October 1983 to 9 January 1984) and that pilot schemes should be conducted and evaluated before considering the general adoption of the proposals. The debate of the CCHMS Committee, which was chaired by Maurice Burrows (later President of the Association of Anaesthetists, 1988-1990). Several of the participants were past or contemporary Members of Council of the Association of Anaesthetists; they included Professor J P Payne, Margaret Heath and Brian Lewis.[166]

The 1984 Reorganisation

The implementation of the Griffiths proposals did not require legislation because it was proposed that the existing administrative tiers of the NHS structure were to survive intact. The Conservative administration were in a strong position having won a landslide victory in the General Election of June 1983. The aggressive ministerial team (Norman Fowler as Secretary of State for Health and Social Security with Kenneth Clarke as Minister for Health) were determined to go ahead with the proposals after the brief period of consultation whatever the opinions of those who were normally consulted.[3] The circular in implementation was published in June 1984.[170]

The policy of general management recommended by Griffiths represented a fundamental political change in the organisation of the NHS, from an administered service to a managed service with central control. It is of interest that the document "Patients First"[171] issued by the Conservative Government when it took Office in 1979, had actually rejected the concept of general management and restated the policy of Aneurin Bevan at the inception of the NHS:-

"It is doctors, dentists and nurses and their colleagues in the other health professions who provide the care and cure of patients and promote the health of the people. It is the purpose of management to support them in giving that service."[2-4,171]

More conservative members of the medical profession saw the Griffiths proposals as a threat to the cherished clinical freedom to treat patients in the way that they considered best. Many doctors welcomed the concept of general management however, but they felt that if general managers were to be appointed they should be medically qualified and drawn from the ranks of the clinicians.

The Griffiths report also proposed other important new initiatives; these were specifically the holding of budgets by clinicians and emphasis on accountability and cost effectiveness. The 1984 reorganisation could have been a success and might have led to a happier service than has resulted from its successor in 1991 with its complicated purchaser-provider split (see below) but, whatever Griffiths intended with respect of involvement of medical clinicians in management, the report was, in the event, a step on the road to the domination of the NHS by nonmedical General Managers (later redesignated "Chief Executives") and the imposition of an overriding market philosophy on a caring service. Competition between hospitals was to replace cooperation.[168]

The failure of the 1984 reorganisation to attract clinicians into general management originated in the decision to impose central control on the way the general management posts at all levels were appointed, and in the nature of the short-term contracts which were offered. The implementing circular for the 1984 reforms set a target for the process of completing the appointments of general managers by 1985. Health Authority Chairmen were charged with "identifying" preferred candidates but the final decision to appoint was to be taken by the Ministers and civil servants at the DHSS. It seems clear that the political objective was to attempt to ensure that the appointment of a reasonable mix of professionals (doctors and nurses) and outsiders (including businessmen, industrialists and retired Army Officers). It was also the first time in the history of the NHS that short-term contracts (usually for three years) with "individual performance review" before renewal, and pay increments related to performance, were introduced for managers. These conditions of employment were stipulated despite the fact that Griffiths had warned against expecting rapid results from the general management revolution.[172] Attempts were made to encourage doctors to become general managers by making special provision for them to be employed part-time in management and return to their clinical posts at the end of their management contracts. There are however real difficulties about the return of clinicians to whole-time consultant practice after even a short term secondment to management which have never been resolved.[173] Management is a challenging task and doctors as a profession have a strong work ethic and readily become overcommitted;[174] even if they intend to work part-time they often find that a progressive reduction in their clinical commitment is necessary, and meanwhile the technical developments in their specialty can easily pass them by; consequently return to full-time clinical employment becomes difficult. There is, however, credence for the argument for "doctors who have had clinical experience and are motivated to move into administration to do so [permanently] and cut their clinical ties altogether"[175] at any level of management other than that of the Clinical Directorate.

The writer believes that it is quite probable that, if long term General Manager appointments for medical clinicians had been properly promoted and attractively financed in 1984, a sufficient number of clinicians might have been attracted by the challenge to make the change to management during the second half of their careers; as a consequence the direction of the NHS might even now be "safe in their hands" and the further upheaval of the 1991 reorganisation introducing the internal market might well have been avoided. Certainly those relatively few clinicians who have been appointed to senior general management or as Health Authority Chairmen in the NHS have been outstandingly successful; for example Professor Cyril Chantler[167] (Professor of Paediatric Pathology and Unit General Manager at Guy's Hospital, London) and Maurice Burrows (President of the Association of Anaesthetists 1988-1990 and Chairman of the Wirral Hospital NHS Trust). Clinicians are intelligent and educated individuals with all the qualities necessary to be good managers who, of necessity, already have considerable practical experience of management by the time that they have had several years experience as clinical consultants,[167] and "at the end of the day" it is not difficult to learn the "language of management" with which the lay managers seek to mystify their activities "at this moment in time"![176] It is a myth put about by lay administrators,[4,164] and to a lesser extent by administrative nurses,[177] who may feel threatened,[178] that doctors do not have the skills to manage. Experience has suggested, in fact, that at the start of general management development (1986) "many managers did not have management skills" either. Both doctors and managers had much to learn![178,179]

Neither administration nor management are ends in themselves. Doctors make good managers because they are both experienced in communicating with people and are also aware of the minutiae of the technicalities and difficulties of caring and treating individual patients.[180-182] It is certainly easier for a doctor to become an effective manager than it is for a manager to become a clinician! The best combination in medical management is for a doctor with clinical experience and some additional training to be assisted by a competent business manager.

In the event, and despite intervention from the centre in an attempt to block in-house appointments, approximately 60% of the General Managers appointed as a result of the 1984 reorganisation had previously been hospital administrators. This was probably partly because of their perceived competence and knowledge of the NHS, but also because of lack of competition from the clinical professions or from candidates outside the service, and because of the low salaries and absence of fringe benefits in comparison with the private sector and the short fixed term conditions of the contracts which were on offer.[2,164] The position in 1986, after most of the appointments had been made, was that at Regional level, amongst 14 General Managers there were nine former NHS administrators, one doctor (a former Regional Medical Officer), one nurse (a former Regional Nursing Officer) and three appointments from outside the NHS; amongst 191 District General Managers, 132 (69%) had been NHS administrators, 16 (8.5%) were doctors, 5 (2.5%) were nurses and there were 36 (19%) appointments from outside the NHS. The latter were mostly businessmen, who were either retired or approaching retirement, or retired members of the armed forces, for whom no doubt, the extra cash would be a useful addition to their pensions. Eight hundred and sixteen Unit General Managers were appointed; 496 (60.5%) were former NHS administrators, 127 (15.5%) were doctors, 77 (9.5%) were nurses and 96 (12%) came from outside the NHS.[2,164] There had been a 5% turnover of general managers by 1987.[164] This was particularly amongst individuals, including those from the armed services, who had been appointed from outside the NHS. This circumstance was probably partly because of the culture shock of joining and trying to organise the (to them) strange world of the NHS, or because of the difficulties of the resource constraints of the period. Over 34% of those who had joined the NHS from outside had left by 1989 in contrast to 17% of those who had been previously employed by the service; amongst the latter must be counted a number of doctors, most of whom were part time, either because of disillusionment, or had resigned on "matters of principle" usually concerned with strained resources.[2]

The successes and failures of the 1984 reorganisation. The 1984 reorganisation could have been a success given more careful planning, more consideration for the workforce, and ultimately more time to develop its potential. It established a direct line of management from a quasi-independent Management Board in the DHSS through Regional and District to Unit, with accountable General Managers at all levels. Unit General Managers were in theory solely responsible for the activities of all personnel within their hospital, whether these activities were in response to initiatives originated by the NHS Management Board, or from local organisation or operational management.

Many General Managers, as noted above, were experienced as NHS administrators in the consensus period (1974-1984) when decisions were collective, but not as managers when decisions had to be theirs and theirs alone. The most successful were those who realised early on that, in the NHS, "management is essentially about persuasion rather than command," and that when a decision has to be made it "will usually be carried through as long as those who have to implement it have been consulted. Leadership implies that those that are led are prepared [in both senses of the word] to follow".[178] Sadly before both the 1984 and 1991 reorganisations these elementary precepts were ignored centrally, and are still (1998) being ignored at operational level, with unfortunate results on the morale of the medical profession. It should not be forgotten that the NHS is unlike the usual commercial organisation in the UK in which the more senior individuals are remote from those serving on the shop floor; in the NHS the senior professionals give direct care to patients throughout their careers.

The preparations for the 1984 reorganisation provided the opportunity for the establishment of the National Health Service Training Authority in 1983 to train NHS managers. It also initiated the development of much needed information on computer technology with which reasonably accurate data on cost and outcome could be deduced based on the 1982 report of the committee of Mrs Edith Korner, Vice Chairman of the South Western Health Authority.[2] It was, however, unfortunate that, though information policy was dictated by the Management Board of the DHSS, the exact aims of the initiative were not well defined, nor was the outcome adequately monitored. Many Authority Chairmen and Chief Executives were not conversant with computer technology and called in management consultants at great expense who had an exaggerated concept of the potential requirements. Disparate and elaborate systems were devised which were incompatible and later became white elephants and had had to be scrapped.[2] The Wessex Health Authority spent twenty million pounds on management consultants and hardware which eventually had to be written off;[183,184] nonetheless the principle of gathering and assessing information was established as was the concept of attempting to obtain "value for money" with a budget based on available information. The systems for gathering information were not well managed and often produced inaccurate results which were hotly disputed, particularly with regard to "performance indicators" such as bed occupancy, average stay in hospital, and return visits to outpatients.[2-4]

There were also difficulties at the centre of the NHS organisation. Griffiths, writing in 1992, confirmed his opinion that the proposals of the Supervisory Board to establish a strategic policy, and a separate Management Board to control day to day operations were "absolutely correct in principle but half-hearted in their implementation. Major policy issues were left uncovered and there was no attempt to establish objectives at the centre".[185] He believed that the first priority should have been "to establish responsibility at local level, and a management structure capable of delivering the tasks of the hospital" and that "systems information and financial management would follow and support the responsibilities but would be clearly secondary to that process".[185] The course adopted in practice was the reverse.

General Managers were given a great deal of latitude in devising the management structures for their units. Some perpetuated the 1982 arrangements even to the extent of retaining a consensus team; others set up a structure which controlled all personnel, including nurses, directly without the intermediate tiers, but retained the Medical Advisory Committee, some enterprising schemes were, however, initiated by a few hospitals in this period which saw the start of the Clinical Directorate at Unit level, including management of devolved budgets with the medical Consultants as Clinical Directors.[164] Prominent amongst these was the major trial at Guy's Hospital, London[179] and the successful schemes managed by anaesthetists such as those of Robert Buckland at the Royal Hampshire County Hospital, Winchester, who supervised a Directorate which included anaesthesia, intensive care, the day surgery unit and the operating theatre,[180] and Ann Naylor (Member of Council of the Association of Anaesthetists 1994) who was in charge of operating theatres at Basildon, Essex after 1986.[181]

These interesting schemes predated the centrally initiated and funded experimental Resource Management Initiative (RMI) introduced in 1986 in trial units. The schemes at Guy's (the so-called "NHS Flagship") and at Winchester were incorporated into the RMI and the others were at the Freeman Hospital, Newcastle upon Tyne, Birkenhead, and Boston, Lincolnshire. There had been an earlier attempt to introduce pilot clinical budgeting schemes at 14 sites in 1983 shortly after the publication of the Griffiths Report. These schemes included specialty budgets and ward budgets administered by nurses, but they often failed because of unreliable and inaccurate information technology (manual ball point pen collection of data instead of by computers). They frequently became a tiresome irrelevance producing irritating theoretical disputes between nurses and medical clinicians, and between nurses with regard to "whose budget" a particular item of equipment should be debited!

The trial 1986 RMI was different. It was based on a defined Clinical Directorate system and was centrally funded by the DHSS chiefly for the provision of administrative back up and computer technology, ultimately to a sum that was more than double that estimated by the DHSS (in the case of Guy's Hospital alone £2.6 million). The BMA and the Royal Colleges and their Faculties lent their support to RMI through the Joint Consultants' Committee (JCC) and the medical profession was promised that the results of RMI would be fully evaluated by the Health Economics Research Group from Brunel University and modified if necessary before RMI was introduced into other areas of the NHS. This promise was not kept. The aims of RMI were to introduce effective budgeting, to develop and maintain a database with diagnostic and therapeutic coding, to establish a management system for recording resources used in treating patients, and to implement effective methods of nurse management.[3]

It should be noted that the most successful clinical directorates are those where, firstly, every medical Clinical Director in a hospital unit is a member of a Hospital Management Board "responsible for the finances and other resources of the unit";[179,180] secondly the medical Clinical Director controls the work and conditions of service of all the personnel of the Directorate including nurses and, in the case of operating theatres, the Operating Department Assistants;[180,181] and thirdly, and most important, the nonmedical Business Manager is directly responsible to the Clinical Director, and not perceived as a "management spy" within the Directorate.[180] It is of particular interest that the concept of having an administrator within a Department of Anaesthesia was successfully pioneered by the Department at the University Hospital of Wales as early as 1981 as part of an experimental programme financed by the DHSS.[182] The final important condition is that there must be adequate administrative secretarial assistance of suitable grades.[178,180] These essential conditions should be regarded as mandatory before an appointment as a Clinical Director is accepted by a member of the medical staff. It is a source of regret that such a situation has not been achieved on far too many occasions and, as a consequence, many Clinical Directors have found that "a major frustration for the doctor in management is the feeling that responsibility has been transferred without adequate authority for fulfilment".[178]

Sources of conflict. The way the 1984 reorganisation was implemented soon led to conflict between the established Civil Servants and the Department of Health, and Victor Paige who had been appointed to head the Management Board. Victor Paige had been a very distinguished Chairman first of the Port of London Authority and then of the National Freight Corporation. He had expected to be left alone to manage the NHS, whereas the Civil Servants were determined to influence his decisions in the light of political policy. Paige resigned abruptly in June 1986. The Board was reconstituted with the Minister of Health as Chairman, (Sir) Leonard Peach (formerly Personnel Director of the business machine company IBM) as Chief Executive, and Sir Roy Griffiths as Vice Chairman.[2,3]

Peach established the system of annual targets and individual personal review for General Managers. The reviews were conducted by the General Manager in the next tier above (Unit by District, District by Region and Region by the Management Board Chief Executive) thus a direct line of management was set up which was parallel to the pre-existing NHS route through the Chairmen and the District Health Authorities. The latter were still in being after 1984 with their broad but appointed membership including local authority representatives, hospital doctors, general practitioners, nurses and the consumer orientated Community Health Councils Medical Advisory Committees were also still active. The Unit General Manager's task was not easy as he was responsible to the centre through the Regional General Manager, through his Chairman who had direct links via the Regional Board to the DHSS, as well as to the District Health Authority with its disparate and often contending vested interests. The main concern of a Unit General Manager was, however, to meet the efficiency and performance targets set for his unit within his budget in order that he could keep his job after the next individual personal review.[2-4,164] Performance initiatives included supplying information on activity to Region which in turn could use the figures to compare the performance of his unit with others and set targets for the following year.[2-4]

Griffiths (1992)[185] states:-

"So by the end of 1987 .... we saw General Managers in position accountable for the performance of their organisation; management systems were introduced with performance standards and performance reviews. There was high emphasis on the improvement in service. Authorities had in many cases reorganised to make their services more responsive and to take responsibility for quality assurance. There were significant trials of management budgeting or resource management of resources through budgeting responsibility against agreed workloads and some improvement to information systems."[185]

This is a reasonable description of the position in the more advanced post-Griffiths Units where pioneer Clinical Directorate schemes had been introduced, but they were a minority. It must be remembered that the Resource Management Initiative and similar schemes had yet to be evaluated and generally adopted. The more usual picture of the General Manager, seen through the eyes of the medical staff, was that of an individual endowed with the power to take executive decisions without reference to the medical staff or anyone else, who had been installed to run the unit under "overwhelming pressures to conform to and accept a narrow finance-driven agenda" dictated from above.[4] The cynical view would be that General Managers could and did take unpopular decisions such as the closure of wards and reduction in staffing levels to keep within their budget, but they also promoted various initiatives which helped "to maintain the impression of substantially pro-active managerial activity"![4] This would be a one-sided assessment however, General Managers did facilitate a number of improvements in the environment in which patients were treated and staff worked. There is also no doubt that having a single person in charge of a unit, who could take and implement a decision over an operational matter on his own account, was a distinct advantage over the previous era of consensus management. The post-Griffiths reorganisation of 1984 could well have been successful if it had been given time to develop, and adequate finance had been provided without being undermined by central refusal to meet pay awards and other impositions, if the contracts of General Managers had been less rigid and short-term and more doctors had been encouraged to take up the appointments, and if uniform Unit organisations had been introduced through the NHS similar to those developed by the pilot Resource Management Initiatives. It was clear by 1988 that "although the Griffiths general management revolution was right in principle it had not been properly implemented."[164,186] It was too late by then, a crisis had developed in the NHS which was to lead to a further and much more radical reorganisation in 1991.[2]

The crisis in the affairs of the NHS 1987-1988.

The boom years of the second Conservative Thatcher administration were coming to an end by the time it was returned to power with a reduced but still substantial majority of 100 in June 1987. There was already mounting discontent about the state of the NHS on the part of both the public and the medical profession. "Doctors were trying to do their best for patients, within what seemed to them ever decreasing resources .... and yet all politicians, academics and managers seemed to do in those days was to point their fingers at them and say they were idle good-for-nothings and the root of all inefficiency in the NHS".[2] It was fortunate for the profession that the public knew where the blame actually lay; the NHS was in fact treating more patients with fewer beds, but the more efficient the medical profession became at increasing the number of patients who were treated, the more the cost, and the more restrictions that were imposed to try to keep within the budget (the so-called "efficiency trap"). Resource restraint, efficiency savings and the adverse effect of RAWP (Resource Allocation Working Party redistribution of resources between Regions) on some Health Regions had all led to cuts, shortages and rationing as demand had outstripped supply.[164] Another burden was the attempt to fund or partially fund pay increases (including those of doctors and nurses) out of putative "efficiency savings".[2] The Government's response was to try to force the system to confront reality by restraining the growth of real resources below the rate warranted.[164]

The ghastly situation is well described by Brian Edwards (Regional General Manager, Trent RHA and Association of Anaesthetists Pinkerton Lecturer 1993) in his book "The National Health Service: a Manager's Tale 1946-1992".[2] General Managers tried desperately to balance their budgets (and thus preserve their jobs after their next individual performance review, and perhaps even receive a bonus for their efforts). Many "budget juggling tactics" were tried.[2] Over 3,500 beds were closed country wide for financial reasons over the winter 1988/1989, service developments and building maintenance were postponed, capital was transferred to revenue accounts, recruitment was frozen, locums were not provided and consequently junior doctors and nurses were overstretched, and the former began to call for a reduction in the 120 hour week some of them were working.[2,187]

A "waiting list initiative" to reduce waiting lists was proclaimed with the nominal provision of £50 million (1996: £75 million) of additional money just before the 1987 General Election; then as now this was a useful propaganda gimmick. In fact such initiatives only compound the situation; for example the West Berkshire Health Authority took 900 low priority patients off the waiting list but had to postpone 3,000 other elective operations to combat a projected "overspend" of £1.3 million (1996: £2 million).[163] The West Berkshire General Manager, who had come from industry towards the end of his career, resigned and appeared on television to protest at the cuts he was being forced to make to try to balance the books.[2] A survey of District Health Authorities by the National Association of Health Authorities was conducted in 1987; only 55% (106) of the 192 DHAs responded but the replies suggested that over 50% were in serious financial trouble. The shortfall was estimated to be £228 million (1996: £340 million).[2,188] The House of Commons Select Committee on Social Services concluded that between 1980 and 1987 the hospital and community health services had been underfunded by £1,325 billion at 1986 prices (1996: £2,067 billion).[2] The staff at the interface with the patients, the only interface which matters, struggled to provide a service under deteriorating physical and financial conditions; after spending 24 hours at King's College Hospital Accident and Emergency Department Tony Delamothe, Assistant Editor of the *British Medical Journal*, wrote in 1987:-

> *"It wasn't "crisis management"; despite the shortage of cubicles, trolleys, chairs, doctors, nurses, cleaners, porters and other ancillary staff. Members of staff never lost their cool, their politeness, and their compassion....*
>
> *I cannot justify to you why my local accident and emergency department should be better equipped than ones I have seen in the Third World, but I am surprised that its facilities are worse."*[189]

Those politicians and senior managers of the period who glibly dismissed the countless protests of the professions both public and private[2] as "shroud waving," and even actively sought to suppress public criticism from within the NHS by doctors and nurses and others,[190] should search their consciences. Those of today's (1998) politicians, senior managers, health commentators and consumer protectionists, who seem to believe that compassion for patients is solely the result of the 1991 reorganisation since they succeeded in "controlling the professionals",[4] should think again. The newspapers it is true, as they often do, attempted to generalise by citing certain specific sensational cases such as the baby in Birmingham whose cardiac operation was postponed five times because of a lack of skilled paediatric intensive care nurses,[2] but the fundamental problem (lack of resources for treating patients and maintaining the modern infrastructure required to treat them in) remained.[191]

The clinicians were doing their bit. The majority had, by 1987, accepted and even approved of the idea of general management as put forward by Griffiths, provided professional advisory input was properly and adequately maintained; they had accepted budgeting control and the need for obtaining "value for money" (though not of cheap solutions at any price) and they had improved clinical efficiency (indeed the "efficiency trap" was partly responsible for the problems of the NHS). The Royal Colleges (including, notably, the Faculty of Anaesthetists) had greatly improved their training requirements and specialist examinations, the profession had begun to institute monitoring procedures, including clinical audit, and a number of them had shown themselves to be efficient managers in the burgeoning clinical directorate initiatives. The patients, the professions, the ancillary staff and the public were justified in looking to the Government for increasing resources. The Government responded by promising cash for the future (£700 million in 1988-1989 and £800 million in 1989-90) but this, of course, did not alleviate the existing crisis; finally an immediate, "one off", £100 million was offered to rescue the DHAs but this was less than half what was required. Professional, parliamentary and public disquiet mounted and there were demonstrations outside the Houses of Parliament and elsewhere by nurses and others. The BMA petitioned the Government and finally on 7 December 1987 the Presidents of, the Royal Colleges of Physicians of London, of Surgeons of England and of Obstetrics and Gynaecology, despite their academic detachment and the charitable status of the Colleges, felt compelled to issue a rare joint statement protesting about the conditions under which the Fellows, Members and trainees were vainly endeavouring to maintain the professional standards which the Royal Colleges required, and calling for a review of the acute hospital services and an exploration of "additional and alternative funding!"[192] The Royal College Presidents had an interview with John Moore, the then Secretary of State for Health and Social Services on 13 January 1988. They believed that their request for an inquiry and increased funds had been sympathetically received, but the Treasury immediately issued a denial that more cash had been promised.[2,193]

A debate in the House of Commons on 19 January 1988 brought forward what was then, and still is in 1998, the familiar rhetoric applauding the achievements of the NHS and the "extra" funds which had recently been injected by the taxpayer, and urging still more effective use of resources. A motion acknowledging these propositions was predictably passed by the large Conservative majority of Members of Parliament.[2,193] The public and professional clamour would not go away however, and Mrs Thatcher, the Prime Minister, defied parliamentary protocol by announcing on the television programme "Panorama" on 25 January 1988 that there would be an internal review within the Cabinet Office which would take place behind closed doors[2,194] Sir Roy Griffiths writing in 1992, has described the initiation of the 1989 review, its conclusions, and what followed, as "an astonishing episode in many ways".[185] He was undoubtedly correct!

The 1988/89 Review and the 1989 White Paper *Working for Patients*.

Tony Kember, spent his entire career from 1956 to 1992 in the service of the NHS starting as Administrative Trainee and rising via Regional General Manager to Communications Adviser to the Department of Health.[3] He tells that:-

> *"The White Paper was written over a period of one year by a small policy group working directly to the Prime Minister (a free-floating "Think Tank" which only leaked intentionally), whose members were distinguished by both their political affiliation and by their ignorance of the day-to-day workings of the NHS. Their work was undertaken in isolation and was surrounded by secrecy .... Neither senior clinicians nor senior managers from the service were directly involved*

at any time...... Only occasional missives were sent across the road to Richmond House [headquarters of the Department of Health and its civil servants] demanding urgent comment on the latest bright idea. It is believed that the Chief Medical Officer, who was the adviser to the whole of the Government and not just to the Department of Health was only consulted intermittently and then only on highly specific and isolated issues...."[3]

We are also told by Sir Roy Griffiths[185] that the review body:-

"started to examine new methods of funding the NHS and after careful consideration moved abruptly from this theme. It then switched to building on the existing management reforms and seeking to inject more competition and choice into the service."[185]

The decision not to consider new means of funding any further was a serious omission, but it was obviously politically motivated.[195] The preservation of a health service "entirely free at the point of use to all" irrespective of income is considered to be axiomatic and written in tablets of stone in the British public and political psyche, as well as in the manifestos of all political parties It would certainly be a brave politician who would seek to reverse this policy, but ultimately the writer believes that someone must grasp the nettle. The concept was a reasonable, if a little ingenuous, policy when Bevan inaugurated the NHS in 1948 (Chapter 5) in the context of medical technology as it then was, but in 1998, in the light of the enormous scientific advances which have occurred, it is fast becoming, or is already, untenable.[196] Almost every other health service in Western Europe is based on state subsidised personal insurance. Such schemes seem to result in more satisfactory funding and better facilities at the point of delivery of the clinical service. The major share of the cost is provided by the state from taxation and added to the direct contribution of the patient which can be covered by private insurance. Brian Edwards, Regional General Manager of Trent Regional Health Authority, whose book "The National Health Service, a managers tale" has already been quoted, suggests that 80%:20% split between state and personal insurance would be reasonable for those who are not indigent or exempted for other reasons.[196] Such a scheme would emphasise the enormous cost of the NHS and its value to the individual patient, and engender a greater respect in the minds of the minority of patients, for example those who do not turn up for booked outpatient appointments, day surgery, or inpatient admission (the suggestion at a committee that patients should be asked to put down a returnable deposit when booked for a specific date is guaranteed to get a rise out of General Managers!). It is interesting that a previous policy "Think Tank" recommended a move to health insurance in 1982 before Griffiths began his inquiry; needless to say the report was hastily "consigned to the dustbin".[196]

During the year which passed between Mrs Thatcher's announcement of her review in January 1988 and the publication of the White Paper *Working for Patients* in January 1989[2-4,195] a much needed governmental reorganisation took place. The mega-ministry Department of Health and Social Security (DHSS) was split into its component parts and once again there was a separate Department of Health (DH) and a Secretary of State for Health of Cabinet rank. Kenneth Clarke, who had earlier been Minister for Health was appointed to that Office.

Most clinicians simply got on with the job of "working for patients" in the prevailing difficult circumstances, and there were further developments in the area of resource management and the introduction of clinical directorate systems; there was also a considerable volume of speculation and advice for the Government and members of the "Think Tank" in many books, professional journals and lay magazines and, in particular, in the columns of the *British Medical Journal* and the *Lancet* (1988).

It is known that Mrs Thatcher became impressed by an essay written for the Nuffield Provincial Trust in 1985 by Professor Alain Enthoven of the Graduate School of Business of Stanford University, California.[2,3,163,164,197] Enthoven's suggestions were, however, very moderate compared with the scheme that emerged after the 1991 report of the review, but they did supply the nucleus of an idea for a "managed" market. Enthoven proposed that the District Health Authorities (DHAs) should continue to be funded on a *per capita* basis adjusted for such demographic matters as sex, age and the mortality of their populations, but that they should "buy" some services by contract from other DHAs for their population if this was financially advantageous. The benefits would be the search for increased efficiency (as in the existing Resource Initiative and Clinical Directorate trials) enhanced by competition between DHAs and economies of scale if some DHAs specialised in the provision of certain services.[2,3,163,164,197] An extension of this idea would be a variation of the American Health Maintenance Organisation (HMO) concept involving the purchase by DHAs of comprehensive services from both General Practitioners and the Hospitals as advocated by (Lord) David Owen.[163] It is of historic interest that the idea of an "internal market" in health provision was apparently excluded from the Conservative election manifesto for the 1987 election as being too politically sensitive, but was included in that of the SDP/Liberal Alliance of which Owen was joint leader.[163]

John Chawner, Chairman of the BMAs Central Consultants and Specialists Committee (CCSC), when interviewed in 1992 in connection with the BMA publication "Leading for Health",[198,199] doubted the validity of the philosophy embraced by some politicians and commentators that funding the NHS was like pouring money into a "bottomless pit". He believed that the demand was not infinite and that a level could be reached if a "hypothecated" tax of about 9% gross national product (GNP) was levied.[199] It is worth emphasising that, although in 1987 the United Kingdom came low (6.1%) in the table of the provision of health expenditure out of the GNP of developed countries (range 4.3%-9.2%, mean 7.5%), the proportion of the provision provided out of public funds (87%) was the fifth highest in a list of 24 developed countries (range 40% to 90%, mean 76%) according to figures supplied by the Organisation for Economical and Cultural Development. Chawner also suggested that hospitals and clinical departments should be reimbursed from a central agency according to each item of service which was undertaken on the basis of defined "diagnostically related groups" (DRG);[197] in such a system patients, guided by their General Practitioners, would be allowed to seek treatment wherever they chose.[3]

It is, indeed, difficult not to conclude that, had time been allowed for the development of the 1984 reorganisation which followed the Griffiths report, and given improvements in cost information and resource management, a system could have been devised which was less confrontational and complex than that which has been put in place after the subsequent 1991 reorganisation, and without the inordinate cost of managerial and administrative expansion which has ensued.[2,200] It is also worth remembering that Sir Roy Griffiths himself "did not believe in bringing large numbers of people in from outside [the NHS]", and that the time required to introduce the type of management changes that he had put forward, would be "a long process". He also paid tribute to the way the medical profession rethought its position after his report was published, and the way in which many doctors had accepted much needed changes in professional practice such as the establishment of clinical directorates and the institution of clinical audit.[185] No time was allowed for the post-Griffiths measures to settle down however before the Government's secret 1988-1989 review was undertaken and published as a White Paper, which implied a commitment to yet another reorganisation of the NHS.

The White Paper *Working for Patients*[201] was launched by Kenneth Clarke, Secretary of State for Health, on 31 January 1989 with all the razzmatazz of a Eurovision song contest at a cost of £1.25 million (1996: £1.7 million).[66] His speech at the Limehouse Studios in London's Docklands scheme was beamed simultaneously in a teleconference to 2,500 doctors, managers and Health Authority Chairmen in Regional Centres throughout the United Kingdom. It was the first attempt at a controlled mass communications exercise throughout the NHS. Managers were to return armed with videos and briefing packs to spread the news throughout the service."[2]

The title of the 1989 White Paper *Working for Patients*[201] was mildly provocative. More senior clinicians in the NHS can be forgiven for wondering what the Government thought they had been doing for up to 40 years past![202] Be that as it may however, Mrs Thatcher, the Prime Minister, in her foreword to the White Paper stated *inter alia* that:-

> "The National Health Service will continue to be available to all, regardless of income, and to be mainly financed out of general taxation. ......We aim to extend patients' choice, to delegate responsibility to where the services are provided and to secure the best value for money."[164,201]

The weakness, as has already been stated above was of course enshrined in the first sentence of this quotation and in the last statement; as Day and Klein of the Centre for Analysis of Social Policy of the University of Bath, wrote in an Editorial in the *British Medical Journal*:-[195]

> "Leaving aside the hyperbole, "Working for Patients" is remarkable

for what it does not say. A policy review launched a year ago in an attempt to devise a new funding system has ended up by saying nothing about how to finance the NHS."[195]

The only way to produce more finance for the service mentioned in *Working for Patients* was to be by promoting "cost effectiveness" to obtain "value for money" by "increased efficiency". There is, however, a limit to what can be squeezed out of a system by this means, and the inevitable consequence must be, and has been, curtailment and rationing of services and a decrease in the universality of the NHS. The result of this approach together with the expressed intention in the White Paper to bring management closer to the patient means that "the onus for action falls heavily on doctors [and managers at the Unit level] though in a way that is electorally fail-safe. If it does not work little lasting damage can be done [to politicians and central management at the Department of Health]",[203] and the doctors and managers at the point of delivery of the service can be blamed for their inefficiency.

The basic structure of the NHS also remained outwardly intact although its actual constitution and function were considerably altered. The political Supervisory Board became the Policy Board and the Management Board became the NHS Management Executive chaired by the Chief Executive Duncan Nichol, the former Mersey Regional General Manager. Regional and District Regional Health Authorities were to remain in name but included Chief Executives as members and were much smaller with politically appointed Chairmen and Non-executive Directors, and without statutory representation of local authorities or Community Health Councils representing consumers, or of medical or nursing staff. The management arrangements for Units (hospitals) managed directly by the DHAs were not clearly defined but, in the event, as the clinical directorate system developed, the old Medical Advisory Committee inevitably became ineffective in influencing the General Manager and many were disbanded; whether or not the Chief Executive meets regularly with the Clinical Directors, who are appointed by him and not elected by their peers, as a clinical management board, or as individuals, or at all, depends on the whim of the Chief Executive or General Manager and his relationship with the medical staff.

The White Paper *Working for Patients* was nominally intended for consultation but, in fact, it outlined the strategic changes in the NHS which the Government had already decided to implement. The White Paper was followed during the next six months by eleven Working Papers on various aspects giving further details. These were supposedly negotiable but, in fact, very little variation was ultimately obtained by professional organisations and trade unions. It was laid down that the necessary preparation was to be completed in time for the reorganisation to be effective from 1 April 1991. This would enable the new system to be established and difficult to reverse before the next General Election due at the end of 1991 or early in 1992.[204] The medical and nursing professions, as well as many civil servants and managers, were united in the opinion that this was far too short a period for adequate changes to be properly organised, let alone for adequate consultations to be undertaken.

The term "purchaser-provider split" was not used in the White Paper but the implication was clear, and the concept was developed in the Working Papers. The system was to be much more complicated than that suggested by Enthoven.[197] Regional Health Authorities (RHA) were to receive funds based on a resident population from the DH, and DHAs were to be funded on a resident population basis to provide services for their notional populations. There were to be two types of hospitals ("provider units"), Directly Managed Units (DMU) (responsible to the DHA but with greater operational freedom of day to day management than hitherto), and NHS Trust Hospitals (larger hospitals or groups with at least 250 beds). The latter, if approved after application to the DH by their General Managers, would have separate legal status and be independent of the DHAs. They would be given considerably greater latitude than the DMUs in the use of funds, in employing staff and determining their conditions and contracts of service and pay rates, in responsibility for assets such as buildings for which they would pay a nominal "rent" to the DH, and which could be disposed of and, if the schemes put forward were approved, the power to borrow money for projects. There would also be two categories of General Practitioners, those whose activities were organised and financed by the DHA, and larger practices (initially with more than 11,000 patients) who could apply (voluntarily) to become "fund holding" practices and, if approved, would have their own independent budgets to purchase some services independently for their patients from providers. The

DHA would be required to purchase certain core services from provider units for all their population however, whether patients were referred from fundholders or non-fundholders, or for patients arriving directly at the Accident and Emergency Departments. These core services were to include accident and emergency services, other immediate admissions, and outpatient and support services. Both DHAs and independent fundholding GPs would in theory be able to purchase services from DMU hospitals in their own or other Districts, from self-governing Trust hospitals, or from Private Hospitals. Purchase of services was to be by contract between purchaser and provider and extra contractual referrals for individual patients a comparative rarity, although fundholding GPs have subsequently proved to have much more flexibility in this area. Other changes were to be the inclusion of General Managers (Chief Executives) on Medical Appointments Boards and Distinction Award Committees, and there was to be five year reviews of individual distinction awards, which would only have become pensionable after three years in the NHS.

Maurice Burrows (then President of the Association of Anaesthetists) made a thoughtful initial assessment of *Working for Patients* and the subsequent working papers in *Anaesthesia News* in June 1989.[206] He drew on his wide experience as a senior officer of the BMA. He gave a cautious welcome to some of the proposals but correctly assessed the possible weaknesses. He welcomed the Government's apparent intention to allow "money to flow to hospitals which treat most patients" to avoid the "efficiency trap", but from the terseness of his four word comment, one suspects that he already feared that, due to the contract system and the duality of the providers (DHAs and fundholding General Practitioners), "patients might follow money" rather than "money follow patients".

Maurice Burrows also foresaw some of the political difficulties that have arisen with self-governing Trust Hospitals. These included, the danger of abandoning nationally agreed rates of pay which might result in the failure to maintain nation-wide standards, and unfairness to the "less entrepreneurial branches of the profession" (including, of course, anaesthesia), the possible disadvantageous effects on training and research, and the need to release medical staff for College and Association business. He welcomed funding for "medical audit" which was, in any case already well established in many departments of anaesthesia. Burrows also stressed the importance of appointing "the best medically trained and qualified applicants for the advertised post", of not causing disadvantage to consultants over 60 who might reasonably have received a higher award under the old regulations, and also of ensuring that, as far as possible, the five year review of awards should be conducted by the same committee that made the original award. A proposed increase in Consultants in the NHS was welcomed but the "obvious link between more surgical posts and more anaesthetic posts" should not be overlooked.[206]

(Sir) Duncan Nichol, former General Manager and Chief Executive of the Mersey Regional Health Authority was a career NHS manager. He was appointed Chief Executive of the National Health Service in January 1989 and became Chairman of the Management Executive the following May. He addressed the Annual Conference of Linkmen of the Association of Anaesthetists at Swansea by invitation on 13 September 1989.[207] He stated that his objective was to review the proposals of *Working for Patients* and their background and to emphasise the advantages which would follow their implementation. He stressed the importance and value of the purchaser-provider split and sought to allay fears that self-governing (Trust) hospitals would be allowed to opt out of the NHS and might only offer profitable services.[207] It is of interest that he also implied that the ideas of the White Paper would be tested well into the 1990s and that cataclysmic change would be avoided![207]

The implementation of the White Paper *Working for Patients*

The Secretary of State for Health (and presumably the Prime Minister, Mrs Thatcher) had other ideas. Kenneth Clarke's frenetic activities have few parallels in British public life; they were autocratic in the extreme and cut across the principles of good management which are so much promoted by management gurus. These include listening to and the getting the good will of the work force; and perhaps even making modifications accordingly.[2,3] The leading academic Sir Maurice Shock (former Rector of Lincoln College Oxford and Chairman of Nuffield Provincial Hospitals Trust) has compared Clarke's campaign to an enemy blitzkrieg in the Second World War and Clarke himself to a Panzer General:-[208,209]

> *"It was blitzkrieg from the right with little consultation, indeed not much discussion with civil servants let alone those outside Whitehall. And there was appropriate accompanying propaganda about the selfish doctors and their grasping trade union [the BMA] and about rights and charters for patients and how the Government would be fighting for them."*[209]

An exercise to control costs without attending to the question of seeking methods of raising additional resources or restricting the scope of the provision of health care was thus represented as a scheme to benefit the consumer despite the "wicked" doctors. It is interesting that Donald W Light,[210] an American commentator, wrote in September 1991, five months after the NHS reorganisation had come into operation on 1 April:-

> *"Do they not know that they [the British Government] were [and are] getting better value for money than any other system in the industrialised world?......Do they not know that experts from other systems marvel at how hard British nurses, technicians and physicians work for so little pay? The level of dedication measurable in services rendered per million pounds of pay provides this government with use of the greatest bargains in the world..... with the cost of the NHS at £45 billion and rising at 2% over inflation the question is why do British leaders think they can treat the nation's ill for a third less than anyone else...Although the government apparently intends the reforms to make the NHS more efficient, their latent function is to transfer the political heat to managers and doctors in the guise of "inefficiency."*[210]

It is impossible not to admire Kenneth Clarke's tenacity however.[211] He pushed his agenda through against the opposition of the substantial majority of the medical and nursing professions, the trade unions of the NHS employees, and the general public. He was aided and abetted by the General Manager organisation set up by the 1984 reorganisation. The Managers had much to learn and organise. New concepts of "pricing contracting for clinical services, capital changes, marketing, business planning, constructing GP fundholding budgets" etc.[2] Opposition to local hospitals who were seeking Trust status was considerable on the part of both public and staff. General Managers prepared glossy brochures "expressing interest" in Trust status in defiance of large majorities on their medical staff committees and their Health Authorities.[2,3] Some statements made by managers in their bids for Trust status were somewhat economical with the truth; for example one of them stated in his application that it "had the approval of senior medical staff", when in fact over 90% of the staff had voted against it and less than 10% (two individuals) in favour (personal recollection)!

The Iraqi invasion of Kuwait and the subsequent Gulf War (August 1990 to February 1991) diverted public attention from the preparations for the reorganisation which was to be initiated on 1 April 1991; but, even before the Gulf crisis began, as legislation to implement the reorganisation came before Parliament and was passed by the overwhelming Government majority, the BMA and the medical profession as a whole, began to accept the inevitable and, as in the past, and in the interest of patients, set themselves pragmatically to make the best of the situation. They were particularly successful in developing the Medical Directorate concept within provider units,[167,168,178-181] but it was unfortunate that the extent of the involvement of the medical profession in the negotiation of contracts with purchasers was very variable.[2,3,211]

Sir Maurice Shock has said that "particularly to be admired is Panzer General Clarke's handling of the decisive weapon, money";[209] certainly though the government had denied extra funds to the NHS for clinical purposes it was able to find a very considerable amount of money to ensure a smooth take off before the unavoidable general election in 1992.[3] Eighty five million pounds was provided in 1989-1990 and £305 million in 1990-1991 to cover the increased number of managers and the increases in their individual pay. The NHS spent only £25 million on general managers pay in 1987 compared with over £251 million in 1991, during which time the number of managers in the NHS rose from 700 to 13,200; as Alan Milburn the MP for Darlington put it, "managers and administrators have taken an extra £550 million from a cash strapped NHS [between 1989 and 1991]. General Practitioners were offered £16,000 per practice for development if they participated in fundholding schemes.[2,3]

A cabinet reshuffle occurred early in November 1990. Kenneth Clarke went off to confront and attempt to reorganise the educational establishment and was replaced by the urbane and scholarly aristocrat William Waldegrave,[211,212] and then, on 28 November 1990, the unthinkable occurred, Margaret Thatcher resigned under pressure from her own colleagues and was replaced by John Major. The time-table so far as the intended reorganisation of the NHS on 1 April 1991 however remained unchanged; Kenneth Clarke had set the juggernaut rolling.[2]

The members of the medical profession had a sneaking admiration for Clarke as a tactician, as soldiers might have for the commander of an enemy army, but, when he departed, "many believed that his negotiating tactics had been unnecessarily provocative" and that his "approach had demoralised and antagonised the profession to an extent that [would] adversely affect the service".[211] He had been particularly ruthless in imposing a new contract on the general practitioners. This had a considerable element of performance related pay geared to achieving "targets" for their practice populations in such matters as vaccinations and preventative diagnostic procedures such as cervical smears. His attitude so far as hospital practitioners was concerned was expressed in an interview with an American journalist towards the end of his tenure of office.[213] He stated that (in the new NHS):-

"The doctor [will become]....... responsible for the performance as a whole of his unit, not just carrying out clinical work and walking away from the rest and moaning because some damned administrator and some politicians are failing to provide the resources he thinks he requires."[213]

Clarke and the Government lauded the principle of consumerism and putting the patients first. He saw himself "as a representative of the consumer" but admitted that "General Practitioners and Health Authorities [his purchasers] are much more informed customers of the services than any patient."[213]

A contrasting comparison can be made between Aneurin Bevan's success in establishing the NHS (Chapter 5) and Kenneth Clarke's success in the confrontational imposition in the 1991 reorganisation.[215] Bevan was for political ministerial responsibility (a bed pan should not fall in the NHS without the Minister knowing about it) whereas Clarke sought to distance politicians from management.[213] Bevan was a leader who saw the value of flexibility and pragmatism in pursuing the main ideal, and of considering the opinions of the work force (including primarily the medical profession) in achieving those ends. Bevan also foresaw a number of the difficulties with which the NHS was, and is still faced with in the nineteen nineties,[214] but the

NHS was invigorated in 1948 with the aid of a medical profession which was generally supportive even if reluctantly so.[216]

William Waldegrave was more courteous and less confrontational as Secretary of State for Health than Kenneth Clarke but he remained unmoved on the principle planks of the reform system. His problem was to ensure a "level playing-field"; every District was required to enter the new contractual system with a clean balance-sheet to ensure a smooth transition. Eighty one million pounds was provided to help authorities with severe deficits, but sadly they were once again forced to close about 4,000 beds prior to the reorganisation and to force a reduction in clinical activity.[2]

The launch of the 1991 reorganisation. The reorganised NHS came into being on 1 April 1991 although, of course, a great number of preparatory measures had also been implemented including the new contract for General Practitioners. There were initially 57 semi-independent Trust Hospitals and 306 fundholding general practitioners. There is no doubt that the transition to the new system was managed with remarkable facility.[217] William Waldegrave bestowed much praise on the General Managers for their "creative and enthusiastic commitment" during the 800 days since the publication of the White Paper in January 1989,[2] but credit should also be given to the clinicians who continued to maintain a dedicated service to patients, which after all is why the NHS exists, despite the financial restrictions and the bureaucratic upheaval of the reorganisation.

The First twelve months after the 1991 Reorganisation, 1 April 1991 to 9 April 1992. It was a coincidence that almost exactly a year elapsed between the inaugural day of the 1991 reforms and the General Election on 9 April 1992. The clinical work of the service and the relentless imposition of the new financial management continued against a background of claim and counter claim of the rival political parties.

The leaders of the Labour Party in opposition pledged that, if returned to power, they would "restore the NHS as a public service giving priority to medical need rather than commercial return". They stated that they would abolish fundholding general practices and Trust hospitals and bring the latter back into the control of the District Health Authorities.[218-220] It was proposed that the purchaser-provider split between the Districts and the provider units (individual hospitals) would remain however, with agreed "service agreements" embodying outputs and standards substituted for "contracts" between them. There would also be additional incentive payments for those providers who exceeded their targets. This would certainly have been an interesting innovation since a feature of the working of the 1974 reorganisation initiated by the Labour Party had been the imposition of cash limits. General Practice ("Primary Care") would retain to some extent the influence it had gained as a purchaser by obliging District to secure the agreement of general practitioners when designing service agreements.

The Liberal Democrats condemned the internal market, this despite the fact that their predecessors the Liberal-SDP Alliance in their 1987 pre-election manifesto had extolled the value of patient choice of hospital and, to that end had recommended that Health Authorities should "buy and sell hospital treatment from each other". The Liberal Democrats in 1992 also proposed to maintain the purchaser-provider split, and like the Labour party supported the concept of "service agreements" instead of contracts.[219-221]

The Liberal Democrats also suggested that specialist training should be aligned with European practice with a single training grade leading to accreditation. The post of Consultant would be abolished and the day to day clinical management of patients in the NHS would fall on teams of accredited specialists. This proposal obviously had its origins in the debate concerning the legality in respect of European Community medical directives of the British use of "Accreditation" as the acknowledgment of the termination of specialist training and accepted passport independent specialist practice as a Consultant; this followed the High Court decision in the Goldstein case (Chapter 8).[220,222-226] It pre-empted the decision of the BMA Junior Doctors Annual Conference to press for a single tier of specialist training in the following June 1992,[223] and the establishment of the Working Group under Kenneth Calman (the Government's Chief Medical Officer) in August 1992.[224] The report of the Calman committee, which was published in May 1993[225,226] went much wider than the question of determining a definition of independent specialist status and has caused a revolution in the organisation of specialist training in the United Kingdom.

The Conservative Government naturally made every effort to demonstrate their conviction that the 1991 reorganisation was progressive and advantageous. William Waldegrave introduced a policy of positively promoting health by preventing disease in line with a policy based on a declaration by the WHO on "Health for All by the Year 2000" issued in 1981.[227] A consultative document was published detailing sixteen possible areas to be targeted, and this was endorsed by the Prime Minister at a conference with leading members of the medical profession. The document and the subsequent consultation resulted in the publication in July 1992, after the April election, of the White paper *"Health of the Nation"* by the new Secretary of State for Health Virginia Bottomley.[2,228-230] This set targets for a reduction in incidents or improvement in management in five areas by the year 2000; these were heart disease and stroke, cancers, mental illness, HIV/AIDS and sexual health, and accidents.[229] A ministerial committee covering eleven government departments was set up with the objective of ensuring that these concepts pervaded government policy. Two omissions highlighted by the political opposition and others were, the absence of a mention of poverty and homelessness as a cause of ill-health, and the refusal of the Government to forbid the advertising of tobacco products in line with European Community policy.[228-230] It must also be pointed out that the positive promotion of health policies was one of Aneurin Bevan's main aims at the inauguration of the NHS. A policy initiative of this kind was welcome and valuable but it could have been promulgated at any time and was not directly a consequence of the 1991 reorganisation despite some attempts to represent it as such.[231-232]

The Patients' Charter was published in October 1991 and distributed to every household in the country. It was claimed that its launch and implementation was made easier by the introduction of the purchaser-provider split in 1991,[233] but it is doubtful if this is entirely justified. It is not reasonable to echo the description of the Director of the Patients' Association which dismissed the Charter as "a rather flabby gelatinous object,"[2] but nonetheless, it did attempt to define the obvious in stating the rights and standards in the delivery of care which an NHS patient could reasonably expect; however, it said nothing about the guarantee of the quality of care. Barbara Stocking, Director of Kings Fund Centre noted that the Charter concentrated "on what the NHS should be doing for the patient, but this is only one side of the bargain" and commented that "people have responsibility for their health care too".[234] Many doctors and nurses, particularly those who work in Accident and Emergency Departments may well feel that a "code of practice for patients" or a "doctors and nurses Charter" was then and still is in 1998, long overdue!

The 1991 Reorganisation had come into being smoothly and quietly.[2] William Waldegrave and Duncan Nichol expected some initial unevenness in the delivery of health care peripherally due to the delegated contracting system but they viewed this pragmatically; they believed[235] that it was:-

> *"better to have people gaining, even if others are not gaining at the same speed, rather than have no improvements on the grounds that it is unfair that anybody should gain."*[235]

Monitoring the 1991 Reorganisation. The reorganised NHS was under the continual scrutiny of the House of Commons Select Committee on Health under its redoubtable Chairman Nicholas Winterton. Winterton was himself something of an anachronism as Chairman. He was one of only two Conservative MPs who had voted against the 1991 reorganisation and he owed his election to the Chairmanship to the support of the opposition MPs on the committee.[236] The self-governing NHS Trusts very quickly came under scrutiny when they started sacking staff and making cuts in May, (Guy's Hospital, London lost 600 jobs and £6.8 million, and Bradford 300 jobs). Chief Executives (including Duncan Nichol) appeared before the Select Committee at intervals during the first year. It must be acknowledged that they acquitted themselves well in defence of the business culture they represented in the face of close questioning.[2,237,238] It must also be said however that the Parliamentary Commissioner (the "Ombudsman") had a less rosy view of the quality of management based on the increasing number of complaints being received in the reorganised NHS; "it is the responsibility of management to manage and all too often it seems to have abdicated its responsibility".[237] One very unfortunate aspect of the 1991 reorganisation, which gave rise to concern, emerged during the Health Committee hearings; it was the refusal of Chief Executives (and even Ministers in answer to Parliamentary questions) to give details of Trust business plans and other financial performance information on the grounds that they were commercially secret;[2,239] as the commentator "Hart" wrote in the *British Medical Journal*:-[239]

> *"Most of the money paid to Trusts comes directly from tax payers; haven't they got a right to see whether the Government has opted for the best buy."*[239]

Winterton wrote a critical report on NHS Trusts which was leaked in advance to the Department of Health and thereafter relegated to an appendix;[236,239] subsequently a Conservative member of the Committee resigned[239] and, following an alteration to the rules relating to the permitted length of service of Members of Parliament on Select Committees after the Conservatives were returned to power in the April 1992 election, Nicholas Winterton was excluded from membership.[236]

The NHS Management Executive took the unusual step of publishing a report on the first six months of the operation of the 1991 reorganisation (1 April to 30 September 1991) in January 1992.[240-243] "The timing of the report [was] not unrelated to the British political calendar as a general election [was] likely before the full years figures [were] available".[242] The Chief Executive Duncan Nichol stated in the report:-

"Changes in the way the NHS is organised ..... are leading to improvements in the quality of care, greater responsiveness to individuals and even better value for money for the growing NHS;"[240,242]

The members of the Radical Statistics Health Group were less sure, however, and, after careful analysis published in the *British Medical Journal,* they concluded:-

"The data presented in "NHS Reforms: the First Six Months" fail to support Duncan Nichol's claim that the changes introduced on 1 April 1991 are leading to improved care, greater responsiveness to individuals and better value for money."[243]

Other commentators believed that:-

"Although the improvements are attributed to the 1991 reforms, they may be related to management changes begun by Sir Roy Griffiths in the 1980s and financial controls put in place over the previous three years."[242]

The Report was however:-

"A reassuring picture of a service that continued on much the same trajectory as in previous years, with an increase in the number of

patients treated and a reduction in long waiting times."[242]

It can further be pointed out that at least two of the stated increases in activity cited were not the result of the 1991 reorganisation. These were the increase in immunisation rates (the result of the new General Practitioner Contract) and the decrease in patients waiting over two years (the result of central funding the waiting list initiative financed directly by the Department of Health which enabled payments to be made to surgeons and anaesthetists for additional lists).

The BMA document "Leading for Health" (the result of a widespread investigation amongst prominent persons concerned with health policy) was published by the BMA in October 1991.[244] This emphasised the importance of public health in its widest sense (including promotion of health education, prevention of disease, poverty, poor housing, etc.), and went on to discuss the various alternative systems for delivering and funding health services. This informative, succinct, and well written document did not, and was never intended, to produce a definitive policy for the British NHS, or to choose between the various alternatives discussed in it; its purpose was "to set an agenda for discussions on health and policy setting". It was an admirable document, which would have been of considerable value in 1988 while discussions on the future of the NHS were being held, but it was too late in 1991 after reorganisation was already in being![242,243] It may be however that the BMA, like many others, expected a Labour victory in the general elections and hoped to influence the development of new policies![245]

The 1992 General Election. April was a good month for the Prime Minister (John Major) to choose to hold an election in 1992 so far as the NHS was concerned. The upbeat report on the first six months of the 1991 reorganisation referred to the period April to September 1991[240,241] and therefore did not cover the period October 1991 to March 1992 when clinical activity had been once again restricted to balance the books of District Health Authorities and the independent NHS Trusts.[246] Fundholding by General Practitioners was being promoted and extolled by the Government, and ministers pointed to the number of applications as a sign of approval for the scheme as such, although the considerable financial inducements to sign up for fundholding were not stressed,[247,248] nor the deterioration in morale due to the conditions of the new contract for all General Practitioners which had predated the reorganisation of the NHS by a year (April 1990).[250,251] Conservatives stressed the improvements in the way patients were treated administratively with regard to waiting times etc on the lines of the Patients' Charter but, as the Chairman of one NHS Trust emphasised, all these improvements could have been achieved before the 1991 reorganisation.[252] The statistics of a centrally initiated waiting list were emphasised but their significance was open to debate. The number of patients waiting over two years fell markedly and those between one and two years to some extent, but it was believed that this was at the expense of those waiting less than one year, and that in some instances minor operations were taking precedence over more serious cases.[242,247,253,254] It was even suggested that some hospitals had declined to put patients on waiting lists at all because they could not be treated for over two years.[253]

Many of the predictable weaknesses due to the nature of the reorganisation were however becoming manifest by the time the election took place in April 1992.[248] First there were the difficulties brought about by having two kinds of "purchasers" (General Practitioner fundholders and District General Practitioners funded by Health Authorities). The fundholders were more flexible and better funded, consequently budgeted money for contracts for non-fundholders ran out and provider hospitals would only accept patients from fundholding practices; the anticipated "two-tier" service thus became a reality.[248,250,255] It was becoming clear that in many cases "patients were following money" rather than "money following patients".

There was also no doubt that the freedom to refer individual patients to hospitals other than those with whom contracts had been made either by non-fundholding General Practitioners or by Hospital Doctors was eroded despite denials by the Minister. These restrictions obviously diminished the patient's choice even when exercised vicariously by the doctor; it is noteworthy that the freedom to make an extra contractual referral was one of the original concepts behind the purchase-provider split.[256,257]

Secrecy in the NHS. Much more unfortunate developments were attempts on the part of General Managers to impose a veil of secrecy over the operations of the NHS (particularly those of the quasi-independent Trust Hospitals) and to deny hospital medical and dental practitioners the right enshrined in paragraph 330 of their nationally negotiated "Terms and conditions of service":-

> *"to be free without the consent of the employing authority, to publish books, articles, etc. and to deliver any lecture or to speak, whether on matters arising out of his or her hospital service or not."*[258]

These attempts at "gagging" both doctors and nurses actually predated the 1991 reorganisation and dated back to the introduction of general management in 1984,[259,260] but the pressure on individuals increased after 1991, often on the grounds that it is necessary to preserve "commercial secrecy".[4,258] Doctors and nurses are the true "patients' advocates"; their first duty is to their patients (although this has been challenged by the Chairman of a NHS Trust who believes that a doctor's first duty is to the organisation in which he works).[260] There is no doubt that the right to speak out publicly when the conditions under which patients are treated are not satisfactory should be preserved. It was unfortunate and short sighted that Health Ministers have left the Management Boards of NHS Trusts free to include gagging clauses in their contracts.[258] An atmosphere of secrecy pervaded all levels of the NHS after the 1991 reorganisation:-

> *"The important meetings of the (now small and politically appointed) policy board, health authorities and trusts all take place in private... with no press, public or community health councils, [or professional or local authority representatives] present."*[261,262]

This surely is an anachronism since one of the main objectives of the 1991 reorganisation was stated to be to make the NHS more accountable to the public!

It was unfortunate in this period also that some managers saw their mission in life as being to "take on the doctors and win".[263] Some hospitals doctors were "suspended" for trivial reasons unconnected with clinical practice.[264] The use of suspension was not new of course. There had been at least 83 instances between 1983 and 1993, and in 80% of cases it had been shown that there was no case to answer and reinstatement has followed.[265] Management do not regard suspension on full pay as a punishment, but merely a measure to ascertain the facts, but the stress imposed on individuals is considerable.[265] This was "macho" management. The period 1991-1992 was also a time when many managers with short term contracts were sacked at short notice by the superiors allegedly in the interests of efficiency (the "clear your desk and leave" phenomenon), and the Chief Executive of the NHS Duncan Nichol felt compelled to intervene and give guidance.[2,266] It was unfortunate that there was an impression that those who were sacked were frequently "the ones closest to the doctors".[267]

Such then was the state of the NHS at the time of the April 1992 General Election. It is doubtful whether very active debate on the NHS had any great effect on the result of the election, but certainly the medical profession and the managers held their breath and pondered on the possibility of a change of Government.[2,268]

The National Health Service 9 April to 31 December 1992.

The election in April 1992 returned the Conservative administration to power with a greatly reduced overall majority of 21.[1] It was, therefore, clear that the implementation of the 1991 reorganisation would be a continuing process.[269]

Virginia Bottomley, a former psychiatric social worker, who had been Junior Minister of Health since 1989, replaced the urbane William Waldegrave as Minister of State for Health, Brian Mawhinney, a PhD in radiation biology, became her deputy as Minister for Health, and Baroness Cumberledge became Health Minister in the House of Lords (she had previously been Chairman of the South West Thames Health Region and had regrettably expressed somewhat antagonistic views about the way Consultant private practice was conducted in the NHS).[231,269-271]

The attitude of the medical profession and the British Medical Association was at first pragmatically conciliatory and there was obviously hope that, in both primary and hospital care, some of the difficulties which had arisen as a result of the hastily introduced 1991 reorganisation would be ironed out.[269-271] Virginia Bottomley met both the BMA General Practitioner General Medical Services Committee (GMSC) and the BMA Central Consultants and Specialists Committee (CCSC) in late September 1992, but she gave little away and made few positive promises to allay legitimate concerns.[272,273] Speaking to the CCSC Virginia Bottomley agreed that there were teething problems in the concept of money following patients (for example restrictions on elective surgery for patients of non-fundholding practices at the end of the financial year) and in the matter of extra-contractual and tertiary referrals between hospitals, but she did not want to create "unrealistic expectations". She was evasive on freedom of speech as enshrined in paragraph 330 of the terms and conditions of, but said that there were no "immediate plans" to interfere with the review body system of determining pay, but could not give a guarantee about what would happen in 10 or 20 years time (in the event this matter has come to the fore considerably earlier than this!) She also foresaw that difficult decisions would have to be taken in implementing recommendations of the then (September 1992) imminently expected Tomlinson report on health care in London, and was "excited" at the opportunity offered by the review of medical training which the Government's Chief Medical Officer was undertaking.[273] Both the latter issues were to occasion considerable debate and became important considerations in 1993.

Conditions in the NHS at the end of 1992 (the year in which the Association of Anaesthetists of Great Britain and Ireland celebrated its Diamond Jubilee) were a cause of considerable anxiety to the medical profession. The pattern had become all too familiar over the previous two or three years as the end of the financial year (April 1993) approached:-

> *"The winter 1992/93 proved bleak for the NHS. First the market seemed to be failing to deliver the goods with hospitals having spent their contract money, beds were closing, operations were postponed until the new financial year and some hospitals were only treating patients from GP budget-holders. The scenario looked like fulfilling fears of the market becoming a two-tier system."*[3]

The folly of trying to create a quasi-market with a divided purchasing element without reviewing the system of restricted funding from general taxation, or reconsidering the extent of the services provided by the NHS, was becoming all too apparent.

Macho management was not dead either and some notable battles with members of the medical and nursing professions on administrative grounds ultimately ended in reinstatement, apologies, successful libel actions and successful claims for unfair dismissal, but not without unnecessary stress and aggravation to the individuals concerned and high cost in legal fees to the tax payer.[258,274-278]

The particular issue of whistleblowing ("going public") by professionals and "gagging" by management had caused considerable controversy. The concern is that medical consultants and senior nurses owe it to their patients to retain the right in the last resort to go public if blatant management failures do not provide satisfactory conditions to enable patients to be properly cared for; however, as Richard Smith the Editor of the *British Medical Journal* noted in an admirable editorial:-

> "......*managers worrying about whistleblowing should concentrate their energies on improving the management in their institutions rather than trying to gag staff. Similarly, staff should insist first on good management and only secondly on the right to blow the whistle - because whistleblowing usually achieves little.*"[279]

If however "the insistence on good management" is ineffective the urge to whistleblow publicly may well become an overwhelming professional duty.[280] Guidelines by the Department of Health issued in June 1993 implied that NHS employees, having exhausted locally established procedures might wish to consult their Member of Parliament in confidence, or, as a last resort, disclose their concern to the media, but warned, ambiguously, that such action "if entered into unjustifiably could result in disciplinary action".[281] MPs protested that so far as reference to MPs was concerned this document infringed the basic democratic rights of the individual, and in November 1993, it was acknowledged by the Department of Health that the NHS should not prevent members of staff contacting MPs at any time.[282] There is no doubt, however, that the Department of Health had moved to restrict freedom of speech by NHS employees partly because of the perceived need for "commercial secrecy" since the 1991 reorganisation. There seems at times to be genuine or politically motivated confusion between the absolute need for "confidentiality" about individual patients, and the desire to keep the operations of the system secret for commercial reasons.[277]

Many working Consultants had sympathy for Unit Managers, most of whom were not medically qualified, who had to "take decisions which frequently had a profound clinical impact", but deplored the confrontational attitude some of them adopted towards highly qualified professionals, and the fact that they ignored the first principle of management which is to exercise leadership; as anyone who has served in the armed forces knows:-

> *"the troops will follow you to the end of the earth provided they consider your ideas sensible, that you are concerned with their welfare and that you will stand by them when the going gets rough. ....It takes a strength of character to say thank you ..... but it might go a long way to improving staff morale."*[283]

The NHS Management Executive Annual Report of December 1992 was upbeat, "All glossy print, beaming bonhomie and looking for all the world like the report of a prosperous company".[284] It left many questions unanswered however, and there was considerable doubt about the interpretation of the statistics on increased activity.[284,285]

A revealing summary of the state of the NHS in the winter 1992-1993 is contained in an open "Letter to Mrs Bottomley" written by R F (Bob) Bury a working Consultant Radiologist, and published in the *British Medical Journal* in March 1993,[286] from which the following extracts are taken:-

> *"Truths which are self evident to those of us who actually work in public services hold novelty value for our masters."*

> *"Even your supporters are becoming alarmed by the destabilising effect of general medical practice fund holding. .... Waiting list initiatives have had exactly the same effect because money was diverted to solve a politically sensitive problem, health care priorities have been distorted so that in some cases cash rather than clinical need dictates who gets treated."*

> *"As for the argument that money would follow patients and so make it possible for hospitals to treat more of them, that was always a non-starter given that the total amount of cash available to purchasers was not going to be increased. ... The purchaser runs out of money before the end of the year. We then start to read the familiar stories of ward closures and idle operating theatres. ......To tell hospital managers that they should have paced themselves to spend the money*

over the whole year is a denial of all the theoretical advantages of a free market. In 1988 the money ran out because of 'inefficiency', and 'bad management' prompting the NHS review. This year [1992-1993] the same problem has arisen as a result of "over trading". Patients refused admission can not be expected to take much comfort of this explanation."

"When Kenneth Clarke first told us of his ideas these and other flaws were so obvious that we assumed that he too ....had spotted the pitfalls and had solutions up his sleeve. We now realise that this was not the case. The NHS did need a kick up the backside and a lot of us were (and still are) far more prepared than you realise to promote any scheme that looks halfway decent. Sadly there was no discussion or consultation, and the present confrontational atmosphere was allowed to develop."

"Please listen to the arguments of those of us who are doing our best to make the new system work."[286]

The attitude of the Association of Anaesthetists to the 1991 reorganisation was pragmatic from the start but its Officers were determined that if Consultants were to be involved in management it was essential that anaesthetists should be amongst them. Consultant Anaesthetists were amongst the first to be successful as Clinical Directors and, in September 1992, a Working Party chaired by the then Honorary Treasurer W R (Bill) MacRae, prepared a very valuable guideline document with the title *NHS Management changes, implications for Anaesthetists*. This booklet largely confined itself to considering in detail the Clinical Directorate level of management emphasising the importance of "one of the specialty's greatest strengths - the unity of working groups of colleagues who stick by jointly agreed local policies which are in the majority interest", but it also contained very valuable advice on terms and conditions of service and, in particular, to recently promoted consultants who could be offered individual contracts by NHS Trusts which, though superficially more remunerative, were in practice, more restrictive.[287]

The Nurses and the 1984 and 1991 NHS Reorganisations

The nursing profession reached its managerial zenith in the era of consensus management after the 1974 Reorganisation; nurses who wished to move from bedside nursing, achieved parity in the management teams at all levels with administrators and doctors; indeed the only route by which a nurse could aspire to promotion or higher salaries was on the managerial ladder. This left more junior staff and married women and others who were dedicated to caring for patients and did not seek promotion, at the bedside.[1-4,163] This situation continued after the 1982 Reorganisation, but was radically changed in 1984 with the advent of General Managers. The latter were given considerable latitude as to how they organised the management structure within Districts and Units. Many of them took direct control of nurse administration. This relegated the District or Unit Nursing Officers to the role of advisers, or even did away with their posts altogether; only six nurses succeeded in moving into higher management by being appointed to District General Management posts, and initially even the Chief Nursing Officer of the Department of Health was excluded from the new NHS Management Board, although this decision was later rescinded under pressure.[2-4,163-164]

It was not surprising that the nursing profession reacted strongly to the 1984 reorganisation proposals and their implementation which followed the Griffiths report. The Royal College of Nursing mounted a spirited and expensive campaign to regain influence at managerial level ("Why is Britain's nursing profession being run by people who do not know their coccyx from their humerus?"). The campaign was largely unsuccessful although it did succeed in the appointment of some additional District Nursing Advisers, it was however a far cry from the days of consensus management.[2-4,163,164]

There were other reasons for mounting anger on the part of the rank and file nursing profession resulting in low morale, many resignations from the profession, and diminishing recruitment.[288] These culminated in a day of action on 3 February 1988 shortly after the Prime Minister (Mrs Thatcher) had announced her secret review of the NHS on the Panorama Television Programme; as the commentator "Scrutator" summarised the situation in the *British Medical Journal* on 6 February 1988:-[289]

> "The position British nurses now find themselves in bears eloquent testimony to the rewards of avoiding action."[289,290]

"The industrial action planned for this week, ranging from protests to a 24 hour strike is ..... provoked not by just self interest - though as nurses pay and conditions are, as Dr. Delamothe describes,[290-295] scandalous - but by acute frustration over deteriorating standards of care in the NHS and the Government's apparent indifference to them."[289]

A P (Tony) Delamothe (Assistant Editor of the *British Medical Journal*) wrote an outstanding series of articles on the "grievances" of the British nursing profession early in 1988.[163,290-296] These were based on interviews with many nurses over the last six months of 1987. The saddest quotation from this series emphasises an aspect of conditions in the NHS which regrettably persist, to the present time:-[295]

"The grievances dealt with in these articles arose from discussions in Aberdeen, London, Manchester, and Nottingham. Such are the current fears within the health service of reprisals that most nurses agreed to speak to me only on condition that they would not be identified: many thanks to them all. Happily such fears do not exist elsewhere and I can acknowledge the assistance of [named Scandinavian and Australian nurses]."[295]

The truth was that, in addition to the decline in managerial status, the 1984 reorganisation threw a heavy extra burden on the nurses at the bedside. The new breed of general managers saw bedside nurses as an easily managed resource. They traded on their strong work ethic for patient care and traditional response of shutting up and getting on with caring for patients whatever the difficulties. Managers were getting bonuses for cutting costs, getting waiting lists shorter and increasing productivity, while cutting back on staff and equipment, "rationalising" support services, and packing more and more patients into overworked wards. Hospital activity in all fields (inpatients, outpatients and, particularly, day cases) rose dramatically without any increase in the number of nursing staff.[288,290-296] The high hopes engendered by the introduction of the Nurses Pay Review Body ("the imposition of a no strike agreement by the back door") had been dashed when the Government failed to implement the Review Body recommendations in 1985 and 1986, and what increases there were came partly from existing hospital budgets. The last circumstance "invariably caused further cuts to services for patients - hence nurses reluctance to push harder for what they think they deserve." The 1987 pay award, 18 days before the date of a general election was called was funded in full.[291] The predominant feminine gender of the nursing profession,[294] when compared with other non-manual workers (e.g. police and firemen)[290] made:-

> "it difficult to counter the assertion that nurses' salaries reflect assumptions that nurses are either single women who will soon leave to get married, confirmed [and dedicated] spinsters who do not need much money, or married women who are working for 'pin money'."[291,294]

The low morale amongst nurses prompted an increase in the exodus from the NHS nursing workforce well above the departures which might be expected due to the "natural" causes of marriage and childbearing.[294] Delamothe produced figures from various well researched sources to show *inter alia* that half of a large sample questioned had "considered" or "seriously considered" giving up nursing in the NHS during the twelve months 1986-1987. Ten per cent of qualified nurses left each year, most nurses left before they were thirty, and nationwide the number of qualified staff in 1986 fell short of the establishment by 10% and in inner London by 20%; between 1981 and 1987 there was a reduction of 29% in the numbers entering basic nurse training, and 21% of these did not join the NHS (13% discontinued training, 2% failed the exams, 2% passed but did not register, and 3% registered but did not join the NHS).[2]

Nursing professionalism in the NHS. The long-term perceived desire to increase the professionalism of nurses, and with it the independent status of the profession, predated the Griffiths report, but was given fresh impetus by the implementation of the 1984 reorganisation which followed. The nursing hierarchy, having had their pretensions to the upper echelons of the NHS management considerably curtailed in 1991, turned their attention to extending the scope and status of clinical nursing and upgrading the academic status of the discipline.

The Nursing Process originated from theories developed in the United States of America in the nineteen sixties.[297-299] The concept made a praiseworthy attempt to change the application of nursing care in the ward area from being task orientated to patient orientated; a "named nurse" responsible for the maintenance of the "daily living activities" of each individual patient. "Daily living activities" are considered to be separate from but complimentary to the tasks performed by the doctor, whose province includes such matters as diagnosis and treatment. The nurses' Project 2000 (see below) involves data collection (history taking), assessment, planning, implementation, evaluation and appropriate individual nursing notes separate from those of the medical team.

The basic principle of the Nursing Process focusing on the individual patient is admirable and the substitution of individual nursing notes for the general ward "Cardex" record, though time consuming when carried on to excess,[297] can be considered to be an advantage.[299] The concept that nursing care can be completely independent of medical care, and the extension of this philosophy that the nurse should be the coordinator of patient care are however naive (rightly "the legal buck stops with the Consultant or principal in general practice to whose care the patient has been entrusted").[297] Particularly embarrassing situations have arisen in recent years; for instance, where nurses have stepped outside their field of specialised knowledge and visited the preoperative patient; they have sometimes erroneously described the nature of the particular procedure which the patient is to expect in the anaesthetic room and even defined the particular anaesthetic which will be administered.

The Nursing Process was unfortunately generally introduced into the NHS in the eighties without adequate discussion with the medical profession.[297] The confrontation which has arisen is not primarily about the Nursing Process itself. It is due to the colossal edifice of jargon and antagonistic rhetoric promoting the independence of nursing which has been built upon it by the leading managerial "union" and the teaching sections of the profession, who are not actively engaged in bedside nursing.[299] This tendency is particularly emphasised by some of the members of the male element in nursing who hold a disproportionate number of administrative posts in relation to their numbers.[294] It is sad that some Nursing Schools (or Colleges) do not always teach what the ward sister would like to see taught and, intentionally or otherwise, indoctrinate a minority of young men and women with a suspicious and confrontational stance towards the medical profession. "Assertiveness" (now apparently praised as a virtue) can so easily develop into aggression! A senior General Practitioner "of vast practical experience" at a seminar on the Nursing Process has some words of comfort for the nursing profession; "It's a phase. You'll get through it".[294] He is probably right, a Norwegian nurse, whose profession went through a similar revolution earlier and with rather less upheaval, including admission to the University system, acknowledged, "I am much happier with my role and want to do that better. We've got a better relation with doctors. ...It's much easier for me now to cooperate, because I've got my own identity as a nurse, and I think it's much easier for the doctors to cooperate too."[295] The emergence of Clinical Directorates within hospitals, the most successful of which are acknowledged to be those where nurses are responsible to a medical Clinical Director, may constitute a step in the right direction.

Regrading 1988 et seq. The Government accepted the Nursing Pay Review Body award in full in April 1988 together with a recommendation that a new grading structure of pay for nurses be adopted and all nurses and midwives in post should be placed in appropriate grades. The new grading structure was designed to provide "a sensible career progression for clinical staff and a proper recognition of the qualifications, skills and wider responsibilities for those who progress to higher grades now or in the future". The system was designed to place the clinical nursing staff, from nursing auxiliaries to senior ward staff, in lettered grades from A to the highest grade of I.[2,3,164,300]

The medical profession enthusiastically welcomed the concept because of its apparent emphasis on the clinical competence, rather than managerial skills. Anaesthetists were particularly pleased because they at first anticipated that at last their highly skilled and competent nursing colleagues in one to one patient management in intensive care, higher dependency and recovery units, and anaesthetic rooms, would get proper recognition of their skills on an individual basis.

It was at first rather naively intended that the regrading process would be completed by 31 October 1988, but the performance of management and senior nursing staff who undertook the regrading left much to be desired.[2] It may be that they had difficulty in accepting the concept that clinical skills might possibly deserve equal remuneration with those of management! Management seemed determined to keep the number of higher grades to a minimum level despite reasonably generous central funding. Particular controversy arose over the allocation of the senior nurse/sister grades F, G, H, and there is apparently no doubt that quotas for advanced grades were covertly introduced by some Health Authorities contrary to the original intention of the scheme.[2] The grading exercise has certainly been unjust in a number of cases,[301] and has consequently "set nurse against nurse, left a bitter legacy of disharmony between nurses and local management, and clogged up the administrative machinery of Authorities for years to come" with appeals to higher authority against local grading decisions.[301] The Royal College of Nursing described grading as " the biggest con that ever was"; by April 1989 over 100,000 appeals had been lodged and there were still about 25,000 pending in April 1993.[23,302] Attempts were made in 1993 by some Health Authorities to "buy out" appeals by one-off cash settlements.[302] It is a sorry story.

Project 2000: A new preparation for practice. Much has been written in recent years about the need for nursing to become a "true profession".[303] This is somewhat perplexing to many British doctors, including the present writer, who have always regarded nursing as the primary complimentary profession to medicine and respected and admired the expertise of its practitioners as such. It is, however, undoubtedly true that in some countries, notably in Australia and Scandinavia, improvement in status for nurses (and by implication their ability to attract higher salaries) has followed entry into the academic field of tertiary education, though it is difficult to understand why the State or General Registered qualification should not be regarded as a better degree or diploma than those offered by universities and polytechnics in some abstruse sociological subjects.[295] A revolution, involving a change from apprenticeship to academic training was recommended for British Nurses by the Briggs Report in 1972. This Committee which had been initiated with the objectives of improving the image of nursing in relation to patient care, which had been somewhat obscured by the Salmon reorganisation (Chapter 8), and of making a career in nursing more attractive to well qualified school leavers. The Briggs report also considered that a necessary first step to achieving this objective was the amalgamation of the various regulatory authorities governing nurse and midwife registration into a single body for the United Kingdom.[303]

Progress was slow, probably mainly because of the cost implications, and possibly because senior nurses achieved influence and satisfaction in management after the 1974 NHS reorganisation. Enabling legislation was passed in 1979 and the United Kingdom Committee of the Central Council for Nursing, Midwifery and Health Visiting (UKCC) came into being in 1983 at a time when recruitment to the nursing profession was again beginning to decline.[4,163,164,289] The UKCC proposal known as Project 2000, aimed at reorganising both the structure and methods of the education of the nursing profession, which contained many of the principles contained in the Briggs report,[303,304] followed in 1986, at a time when there was renewed interest in clinical nursing following the 1984 reorganisation.[4,163,164,289,293,304,305]

A few universities had run degree courses for nurses from the nineteen sixties onwards, but the number trained in this way was small and, on the whole, those who had remained in nursing had gone into the higher echelons of nurse management. Project 2000 proposed that all nursing students would base their training in institutions of higher education and, instead of spending 80% of their time on the wards as "pairs of hands", they would spend only about 20% of it in supernumerary "placements". The course for all nurses leading to the grade of "Registered Practitioner" was to be an 18 month foundation programme followed by an 18 month programme in either nursing of the adult, the child, the mentally handicapped or the mentally ill. The practical (State) Enrolled Nurse (SEN) qualification would be discontinued and the Registered Practitioner would undertake the duties of both the old (State) "Registered" or "Registered General" Nurse (SRN or RGN) and the "Enrolled" grades. Registered Practitioner nurses could then go on to take further training to become Registered Midwives, or undertake specialist courses to qualify as Specialist Practitioners.

There would in addition be "Helpers" or Nursing Auxiliaries (to be known as Health Care Assistants or HCAs) in the nursing team trained and assessed "in house" in the National Vocational Qualification (NVQ) scheme introduced in 1985.[306]

The Government took time before they formally endorsed, and finally implemented the Project 2000 scheme,[307,308] chiefly because of the financial implications. Insufficient funds were allocated and serious doubts about its viability were raised at the end of 1992 when the National Audit Office declared, after £209 million had been spent on the initial pilot projects, that it had proved to be a "radical and costly" enterprise, and raised doubts about its financial planning. Kember and Macpherson assert in their perceptive book published in 1994 that, the execution of the scheme "like that of the clinical regrading exercise of 1988 was another sorry tale of central mismanagement".[3] The scheme went ahead however, nursing schools amalgamated and became associated with institutions of further education (not without imposing considerable difficulties for integration of Nursing Tutors in post),[309] student nurses became "students" in the real sense of the word (they became supernumerary during their clinical "placements" and were funded by bursaries instead of salaries). The new student nurses did not necessarily find this change of status an advantage! The new business minded NHS hospitals promptly put up living-in rents in nurses homes to "economic" levels because the students were no longer part of the active work force, and there were travel expenses to be met to the fewer merged training colleges.[307,310,311]

The first Project 2000 nurses from the original pilot schemes received their RN (Dip HE) qualification (Registered Nurse with Diploma in Health Education) during the second half of 1992.[308,312]

There is little doubt that the nurses central council who originated Project 2000 envisaged it as a means of conferring academic status on the bedside nurse:-

> *"This new nurse will continue to work directly with patients and clients once qualified rather than be solely involved in supervising others and to decrease the present dependence on a continually changing population of unqualified staff and those undergoing training."*[305]

Even at the time the Government accepted the project in principle, however, it was obvious that they and the Department of Health and its managers saw things very differently.[307] They soon realised that Project 2000 might be a way of cutting costs with the prospect of "the emergence of a much smaller professional elite educated in the new system to supervise an army of helpers (in house trained, Health Care Assistants or HCAs)".[3,4,307,308] Many academic commentators also saw Project 2000 as an attempt to sharpen the distinction between those undertaking professional nursing and those engaged solely in basic care.[313] There was a prediction that "the rise in the shortfall [to nursing] of 3000 entrants [due to a demographic fall in school leavers] in 1994 without Project 2000 .... to 16,000 with it" (due to student nurses becoming supernumeraries) might "bring the NHS to its knees",[314] and this eventuality has only been avoided by the dilution of the ward nursing staff ("skill mix") by HCAs.[315] It is difficult to see how the desired principle of one to one qualified nurse to every patient can become a reality in such circumstances. There is even a "suspicion" that, since the £500 million or more already spent on Project 2000 has not been "ring fenced" (specifically dedicated), the portion allotted for staff replacements "has simply been redirected to other areas by some hard up [NHS] Trusts".[316]

Some management texts even see the emergence of the "diploma nurse" and the introduction of National Vocational Qualifications for HCAs, as "eroding" the worth of the previous nurse qualifications (SRN and RGN) and making "it difficult to see the distinction between the types of peripheral workers sustained. This could force the cost of such workers downwards...."![4] If, as is the case in Norway, schools for nurse auxiliaries with one year courses should be started,[295] the discontinued (State) Enrolled Nurse (SEN) strata of nursing may well be reinvented under another name!

There is also criticism of the content of the educational material being imported by the Project 2000 Training. Professor Roger Dyson (Director of the Clinical Management Unit of Keele University) has been reported as contending that nurses are being trained to see their future as primary practitioner nurses in General Practice,[301] community nursing or in Accident and Emergency Departments,[317,318] and that the future needs of hospital nursing are being ignored. This, or course, is hotly contested by nurse educationalists.[317] It must be admitted, however, that the anonymous triumphalism and confrontational attitude of some Project 2000 student nurses (of which the following is a sample) gives pause for thought:-

> "Project 2000 is taking caring individuals and preparing them to be successful in the role of patient advocates."

"Project 2000 is arming us with what we will need for such change; communication skills, presentation skills, awareness of social and public policy, of culture and ethnicity."[319]

It seems to be certain that nurses who "may not actually mix with staff of their home hospital until over halfway through their training"[320] need all the assistance that is proposed for them when they come on the wards as Registered Nurses![312]

It is also to be hoped that adequate courses will be developed, and adequate remuneration will be forthcoming, for the much needed Specialist Practitioner nursing grade for work in Intensive Care Units and similar situations. This emphasis on the practitioner nurse has, of course, potential implications for anaesthetists. The idea of the supposedly "cheaper" option of employing nurse anaesthetists seems to be never far from the minds of some health economists and NHS Trust managers.[321] These protagonists seem to have little concept of what physician anaesthetists actually do both inside and outside the operating theatre, or of the length of training required to graduate as a nurse anaesthetist (an extra three years in Sweden), or of the expense of setting up schools of nurse anaesthesia, or the requirement of physician anaesthetists to instruct and supervise nurse anaesthetists, or of the limitations imposed by the pattern of nursing shifts.[322,323] Once again however in the nineteen nineties the issue of nurse anaesthetists is being raised because there is a shortage of physician anaesthetists of the required grades as a result of the curtailment of junior doctors' hours and the new postgraduate medical education requirements.

The business of the Association 1983-1992

The central event in the life of the Association of Anaesthetists of Great Britain and Ireland in the decade between the celebration of the Golden Jubilee of the Association in 1982 and its Diamond Jubilee in 1992 was the establishment of its headquarters in a separate building in the elegant Georgian house at 9 Bedford Square, London. The realisation of the ambition of the Association to occupy its own building has enabled its advisory service to members to be considerably rationalised and improved, its educational activities to be greatly expanded, and its medicopolitical function to be considerably enhanced.

The constitution, committee structure and electoral procedures and financial status of the Association of Anaesthetists were fully established as the result of the reorganisation which had taken place in the seventies. One further major step, the incorporation of the Association as a Company limited by guarantee under the Companies Act proved to be necessary and this was achieved in 1985.

The final year of the decade under review also saw the foundation of an independent Royal College of Anaesthetists; the establishment of which the Association had advocated for a number of years.

Membership 1982 to 1995

The overall membership of the Association of Anaesthetists rose steadily by over 34% (from 4,434 in 1982 to 5,930 in 1992). The Junior Anaesthetists Group (after April 1991 Group of Anaesthetists in Training) had increased its membership by 51% (1982:1,293 and 1992: 1,958) and its proportion of the voting membership of the Association (Overseas and Honorary categories being excluded from voting) rose from 39% to 44%. Overseas (nonvoting) membership had, however declined by some 10% (1982:816 and 1992:739);[324,325] this may reflect the increasing number and status of other national societies, but it might also have been influenced by the policy of a disproportionate increase in subscription rates in real terms of over 45% during the decade: from £40 in 1982 (1996: £75) to £110 (1996: £120) in 1992.[324,326] A decision was taken to freeze the Overseas Membership subscription to £110 in 1992; nonetheless the number of Overseas Members has continued to decline (1997: 564).

Nine Bedford Square, London WC1. A Headquarters for the Association of Anaesthetists of Great Britain and Ireland

The search for premises for the Association had its origins in the protracted discussions concerning the possibility of the formation of an independent Royal College of Anaesthetists during the Presidencies of Philip Helliwell, Cyril Scurr and Stanley Mason (Chapter 8); at that time, in addition to a desire to provide a worthy headquarters for the Association of Anaesthetists and British anaesthesia, little progress was being made on the College front, and there was a perception that it might be desirable to form a separate College, independent of the Faculty of Anaesthetists in a separate building from the Royal College of Surgeons in Lincoln's Inn Fields.

A resolution was passed at the 1977 Annual General Meeting during Cyril Scurr's Presidency authorising the Officers to investigate the possibility of purchasing premises for the Association and, if necessary to raise a mortgage or loan not exceeding £200,000 (1996: £840,000).

The resolutions passed by the Faculty in May 1980 indicated that its Board were at least actively "exploring" the possibility of "autonomous" Collegiate status. The perception that it might be desirable for the Association of Anaesthetists to take the drastic action of forming a rival College therefore receded in the eighties, but, nonetheless, as Derek Wylie has written:

> *"the rapid development of the specialty of anaesthesia had greatly increased the role of the Association [of Anaesthetists] in the medical and political aspirations of anaesthetists throughout the United Kingdom and Ireland, and it was becoming evident that the then offices in Tavistock House [BMA Headquarters] would soon provide inadequate accommodation for the necessary administration."*[328]

Wylie's proposal that the Officers should search actively for new premises was agreed in October 1981. The estate agents Hillier and Parker were engaged to assist in the search, and two properties were considered but rejected in 1982.

Michael Vickers, on assuming the Office of President in October 1982 invited Derek Wylie to continue the active search for suitable premises. It was considered at that time that the upper limit which the Association funds could bear for a purchase price was £300,000 (1996 equivalent £564,000).[328]

Wylie, while walking through Bedford Square early in 1983 noted that a row of houses on the east side of the Square were for sale by the building developers Tarmac Properties South Ltd.[328,329] Number 9, like the adjacent houses, was in a very dilapidated state, but it had enough accommodation for the requirements of the Association of Anaesthetists and had charm and potential. The house, though a Georgian Grade 1 listed building, was not precluded from use as the headquarters of a professional association, indeed it had been the offices of the Institute of Electronic and Radio Engineers until the mid nineteen seventies. Derek Wylie took expert advice which was favourable. It was agreed that the asking price of £500,000 (1996: £900,000) might make it "a bargain for anyone who wanted a period house of historic interest and could afford the necessary restorations"; sadly, however, Wylie concluded that the price and the potential cost of renovations were beyond the resources of the Association of Anaesthetists at that time.[328]

Maurice M Burrows (at that time Honorary Treasurer elect) also noticed that the house was for sale some months later and called the attention of the Officers of the Association to its possible suitability. The resources available to the Association had meanwhile improved considerably, in part due to the surplus generated by the 1982 Sixth European Congress of Anaesthesiology (Chapter 8). The Officers estimated that the total cost and refurbishment charge, including professional fees would amount to approximately £1,000,000 (1996: £1,800,000). It was considered that, though the cost of the building could be met from Association capital funds, a proportion of the restoration and refurbishment would necessitate an appeal to the membership and to friends of the specialty of anaesthesia.[328,329]

One other property came on the market in the late summer of 1983 which could have been purchased within the monies allocated for the purpose. The building was in Great Russell Street opposite the headquarters of the Trades Union Council. The property had been fully restored for unrestricted use as potential offices and had adequate accommodation. Its acquisition would have meant that the Association of Anaesthetists could have achieved its objective immediately, but the executive officers decided that "as a building it had no great charm and it was in a location that would not have been appropriate for our headquarters".[328] The present writer was Vice President but not yet President elect, and was contemplating honourable retirement from active participation as a member of the Council of the Association at the time the two properties came under consideration; he recollects that, although he greatly admired the courage and enthusiasm of the President (Michael Vickers) and the then Honorary Treasurer (Michael Rosen) he himself had grave doubts about the wisdom of the decision to choose the internally derelict 9 Bedford Square. If the decision had been left to the writer alone he would probably have opted for the more cautious and less expensive line of action and chosen the ready made building in Great Russell Street! How mistaken that decision would have been!

The decision to negotiate for 9 Bedford Square was finally taken at the Council Meeting of the Association of Anaesthetists held at the Gosforth Park Hotel during the Annual Scientific Meeting at Newcastle upon Tyne on 22 September 1983, after the resource options available had been exhaustively debated. The Council agreed:-

"that they supported the decision of the Advisory Committee to authorise an agent to negotiate on behalf of the Association, to a total purchase price and refurbishment charge, including professional fees, of £1,000,000 [1996: £1,800,000]."

This decision was communicated to the Annual General Meeting which followed later in the day.[328,330]

The purchase of 9 Bedford Square. The negotiations for the purchase of the 125 year lease of 9 Bedford Square were fruitful; in the event the price paid was £400,000 (1996: £684,000) which was a 20% reduction on the original asking price.[328] The appointed agents were Messrs Healey and Baker of London, W1, (Council Minutes 7.10.1983).[27,331] The contract was signed early in April 1984 (Council Minutes 13.4.1984)[27] after some delay for necessary structural surveys and planning permissions. (Council Minutes 2.12.1983).[27]

There had also been a limit to the time the vendors were prepared to wait for signatures on the contract. An unacceptable delay might have arisen, or the sale might even have been lost because the British Museum, who held the ground lease from the Bedford Estates, were unwilling to assign it to an unincorporated body, which the Association of Anaesthetists still was in 1984 because Council had decided in 1973 that there would be no advantage in incorporation under the Companies Act at that particular time (Chapter 8); this was before the purchase of premises was under consideration. The problem was solved by the initiative of two of the three Trustees of the Association of Anaesthetists, Michael Vickers, the reigning President, and his predecessor as President W Derek Wylie, who agreed to sign the contract; legally this was on their own financial responsibility even though the Council passed a resolution agreeing to indemnify them (Council Minutes 2.12.1983). The third Trustee (Douglas Howat) had not been closely concerned with the mechanics of the proposed purchase of 9 Bedford Square and felt unable to accept such a heavy financial liability without indemnity insurance; understandably he resigned before the contract was signed (Council Minutes 17.2.1984).[27,329] Stanley Mason was elected as the third Trustee at the 1984 Annual General Meeting.[332]

A change in the legal status of the Association of Anaesthetists. The Association of Anaesthetists of Great Britain and Ireland and the renamed Education and Research Trust became separate "companies limited by guarantee and not having share capitals" in April 1985, with the Education and Research Trust also having charitable status. The Members of Council for the time being became Directors of both companies. The "land and buildings" assets of the Association are vested approximately equally in the two companies, the total being currently (1998) nearly £1,000,000 according to the Annual Directors Report and Financial Statements.[333]

The history of Bedford Square and Number 9 has been researched by the historian Graham Tite and recorded in a volume commissioned by the Association of Anaesthetists,[334] and by C A Fuge (Consultant Anaesthetist, Bath).[335] There are interesting connections with the medical profession.

There is a tradition that the 4th Duke of Bedford envisaged the classical facades of Bedford Square as an echo of the style of Bath, which was a city with which he was familiar from his visits in search of relief for his gout; be that as it may the 4th Duke died in 1771 and it was left to the Dowager Duchess, the guardian of his grandson the 5th Duke, who was a minor at the time, to issue the building leases. The Square was built between 1775 and 1780. The designs are attributed to the architect Thomas Leverton (1743-1824), who later became an early resident in the Square, and the building contractors were Robert Grews and William Scott.[334]

Bedford Square became a prestigious address for politicians and eminent professional men, and particularly for leading members of the medical profession; by 1841 there were 41 physicians and surgeons resident in the area of Bedford Square; at the time there were only 14 registered as living in

Harley Street. Thomas Wakley (1795-1862), the exuberant founder editor of the *Lancet* in 1823 was resident at No 35.[335,336]

The head of the household in Number 9 in the mid eighteen forties to the eighteen sixties (spanning the years in which ether and chloroform anaesthesia were introduced in the United Kingdom and accepted into medical practice) was Clement Hue, MD, FRCP the cantankerous Senior Physician to St Bartholomew's Hospital.[334,337] The most prominent Lord Chancellor of the nineteenth century John Scott, First Earl of Eldon (1751-1838) resided at Number 6 Bedford Square.[338] Wakley published in the *Lancet* without permission, lectures delivered by the staff at St Bartholomew's Hospital to the students, including those of Hue. A legal dispute followed which was adjudicated upon by Lord Eldon![335-338]

Gower Street, which runs into the northern corner of Bedford Square was the scene of the first use of ether in England by the dentist James Robinson for a dental extraction at the house of his friend Dr Boott on 10 December 1846 and, on 21 December 1846, of the first amputation under ether by the surgeon Robert Liston at the North London (now University College) Hospital; an event which led on to the general acceptance of general anaesthesia in the United Kingdom.[339]

The physician James Elliotson (1791-1868) had experimented with hypnotism (mesmerism) and advocated its use to relieve the pain of surgery at the same hospital in the years immediately preceding the introduction of anaesthesia; unfortunately his enthusiasm for the use of mesmerism in the treatment of disease in general was obsessive. Wakley was vociferous in his opposition and regarded mesmerism as humbug. An experimental session in Wakley's house in Bedford Square in reality proved nothing, but it discredited Elliotson who was forced to resign from the North London (University College) Hospital in 1838. He then founded the London Mesmeric Infirmary "for the cure of diseases and the prevention of pain in surgery" in 1850 in 9 Bedford Street (renamed Bayley Street in 1878), which joins the west corner of Bedford Square with Tottenham Court Road;[335,340] as Fuge remarked in 1986. "It seems appropriate that the new centre for anaesthesia should be established in a part of London which has historical connections with the evolution of anaesthesia".[335]

The restoration of the interior of 9 Bedford Square began in earnest once the contract was signed. The architects were Shankland Cox, the builders Elliot-Layford, the engineers Price and Myers, the quantity surveyors Bucknall, Austin, and Partners, and the interior designers Christopher Rowley. Great care had to be exercised because of the Grade 1 listed status of the building; some difficulties were experienced with the Greater London Council Historic Buildings Department over double glazing but these were overcome on appeal (Committee Minutes 5.10.1984). There was a delay of some 12 weeks on the completion of the building contract. This was partly due to a necessary survey to eliminate the possibility of dry rot in the panelling in the Council Room (Council Minutes 1.2.1985). The building decorated and completed but not yet furnished, was ready for occupation by September 1985 (Council Minutes 4.10.1985. Annual Report 1984-1985).[27,341]

The move to 9 Bedford Square. The last Council Meeting in the suite of offices in BMA House was held on 4 October 1985.[27] It fell to the writer as President, the Honorary Secretary Michael Inman (Plymouth), the Assistant Honorary Secretary Peter Morris (Manchester), and the Administrative Secretary Miss Ann Muir (see below) with her small staff of two to organise, and to a certain extent personally physically achieve, the move to 9 Bedford Square on 16 November 1985 before the lease of the old suite of offices in BMA House terminated on 31 December 1985. Michael Inman's resourceful contribution should particularly be appreciated; he is probably the only person to have slept overnight on the job in the building since it became the headquarters of the Association of Anaesthetists!

The policy adopted by the Officers and Council was that the building should first function as an administrative headquarters, much as had been the case at BMA House, and then an ambitious programme of furnishing and academic and social expansion should gradually follow as money from the appeal fund for furnishing and academic development became available.[341]

The possessions of the Association of Anaesthetists at that time were indeed modest; just the all important filing cabinets and their contents, a couple of electric typewriters, the utilitarian Council table and its accompanying chairs, the framed grant of arms, and the book case housing the Bryn Thomas collection of historic books.[324] One was reminded of the first move of a young married couple from a small rented flat into their first house; only in this case the step up was even more emphasised by the elegance of the new surroundings, and there was little "do-it-yourself" to be done other than odd tasks such as the lengthening of electric flexes and the hanging of one or two pictures. Part time domestic staff were organised to do cleaning and washing up, and a visit to the John Lewis department store by Michael Inman with his credit card produced the necessary domestic equipment and a vital tool box.

The administrative functions of the Association went on without interruption and the exciting task began of furnishing the building and expanding the work of the organisation. The first Council Meeting at 9 Bedford Square was held on 6 December 1985 followed by the Annual Council Dinner.[27]

The Appeal for furnishing 9 Bedford Square was officially launched at the Annual Scientific Meeting at the University of Exeter in 1984[341,342] but, before that, Members of Council had already responded generously with covenants, and also a donation of £100 (1996: £170) from the Edinburgh and East of Scotland Society of Anaesthetists had been received (Council Minutes 17.2.1984 and 4.6.1984).[27] The funds required for the purchase and refurbishment of the fabric of the actual building at 9 Bedford Square were provided from the existing resources of the Association of Anaesthetists, though at one time there was a need for an "internal loan" from the Research and Education Fund to the General Fund.[341] The money raised by the Appeal was devoted solely for furnishing the new headquarters in an appropriate manner.[342,343]

The Chairman of the Appeal was Sir Cecil Montacute Clothier (Council Minutes 4.6.1984),[27] who had continued to take a very active interest in the Association after he had delivered his outstanding John Snow Lecture in 1980 (Chapter 8), and patrons included Sir John (Lord) Butterfield (Regius Professor of Physic, University of Cambridge 1976-1987), Sir Ivan Magill (doyen of British anaesthetists),[345] Sir Geoffrey Organe (President of the Association of Anaesthetists 1953-1956),[346] Professor E M Papper (United States), Professor T Gilmartin (Royal College of Surgeons in Ireland),[347] and Lord Porritt (President of the Royal College of Surgeons of England 1960-1963 and an Honorary Fellow of the Faculty of Anaesthetists).[348]

The driving force behind the Appeal was, however, the Vice Chairman of the Committee Michael Rosen, who was at that time President Elect of the Association, Chairman of the Finance Committee and Chairman of the Furnishing Working Party for 9 Bedford Square.[341-344] His infectious enthusiasm successfully obtained donations from individuals, charitable organisations and commercial firms; indeed his expertise can be compared with that of that prince of fund raisers John Morton (1420-1500), Lord Chancellor to Henry VII. Morton repeatedly extracted money for the Royal coffers with equal facility from the overtly well off and cannily parsimonious by wielding the alternate verbal prongs of his legendary "Morton's Fork" with words carefully tailored to the ears of each individual![349]

The Appeal aimed to raise £600,000 (1996: £960,000) by one year after the building was occupied by the Association, and to spend the money as it was raised on selected good quality reproduction Georgian furniture to match the building. This objective was exceeded; in fact over £700,000 (1996: £1,120,000) was raised from all sources (Council Minutes 31.10.1986).[27] The Appeal was closed at a resolution at the 1986 Annual General Meeting when Michael Rosen's outstanding contribution was acknowledged with enthusiasm.

The members of the Association of Anaesthetists contributed £270,000 (1996: £434,000) (Council Minutes 31.10.1986)[27] mainly by deed of covenant, but there was some disappointment on the part of the Council concerning the number of individual Members who contributed to this total. There was a perceived reluctance at the time amongst some Members of the Association living at a distance from London, that 9 Bedford Square was likely to become simply a club house for those living in the metropolis, and the home counties;[342] in the event however the greatest benefits for members have been the expansion in administrative activity which has enabled the medicopolitical and educational aspects of the work of the Association to be extended. The highly successful and oversubscribed seminar programme (also inspired by Michael Rosen) has enabled many hundreds of members to attend valuable and enjoyable meetings in elegant surroundings, accompanied by admirable catering arrangements, and consequently to appreciate that 9 Bedford Square is a working centre for anaesthesia and a pleasant place to visit. It is believed that few active Members, even those from more distant points of the United

Kingdom and Ireland, now feel that the house was not one of the best investments ever made by the Association of Anaesthetists.

The names of the founder donors of the Appeal are recorded in a commemorative book which is kept at 9 Bedford Square.[344] The Board of the *British Journal of Anaesthesia* was an early contributor and the Library is named after the journal.[341] A number of charitable and commercial firms made substantial contributions. They included the Wolfson Foundation, the Wellcome Foundation, Abbott Laboratories, Dräger, Portex, the British Oxygen Company, Janssen Pharmaceuticals and Imperial Chemical Industries.[344] Major contributing organisations were commemorated by naming suites and rooms in their honour and Council Minutes 6.12.1985, 4.4.1986 and 31.10.1986).[27,350,351] The donations of many individuals, anaesthesia societies and groups are commemorated on plaques on the backs of chairs in the Council (Dräger) Room.

A number of special objects have been donated; amongst these are the beautiful sculpture of mother and child by Jonah Jones donated by the Obstetric Anaesthetists' Association which is now in the entrance hall, the picture of the outback from the Australian Society of Anaesthetists, the Maori axe from the New Zealand Society, and the model loon (waterfowl) presented by the Canadians.[341,352]

The portrait of the Founder President Henry Featherstone which hangs in the entrance hall was painted from a photograph by David Griffiths of Cardiff. It was presented to the Association of Anaesthetists by the Board of the Faculty (now Royal College) of Anaesthetists (Council Minutes 31.10.1986).[27,353]

The decision to have the portraits of living former Presidents painted by contemporary artists at the expense of the Association itself was more controversial (Council Minutes 6.12.1985 and 31.10.1986),[27] but on the whole it has been proved to be in keeping with the use of the house as the headquarters of a professional organisation, and subsequent Presidents have also been painted. Portrait photographs of all past Presidents are hung in the British Journal of Anaesthesia Library.

Several silver items have been presented to the Association by former Presidents and others and grace the table on formal occasions. They include a three piece cruet (Mason: President 1978-1980), a sweet dish (Wylie: President 1980-1982), a bon bon dish (Boulton: President 1984-1986), a sugar sifter (Rosen: President 1986-1988), a candelabrum (Burrows: President 1988-1990), a tea caddy, a pair of wine coasters and a vase (Baskett: President 1990-1992), a Scottish quaich (MacRae: President 1992-1994), two chamber candlesticks modified as wine coasters (Howat: Honorary Treasurer 1969-1974, Vice President 1975-1976), a silver Armada dish (Miss Ann Muir, Honorary Member 1992), a silver jug (G A D Rees, Cardiff) and a silver dish P B Murphy.

The official opening of 9 Bedford Square as the Headquarters of the Association of Anaesthetists of Great Britain and Ireland, by HRH Princess Margaret, Countess of Snowdon, took place on 9 July 1987.[350,354] It was an outstandingly successful occasion.

Her Royal Highness was met on the steps of 9 Bedford Square by the President Professor Michael Rosen, who introduced her to his wife, Mrs Sally Rosen, to the Dean of the Faculty of Anaesthetists Aileen Adams, and to the President Elect Maurice Burrows and his wife Mrs Sylvia Burrows. Princess Margaret then visited the Janssen reception suite on the ground floor of 9 Bedford Square and the Portex Seminar Room and the Dräger Council Room on the first floor; in these rooms she met the Officers of the Association and many representatives of the organisations who had contributed so generously to furnishing the building, and also saw a selection of items from the archives of the Association and the Charles King collection of historic apparatus.[350]

Her Royal Highness next crossed to the gardens in the centre of Bedford Square where the Bedford Estates had given permission for a very large marquee to be erected which accommodated some 500 members, guests and friends of the Association of Anaesthetists; here the President made a short speech and Princess Margaret unveiled the commemorative plaque which is now mounted in the hall of Number 9. Professor Rosen then announced that Her Royal Highness had also graciously consented to become the Patron of the Association and presented her with a Certificate of Patronage and an engraved jardinière depicting both the house and the coat of arms of the Association of Anaesthetists.[350]

Princess Margaret thereafter spent considerable time moving amongst the guests and examining various exhibits depicting the work of the Association. She met amongst many others Sir Robert Macintosh [355] and the Presidents of the American and Australian Societies of Anaesthetists. It was a memorable occasion to which the charm of the new Patron of the Association of Anaesthetists contributed so much, and it heralded a new era of expansions and further achievement for the Association.[350,354,356]

The interior of Nine Bedford Square and its organisation as a Headquarters of the Association

The rooms which Princess Margaret visited on the ground and first floors on the opening day were the original principal reception rooms of Number Nine.[334,350,354] They are almost unique amongst the houses in Bedford Square because of the preservation of the exceptionally high quality original plasterwork. This was the work of Robert Philips of St Marylebone, who was also one of the signatories to the original building lease and was a contemporary of Robert Adam.[334,357] The two ground floor rooms (the original dining room and morning room of the residence) had been made into a single room running from the front to the back of the house at some time in the past, long before the Association of Anaesthetists purchased the property; fortunately, the planning authorities did not require the Association to restore the wall in its original position despite the Grade 1 listing of the building! The long elegantly panelled double (Janssen) room that has resulted from the removal of the wall extends from the front to back of the building and has large windows at either end. The room now has two fireplaces which are the central feature of separate sitting areas practically out of earshot of each other. These areas are furnished with sofas and coffee tables. There is one of Robert Philip's graceful plaster figure reliefs on the wall above each fireplace and another over the door of the former dining room. Those in the Dining Room area depict love and merry making![357]

It is of interest that this room, unique in the Square because of the removal of the wall, originally attracted the attention of the Honorary Officers as a possible lecture room (personal recollection); in the event however, so far as can be remembered, it has only been used once for this purpose.[351] The room was temporarily used for the main office of the Association of Anaesthetists when the small secretariat first moved into the building but, when the number of staff increased they moved to the rooms on the second floor leaving only the desk for the Administrative Secretary Miss Ann Muir as the welcoming chatelaine of the house in the principal and elegant reception room (Council Minutes 31.10.1986), Sally Jenner (now Mrs Collins) who succeeded Miss Muir in 1992, and Mrs Lesley Ogg who followed her in 1996 have continued the practice of working in the room. This ensures a warm and informal but well informed reception for Officers, Members of the Association and visitors alike. The principal use of the room is for informal discussions between officers, members and other visitors, as an assembly room for lunch before Council meetings for all its thirty odd members, and for other social functions.

The staircase of 9 Bedford Square is a spectacular feature enhanced as it is by the lantern light fittings donated by the interior decorators Christopher Rowley, and the portraits of Past Presidents are arranged on the outer wall of the spiral.

The two rooms on the first floor are separated by intervening double doors, which, when open, convert the whole of the first floor into a large T shaped area. These two rooms were originally the "state" reception rooms of the house (the principle reception room and the adjacent drawing room overlooking Bedford Square). They are now used as the (Portex) Seminar and Committee Room and the (Dräger) Council Room. Both rooms have elegant and original plasterwork ceilings. The ceiling in the Council Room representing the "four seasons" is particularly outstanding. Each room is enhanced by a modern reproduction chandelier of appropriate classical design. The nineteenth century lime washed bleached panelling in the Council Room has been stripped of its dark varnish and restored to its original colour. The silver grey oak panelling and the full range of windows on the outer wall, contributes to the formation of a delightfully light Council Room.[357]

The Council Room houses the magnificent specially designed and custom made Council table presented to the Association by Abbott Laboratories, and made by the skilled craftsmen of William Tillman Ltd of Sevenoaks, who also made several other items of furniture for the building. The table is built as a series of free-standing units which may be joined together as a unity, arranged in a variety of different configurations, or used individually. The Council Room doubles as a small lecture room. The audio-visual apparatus was donated by British Petroleum.

The interior of Nine Bedford Square and it's organisation as a Headquarters of the Association

The Council Suite on the first floor is eminently suited as the self-contained location for the seminars which have become such a feature of the educational activities of Bedford Square; the seminar participants are able to adjourn from the Dräger Council (lecture) room to the adjoining (Portex) room for buffet luncheon.

The rooms on the second floor constitute the Wolfson suite. This is composed of the British Journal of Anaesthesia Library at the rear of the building overlooking the Senate House of the University of London, and the general and finance offices at the front, overlooking Bedford Square.

The Wellcome Foundation room at the rear of the third floor is a pleasantly furnished discussion room for small groups and committees and for individuals to work and study quietly. The large front office houses the desks of the British Oxygen Company (now Ohmeda) Educational Coordinator, the Seminar Organiser, the secretary who deals with the Group of Anaesthetists in Training and the specialist societies (some of whom including the Intensive Care Society, the Pain Society and the Obstetric Anaesthetists Society have rented facilities from the Association of Anaesthetists), and the desk-top publication facilities.

The well-equipped catering kitchen is in the basement from which excellent buffet lunches and dinners are provided by caterers headed by Mrs Barbara Whitehouse for the official functions of the Association.

The BOC Museum of Historical Apparatus is also located in the basement and the back door opens on to the attractive garden area originally financed by Tricomed Ltd in 1988 but since 1993 maintained by Penlon Ltd.[378]

All in all 9 Bedford Square is a fitting Headquarters for the busy professional and social activities of the Association of Anaesthetists.

There is not, unfortunately, room in the house for space to be set aside for club facilities, which perhaps some members rather optimistically imagined might be provided at the time of its purchase.[342] Many individual anaesthetists both from the United Kingdom and overseas visit the building however. They can enjoy a warm welcome and an informal chat and a cup of coffee in elegant surroundings with any of the Officers who may be about their business in the building, and the staff, who are always present during working hours, and perhaps visit the Museum. Space can also always be found for a member to relax, write or read in the library, and several hundred members have now attended the very successful and intimate seminar programmes which were initiated at the suggestion of Michael Rosen.

Computerisation at 9 Bedford Square. The move to the new house afforded an opportunity for the Association to enter the computer age. W R MacRae, aided successively by the technical advisers John Mortlake and Andrew Rigby has been primarily responsible over the years for masterminding the development of the efficient interlinked system which now serves the Association offices.[341]

The Historical Resources of the Association of Anaesthetists of Great Britain and Ireland

The BOC Museum of historical anaesthetic apparatus. The British Oxygen Company (BOC) generously donated the handsome illuminated showcases in the Museum and Charles King's association with both the collection and the BOC are commemorated on an attractive montage at the entrance of the Museum.[358-561]

The original collection donated by Charles King (Chapter 6) has been considerably extended by donation and purchase and, although the space allocated for the Museum at 9 Bedford Square is generous, it would not be possible to display all the items at any one time unless several other large rooms were taken over! Much of the holding is therefore preserved in a store at Woolwich. The policy has been adopted of changing the exhibition each year. Visitors paying an annual pilgrimage to the Museum between January and November during the last several years have been able to study the origins of anaesthesia and analgesia for obstetrics, the life and work of Sir Ivan Magill, KCVO,[345] dental anaesthesia, artificial ventilation, the original Charles King collection, anaesthesia in war time, a display of recent acquisitions and the history of nitrous oxide anaesthesia.[360] A special exhibit commemorating the one hundred and fiftieth anniversary of the introduction of ether anaesthesia was mounted in 1996 and one for chloroform for 1997.

The British Journal of Anaesthesia Library is based on the Bryn Thomas Collection of Books and Pamphlets. This collection had been acquired by the Association of Anaesthetists in 1979 after the death of K Bryn Thomas who had been an international acknowledged medical historian and a Consultant Anaesthetist to the Royal Berkshire Hospital.[324,361] The decision was taken early on to develop the library as a unique historical resource of material concerned with anaesthesia and resuscitation, and not to attempt the impossible task of creating an adequate reference library as that function is already well served by other institutions in London, notably the Royal Society of Medicine and the British Medical Association; like the collection of historical apparatus, the historical library has been considerably extended by donation and purchase.[325,361,365]

The audio-visual section of the library is probably unique. A large number of historic films have been collected and video-taped by Ian McLellan and a basic catalogue prepared. This includes an indication of the persons involved (many of them famous anaesthetists of the past) and the topics covered by each film.[325,363-365] Selections from this archive have been a feature in the exhibition area of a number of Association Scientific meetings.

Archival material includes past Minute Books, Annual Reports, a considerable number of photographs and a few deposited archives of former Officers and Members of the Association of Anaesthetists and others associated with the specialty of anaesthesia.[361]

Care and supervision of the collections. The present writer, then completing his term as Editor of *Anaesthesia*, was asked to coordinate the care and cataloguing of historical equipment and books in 1981 and, at about the same time David Wilkinson (St Bartholomew's Hospital, London,) was appointed Honorary Curator of the Charles King Collection (then at the Royal College of Surgeons, Lincoln's Inn Fields). Ian McLellan (Leicester) was recruited to take charge of the Bryn Thomas Collection of Historic Books which had recently been acquired and housed in the Association of Anaesthetists Council Room in the suite at BMA House;[324,359] in 1982 the writer was appointed Honorary Archivist and the appointments of David Wilkinson as Curator and Ian McLellan as Honorary Librarian were confirmed.[366] Little more could be done beyond cataloguing and caring for the apparatus and books until the Association of Anaesthetists moved into 9 Bedford Square in 1985. It then became clear that professional help would be required to organise, care for, and exhibit the collections of the Association, and to prepare a state of the art computer catalogue; to this end, and with the aid of a generous grant from Imperial Chemical Industries, Audrey Eccles PhD was appointed as ICI Archivist-Librarian, on a self-employed sessional contract basis, but devoting the major part of her week to the Association of Anaesthetists, and she started work in January 1987.[359] Audrey Eccles was a professional archivist but she rapidly set about acquiring skills as a museum curator and librarian. The BOC Museum was opened in July 1987 with an exhibition illustrating the history of analgesia and anaesthesia for obstetrics, which was a subject upon which she had previously contributed to the literature (Council Minutes 23.10.1987).[27]

Audrey Eccles continued in post as Archivist-Librarian until July 1994. The 1993-1994 Report of Council paid tribute to "the professionalism and enthusiasm with which she had successfully tackled the task of organising the historical resources of the Association of Anaesthetists; computerised control systems for archival museum and library holdings of the Association have been established and the collections catalogued in detail". The Report also thanked her for being "responsible for obtaining and collating historical information for many members and outside bodies and individuals."[366]

The Museum Archives and, Library Committee was constituted as a Working Party in 1988,[362] as a Council Sub-committee in 1989,[363] and as a full Standing Committee in 1990.[364] Close relations have been maintained with the Science Museum, South Kensington and a number of other collections. Dr Ghislaine Lawrence (Senior Curator for Life Sciences of the Science Museum) is the Honorary Curatorial Adviser to the Association.[325,364,365]

The present writer retired as Honorary Archivist in 1994 and was succeeded by David Wilkinson. Anna-Maria Rollin (Epsom) succeeded David Wilkinson as Curator of the Museum. Andrew Griffin, Archivist to St Bartholomew's Trust undertakes the management of the historical resources on a consultancy basis (Council Minutes 2.6.1995).

The expansion in the educational activities of the Association after the move to 9 Bedford Square in 1985

Prior to 1986 the Association of Anaesthetists was organising two major scientific programmes each year, at the Annual Meeting in September and at the Annual Meeting of the Junior Anaesthetists Group in April. The Postgraduate Study Day which the Association of Anaesthetists had initiated and organised in conjunction with the Faculty of Anaesthetists at the time of the European Congress of Anaesthesiology in 1982 (Chapter 8) had also become, and has continued to be, a popular annual event. It has been administered by the Association and Faculty (now Royal College) alternatively in 3 year stints.[366] The 1995 meeting (now known as the Continuing Medical Education Day) attracted over 300 registrants.

The occupation of 9 Bedford Square at the end of 1985 presented the opportunity for the enlargement of the educational activities of the Association of Anaesthetists and the expansion and accommodation of the secretarial staff to support them. A particularly successful initiative was the introduction of the Seminar programme in 1986, and the Winter Meeting in January 1987. Both these programmes were inspired by Michael Rosen (President 1986-1988).

The Seminar programme at 9 Bedford Square began in 1986. The first floor suite consisting of the Council Room and adjoining Committee Room is an ideal self-contained suite for meetings of 30 to 35 members. The intimate nature of the gatherings, as well as the informal atmosphere of the luncheon and tea breaks, give ample opportunity for participants to question and converse with the lecturers who are experts on the particular field chosen for the seminar, and the timing (10.30 am to 4.00 pm) enables most registrants to leave and return home to destinations in the United Kingdom and Ireland within one working day.[356,368]

The Trustees of the Anaesthetists' Academic Foundation granted the sum of £15,000 (1996: £23,000) at the start of the scheme (Council Minutes 31.10.1986).[27] Three experimental seminars were held in 1986 on "the conduct of private practice", "the management of head injuries" and "analgesia for the neonate"; they were highly successful and oversubscribed.[362,369] The programme was formalised for 1987 with John Searle (Exeter; later Vice President 1992-1994) acting as Seminar organiser working with Professor Graham Smith of Leicester (Chairman of the Education and Research Committee).

The increased educational activity coincided with the appointment to the secretariat of Mrs Catherine Goff as BOC Educational Coordinator with responsibility for the administration of the educational activities of the Association (Council Minutes 31.10.1986).[27,356] The salary of the Educational Coordinator was financed by a very generous grant from the British Oxygen Company (now Ohmeda). This Company, together with other companies including Eli Lilly, also altruistically sponsored seminars without being in any way involved in the choice of subject matter.[356] An "extensive range" of seminars took place in 1987, in 1988 22 were held, and by 1994 there were 35.[356,362,366] The seminar programme has continued to be very popular and many individual seminars are oversubscribed and have to be repeated. The subjects covered are very diverse and include an increasing number of managerial topics in addition to pharmacological and clinical subjects. The History Seminar was first held in 1988.[370] It was unique in being an evening seminar. It included tea and a buffet dinner. It has become an annual event to which members can invite non-medical guests, including spouses and older children, to enjoy the elegance of 9 Bedford Square, and subject matter of general, if specialised, interest.

The seminar programme as a whole has a net financial deficit despite some continued commercial sponsorship, but Council has no intention of modifying this popular service to Members. All must feel a sense of gratitude to the many individual members who have organised seminars, as well as those who have been successively been responsible for the overall organisation (John Searle (Exeter), Tony Wildsmith (Edinburgh), Alan Aitkenhead (Nottingham) and John Sear (Oxford).

The Winter Scientific Meeting and Technical Exhibition was first held on Friday and Saturday 15 and 16 January 1988 at the Royal College of Surgeons of England, Lincoln's Inn Fields with the Annual Winter Dinner at the Waldorf Hotel, Aldwych taking place on Friday 15th 1988.[356,362,371] Both events were highly successful. The meeting obviously met a need at a time of the year when generally there is minimal academic activity after Christmas

The expansion in the educational activities of the Association after the move to 9 Bedford Square in 1985

and, (dare one say it) when accompanying persons can take their credit cards to the January sales in London.[372]

The first meeting was noteworthy for the rapidity with which it was conceived and arranged. It was first suggested to the Education and Research Committee by President Michael Rosen in December 1986 and decided upon as a practical proposition in April 1987, the programme was arranged by June 1987 and the meeting took place in January 1988. The success of the meeting owed a great deal to the efforts of Graham Smith (Professor of Anaesthetics at Leicester) then Chairman of the Education Committee, and to Peter Morris (Manchester) and Mrs Catherine Goff (BOC Educational Coordinator). Ralph Vaughan organised the technical exhibition in the difficult architectural conditions of the Royal College of Surgeons.[362,371]

The Winter Meeting has become a highly successful annual event. It was held again in the Royal College of Surgeons, Lincoln's Inn Fields in 1989 and 1990[363,364,372,373] and in 1991 and 1992[374,375] and thereafter up to the present time (1998)[376,377] at the Queen Elizabeth II Conference Centre, Westminster where a much larger and profitable trade exhibition can be organised to offset additional costs (Advisory Minutes 12.1.1990).[325] It became the custom since 1991 (with the exception of the 1992 Jubilee Winter meeting) for one of the specialist societies of anaesthesia to arrange and present a lecture session at the Winter Meeting. The first to do so in 1991 was the Paediatric Anaesthetists Association.[365] The 1992 Winter Meeting was utilised as the principal event to mark the Diamond Jubilee of the Association.[325]

Radiometer Ltd provided financial support for a lecture at the Winter Meeting in 1989 which was delivered by Professor John Severinghaus of San Francisco on "the history and current status of oximetry", on which subject he is a world authority. Radiometer Ltd were willing to fund the 1990 lecture also but did not agree to the choice of lecturer made by the Education and Research Committee. Council found that it was not possible to accept sponsorship in these circumstances (Council Minutes 2.6.1989). BOC Health Care Ltd then agreed to sponsor the Winter Meeting Lectureship. John F Nunn, who had been awarded the first Sir Ivan Magill Medal for innovation in 1988 (see below), agreed to speak at what was very short notice for such a task; characteristically he delivered an outstanding lecture on "the air we breathe".[373] BOC (now Ohmeda) Health Care have continued to sponsor this lecture at the Winter Scientific Meeting[376,377] and registrants have enjoyed a series of particularly erudite presentations on topics by leading authorities. The 1991 lecture was given by Professor W B Runciman (Adelaide, South Australia) on "Balancing cost, benefit and risk; the major challenge of the future", the 1992 lecture at the Jubilee meeting by Professor Sir Keith Sykes on "Clinical measurement and clinical care".

Informative publications from 9 Bedford Square

The move to 9 Bedford Square accompanied by an increase in secretarial staff and improved facilities (including desk-top publishing) enabled the Association to considerably increase its publication of educational material.

The booklet series of informative pamphlets in glossy covers has a double purpose; first they formulate an acceptable standard of contemporary practice (organisational as well as overtly clinical), and secondly they provide a well produced and authoritative text which can be used as a basis for persuading NHS managers to provide acceptable safe, adequate and modern conditions for patient care.

The production of each pamphlet entails a considerable amount of work on the part of a specially appointed Working Party of Members of Council, which seeks views of other experts. Some of the pamphlets have been compiled by joint working parties with other bodies such as the Royal College of Anaesthetists, and all of them are subjected to the closest scrutiny and criticism by the Advisory Committee and the Council itself before the definitive version is published.

The Association of Anaesthetists had, of course, produced some pamphlets for the assistance and guidance of its members prior to the move to 9 Bedford Square at the end of 1985. The most influential of these has undoubtedly been that on "Workload for Consultant Anaesthetists". This was originally produced in 1975 and revised in 1980, 1983, 1990, 1991 and 1997 at the time of alterations in the NHS Consultant Contract. This has been widely accepted by employing authorities as well as the profession to ensure that newly appointed consultants are offered reasonably balanced programmes of contractual obligations both inside and outside the operating theatre. Other early pamphlets were, in 1981 on "the use of controlled drugs in operating theatres" (the sensible recommendations of which were not universally adopted in the NHS), in 1983 on the (required) "Anaesthetic staffing of a district general hospital" and, in 1984, on "the implications of reductions in junior staff and the consultant only hospital", both of which were produced in response to the 1981 Report from the Social Service Committee on Medical Education (the Short Report);[379] this advocated a reduction in the number of registrars in training to correct the perceived distorted career structure in hospital medicine. A pamphlet was produced in 1984 on "the responsibilities of consultants for non-consultant career grade staff in isolated units in the NHS"; and another in 1985 on "professional references in the National Health Service". Nearly all these helpful early documents were influenced by the participation and perceptiveness of Michael Vickers.

The titles of booklets issued by the Association of Anaesthetists since the move to 9 Bedford Square in 1985 provide a valuable historical overview of the administrative and clinical problems of anaesthetists in the United Kingdom and Ireland, which have arisen and been considered by the Council of the Association, amongst many other matters, during the late eighties and early nineties:

1987   "Anaesthetic services for obstetrics. A plan for the future with special reference to smaller obstetric units."
(Prepared by the Association of Anaesthetists in association with the Obstetric Anaesthetists Association.)

1988   "Guidance on the conduct for private anaesthetic practice. Intensive Care services. Provision for the future."
"Guidelines on duties of Chairmen of Divisions."
"Assistance for anaesthetists."
"Recommendations on standards of monitoring."
(Reprinted 1989. Revised 1994.)

1989   "Efficiency of theatre services."
(Prepared by the Association of Anaesthetists and the Association of Surgeons of Great Britain and Ireland in consultation with nine other specialist surgical associations.)

"Consultant-Trainee relationships. A guide for Consultants."
"Anaesthesia in Ireland. The provision of a safe service."

1990 "Anaphylactic reactions associated with anaesthesia."
"Checklist for anaesthetic machines. A recommended procedure based on the use of an oxygen analyser."
"Guidance on the conduct of private anaesthetic practice."
"Your anaesthetic. Some questions answered."
(*A guide for patients. See also 1992.*)
"Working load of Consultant Anaesthetists."
(*Prepared in association with the (Royal) College of Anaesthetists with supplement in 1991.*)

1991 "The High Dependency Unit. Acute care in the future."
"The role of the anaesthetist in the Emergency Service."
"Workload for Consultant Anaesthetists in Ireland."

1992 "NHS management changes. Implications for anaesthetists."
"Department of Anaesthesia. Secretariat and accommodation."
"HIV and other blood borne viruses. Guidance for anaesthetists."
"Anaesthesia patients' guides." (*Prepared in association with the Northern Regional Health Authority. Replaces "Your Anaesthetic" 1990.*)

1993 "Immediate postanaesthetic recovery."
"Non-consultant career grade anaesthetists."
"Anaesthetists and non-acute pain management."
(*Prepared in association with the Royal College of Anaesthetists and the Pain Society.*)

1994 "Anaesthetic related equipment. Purchase, maintenance and replacement." "Recommendations for standards of monitoring during anaesthesia and recovery." (*Revised. See 1988.*) "Day care surgery. The anaesthetists role in promoting high quality care."

1995	"Surgery and general anaesthesia in general practice premises." (*Prepared in association with the Royal College of Anaesthetists and the Association of Surgeons of Great Britain and Ireland; with comments by the Royal College of General Practitioners.*). "Anaesthesia. The role of non-medical personnel." "Controlled drugs security and distribution within the operating theatre suite." "Suspected anaphylactic reactions associated with anaesthesia; revised edition."
1996	"Anaesthesia in Great Britain and Ireland: a physician only service." "Recommendations for the transfer of patients with acute head injuries to neurosurgical units." *(Prepared in association with the Neuro-anaesthesia Society of Great Britain and Ireland.)*
1997	"Checklist for Anaesthetic Apparatus 2." "Stress in Anaesthesia." "Guidance on contracts and workload for Consultant Anaesthetists." "Anaesthesia and anaesthetists: information for patients and their relatives." "Suspected anaphylactic reactions associated with anaesthesia 2." *(Prepared in association with the British Society of Allergy and Clinical Immunology.)* "Provision of pain services." *(Prepared in association with the Pain Society.)*
1998	"Risk management." "Your career in anaesthetics." "Good practice; a guide for Departments of Anaesthesia." *(Prepared in Association with the Royal College of Anaesthetists.)* "Guide lines for the management of a malignant hyperthermia crisis."

(In association with the British Malignant Hyperthermia Association.)

The booklet *"Anaesthetic services for obstetrics: a plan for the future"* (1987) recommended "the closure of small isolated obstetric units without adequate cover by trained anaesthetists or paediatricians." This caused considerable controversy and correspondence (*Anaesthesia News* 1988 Nos 10, 13, 14, 15, 16). General practitioners defended their small units[380-382] and the National Childbirth Trust and others requested amendments but, on the whole, the evidence in the interest of safety are irrefutable and was expressed succinctly by Michael Rosen,[383,384] and Council supported him (Council Minutes 17.6.1988). The Report in fact led to the closure of a number of isolated general practitioner units. The present writer, after experience of several near or actual tragedies soon after qualification in the late nineteen forties, has always believed that one of the more progressive developments in the provision of health care in his professional lifetime was the move to ensure that all births occur in hospital, or in general practitioner or midwife administered units located within the general hospital complex, where emergency care and modern analgesia techniques are to hand. This is especially the case bearing in mind the increased expectations of an invariably successful delivery by the public in recent years. Current pressure to reverse the trend away from the hospital unit, and especially to promote domiciliary midwifery again, would seem to be misguided;[385-388] moreover, however much the standards of antenatal care have improved in recent years, emergencies still occur, and an appreciable number of patients who believe that they can go through the experience without undue pain change their minds and request specialist analgesic techniques.

The Secretariat of the Association 1983-1995

The Secretarial staff which moved to 9 Bedford Square with the Association of Anaesthetists in November 1985 was composed of three long serving members (Miss Ann Muir, Administrative Secretary since 1973, Mrs Betty Tyler, clerical assistant since 1981 and Mrs Pat (Jasmine) Plant, Financial Assistant since 1982); by 1992 there were six staff members.[325] Mrs Catherine

Goff (BOC Educational Coordinator) joined the administrative staff during 1986, and Dr Audrey Eccles (ICI Archivist-Librarian) was appointed in 1987 and retired in 1994.[356] The staff was further augmented by the arrival of Lyn Hunt (later Mrs Frimpong) in 1988. Mrs Goff retired for domestic reasons in 1988 after a very successful period as the first BOC Educational Coordinator and was succeeded by Mrs Lesley Ogg.[362] Mrs Ray Richard was Minute Secretary from 1988 to 1990 when Sally Jenner (now Mrs Collins) succeeded her.[364] Miss Jacqui Wallace was in charge particularly of the desk-top publishing from 1991-1993.[365,391]

Miss Ann Hermione Muir. Nineteen ninety two saw the end of an era. Miss Ann Muir retired after nineteen years of devoted service to the Association of Anaesthetists as Administrative Secretary.[389-392] Mrs Betty Tyler her assistant for nearly a decade retired the following year. Sally Jenner (now Mrs Collins) succeeded Miss Muir and maintained the standards of warmth, friendliness and effectiveness associated with the administration at 9 Bedford Square as has Mrs Lesley Ogg who was appointed to take over from Mrs Collins in 1996.

Miss Muir originated from the fiercely independent border town of Berwick on Tweed whose citizens are renowned for their resourcefulness. She joined the Association of Anaesthetists after a varied and versatile early administrative career embracing amongst other things, advertising, public relations, travel and architecture, but it was, in fact her love of music and her appointment as Secretary to the Music Club of London that brought her to the attention of the then Honorary Secretary of the Association of Anaesthetists (Michael Coplans 1970-1972), who proposed her as the successor of the retiring Miss Joyce Baxter.

Miss Muir joined the Association towards the end of the Presidential term of office of J Alfred Lee in 1973 and looked after its officers through the nine succeeding presidencies, from Philip Helliwell[393] to Peter Baskett; in the process she supported and guided the activities of ten Honorary Secretaries, four Honorary Treasurers, three Editors of *Anaesthesia* and over 100 Council members. She saw the Association through the years of its greatest rate of development, and from a one room office to an elegant headquarters over which she presided not only with efficiency but also with great warmth and friendliness, always looking after the needs of the membership no matter how small or how great;[389] as Peter Baskett (President) and Ed Charlton (Honorary Secretary) wrote in *Anaesthesia News* shortly before her retirement "to the majority of members, to our brother and sister organisations, to our partners in the technical and pharmaceutical industry, Ann Muir is the Association of Anaesthetists. She is the ultimate charming and efficient link-person who has been a wonderful ambassadress for the Association".[390]

Election to Honorary Membership of the Association of Anaesthetists at the 1992 Annual General Meeting at Bournemouth was a fitting and well deserved tribute to her long and devoted service.[391,392]

The secretarial staff in 1996 was composed of six very willing and hard working members:- Mrs Ogg (Administrative Manager), Mrs Plant (Finance), Mrs Louise Watts (Ohmeda Educational Coordinator) and Miss Sarah Loader, Miss Sally Marsh, Mrs Karungari Murira with Mrs Wendy Nicholson as housekeeper.

Association Honours 1983-1996

The Sir Ivan Magill Gold Medal for innovation in anaesthesia. Sir Ivan Magill, KCVO (Founder Member 1932, Honorary Member 1956, John Snow Silver Medallist 1958,[345] one of the great British pioneers of modern anaesthesia died in 1986 in his ninety eighth year.[345] Council decided to honour the centenary of his birth with a commemorative meeting, the commissioning of a posthumous portrait, and the inauguration of a gold medal for occasional award for exceptionally outstanding innovations in anaesthesia (Council Minutes 6.3.1987).[27] The sum of £1000 which Sir Ivan had bequeathed to the Association of Anaesthetists, was put towards the fund initiated for the striking of the first medal (Council Minutes 5.6.1987 and 4.12.1987).[27] The medal is struck in gold. It is $2^{1}/_{2}$ inches (6.34 cms) in diameter and has a relief portrait of Sir Ivan on the obverse and may be worn round the neck.

The first award of the gold medal was made to John Francis Nunn (Head of the Division of Anaesthesia Medical Research Council Clinical Research Centre, Harrow 1968-1991, Professor of Anaesthesia University of Leeds 1964-1968, Dean of the Faculty of Anaesthesia 1979-1982, Vice President of the Association of Anaesthetists 1968-1990) at the Commemorative Dinner on 22 July 1988, after the Magill centenary meeting. This award was richly deserved. John Nunn's contribution to applied respiratory physiology, academic anaesthesia, and medical administration have been uniquely outstanding and recognised worldwide.

The Magill Gold Medal was awarded to Michael Rosen in 1993 who had played such an important part in the development of both the Association of Anaesthetists and the Royal College of Anaesthetists.[366] A third award was made to Archie (A I J) Brain in 1995 in recognition of the invention of the laryngeal mask which has changed the face of anaesthetic practice worldwide in such a remarkably short time (*Anaesthesia News* 1996; No 102: January).

John Snow Silver Medals were awarded between 1983 and 1996 to five former Presidents of the Association of Anaesthetists (Cyril Scurr, CBE, LVO, Philip Helliwell,[393] W Derek Wylie, Michael Vickers and Tom Boulton), and to six other distinguished British anaesthetists (Professor Thomas Gilmartin, doyen of anaesthesia in the Republic of Ireland and first Dean of the Irish Faculty),[394] Sir Gordon Robson (Dean of the Faculty of Anaesthetists 1973-1976 and Adviser to the Chief Medical Officer), Gordon Jackson Rees (the veteran Liverpool paediatric anaesthetist), to Sir Keith Sykes (Nuffield Professor of Anaesthetics, Oxford and Adviser to the Chief Medical Officer), John Zorab (President of the World Federation of Societies of Anaesthetics) and John Lunn (Editor of *Anaesthesia* and an initiator of successive confidential inquiries into peri-operative deaths).

The Pask Certificate of Honour was awarded thirty five times during the period 1983-1996. The broad categories envisaged when the award was instituted in 1975 (Chapter 8) were adhered to. The awards included those to members of the Association of Anaesthetists for particular acts of gallantry, or in recognition of specific tasks performed on behalf on the Association as well as nonmedical employees of both the National Health Service and industry who had given particular support to the Association and to its Standing Committees, and to Officers of other national societies with which the Association had held joint meetings. A unique certificate was awarded to the Ministry of Defence in 1983 in recognition of the services of the 14 anaesthetists from the medical services of the Army and Navy who had served in the Falklands War in 1982. Each individual medical officer received a copy of the award at the 1983 Annual Dinner at Newcastle upon Tyne.

Honorary Membership was granted "with acclaim" to thirty-eight recipients at Annual General Meetings in the period 1983-1996. Twenty-six of them were British anaesthetists and, with the exception of Doreen Vermeulen-Cranch, CBE, who had spent her working life in Holland, and Barbara Weaver, the veterinary anaesthetist, all had been Members of Council. Many of them had been Officers, including seven former Presidents, and the list included five Deans of the Faculty of Anaesthetists of the Royal College of Surgeons of England and two Deans of the Irish Faculty.

Four prominent medical men from other disciplines who had been concerned with the affairs of the Association of Anaesthetists were honoured; Herman Lehmann, the Professor of Biochemistry at Cambridge who advised the journal *Anaesthesia* for many years, Professor Kenneth Rawnsley, CBE who had had much to do with the "help for the sick doctor" scheme, Lord Smith of Marlowe, President of the Royal College of Surgeons of England 1973-1977 and Douglas Chamberlain, CBE, President of the British Cardiac Society.[375]

Four non-medical Honorary Members were elected, Sir Cecil Montacute Clothier, KCB, Robert J Maxwell (Chairman of the King's Fund), W W Mapleson (Professor of the Physics of Anaesthetics, Cardiff) [396] and Miss Ann Muir.

Four world leaders in anaesthesia also became Honorary Members (M H Holmdahl of Sweden, Carlos Parsloe of Brazil, Otto Mayrhofer of Germany and Henning Ruben of Denmark).

The Journal *Anaesthesia* 1983-1996

The succession of John Lunn of Cardiff to the Editorship in 1982 heralded the beginning of a decade which saw considerable changes in the nature and content of the journal. It had become clear by the early nineteen eighties that, important though they were, the number of pages in each issue of *Anaesthesia* necessarily devoted to purely domestic issues of interest to British anaesthetists in general, and Members of the Association in particular, was disproportionately not compatible with the growing scientific status of the journal. The sections devoted to "News and Notices" were "to some extent rationalised and thereby abbreviated" from 1983 onwards and this "led to a restriction on the length of reports about specialist society meetings". This was not altogether popular[356] but it paid a dividend in providing space to attract still more eminent authors both from the home countries and overseas, thus allowing increased space for the quality scientific material to be published.[369] The publication of *Anaesthesia News* (separate though circulated with *Anaesthesia* to the membership resident in the United Kingdom and Ireland) has gone a long way towards satisfying the essential need to publish domestic news and views (see below).[356]

Personnel. Philip Helliwell[393] retired as chairman of the Editorial Board in December 1987 after 14 years of devoted service and wise guidance;[362] thereafter the chairmanship has been undertaken by the reigning President of the Association of Anaesthetists.

The panel advisors of eminent members of the medical profession who were not anaesthetists were disbanded in 1983 after several retirements. It was felt that as "the breadth of knowledge of the editors had increased over the years" and they were well able in general to assess the importance of the disciplines in their relationship to the specialty of (the) anaesthesia and to seek *ad hoc* assistance if it was required. Herman Lehmann (Professor of Biochemistry at Cambridge) whose work had had a particularly close relationship with anaesthesia was elected to Honorary Membership.

John Lunn (Cardiff, Vice President 1991-1993) concluded his ten year term as Editor of *Anaesthesia* in 1990 after a successful and productive 17 years of association with the journal as Assistant Editor, Associate Editor and Editor. He was succeeded by Maldwyn Morgan of the Royal Postgraduate Medical School who had been Associate Editor since 1988 and who continued to develop the international scientific status of the journal while retaining some of its popular features, including its generous correspondence pages.[362,364]

A number of well known anaesthetists contributed their expertise as Assistant Editors during the period 1983-1996 (Annual Reports 1983-1995):- A P Adams (1976-1983: Professor, Guy's Hospital, London), M Morgan (1979-1990: Royal Postgraduate Medical School; appointed Editor 1991),

I Corall (1980-1985: King's College Hospital, London), C E Blogg (1982-1987: Oxford), R Greenbaum (1983-1992: University College Hospital, London), R M Jones (1985-1989: Guy's Hospital, London; later Professor St Mary's Hospital, London), A R Aitkenhead (1987-1994: Leicester, later Professor Nottingham), D E F Newton (appointed 1989: Harrow), Rosemary A. Mason (appointed 1990: Swansea), M Harmer (1991: Cardiff), J P H Fee (1992: Belfast), D G Bogod (1994: Nottingham), W Harrop-Griffiths (1996: St Mary's, London).

The particular contributions of a number of others whose services to anaesthesia were invaluable extending well into the eighties and nineties was described in Chapter 8.

The format of *Anaesthesia* underwent a major change in 1988 (volume 43) when its page size was increased to A4 following the example set by a number of its contemporaries.[363] Many subscribers and libraries regretted the demise of the familiar small sized, dumpy and compact monthly numbers which stood upright on the bookshelf without flopping over even when not bound! The Editor of the day (John Lunn), while sympathising with librarians and others who had somehow to increase the vertical height between shelves, bluntly and tersely described the change as "inevitable".[395] He might also have remarked that the "inevitability" was partly the result of the relentless march of technology which generally promotes uniformity at the expense of individuality!

There are undoubted advantages however. The 1988 volume (43) (excluding the valuable but commercially sponsored supplement circulated with it) when compared with that of 1987 (42) accommodated over 30% more words to each double column page at the expense of less than a 20% reduction in the number of pages, thus providing still more space for the greatly increased number of excellent scientific articles which were being received.

Publication. Academic Press continued to publish *Anaesthesia* under contract on behalf of the Association throughout the nineteen eighties and into the nineties. Contracts were renewed in 1985[341] and 1990.[363] The financial success of this partnership was reviewed in Chapter 7 and the professionalism of Academic Press and the high standard of production achieved were greatly appreciated; once again, however, as the result of a purely commercial bid, Blackwell Scientific Publications once more took over the publication of *Anaesthesia* from January 1997.

Anaesthesia News

Anaesthesia News was first published in broad sheet newspaper style in April 1987 and circulated with copies of *Anaesthesia* to Members of the Association.[356,397] *Anaesthesia News* was designed "as a separate and expanded section of the journal *Anaesthesia* " to publish "Important announcements by the Association, by its subgroups, and by other specialist organisations as well as a diary of national events (meetings of regional societies etc.)". The Editorial Board of *Anaesthesia* hoped that the publication would meet the criticisms of those Members of the Association who felt that *Anaesthesia* had not been publishing sufficient information about current events. *Anaesthesia News* was also intended "to give a new opportunity for readers to contribute in a number of less formal ways than scientific and clinical articles" including "more light hearted contributions".[397] *Anaesthesia News* has succeeded in fulfilling those objectives; besides providing news, reports of meetings etc., its articles, particularly on medicopolitical subjects, have stimulated considerable debate in its correspondence columns, and its occasional light-hearted humour is appreciated by all but the most serious of its readership!

Anaesthesia News was first mentioned in Council on 31 October 1986 as an approved recommendation from the Advisory Committee held on 10 October 1986 (Council Minutes 31.10.1986). The minute is brief but there is little doubt that the circulation earlier in 1986 of the new publication *Today's Anaesthetist* (supported by advertising and free to anaesthetists) had caused some concern and acted as something of a stimulus to the birth of *Anaesthesia News*. This free journal had to some extent filled the gap left by the reduction of reports on meetings of anaesthetists in the "News and Notices" section of *Anaesthesia* (personal recollection). The Officers need not have worried however; as things have turned out there seems to be room for both publications, particularly in the field of light hearted articles to relieve the encircling gloom, stimulating correspondence pages, and serious reports of meetings and of service overseas and in unusual circumstances.

Anaesthesia News remained directly the responsibility of the Editorial Board of *Anaesthesia* until 1989 when a separate Management Board was formed, but its distribution continues to be limited to the Membership of the Association of Anaesthetists. The format was changed from broadsheet to a more manageable tabloid during 1990.[365]

John N Horton (Cardiff) was the Editor of *Anaesthesia News* from its inception in 1987 to December 1992 when J E (Ed) Charlton (Newcastle upon Tyne) took over. John Horton was awarded a well deserved Pask Certificate of Honour at the 1992 Annual General Meeting.[392]

The Linkman Organisation 1983-1992

The Linkman Organisation, was initiated as a two-way system of communication (Chapter 8). It was intended that the Officers would be able to rapidly sound out grass root opinion on a particular issue without having to mail every member of the Association of Anaesthetists, and, reciprocally, Council would be able to disseminate news and its views on particular issues throughout the domestic membership by means of its 285 regional Linkmen - including one for the Channel Islands and one for the Republic of Ireland. Regional Irish Republic Linkmen also now communicate directly with the Irish Standing Committee (see below).[366]

The first Linkman conference was held in 1976 on the day preceding the Annual Meeting at the Tara Hotel, London. Linkman Conferences have been held annually ever since. Separate detailed reports of the meetings have appeared in *Anaesthesia* each year (*Anaesthesia* 1977-1995; volumes 32-50) with the exception of the 1992 meeting (*Anaesthesia* 1993; volume 48), and the meetings have also been reported in the "Annual Reports of Council".

The Linkman organisation was used to obtain opinions of the membership on a variety of topics in the first few years of its existence. The views expressed were very useful and were taken into consideration in forming Association policy, but the use of this function gradually declined. Attendance at the Linkman Conference fell from 88% of Linkmen (250 out of 285) in 1977 and 70% in 1978, to 39% in 1979, and averaged 130.

Michael Vickers, one of the initiators of the Linkman scheme, reviewed the function of the organisation in a perceptive article in *Anaesthesia News* in

January 1988.[398] He considered that the scheme was not fulfilling its full potential or being used effectively by the Officers in the way the originators had intended.[398] He believed that a significant number of Linkmen were not always passing on the material they received from the Honorary Secretary to their constituents. There is certainly a difference in motivation between that required when a Linkman is asked to canvas opinions of his members on a particular issue, and being a mere postman for material fed from the centre. Vickers also believed, probably correctly, that some Linkmen, having been in office since the inception of the scheme, appreciated the special relationship of being in the confidence of the Officers and Council, and enjoyed the exclusive nature of the lively Annual Conference of Linkmen and the social contact that went with it, without necessarily continuing to fulfil the communicative functions originally intended; in such circumstances it was likely that the views they expressed at the conferences were their own, rather than a distillation of those of their colleagues.[398]

Difficulties encountered in contacting Linkmen and gaining their cooperation were confirmed during the recruitment of volunteers for a sample survey of Anaesthetic Practice. This investigation was commissioned by the Association of Anaesthetists and was supported by Ohmeda and Dräger Medical. It involved obtaining details of 25 personally administered anaesthetics by individual volunteer anaesthetists as a basis for future studies in morbidity.[399,400] The survey took place and a report was ultimately published and was circulated to Linkmen. It is an interesting document capturing an expression of practice at that particular time but, as the authors readily acknowledge, it is difficult to draw conclusions from it because of the incomplete nature of the data.

Anna-Maria Rollin (Epsom) describing herself in 1988 as a "Linkman in a very small district" (but later (1990 onwards) a prominent Council Member and a Vice President of the Association) echoed and confirmed many of Michael Vickers misgivings in a letter to *Anaesthesia News*.[401] She criticised the dated nature of much of the information sent to her as a Linkman, and sometimes found it a little patronising. Anna-Maria believed that some of the documents issued by Council envisaged Utopia but were "sadly remote from the working reality of most anaesthetists' lives", but she, nonetheless, acknowledged that "these documents can be excellent ammunition against intransigent administrators (or even colleagues)". She was, however, enthusiastic about the Linkman Conference which not only conveyed information but initiated valuable contacts and was socially a "jolly affair".[401] Paul Cartwright from Derby, also later a Council Member, supported Anna-Maria, and even wondered whether the introduction of the publication *Anaesthesia News* each month had not taken over the function of the Linkmen.[402]

Regeneration. The Officers and Council were aware of the criticisms of the Linkman Organisation even before the publication of the article by Michael Vickers in January 1988.[398] A review of the list of Linkmen had been instituted during 1987 and they had been asked for information on the levels of assistance for anaesthetists and the provision of high dependency care prior to the production of booklets on these topics.[356] W R MacRae produced a discussion document for the consideration of Council in March 1988 (Council Minutes 4.3.1988). MacRae recommended that a senior elected member of Council should be appointed as Linkman Coordinator and, specifically, that holders of the Assistant Honorary Treasurer's post should have this responsibility in future. This actually pre-empted a suggestion subsequently made by Anna-Maria Rollin in her letter to *Anaesthesia News* in May 1988.[401] The Coordinator was to have special "responsibility for ensuring that Linkmen were kept informed of the activities of Council, and initiatives, seminars and matters of current interest in the specialty, at an early stage". Full use was to be made of *Anaesthesia News,* and "the term of office of Linkmen was to be limited to 3 years, renewable only for a further period of 3 years". A special Linkman tie was also to be made available (Council Minutes 4.3.1988). This last recommendation has never been implemented; one may be forgiven for wondering whether such an adornment would be universally approved in the present anti-elitist age, especially as Council itself does not have such a tie!

The Linkmen were requested to provide further information on specific topics during 1988 and Ed Charlton, the incoming Assistant Honorary Treasurer, was appointed as Linkman Coordinator.[362]

Michael Vickers attended the 1988 Linkman Conference as an observer in the following September. He was somewhat critical of the format of the meeting, particularly of the length of time taken up by speakers from the platform, but he concluded, "My overall verdict, then, on the Linkman Conference as a functioning organism of the Association of Anaesthetists; alive, but perhaps not kicking hard enough".[363,403]

The minor mid-life crisis of the Linkman Organisation, the re-evaluation of its *modus operandi*, and the commission given to Ed Charlton and his successors, has gone a long way to revitalising the system as an arm of the Association. There is now a continued interchange of ideas between the Officers and the Linkmen as the reports published in *Anaesthesia* testify. The Annual Linkman Conference is a particularly important event in the yearly calendar. The attendance was not below 200 (70%) in the next five years and was even as high as 236 (83%) (Annual Linkman Conference Reports 1989-1995).

The Junior Anaesthetists' Group (from April 1991 the Group of Anaesthetists in Training)

Nomenclature. The original title of the "Registrars' group" when its constitution was agreed in 1968 was "The Committee of Associates in Training" but, when the Associates in Training achieved full voting rights in 1970, the Group was renamed and became the "Junior Anaesthetists' Group" (JAG). Several successive generations of JAG Committee members appeared to be rather fond of this title and its acronym, despite various suggestions from time to time from individual members of the Group and some Officers of the Association that it was becoming outdated (personal recollection); by the early nineties the perceived implications of the word "junior" were found to be unacceptable and a reversion to the original nomenclature of "in training" and "trainee" was considered to be more politically correct "for mature doctors of 30 years of age and upwards who would be middle management with considerable responsibilities in any other sphere".[404] The designation "associates" was no longer applicable either; however, as members of the JAG had full voting rights, the title "Group of Anaesthetists in Training", (GAT) was consequently adopted.[405-407] This change was welcomed as "a major advance", and "in recognition of a group of highly trained professionals" and it was endorsed in the 1990-1991 Annual Report of Council.[365] There must remain some doubts about the semantics however! A "junior" can mean merely that the individual is just younger than someone else and not necessarily less independent than, or subject to, a "senior" colleague, whereas a "trainee" must by definition have that relationship! Is it possible that the "trainees" of 1970 preferred the change to "junior" for exactly the opposite reasons that their successors of 1991 wished to reverse the process?

Communication. The GAT Committee has two essential functions. The first is to assess the groundswell of opinion of anaesthetists in training and to convey that information to the Council of the Association of Anaesthetists and to the various committees on which it is represented. The second is to convey information about opinions and policies of the governmental and professional bodies to the anaesthetists in training. If these objectives are to be achieved it is essential, first that members of the GAT committee sit on as many important committees as possible, and second that there is an adequate mechanism for two way communication with trainee anaesthetists.

Representation. The writer was in a fortunate position while enjoying the privilege of being the representative of Council on the JAG (GAT) committee from 1976-1985. He was an Officer of the Association of Anaesthetists but without direct responsibility for the day to day administration of the Association itself; he was also a Board Member of the Faculty of Anaesthetists. He was thus able to devote very considerable attention to encouraging the acceptance of the participation of trainee anaesthetists in the committees of both organisations.[405] The trend has continued; now, in 1998, the GAT Committee, besides being represented on Council of the Association of Anaesthetists as voting members by its Chairman and Honorary Secretary and on the Advisory Committee by the Chairman, is also represented on the Education and Research Committee, the Safety Committee and the International Relations Committee of the Association of Anaesthetists and the Editorial Board of *Anaesthesia* as well as on almost all Association Working Parties. The GAT Committee also has a representative on the Training Committee of the Royal College of Anaesthetists (formerly the Joint Committee for the Higher Training of Anaesthetists), the Anaesthetic Section of the Royal Society of Medicine, the Anaesthetic Subcommittee of the Central Consultants and Specialists Committee of the BMA, and the Royal College of Anaesthetists Education Committee, and has an "observer" on the Council of the Royal College of Anaesthetists. Susan Geddes (Chairman of GAT 1993-1994) has emphasised that "the presence of GAT Committee members at these meetings is not a public relations exercise. There is now a genuine interest in the welfare of trainees at the Association and the Royal College and we receive a sympathetic hearing for our views". All this activity has necessitated the expansion of the GAT Committee to nine members.[407]

The Junior Linkman Scheme. Communication between the GAT Committee and the Trainee membership had always presented difficulties. An attempt was made to initiate a separate Junior Linkman scheme in 1977 shortly after the senior Linkman scheme was organised, but it was rejected. This was, partly because of expense, and partly because it was believed that Senior Linkmen could and would disseminate information to juniors. Three JAG Newsletters were produced and sent to Senior Linkmen but only one quarter of those present at the 1978 JAG Annual General Meeting had seen them. *Anaesthesia* also began to publish a separate section devoted to the affairs of JAG in 1977. Despite these measures, however, communication with the "grass roots" continued to be difficult.

The Junior Linkman Scheme was finally initiated during 1984, and 60 Junior Linkmen were present at their first conference the day before the GAT Annual General Meeting at Manchester in March 1985.[341,405] The Junior Linkman Scheme was rather slow in gaining momentum at first. Thirty-seven Junior Linkmen attended their conference before the JAG Annual Meeting in 1986, only 18 out of 40 in post in 1988 and 32 out of a possible 52 in 1989.[405]

Michael Vickers who had been responsible for promoting the Junior Linkman Scheme during his presidential term reviewed the workings and uncertainties of administering the Junior Anaesthetists' Group in March 1988 in one of his cogent articles in *Anaesthesia News*.[404] He pointed out that, in many ways, it is much more difficult to be an effective honorary officer responsible for organising the Junior Group than it is to be an Association Officer responsible for organising the Association of Anaesthetists as a whole. This is because of the sense of impermanence resulting from a constituency which is constantly changing due to promotion to consultant rank. Vickers stressed that, because of this fluid situation, there is a special need for a senior figure on Council acceptable to the GAT Committee to attend their deliberations "to advise them what was possible and how to go about it" and to "help present their case in Council". It is also desirable if continuity is to be maintained that the senior Council Member on the GAT Committee should retain that responsibility for some years. This need for continuity was rather forgotten during the mid eighties, but was remedied when Peter Morris took over the responsibility in 1988. Morris has been succeeded by two Honorary Secretaries of the Association who were past members of the Junior Anaesthetists Group (Ralph Vaughan and David Saunders).[405]

Vickers also drew attention to "the thread of anxiety which is common to trainees of all medical organisations, and which particularly affects those who are persuaded to speak for them, namely that they will be subtly victimised as troublemakers at worst or awkward individuals at best".[404] They fear that participation in medical politics may delay their promotion to consultant rank. The present writer (despite the contrary views of others)[408] agrees with Vickers that there is no real basis for the anxiety - quite the opposite.[404] This is especially so nowadays since, as has already been pointed out, so far as the Association of Anaesthetists is concerned, GAT committee members express their views from within the Council and its committees and the committees of the Royal College of Anaesthetists, and not as agitators from outside. This was not always the case, nor is it yet universal within medical organisations; so far as JAG (GAT) is concerned it has often been a source of pleasure and satisfaction to welcome former members of the Committee returning to Council as senior Members or Officers.

All these factors probably played a part in the initial reluctance of peripheral trainees to allow their names to go forward as Junior Linkmen. Further evidence of difficulties in communication was the disappointing entry for the Registrar's Prize (Council Minutes 4.3.1988).

A vigorous campaign to promote GAT and to recruit GAT Linkmen, both by word of mouth by the committee members themselves, and in *Anaesthesia News*, was undertaken during late 1988 and throughout 1989. Twelve entries for the Registrar's Prize were received for the April 1989 Annual Meeting of GAT of which five were selected for presentation (Council Minutes 14.4.1989).[364]

A most important innovation for raising awareness of the importance of GAT and of encouraging the Linkmen was the introduction of the GAT

The Junior Anaesthetists' Group (from April 1991 the Group of Anaesthetists in Training)

Linkman Seminar in October 1989 on the day before the annual Association of Anaesthetists and College of Anaesthetists Postgraduate Study Day at 9 Bedford Square; this was followed by a dinner at the Royal Society of Medicine. The seminar and dinner have been repeated annually and have become increasingly popular, the subjects discussed at these seminars have been of an administrative rather than a clinical nature, ("Resource Management" 1989, "Audit in Anaesthesia" 1990, "Presentation" 1991, "Anaesthetic business" 1992).[325,363,364,392,405] There were 156 GAT Linkmen by the end of 1992.[325]

Publications. The GAT Committee has played a full part in the expanded programme of practical booklets which the Association has produced since it moved to 9 Bedford Square; of particular interest have been those on "Registrars in Anaesthesia", "Consultant-trainee relationships: a guide for consultants" and "Guidelines on the duties of Chairmen of Divisions". The JAG Committee also revised the "Career Guide for Anaesthetists" in 1985.[405]

A project undertaken in the eighties was a "Handbook for Trainee Anaesthetists".[409] This was produced in 1991 after a gestation period of several years.[405] The publication provided much useful information on training and planning a career in anaesthesia. It also gave information about the organisations related to the specialty. The Handbook was greatly improved and expanded as the "Group of Anaesthetists in Training Yearbook 1993/1994.[406] This contained, in addition to purely informative material, a number of authoritative, well written, interesting and very readable articles by selected eminent authors on various aspects of a career in anaesthesia and the organisation of the National Health Service. The Editors of the GAT Yearbook 1993/1994[406] (Alexander Goodwin and Colin Berry the Editor of its successor the GAT Yearbook 1995)[407] are to be congratulated on two such excellent publications. One notes with interest that both started their careers in the Royal Navy.

The Annual Meetings for Junior (Trainee) Anaesthetists gained steadily in popularity throughout the eighties and early nineties and after the establishment of the Linkman Scheme. The series culminated in the Silver Jubilee Meeting of its group 1 to 3 April 1992 at Bristol.[325,405,410] The venues of the meetings between 1983 and 1996 were (with number of registrants in brackets):- 1983, Leeds (260): 1984, Edinburgh (324): 1985, Manchester (not recorded!): 1986, Cardiff (230): 1987, Belfast (160): 1988, Nottingham (200): 1989, Keele (210): 1990, Glasgow (333): 1991, Oxford (350): 1992, Bristol (over 300): 1993, Sheffield (350): 1994, Newcastle Upon Tyne (360): 1995, Leicester (392): 1996, Cambridge (340).[366,392,405,420]

The Silver Jubilee Meeting in Bristol (1-3 April 1992)[410] happily took place in the year the Association as a whole celebrated its Diamond Jubilee in London during preceding January.[411] This particular JAG/GAT meeting was by common consent an outstanding success, scientifically, politically and socially. The Bristol Humphry Davy University Department of Anaesthetics produced a plethora of excellent speakers including its Professor, Cedric Prys-Roberts, who was destined to become the second President of the Royal College of Anaesthetists in 1995. The Pinkerton Memorial Lecture was given by John Zorab (the reigning President of the WFSA). The Annual Dinner of the Group was held in the magnificent setting of the Bristol Council House. It was particularly noteworthy for the presence of 10 out of 16 previous Chairmen of the JAG (GAT) who were presented with Past Chairmen's badges by the reigning Chairman Elizabeth (Liz) Spencer.[325,410] This meeting was in fact permeated by the enthusiasm of Liz Spencer, who as Honorary Secretary (1990-1991) and Chairman (1991-1993) of GAT did so much to lead the Group of Anaesthetists in Training to fresh heights of achievement. The production by Liz Spencer of *Her History of the Group of Anaesthetists in Training*,[405] and the success of the visit of the leaders of the GAT Committee when they met their counterparts in Ireland (see below) are further examples of important initiatives by GAT.

The number of Trainee Members rose steadily between 1982 (1293)[324] to the end of 1994 (2112)[366] when they represented 45% of the voting membership (ordinary plus trainee members) but, by the end of 1995, it had fallen to 1860 (36% of the voting membership) in a year when the Ordinary Membership had risen to an all time high of 3271.[420] This certainly reflected consultant expansion mopping up the available Senior Registrar cadre.

The Irish question

The Association of Anaesthetists was founded in 1932 when the conditions under which anaesthetists were employed had a common origin, and were largely similar in the United Kingdom and the then Irish Free State (Eire,

1937), which was then still loosely a part of the British Commonwealth (Republic of Ireland, 1949). The income of medical specialists in both countries at that time was mainly derived from private patients while public patients were treated free of charge. It was not therefore surprising that the Association of Anaesthetists of Great Britain and Ireland should be founded to further the development of the specialty for the benefit of patients and anaesthetists in both the United Kingdom and the *de facto* independent republican Southern Ireland.

The system of health provision remained basically unchanged in the two countries until the establishment in 1948 of the National Health Service in the United Kingdom which is based on taxation, but free for all at the point of use. The state health service in the Republic developed more slowly, and paradoxically lacked the political stimulus resulting from national participation in the Second World War (Chapter 5), during which the Republic of Ireland was officially neutral although a great number of individual Irishmen joined the British Armed Forces; however clinical expertise progressed in parallel with that in the United Kingdom. Sessional payment arrangements for physicians working in public hospitals with pension and other employment rights were first introduced in 1981 under the terms of a "common contract". About 40% of the Irish population had become entitled to free state-sponsored health care, and the rest of the population are now eligible for care in public hospitals on payment of a graduated means tested levy. The only body authorised to provide private health insurance is the state-sponsored Voluntary Health Insurance Board (VHI) which was set up in 1957 and to which about 30% of the population now belong (personal communication John Cahill).[412-414]

The problems of providing uniform health care in the Irish Republic stem partly from the sparse population of the country (3.5 million compared with some 60 million in the United Kingdom), and the number of small acute general hospitals outside the main conurbations, with a relatively low turnover of patients. The latter are difficult to staff and have establishments for only one or two consultant anaesthetists. This situation has led to the concentration of facilities for modern advanced medical techniques in larger centres for economic reasons, and there is therefore an increasing need to transport patients to the centres under medical escorts; these are often provided by anaesthetists.[412,414] There are approximately 200 consultants and about the same number of trainees in the Republic of Ireland; there are no other grades (personal communication John Cahill).[416] It is clear that anaesthetists in Ireland have been undervalued, under resourced, and under represented over the years.[413,414]

The Association Standing Committee for the Republic of Ireland was established on 16 January 1988. This was at a critical time when the Irish Government was considering fresh plans to develop and rationalise the health service of the Republic and, to begin the long awaited review of the first "common contract" for consultants.[362,413,414]

The Irish Standing Committee consists of a representative from each of the eight Health Board Areas of the Republic, and a representative of the (Irish) Senior Registrar Group, together with the Executive Officers of the Association *ex officio* and the Dean of the Faculty of Anaesthetists of the Royal College of Surgeons in Ireland as a coopted member. The Convenor and Honorary Secretary of the Committee are elected from amongst the elected Members of the Committee. The first Convenor was D Riordan and the first Honorary Secretary P J Breen.[362] The purpose of the Committee is to pursue the medicopolitical objectives which are denied to the Faculty of Anaesthetists of the Royal College of Surgeons in Ireland under its Charter provisions.[414]

The Committee began work immediately on a document designed to define the state of Irish anaesthesia and to suggest possible solutions to the problems.[414] The aims of the Irish Standing Committee as expressed in the report, are threefold:-

1. To emphasise the importance of anaesthesia and anaesthetists in the provision of modern medical care.

2. To highlight deficiencies in the health service in Ireland in relation to the provision of a safe modern anaesthetic service.

3. To indicate how these deficiencies may be rectified to ensure that a safe and comprehensive anaesthetic service is available to communities throughout the country.[414]

The Report, published in 1991, was comprehensive and starkly realistic;

it was commended to the Irish Minister of Health, his Departmental officials and the Health Boards to study and to give serious consideration to its contents.[414] It emphasised that the attitude of hospital administrators to the specialty of anaesthesia and its problems left much to be desired. This was apparently due to a lack of knowledge of the scope of the specialty and its expanding role in the evolution of a modern hospital service. This had led to a lack of consultation concerning the facilities and services required by anaesthetists in the practice of their specialty. It is, for example, noteworthy that the report recommends the elementary proposal for a National Adviser in Anaesthetics to the (Irish) Department of Health, which was a provision which had been made since the nineteen forties in the United Kingdom. It should be noted however that W S (Billy) Wren (Dublin, Vice President of the Association of Anaesthetists 1976-1978) was appointed Adviser on Hospital Services to the (Irish) Ministry of Health in 1990 to advise on all medical specialties (John Cahill personal communication). The particular problems of staffing and retaining staff in the smaller units were emphasised in the Report, as were the need of proper provision and funding of such matters as minimal standards for monitoring, postoperative recovery and intensive care. Much useful reference was made in preparing the report to the administrative and clinical documents previously published by the Association of Anaesthetists. Subsequent documents have considered the establishment of standards for the workload of Consultant Anaesthetists in Ireland (1991),[415] and have surveyed the manpower situation in the Republic[416] and emphasised the need for better staffing and provision of Intensive Care Units in Irish hospitals.[417]

Fees in private practice in Ireland. The payments, offered by the monopoly VHI to patients to cover the anaesthetists' fees in private practice in Ireland were not sufficient to cover an adequate reimbursement for the professional skills involved (in 1988 the payment was only from £26 (1996: £37) to £75 (1996: £107) for the most complex procedures). The newly formed Standing Committee recommended in March 1988 that fees should be based on the guidelines prepared by the Association of Anaesthetists for the United Kingdom, and that the patient should be expected to make up the balance. Many Consultant Anaesthetists in the Republic adopted this policy and, although this represented a considerable increase in their financial contribution, the majority of patients appeared to consider the increase in fee reasonable. The VHI took the opportunity presented by the introduction of a new tax law on the withholding of tax to pay fees directly to consultants, thus necessitating the need for the "balance billing" of the patient for the shortfall.[413] The VHI next generated considerable opposition by proposing that anaesthetists should sign an undertaking not to charge fees at a higher rate than an improved schedule.[365] It was estimated in 1994 by a survey of private practice conducted by the Standing Committee, that less than 20% of private practice was carried out by anaesthetists who held contracts with the VHI, and that the latest offer of the VHI was "inadequate".[366,419] The practice of "balance billing" continued and ensured a high profile of the dispute with the VHI.[419] A provisional but not an entirely satisfactory arrangement, (particularly in respect of benefits for work in intensive care) was agreed in October 1994 to run until March 1997, but Consultants were advised "not to dismantle their balance billing systems ... yet". The agreement represented considerable progress however, and was a compliment to the Association, the Irish Standing Committee and the solidarity of Irish Anaesthetists.[420,421]

Association meetings in Ireland. The initial result of the deliberations on the provision of services in the Republic of Ireland and the negotiations with VHI were discussed at a meeting of the Standing Committee in Dublin on 25 June 1988,[362] and the next day Maurice Burrows, then President Elect of the Association of Anaesthetists, spoke to an open meeting of 24 members of the Association, who were present as Linkmen representing some 130 anaesthetists. The initial work of the Standing Committee was welcomed and discussed.[413]

The Irish Standing Committee meets formally on three occasions each year. The Senior Executive Officers of the Association have continued to attend the yearly November meetings of the Committee in succeeding years.[325,363-366] Special Open Meetings for all anaesthetists in Ireland to discuss VHI proposals were held in January 1990, February 1993, and October 1994 (personal communication J Cahill).[364] The meeting of the Standing Committee in November 1991 was followed next day by an Open Forum and Seminar attended by 80 members. This was popular and has been repeated as a successful and very lively annual event (*Anaesthesia News* 1996; No **104**: March).

The Introduction of the Standing Committee for the Republic of Ireland in 1988 was a much needed innovation to strengthen the consideration of the medicopolitical aspects of anaesthesia in the Republic. The support of the Association of Anaesthetists as a whole strengthens its aims. The election to the Council in 1992 of John Cahill, Honorary Secretary of the Irish Standing Committee by the general electorate of the Association was a personal compliment to him for his very considerable efforts on behalf of both Irish and the United Kingdom anaesthesia. It also reflects the growing strength of the influence of the Association of Anaesthetists in Ireland, and an increase in membership from the Republic which has risen considerably and in 1995 stood at 189 (Association Records).

The Irish Senior Registrar Group was founded in 1981. It has had a representative on the Medical Advisory Committee of the Irish Faculty of Anaesthetists since shortly after the Group was founded, and since 1982 it has had a representative (either elected or coopted) on the Committee of the United Kingdom Junior Anaesthetists' Group (JAG now Group of Anaesthetists in Training, GAT). The Officers of the GAT Committee attended the Annual Meeting of the Irish Senior Registrar Group held at the Royal College of Surgeons in Ireland in Dublin in December 1992. E M (Liz) Spencer (Chairman) and Susan Geddes (Honorary Secretary) gave papers to over 100 trainees on the work of GAT and its Committee, and they had a useful exchange of views with the Irish Senior Registrars' Committee (John Cahill personal communication).[419] An interesting difference between United Kingdom Senior Registrar posts and those in the Republic is that the latter are finite and end with accreditation; many accredited Senior Registrars consequently find it necessary to work in the United States and elsewhere while awaiting consultant posts in the Republic of Ireland. There is a possibility that a similar situation might arise in the United Kingdom as a result of the Calman proposals on higher training![419]

The relationship of the Specialist Anaesthetic Societies to the Association of Anaesthetists of Great Britain and Ireland

The last three decades have witnessed increasing specialisation and very considerable extension of the role of anaesthetists. Specialisation has resulted in the foundation of many specialist anaesthetic societies as well as other organisations in disciplines such as intensive care in which individuals or groups of anaesthetists play an important part. The first in the field was probably the Society for the Advancement of Anaesthesia in Dentistry (1957). Membership is open to both dental and medical practitioners, but is predominantly dental; however its limitations with regard to techniques and its controversial medicopolitical nature did not enable it to be generally accepted by medically qualified anaesthetists at the time. The second organisation to be founded was the Anaesthetic Research Group in 1958, which became the Anaesthetic Research Society in 1970. This Society is not, of course, primarily directly clinically orientated and it is consequently, and rightly, selective in its membership.

The first British medical clinical specialist anaesthetic organisation to be formed was the Neuroanaesthetists Travelling Club which was formed in 1963 and became the in 1993. There have followed:- The Association of Veterinary Anaesthetists (1964), The Pain Society (multidisciplinary: 1967), The Obstetric Anaesthetists Association (1969), The Intensive Care Society (multidisciplinary: 1970), The Association of Paediatric Anaesthetists (1973), The Association of Dental Anaesthetists (medical and dental: 1976), The Society of Anaesthetists of the British Forces in Germany (which was founded in 1977 and became the Tri-service Anaesthetic Society in 1991), The British Association of Immediate Care (multidisciplinary: 1977), The Great Britain and Ireland Committee of the European Society of Regional Anaesthesia (1980), The Resuscitation Council of the United Kingdom (multidisciplinary: 1981), Plastic Surgery and Burns Anaesthetists (1982), The Society of Naval Anaesthetists (1982), The Association of Cardiothoracic Anaesthetists (1984), The British Malignant Hyperthermia Association (multidisciplinary: 1984), The History of Anaesthesia Society (multidisciplinary: 1986), The (multidisciplinary: 1987), The Society for Computing Technology in Anaesthesia (1987), The Age Anaesthesia Society (1988), and The Scottish Intensive Care Society (1991). All of these bodies are naturally motivated by a desire to improve the standards of practice in their own particular spheres. Most of them acknowledge that anaesthesia is not yet rigidly divided into specialties as, for example, is surgery, and they recognise that, in general hospitals, and particularly in emergency practice, anaesthetists may be called upon to administer anaesthesia or undertake intensive care for the patients of surgical specialties other than those with which the individual anaesthetist is routinely concerned. Such organisations are usually prepared to elect to membership those whose main interest is not necessarily in the particular specialty, but who seek information about others. A few societies, such as The Association of Paediatric Anaesthetists and, until recent years, The Intensive Care Society limit membership to those who have a majority sessional interest in the specialty concerned.

Honorary Secretaries of the Association of Anaesthetists of Great Britain and Ireland began to express concern at the proliferation and the uncoordinated overlapping of the increasing number of meetings of both Regional and Specialist societies in the nineteen seventies, and various attempts were made to keep a register of dates at the offices of the Association.[422] The journal *Anaesthesia* also started to advertise the dates of meetings of the regional and specialist societies as far in advance as possible, and Adrian Padfield of Sheffield collated a diary of National and Local Events in *Anaesthesia* from 1974 onwards. *Anaesthesia News* has taken on this responsibility and has published a comprehensive "Calendar of Events" since 1987.

Michael Vickers gave credence to the anxiety which had been expressed "over the political activities of some of the specialist anaesthetic societies" at his first Council Meeting as President (Council Minutes 3.12.1982).[423] There was a feeling that the specialty of anaesthesia should endeavour to speak with one voice, especially when giving advice to the Department of Health or its Regional components and other organisations (personal recollection). It was agreed that officers of the various specialist societies should be invited to meet the Officers of the Association of Anaesthetists "to permit a general discussion on topics of interest".[424]

The first meeting between representatives of the officers of the Association of Anaesthetists and representatives of the Specialist Anaesthetic Societies was in May 1983 (Council Minutes 3.6.1983).[423] It was deemed to be "very successful" in promoting closer liaison between the Association of Anaesthetists and the specialist Societies (Annual Report 1983).[424] Another meeting was held in October 1983 (Annual Report 1984)[331] and thereafter the meeting between the Specialist Societies and the Officers of the Association of Anaesthetists became an annual event. The Intensive Care Society withdrew from attendance at the meetings after the 1985 meeting (Specialist Society

Meeting minutes 14.11.1986). This was probably because of its multidisciplinary composition, which its Council has always been at pains to emphasise even though 80% or more of its members are anaesthetists; however they began to send a representative once more in 1993 (Specialist Society Meeting minutes 12.11.1993). The Association of Professors of Anaesthesia also considered that their attendance would be "inappropriate", presumably because of the political nature of some of the matters under discussion (Specialist Society Meeting minutes 14.11.1986).

The meetings have proved to be very worthwhile. The specialist societies have maintained their independence but they have the opportunity to outline their activities and to present their problems and discuss them with others in similar situations. The Officers of the Association of Anaesthetists, for their part, are able to glean much valuable information, as well as to explain their policies and both to advise and help in resolving difficulties. Discussion at the Annual Meeting with Specialist Societies has also, to some extent, resulted in coordination of the dates of Association and specialist meetings.

Educational Collaboration between the Association of Anaesthetists and the Specialist Societies. The specialist societies have cooperated in the production of a number of the pamphlets on specialist subjects published by the Association of Anaesthetists in recent years and, more recently, they have very successfully collaborated with the Association in organising and presenting lecture sessions to a wider audience at the now well established Winter Scientific Meetings each January. The Association of Paediatric Anaesthetists contributed an excellent programme in 1991,[365] a specialist session was not organised in 1992 as the whole Winter Meeting was organised as the Diamond Jubilee Meeting of the Association of Anaesthetists,[325,365] but sessions were presented by the Association of Cardiothoracic Anaesthetists in 1993, by the Association of Dental Anaesthetists in 1994, by the Age Anaesthesia Association in 1995, and the History of Anaesthesia Society organised the session at the January 1996 Winter Meeting.[391,420] A further development is the inauguration of a Consultant Update Day on the Thursday before the Annual Winter Meeting, to which two specialist societies contribute sessions on topics "chosen to be of interest to the general anaesthetist who may be required to deal with specialist problems when on call". The Obstetric Anaesthetist Association and the Neuroanaesthesia Society produced programmes on these lines for 1996.[420,425]

Further development of academic anaesthesia in the United Kingdom and Ireland

A number of new Professorial Chairs were established between 1970 and 1995 to join those already in existence at the end of 1969. These were:- at the United Medical and Dental School of Guys and St Thomas' Hospital, London A P (Tony) Adams, and at Leicester (Graham Smith) in 1979, at Nottingham in 1986 (J W Downing until 1988 and then A R Aitkenhead), at St Mary's Hospital, London (R M Jones), University College, Dublin (D A Moriarty), and Galway, Republic of Ireland (P Keane) in 1990, at Cambridge (J. Gareth Jones) in 1991 at St George's Hospital, London (G M Hall) in 1992 and at Dundee (J A W (Tony) Wildsmith) in 1995.

Alastair A Spence was appointed to the Professorial Chair at Edinburgh when it was established in 1984. Peter Hutton became Professor of Anaesthesia at Birmingham in 1986, after the Chair had been in abeyance since the early retirement of Professor John Robinson in 1983. This was during the attempts by the relatively newly elected Conservative government to ruthlessly impose "cost saving" cuts on academic departments of all disciplines in common with every other area of industrial and public expenditure, apparently regardless of the social and cultural consequences. It seemed, too, at the time that the all too few Academic Departments of Anaesthesia being relatively recently established were being singled out as candidates for possible closure. The Council of the Association of Anaesthetists, in concert with the Faculty of Anaesthetists, "communicated its grave concern" over projected cuts in academic departments of anaesthesia to the Chief Medical Officer, the DHSS, the Committee of Vice Chancellors and Principals of Universities in the United Kingdom, the University Grants Committee and the Department of Education and Science![324]

A (Tony) Cunningham became Professor of Anaesthesia at the Royal College of Surgeons in Ireland in 1986 and Leo Strunin returned from Canada, where he had been Professor of Anaesthesia at Calgary, to become Professor of Anaesthesia at the (now Royal) London Hospital and the Hunterian Institute of the Royal College of Surgeons of England in 1992, after an interregnum since the retirement of Professor J P (Jimmy) Payne in 1987. Jimmy Payne had held the appointment at the Royal College of Surgeons for 24 years. The original Chair at the Royal College of Surgeons had been endowed by the British Oxygen Company (now Ohmeda) in 1957, and the same firm increased its sponsorship to £85,000 per annum for 10 years in 1987.[426]

Education and Research 1983-1995

The Research and Education Committee became the Education and Research Committee, as the managing committee of the activities of the Education and Research Trust, during 1985 when the Association of Anaesthetists and the Trust (a Registered Charity) were incorporated as separate registered companies (Annual Report 1986).[369] The variable covenant arrangements under which surpluses from the running of the Association were handed over for Research and Education have continued.

Education. The reversal of the terms "Research" and "Education" in the trust title reflected the increasing emphasis on the educational responsibilities of the Committee. These became progressively greater due to the additional number of educational meetings for which programmes had to be organised; in particular, following the introduction of the extensive and popular Seminar Programme.

Research. Council took the generous decision in 1985 that, despite the considerable demands on the resources of the Association of Anaesthetists connected with the purchase of the new headquarters at 9 Bedford Square at that time, the considerable expenditure on research (over £30,000: 1996: £48,000) should not be reduced.[341] The contribution which the Association of Anaesthetists is able to make from its own resources towards funding research is significant, but it is, of course, comparatively small compared with the sums expended by the Government, industry and charitable trusts.[427] It is however important that the Association of Anaesthetists, the Royal College of Anaesthetists and other professional organisations connected with the specialty, such as the *British Journal of Anaesthesia* should make their own worthwhile contributions. This is not only beneficial but also demonstrates to the Government and potentially generous charitable donors that the specialty is prepared to contribute independently to the development of anaesthesia. This has become doubly important at the present time (1998) as recent changes in the way Government research grants are made in the United Kingdom have created particular potential problems for the funding of anaesthetic research.[427]

Applications for research and travel grants are very carefully reviewed and assessed. Concern was expressed in the 1989 Annual Report about the quality of some of the applications,[363] and a useful document defining the policy of the Association of Anaesthetists in granting financial awards to its Members was issued in October 1990.[428] The document emphasises in its introduction that the Association of Anaesthetists is concerned to "encourage Members to participate in research to increase knowledge, to improve the standard of anaesthesia, and also to enhance the standing of the specialty", as well as to enable Members to visit centres of excellence to increase their expertise in clinical work, teaching, and research so that there may be benefit to Members, trainees and patients at home, as well as to "assist with travel to developing countries to participate in teaching with the aim of improving standards of care".[428]

The Association of Anaesthetists Research Fellowship[428] has gained steadily in importance and prestige. Geraldine O'Sullivan completed her work for her MD thesis in March 1984 (Annual Report 1984).[331] Fiona MacLennan (Aberdeen) was appointed to the vacancy from eight applicants to study lung water in pregnancy in 1984[331] but resigned in 1985.[341] Angela Cooper (Cambridge) was appointed to the Association Research Fellowship in 1986 from amongst five applicants to study induced hypertension during neurosurgical operations (Annual Report 1987).[356] Fourteen applications were received for the Fellowship in 1988 and Patrick Armstrong studied nitrous oxide and urinary formiminoglutamic acid under the direction of Professor A A Spence at Edinburgh.[363] Six applications were received in 1990 but an appointment was not recommended[364] and the Fellowship was readvertised. Nineteen applications were received in 1991 and Jane Peutrell of Bristol was appointed.[325] She completed her research into postoperative analgesia in paediatric practice in 1993 and was succeeded by Keith Allman at Oxford in 1994 who undertook a study on the highly topical subject of "clinical and experimental studies on the effect of blocking the nitric oxide/ cyclic GMP pathway in sepsis".[366]

Grants for Research Projects. The number of grants increased in frequency after the suggestion by Alastair Spence (then Chairman of the

Research and Education Committee) that the maximum sum available should be advanced to £5,000 for each project was adopted in 1979. Forty three grants were made between 1983 and 1995; for example in 1992 £17,689 was dispersed in this way amongst four applicants.[325] Most of the grants between 1992 and 1995 were between £4,000 and £5,000; as the purchasing power of £5,000 in 1979 is only £2,400 in 1995 there may be a case for increasing the maximum grant!

Travel grants from the budget of the Education and Research Committee continued to be generously funded during the period 1983-1992.[428] These grants are made for supporting or extending short time visits directed towards research or study or to undertake teaching, whether within the United Kingdom or the Republic of Ireland or overseas, but they are not available for travel for the purpose of taking up appointments abroad or for attendance at congresses or meetings of learned societies. The maximum grant available was gradually increased in real terms from £250 in 1983 to £750 in 1991.[341,365] Thirty-three grants were made in this category between 1983 and 1995.

Educational awards for visits to Third World Countries.[428] There was a quickening interest in providing education in developing countries in the nineteen eighties (see below). The Association of Anaesthetists responded in 1986 by making grants available to support those who were prepared to go abroad for periods (normally not less than one year) to assist in teaching anaesthesia overseas.[369,428]

The Baxter (Travenol) Travelling Fellowship award was instituted in 1983. This award of £2,500 each year was generously funded by Baxter Health Care after several other awards made by industry had been discontinued.[424] It enables a Member of the Association to travel within the United Kingdom or abroad to study new applications of intravenous fluid therapy and subsequently make a written report. The uptake of this award was disappointing in the earlier years but after a reminder in the 1987 Annual Report[356] it has been awarded regularly.

Research grants from the British United Provident Association. The Research Committee also "initiated and co-ordinated an approach to BUPA (the private health insurers) to fund research in anaesthesia" in the form of a Fellowship through the College of Anaesthetists in 1988.[362,427]

The work of the Education and Research Committee is of great importance to the Association of Anaesthetists and has become time consuming for its members and a very exacting responsibility for its Chairman. The Association has been fortunate in having a succession of academically experienced and dedicated Chairmen in post during the period of expansion in the eighties and into the nineties:- Alastair Spence (1979-1980), John Norman (1980-1982), Jean Lumley (1982-1984), E A (Ed) Cooper (1984-1985), Graham Smith (1985-1987), Walter Nimmo (1987-1989), Tony Wildsmith (1989-1991), Alan Aitkenhead (1991-1995), John Sear (1996), and Rajinder Mirakhur (1997).

International relations 1983-1995

The International Relations Committee of the Association of Anaesthetists as now constituted in 1998 includes, in addition to the Officers of the Association and a member of the committee of the Group of Anaesthetists in Training (GAT), representatives from the WFSA and World Anaesthesia.[420]

The International Relations Committee also sends its minutes to a number of organisations whose representatives attend its meetings from time to time when particular matters are under discussion.[420] These organisations with which it liaises, and which frequently seek its advice, particularly in the nomination of individuals for service overseas, now include the important United Kingdom funding organisations the Overseas Development Agency (ODA) and the British Council, as well as the Bureau for Overseas Medical Service, the Inter-Varsity Council, the Committee for International Co-operation in Higher Education, Voluntary Service Overseas and the appropriate Health Resources and Technologies Action Group.[420] This list of multiple connections re-emphasises the further development of the role of the International Relations Committee as a coordinating body for British aid to the Third World in the field of education and training in anaesthesia which was established in the late seventies. The membership of the Committee over the years has included most of those senior anaesthetists who are particularly dedicated to the cause of improving the standard of anaesthetic provision in Third World Countries. Prominent amongst this group are John Zorab, Roger Eltringham of Gloucester, [429] Michael Inman (Plymouth) - all three of whom have been Chairman of the International Relations Committee - as well as

Michael Dobson of Oxford, and Iain Wilson (Exeter). These individuals are amongst anaesthetists who have served abroad in the past for periods of months or years and, although they now have senior responsibilities in the British National Health Service, they are still prepared to go overseas as course organisers and lecturers for short periods in the time that each is able to spare from his commitments in the United Kingdom and Ireland. They have been amongst those who have inspired younger British anaesthetists (mainly those in the immediate postfellowship years) to have the courage and enterprise to establish training programmes by joining (and in some cases establishing) departments of anaesthesia in developing countries.[362,429,430]

Some of these schemes have been made possible by the active participation of the International Relations Committee, and others, which have been independently arranged with its cognisance and encouragement (R J Eltringham personal communication and Annual Reports 1983-1985). In addition to those whose work has already been recorded the following should certainly be mentioned:-

1. The successive appointments as lecturers, (funded by the ODA with contributions by the Association of Anaesthetists), of J R Sinclair (now Consultant at Truro) and I H Wilson (now Consultant at Exeter) to Lusaka, Zambia over a period of four years.[341,362,366]

2. The programme sustained by visiting lecturers and technicians in Kathmandu, Nepal under the supervision of Michael Inman (Plymouth) and Roger Maltby (Alberta, Canada and an Overseas Member). This scheme has been partially funded by the ODA. It has resulted in the inauguration of a local Diploma in Anaesthetics. The lecturers who have been involved in the programme have included Andrew Tomlinson (Consultant at Stoke on Trent), Timothy Jack (Consultant at Leeds and later at Oxford), Michael Carter (Senior Registrar at the Middlesex Hospital and now Consultant at Luton),[430] and Michael Mowbray Senior Registrar and later Consultant at Nottingham). The scheme has also included the secondment of Nepalese anaesthetists to the United Kingdom for training under the Overseas Doctors Training Scheme (ODTS).[331,341,356,366,369]

3. The successive secondments over five years of two paediatric anaesthetists Angela Barlow (then of Manchester now in Vietnam) and Celia Allison then living in Rotterdam.

4. The highly productive link between the Humphry Davy Department of Anaesthetics of the University of Bristol and Khartoum which was sponsored by the British Council following the visit of J A (Tony) Bennett in 1979, and in the success of which Professor Cedric Prys-Roberts (Bristol) and Andrew Black (Bristol) played such leading parts. This ambitious undertaking included the constant supply of teams of lecturers extending over some seven years, and the training of Sudanese doctors in the United Kingdom in the ODTS scheme. It has also resulted in the establishment of a locally staffed postgraduate course and a Mastership in Medicine degree in Anaesthesia.[332,341,366]

5. The continuing training programme conducted in Uganda by the veteran missionary Patricia Coyle in sometimes very difficult political circumstances.[356, 369]

6. The appointment funded by the ODA of Paul Fenton (King's College Hospital, London) to Malawi in 1987 on a six month contract,[356] where he continues to serve to this day (1996)!

7. The one year appointment initially funded by the ODA of Richard Page (now a Consultant in Truro), and Ben O'Donohoe (now Consultant in Carmarthen) to Ghana where a successful training programme was established.[356]

8. The successive appointments of Martin Coates (Plymouth) and Nigel Puttick (Middlesborough) to Fiji funded by the ODA.[363,365]

9. The Lectureships of Michael Dudley (now Consultant in Accident and Emergency at the Royal Hallamshire Hospital, Sheffield) and Katrina O'Sullivan (Dublin) who was funded by the Irish

Aid Organisation to Tanzania.[356]

10. The Senior Lectureship by William Casey (Gloucester) in Nigeria funded by the ODA.

Lecture courses and the WFSA Refresher Course Scheme. Lectureships were funded by the British Council and the ODA and other organisations on request over the years, for example an obstetric anaesthesia team consisting of Jeffrey Selwyn Crawford (Birmingham, 1923-1938),[431] Donald Moir (Glasgow) and Trevor Thomas (Bristol) went to Thailand in 1984.[331] The WFSA began a programme of Refresher Courses in many parts of the world form the mid eighties onwards in which many anaesthetists from the United Kingdom have participated. This scheme was doubtless stimulated by the presence of John Zorab (Bristol) in the inner councils of the WFSA!

The first WFSA Course was held in Nairobi, Kenya by Roger Eltringham.[356,369] Nearly 50 of these courses had been held up to the end of 1995 and a full programme has taken place in 1996, mainly in Africa, but also, since the end of the Cold War in Russia and Eastern Europe, Richard Jack (Slough and the Royal Postgraduate Medical School) has been particularly concerned with courses in Russia and John Lythe of Plymouth has organised and partially funded a course in Romania. Locations have included:- Kenya, Sudan, Ghana, Uganda, Zambia, Malawi, Nigeria, Zimbabwe, Tanzania, Botswana, Mauritius, Russia, Romania and Sri Lanka (personal communications Roger Eltringham).[325,365,392]

Funding has come from a variety of sources, including the WFSA, ODA, and British Council, the Aid Agency of the Republic of Ireland, the American Association of Anesthesiologists (which established a reciprocal committee to that of the Association of anaesthetists of Great Britain and Ireland in 1990),[364] the Dutch and German Societies of Anaesthesia, and industrial firms including Abott Laboratories and Viggo. A number of speakers, particularly from the United States have paid their own expenses.

A major development occurred in 1991 when the council of the Association of Anaesthetists accepted the recommendation of the International Relations Committee under the Chairmanship of S Morrell Lyons (later

President 1994-1996) to invite National, Regional and Specialist Societies to collaborate with the Association of Anaesthetists in funding lectures on WFSA refresher courses.[365] This scheme has been very successful. Lecturers were jointly sponsored between 1991 and 1996 to the WFSA Refresher Courses by the Association of Anaesthetists and the Society of Anaesthetists of the South Western Region, the Scottish Society of Anaesthetists, the Plastic Surgery and Burns Anaesthetists, the Northern Ireland Society of Anaesthetists, the Southern Society of Anaesthetists, the Obstetric Anaesthetists Association, the Sheffield and East Midlands Society, the Society of Anaesthetists of Wales, the South of Ireland Society of Anaesthetists, the European Society of Regional Anaesthesia (British and Irish section) and the Anaesthetic Section of the Royal Society of Medicine.[325,365, 366,392,421]

Seminars on the provision of aid to developing countries have been included in the educational programme at 9 Bedford Square,[325,362] and the Association produced a useful document containing Guidelines for Overseas Lecturers to Developing Countries in 1993.[432] The Group of Anaesthetists in Training has also compiled a database of information, contacts and posts abroad.[325,391]

Other educational activities in the United Kingdom have developed in the eighties in line with the general increasing interest in training and service in developing countries. The Nuffield Department of Anaesthetics at Oxford inaugurated the Courses in Anaesthesia for Difficult Situations and Developing Countries in 1981 shortly after the arrival of (Sir) Keith Sykes as Professor and these have continued to be organised annually by Michael Dobson and Gordon Paterson. This residential course at St Catherine's College has been fortunate in recruiting speakers with considerable and varied experience, as well as a wide cross section of registrants, including representatives of the armed forces of the United States and a number of those who already have overseas experience. It was a source of satisfaction to organisers that the first course was attended by Emeritus Professor Sir Robert Macintosh, the first Nuffield Professor, who had had wide experience of both military and developing country anaesthesia, and that he continued to show an interest until his death in 1989.

The Oxford Course has proved to be very popular but the number who can register is limited due to its residential nature. A parallel annual non-residential course was started in 1986 at Frenchay Hospital, Bristol by John Zorab, Peter Baskett and John Carter, which has been equally successful year by year.[369]

"World Anaesthesia" was founded by Michael Dobson after a Study Day at Oxford in 1984. It is an "informal group of interested and informed anaesthetists who wish to contribute to training in anaesthesia in the Third World".[331] It now (1998) has a membership of nearly 700 and publishes a regular Newsletter (R J. Eltringham personal communication). Michael Dobson has also written a book (*Anaesthesia in a District Hospital*) for developing countries under the auspices of the World Health Organisation.

Update in Anaesthesia is an add-on educational journal supported by the WFSA which was started by Iain Wilson (Truro). It proved remarkably popular and now has a circulation of 300 copies distributed in over 80 countries. (R J Eltringham personal communication).

Eastern Europe. The cultural exchange with East Germany (Chapter 8) continued in the eighties until the destruction of the Berlin Wall and the unification of Germany in 1989. A visit by Dr Ingrid Bergman following Clifford Franklin's visit to East Germany in 1984 was delayed until 1986 and reciprocated by Roger Eltringham in the same year,[369] and Professor Benad of Rostock and Elizabeth Bradshaw (Council Member) exchanged visits in 1987.[356]

The Group of Anaesthetists in Training (GAT) took a new initiative in 1993 when they invited two trainee colleagues from Poland to their Annual General Meeting at Sheffield. Two Romanians attended the GAT Annual Meeting in 1994 and, in 1995 two Lithuanians were present and spent two weeks in the United Kingdom visiting departments in London, Cardiff and Sheffield and other centres in the Untied Kingdom.[366,424,433, 434]

There is no doubt that the reputation of British and Irish anaesthesia abroad has been enhanced by these programmes, but the benefit is by no means one sided; those who have participated, both seniors and juniors, have gained immeasurably by their experiences and contacts with colleagues in other countries.[430] It is to be hoped that the benefit to the British National

Health Service itself of developing the professional and cultural outlook of individuals by service abroad, during training or as part of continuing medical education will not be entirely forgotten, under the new structured training for specialists following the Calman Report![226]

Outpatient dental anaesthesia and the Poswillo Report (1990)

It is apparent from previous chapters that one of the longest running problems with which the Association has had to deal throughout its history has been that of outpatient dental anaesthesia, and latterly of sedation, carried out on the unintubated patient. The subject has also been the cause of unfortunate dissension between specialist anaesthetists and their medical and dental general practitioner colleagues (Chapter 8).

The number of deaths associated with British outpatient dental practice, whether in general dental practice, in the Community Dental Service or in hospital outpatient departments, has never been large; it was calculated at being perhaps one in 250,000 anaesthetics in 1986. The number of outpatient dental anaesthetics administered has also fallen steadily during the last three decades, and especially since the guidelines issued by the General Dental Council in 1983 (Chapter 8).[435,436] These facts were confirmed by two further surveys supported by the Association of Anaesthetists and conducted by Michael Coplans (St George's Hospital, London) and Professor Curson (King's College Hospital Dental School) for the decades 1970-1979 and 1980-1989.[437,438]

Even one death in this area of minor surgery in outpatient dental practice is however of considerable concern. A limited survey of general dental practitioner surgeons conducted in 1988 suggested that, although provision of facilities for general anaesthesia and equipment for resuscitation had improved since a more detailed survey by a group with the same principal author in 1976, there was still a dearth of monitoring apparatus.[439] The public and their Members of Parliament, prompted by zealous reporting in the newspaper and on the radio and television, of the few deaths that did occur, inevitably led to a demand for an inquiry. The Expert Working Party was consequently set up in October 1989 by the DH under the Chairmanship of Professor David Poswillo (Professor of Oral and Dental Surgery at the United Medical and Dental School of Guy's and St Thomas' Hospitals).[440] The Expert

Working Party was charged with reporting on the need for use of general anaesthesia and sedation in outpatient dental surgery and to develop guidelines for the safe use of these techniques; it was also required to make recommendations for the need for undergraduate, vocational and continuing education of dental and medical practitioners in general anaesthesia and sedation; with the usual flurry of activity beloved by politicians when they want to be seen to be "doing something", the Expert Working Party was asked to report in an extraordinarily short time, by 31 March 1990. This deadline presented a considerable challenge to both the Working Party itself and to the organisations (including the Association of Anaesthetists) who were called upon to give evidence.[436,440,441]

The Association of Anaesthetists formed a Working Group chaired by Professor A P (Tony) Adams (Guys Hospital) and composed of representatives from the Association of Anaesthetists, the Association of Dental Anaesthetists and the College of Anaesthetists (Council Minutes 8.12.1990),[441] and commendably it expressed its views in the form of a letter by the DH deadline of 26 January 1990. The group stressed in their evidence that standards of anaesthetic practice in general dental surgeries (including monitoring) should be the same as in hospital, and that verbal communication with the patient must be maintained during sedation techniques. They also expressed the view that dentists should no longer receive training in general anaesthesia (Council Minutes 2.2.1990).[364,441]

The Expert Working Party itself also met their prescribed deadline and the "Poswillo Report" was received by the Department of Health by the end of March 1990;[442,443] however, despite extensive leaks, some of which were "misinformed" it was not published until 30 November 1990, and then only after considerable and continuous pressure from the professional organisations concerned. It now appears that the reason for the delay was due to Government anxiety over the financial implications of some of the recommendations of the Report.[436, 440]

The recommendations of the Poswillo Report were particularly and succinctly expressed and left no doubt as to their implications.[436,440,444] The Expert Working Party, probably wisely, did not, as some had predicted, propose that dental surgeons should cease to administer general anaesthesia, nor that general anaesthesia should cease to be administered outside hospitals or specially equipped centralised clinics, but its recommendations pointed the way to those consequences.

The Report stated unequivocally that general anaesthesia should be avoided whenever possible and sedation techniques (intravenous and inhalation) used in preference. It made strong (and necessarily expensive) proposals with regard to the mandatory availability of monitoring for general anaesthesia. These were in accordance with the guidelines issued by the Association of Anaesthetists in 1988;[145] wherever general anaesthesia was administered an electrocardiograph, a pulse oximeter and non-invasive blood pressure measurement should be regarded as mandatory, and in addition, when intubation was to be undertaken, a capnograph. So far as intravenous sedation was concerned the use of a pulse oximeter and inhaled supplementary oxygen should be mandatory.[442]

The Report boldly recommended that dental undergraduate training should no longer require proficiency in general anaesthesia. Dental undergraduates should however be exposed to and have practical experience of administering sedation techniques and working under their influence. It was regarded as essential that both doctors and dentists who wished to administer general anaesthesia or sedation should have postgraduate training, and that the staff participating in procedures involving general anaesthesia or sedation should be appropriately trained in their supporting role. Doctors and dental surgeons with knowledge and experience should be allowed to continue to do so, but only if they could satisfy the (now Royal) College of Anaesthetists that they were competent and, in the future they should be reassessed periodically.[442]

It was also recommended that all dental surgeons and members of their teams in general practice surgeries should be trained in, and have continuing practice sessions in, resuscitation, whether or not general anaesthesia or sedation was undertaken in their practices, that all dental surgeons should be proficient in venepuncture, and that prescribed resuscitation equipment and a prescribed list of drugs should be available in dental surgeries.[436,440-444]

These were indeed sweeping proposals; they dismissed the long cherished concept that a dental surgeon on qualification should be regarded as competent to administer general anaesthesia without further training, they proposed mandatory standards for the facilities and equipment which should be available when general anaesthesia or sedation was to be practised, and they introduced the requirement that dental surgeons and their staff should be trained and equipped to resuscitate any patient who collapsed from dangerous conditions whether related or unrelated to general anaesthesia or sedation. One further important point was that Poswillo recommended that Health Authorities should be responsible for ensuring that there were sufficient Consultant dental anaesthetic services to meet the need in their Districts.[441,442]

The Association of Anaesthetists of Great Britain and Ireland and the (now Royal) College of Anaesthetists welcomed the Report. There were generally approving editorials in the *British Medical Journal*,[436] the *British Dental Journal*.[440] The Society for the Advancement of Anaesthesia in Dentistry (SAAD) gave cautious support, although they disagreed with certain details, notably the definition of "simple sedation" which was defined as being with nitrous oxide and oxygen or the injection of a single agent intravenously.[445] All these commentators expressed anxiety over the question of the cost and funding. The President of the General Dental Council, prior to initiating discussion with his Council, stressed the need for safety in the practice of anaesthesia and sedation and predicted changes in the Council's guidance.[446]

A number of dental practitioners did not wait for the probable endorsement of the report by the Department of Health and the General Dental Council and ceased to offer general anaesthesia in their practices. They arranged to transfer their cases (mainly children) to Hospital Dental Outpatient Departments, where the existed, or the Community Dental Services Clinics.[447]

Many medical and dental anaesthetists foresaw the demise of the use of general anaesthesia in general dental practice and the phasing out of dental surgeons as anaesthetists.[447-451] There was certainly a contrast between the titles of the Editorials in the *British Dental Journal* in January 1991 shortly after the Poswillo Report was published ("Reprieve for Dental General Anaesthesia"),[440] and that in the same journal in the following December ("Poswillo: The beginning of the end?")[450] shortly after the Department of Health accepted the recommendations of the report over a year after it was published, but without any indications that additional funds would be provided to implement it.[449,451]

The Government finally announced in 1992 that £9 million would be made available to Health Authorities in England[452] and £1.2 million to those in Scotland.[453] It was left to the Health Authorities to divide the money between general dental practices, hospitals and community service clinics in order to meet their local obligations to provide for general outpatient anaesthesia.[442]

The General Dental Council pledged itself to "do its utmost" to ensure that the principal recommendations of the Poswillo Report were carried forward in May 1992, and it issued revised ethical guidance on the use of general anaesthesia and sedation in a new edition of its publication Professional Conduct and Fitness to Practice, in accordance with the Report. The recognition of the need for "appropriate postgraduate training" in anaesthesia and sedation techniques for dental graduates represented a significant advance in policy. One important difference from the Poswillo recommendations was that the guidance did not outlaw the use of more than one drug in intravenous sedation techniques, provided "continuously-acting monitoring devices" and a defibrillator were available.[454]

The present writer in his Presidential Address to the Society for the Advancement of Anaesthesia in Dentistry (SAAD) in 1980 which was entitled "The rise and fall of anaesthesia in the dental chair" stated that he had:-

"reached the inevitable conclusion that full general anaesthesia 'in the chair' will give way to psychological and pharmacological techniques of analgesia and sedation short of full general anaesthesia.....Such outpatient general anaesthesia as is required being treated with the respect it deserves and will be practised in properly equipped day or half day units."[455]

This prophecy is not far from the truth in 1998 if the expression "properly equipped day or half day units" can be deemed to include those fully equipped and staffed clinics and specialist general dental practices which have been brought up to the Poswillo standard and have specialised in anaesthesia. Such clinics and general dental practices now take general anaesthetic cases on referral from other General Dental Practitioners.[456]

The reduction of the use of general anaesthesia was further accelerated by the acceptance by the British Dental Association in July 1990 of a new NHS Dentists' Contract with the Government. This involved a partial continuing care element for the dental profession. The negotiators (the General Dental Services Committee of the British Dental Association) accepted the contract despite the rejection of the draft contract in a referendum by rank and file "high street" dental surgeons, and the contract was implemented the following October.[457] Many dental surgeons began to move into the independent private sector or, at least to decline to take on more adult NHS patients. The extent to which this occurred immediately is disputed but there was certainly a greater tendency to "go private" in the south of England than in the North.[458] The new continuing care scheme with its capitation fee was more successful than the Government anticipated however, and in July 1992 the DH announced its intention of imposing a 7% pay cut for general practitioner dental surgeons to "claw back" the excess expenditure. This somewhat cavalier action has resulted in a further move into the independent sector.[459,460] The move to independent practice does not, of itself, necessitate a reduction in the use of general anaesthesia for occasional cases, but the provision of full Poswillo facilities for general anaesthesia, which must still apply for professional and legal reasons, is an expensive item for a private practitioner. Such evidence as is available suggests that there has been a considerable further fall in the number of general dental practices offering treatment under general anaesthesia since the publication of the Poswillo Report in 1991, (for example nearly 50% of 73 practices in the Manchester area were offering a general anaesthetic service under the NHS in 1991 but, in 1993 only 8% (6 of 72 practices) were doing so).[461] There are also indications of some increase in general dental practitioner referrals (mainly children) for general anaesthesia to dental hospital outpatient departments,[462] Community Dental Service Clinics and specialist dental anaesthetic practices.

A survey undertaken amongst Consultant Anaesthetists of less than seven years standing and Senior Registrars which was conducted in 1993 in the Mersey Region is of interest.[463] Eleven of 46 Consultants practised 'Chair' general anaesthesia; the majority of sessions were in Community Service dental centres and more patients were anaesthetised in them than in general dental practice; of 71 anaesthetists (young Consultants and Senior Registrars),

52 felt that chair dental anaesthesia was acceptable in centres conforming to Poswillo standards, 16 believed that it should be confined to a hospital environment, and three felt that it should not be undertaken at all.[463]

A few established general and medical dental surgeon anaesthetists have undergone assessment and certification courses for a Non-Consultant Register of dental anaesthetists,[464] but provision for postgraduate training in general anaesthesia or sedation for general practitioners of either discipline from scratch is still under consideration by the General Dental Council and the other bodies concerned. It seems probable that the practice of general anaesthesia for dental outpatients as far as it is required, will become the responsibility of Consultant Anaesthetists working in properly equipped Community Service or private clinics or in the hospital environment, as was proposed by Alastair Spence in 1993 when he was President of the Royal College of Anaesthetists.[465]

The Manchester study also records a fall in the availability of the provision of sedation under the NHS contract; in 1991 over 90% of the then 73 existing practices were offering sedation, but by 1993, only 37.5% (8 of the by then 72 practices in the area were employing both intravenous sedation and relative analgesia, 17 intravenous sedation only, and two "relative analgesia" with nitrous oxide only).[461] This probably reflects the situation generally in NHS practice; however, the position with regard to sedation in independent practice is different from that relating to general anaesthesia. It is likely that the partial or total shift of individual practices to the private sector has been accompanied by the continuing or even increasing use of sedation. There are obvious drawbacks to the use of sedation techniques in a busy NHS practice and it is time consuming. Many "mixed" NHS and independent practices offer sedation on a private basis only. The General Dental Council guidelines,[454] though making adequate provision for monitoring, are naturally rather less stringent for conscious sedation techniques than they are for general anaesthesia. The guidelines also sanction the practice of sedation by the trained operator with trained assistance, although there is anecdotal evidence that dental surgeons are increasingly calling upon Consultant Anaesthetists to conduct sedation in the independent sector.

It may be that, on the other hand, the more relaxed conditions of independent practice will lead to a diminution in the use of sedation in favour of the study and practice of what is termed psychological "behaviour control", or in more traditional terms, a good old fashioned "chairside manner"! *Note: Additional guidelines issued by the General Dental Council in 1998 limit the administration of general anaesthesia to medically qualified specialist anaesthetists.* [459]

NHS fees for dental outpatient general anaesthesia.

It has already been noticed that, with the diminution in the number of NHS general anaesthesia cases, the dental anaesthetic fee issue, which had previously been such a preoccupation of the Association of Anaesthetists over decades gradually became to be of less major importance as the eighties progressed. The Anaesthetic Sub-Committee of the BMA CCHMS gave a "cautious welcome" to a 33% rise in fees for anaesthesia in general dental practice in 1986 but remained "concerned at the overall low level of the fees".[369]

Anaesthetists' fees for Community Dental Sessions to which many patients are now referred are not exactly generous either. Two Consultant Anaesthetists calculated that, in 1994, the overall rewards given to the patients by parents acting vicariously for the "tooth fairy" in their area (average £1 per deciduous tooth tax free with no expenses to pay), is better than their own sessional remuneration (£87 before tax to include travelling for a session of up to 12 cases)![466]

Many of the problems and restrictions concerning the payment of NHS anaesthetic fees to medical anaesthetists arise because the fees are paid to the Dentist out of Dental Funds, but despite many representations to the Department of Health nothing has been changed. This now anomalous arrangement has its origins in the days before the NHS when the dentist paid the anaesthetist for his services; today the anaesthetist is an independent practitioner and not the employee of the dental surgeon. The payment of anaesthetists' fees via the surgeon in independent practice has been generally discontinued, and there is no reason why the position should not also be remedied in the NHS dental surgery.

It must also be a cause for concern and illustrative of the perceived relationship between the dental surgeon and anaesthetists in some quarters, that in a recent controversial disciplinary case, both the dental surgeon and the anaesthetist were censured by their respective professional conduct committees for failure to gain adequate consent for a procedure designed to obtain proper pain relief, which might reasonably be considered to be the sole responsibility of the anaesthetist.[467] One must have sympathy with the dentist, but the decision was taken because the Dental Surgeon was deemed to be "in charge" of the activities of his Consultant Anaesthetist colleague. Many will find it unacceptable that the dentist should be required to shoulder a share of the blame.

The unexpected hazard fee (Code 2431) was introduced to replace the "special anaesthetic fee" for difficult cases available under the old dental contract when the new contract was introduced in October 1990.[468] This caused considerable disquiet amongst dental anaesthetists.[469] The special anaesthetic fee had been paid if it was judged *in advance* of the anaesthetic that there was a condition (such as gross obesity or a history of asthma), or a special circumstance (such as an anticipated abnormally lengthy dental procedure), such that "special skill" might be required to avoid a complication or to treat one if it arose; however the new unexpected hazard fee was only to be paid *after* the event if a complication actually arose and was proved to be hazardous.[468,469] The interpretation of the circumstances which would allow the payment of the former special anaesthetic fee to be paid had been fairly liberal since the conditions under which it was to be paid were eased in 1975; it has even been stated that effectively some anaesthetists administering anaesthetics for lengthy procedures, or in the face of potentially dangerous medical conditions had taken a 20% cut overnight with the introduction of the unexpected hazard fee.[470] Other experienced anaesthetists were of the opinion that this "reversal of previous policy .... effectively rewards the cavalier anaesthetist at the expense of the cautious and conscientious practitioner who foresees and prevents possible hazards."[469] Others felt that the act of making a claim might lead to allegations of incompetence, and yet others pointed out the bureaucratic difficulties involved in applying for the fee. There was certainly considerable dispute about what sort of event constitutes an "unexpected hazard" between many consultants and the Dental Practice Board and their expert advisers.[471,472] The matter was taken to judicial review and the decision of the Dental Practice Board to refuse to authorise the unexpected hazard fee in a particular case was quashed. The High Court declared that "the words unexpected hazard mean a hazard which an anaesthetist, knowing the medical history and condition of the patient, would, before administering the anaesthetic, consider what was likely to occur during either the anaesthetic or the recovery state". It was a Pyrrhic victory! The authorities had deleted the "unexpected hazard" item from the remuneration scale before the judicial review took place![468,470]

Private (Independent) Practice 1983-1995 and the Report of the Monopoly and Mergers Commission 1994.

The economic boom of the Thatcher years in the mid nineteen eighties resulted in an increase in the number of people who were privately insured (many of their premiums being paid for by employers as a "perk") and there was as a result, a proliferation of health insurers and private hospitals, many of which were owned by the insurers themselves.[473-477] This increase in independent health provision was encouraged by the Government, but the depression of the late eighties and the early nineties has led to considerable retrenchment. This fact, coupled with an increase in the number of claims per insured person potentially affected the profits of the health insurers, and there were startling increases in their premiums (sometimes amounting to as much as 30% in a single year), and an increase in the pressure by the insurers on the medical profession to cut costs and reduce or contain legitimate increases in fees even if they are in line with rises in the cost of living. The fees of anaesthetists have been particularly disadvantaged as, even before the recession there was a perceived need to make them more proportionately comparable to those paid to their surgical colleagues. The objective of the Association of Anaesthetists has consistently been to secure 30% of the global sum offered by medical insurers to cover both the surgical and the anaesthetic fee. This is estimated to reflect the concept, established in the NHS since its inception, that all medical specialists, irrespective of discipline should be paid the same amount per unit time spent with the patient, whether in consultation or administering therapy.[364,478]

The Annual Reports of the Council of the Association of Anaesthetists[331,341,363-366] and of the Linkman Conferences[342-344] throughout the nineteen eighties contain reports of repeated requests to the medical insurers (particularly to BUPA which had the largest share of the health insurance market; 59% in 1985 and 45% in 1994)[477] asking them to abandon the practice of offering a global benefit to cover the fees of both surgeon and anaesthetist. Private Patient Plan (PPP) the second largest private health insurer (25% in 1985, 27% in 1995)[477] opted not to issue a list of payment rates for professional fees and paid "reasonable charges". The Directors of PPP asserted in 1992 that "most specialists charge reasonable fees".[473]

The Association of Anaesthetists of Great Britain and Ireland was the first medical organisation to issue guidelines setting out recommendations for private fees in 1981. They took effect from January 1982 and were updated every two years in line with inflation until January 1990.[363] These guidelines were, by common consent, helpful to anaesthetists (especially for newly appointed consultants setting up in independent practice) and to patients and surgeons alike. The BMA followed suit in 1989, in response to a request from its Annual Representatives Meeting, by publishing "Private Consultant Work, BMA Guidelines". This contained what was considered to be reasonable charges for some 1500 procedures as guidance for Consultants.[473] It was unfortunate that the BMA apparently ignored the advice of its specialist advisers in anaesthesia in compiling their publication. The BMA proposals were unrelated to those of the Association of Anaesthetists, and the Council of the Association consequently recommended that they should be ignored.[479] BUPA, without warning or prior negotiation then introduced a table of benefit levels based on the BMA guidelines. This proposed large increases for physicians and surgeons but effectively decreased the benefits payable to anaesthetists; after the "strongest possible recommendations" from the Association of Anaesthetists, the Association scale was adapted by BUPA for "minor" procedures, but the benefits available for "intermediate", "major" and "complex" fee levels were not raised to meet the Association of Anaesthetists' guideline levels.[364,478]

The BMA welcomed the cooperation of the Association of Anaesthetists in preparing a second revised edition of its guideline document which, after a delay of two months due to the revision of the anaesthetic section, was published in December 1990. The Committee of the Association of Anaesthetists regarded the revised levels of the BMA recommended fees as being "fair and reasonable" and Council then recommended adherence to its provisions to the membership until 31 March 1992 when a further revision would take place.[479,480]

All the Provident Societies reimbursed the level of fees recommended by the BMA Guidelines except for the Directors of BUPA who continued their active opposition and left a gap between the benefit provided and the BMA Guideline fee, which the patient either had to meet or the anaesthetist had to forego.[365,479]

The discussion dealing with independent practice at the 1991 Linkman Conference was certainly lively and outspoken. The contents of a letter from the Director of Strategic Services of BUPA provoked a "brief but pointed discussion", which made it clear that there was no support for his views, and the Honorary Secretary "was given a mandate to inform him fully of the opinion of the Linkman Conference"![479]

The next move on the part of BUPA was to ask the Committee of the Association of Anaesthetists to "rank scale" the anaesthetists' list in the benefit schedule.[479] This was done but, despite warnings from the Association of Anaesthetists concerning the value of this list, BUPA used the information to issue a new scale of benefit levels in February 1992. These proposed reductions in many categories. BUPA stated that the list was prepared after "discussions with the Association of Anaesthetists". Some of the decreases were remedied after a price revision, but they did not bring the levels up to those recommended in the BMA guidelines.[325]

The writer, because of his particular commitments, both clinical and otherwise, did not practice in the independent sector for the greater part of his Consultant career (after 1961 in fact); he therefore feels that he is in a position to comment without bias. The professional private medical fees generally, and especially private anaesthetic fees, are not exorbitant and bear favourable comparison with fees charged by other professionals (lawyers and accountants for example), or indeed, with the present day "call out" charges of domestic plumbers and electricians![473] BUPA would have been fairer to emphasise to patients that their contribution was a "benefit", proportionate to the premium which the patient has paid, which would not necessarily cover the whole fee as do some other health insurance companies, rather than denigrate the consultants for overcharging.[480]

The Association of Anaesthetists has adopted a very responsible attitude over the years in advising its Members about practice in the private sector.

This advice is encapsulated in its document "Guidance on the conduct of private anaesthetic practice".[481] This pamphlet suggests that, with common consent, many para-anaesthetic services such as preoperative assessment and treatment and postoperative care, including pain control other than the use of epidurals, which might otherwise reasonably be considered to be liable to attract a separate charge, should be included within the fee for the anaesthetic itself.[365,478,481]

The Committee and the Council of the Association has, consistently and correctly, advised members to discuss their fees with the patient in advance and to point out that the insurance benefit may not completely cover the charge leaving a shortfall which will have to be made up by the patient, and then to charge the appropriate fee.[477,481,482] It is obvious however, that such a course of action may be embarrassing, especially in the face of propaganda about "greedy" consultants. It is not therefore really surprising that many anaesthetists charge only according to the provision made by the health insurer, despite the possible medicopolitical consequences of doing so, as has emerged since the reference Monopolies and Mergers Commission (see below).[482]

It is difficult to escape the conclusion that the basic reason for the attempt to contain justifiable increases in professional medical fees, which in fact had not risen in real terms, was basically economic, with the objective of rebuilding operational surpluses which had been depleted by the recession and loss of market share.[476] The downward pressure on surgical and anaesthetic fees was seen to be an easy option compared with attempting to limit expenditure in the private hospitals and, despite denials to the contrary, it is probable that anaesthesia was perceived as an easy target because of an apparently archaic conception of the value of its skills and responsibilities.[483,484] An article in the *Evening Standard* of 25 March 1993 reported that BUPA had returned to "tip-top shape after boosting profits from £1.3 million to £3.6 million in 1992". Subscription revenue had gone up 7% while there was only a modest rise in benefits paid (up £2 million; at £720 million).[485]

The Private Medical Services Monopoly Enquiry was initiated by a reference to the Monopolies and Mergers Commission (MMC) by the Director of Fair Trading in September 1992. This required the Commission to consider the provision of private medical services. The MMC stated that its investigation did not arise from any particular complaint but that they had a "duty to monitor various guidelines".[473] It quickly emerged that, despite its comprehensive title, the enquiry would not be concerned with possible monopolistic activities amongst private hospital owners, which included a number owned by insurers themselves, even those with a large share of the market, or amongst medical insurers as such.[473] The investigation was prompted by the BMA guidelines and its purpose was to investigate how consultants set their charges. The process included examination of group practice arrangements, the proper organisation which the Association had actively promoted in seminars at 9 Bedford Square, and other meetings and in its pamphlet on the conduct of private practice.[325,344,363,369,481,486]

The reference to the MMC presaged a very challenging and active year for the Committee and the Council of the Association. This was particularly so in view of the intensified negative propaganda put out by BUPA to its subscribers suggesting that anaesthetists were overcharging for their services. A questionnaire was circulated to Linkmen, wide ranging discussions were held with the MMC, written evidence, including evidence about the advantages of group practice was presented after it had been appraised by the solicitors of the Association (Hempsons), and a Solicitor and Counsel accompanied the Officers who gave oral evidence to the Commission.[366,387]

The MMC presented its 300 page report to the Secretary of State for Trade and Industry in February 1994.[366,488-490] The MMC had the responsibility of deciding, firstly whether a monopoly existed, and secondly, if it did, whether it was against the public interest. The conclusion of the MMC that a monopoly "existed and was against the public interest due to the publication of the BMA guidelines". This seemed strange from a common sense point of view, especially bearing in mind that guidelines were merely advisory and represented what a Consultant *might* reasonably charge for particular services. The MMC recommendations can no doubt be justified in the light of the particular way the Fair Trading Act is worded however. The Act asserts that a "complex monopoly" exists "if a group of two or more persons .... restrict or distort competition in connection with the supply of goods or services". The MMC had conducted an enquiry and found that, of Consultants questioned, 6,600 NHS consultants fixed their charges with reference to the BUPA maximum benefit list, but only 3,600 by the BMA guidelines;[487,488]

nonetheless this was sufficient to establish that there was a complex monopoly within the definitions of the Act.[473] The MMC held that the use of the BMA guidelines was against the public interest because it was considered that the use of the guidelines artificially operated to raise charges for those Consultants who used them. The MMC were however of the opinion that BUPA as insurers could legitimately be permitted to tell the public the extent of the benefits they would receive in particular circumstances under the terms of their policies.[488, 489]

The BMA described the report as "perverse" but they gave a voluntary undertaking not to publish further revised guidelines before they were ordered to do so; however, the MMC had also stated that it would not be "sensible or practicable to prohibit Consultants from fixing their charges by reference to the BMA guidelines" (plus, of course, an update for inflation on the last permitted BMA recommendations). The MMC did not find that there was any widespread abuse of group practice provisions either. The Association of Anaesthetists therefore continues to recommend that Consultants make sure that their accounts are "transparent" (that is that they indicate the elements which make up the total charge), that the patient is made aware of the fee before the procedure is undertaken, and that a scale of likely fees is made available to surgeons and administrators of private hospitals.[489]

The publication of the MMC Report was unfortunately the occasion of various triumphalist statements in the lay press by the executives of some insurers which included phrases such as "going after" and "cracking down" on Consultants being used.[491] It is fortunate that some companies take a more conciliatory attitude.[492] Downward pressure on fees by some insurers continues however.[490] The ever vigilant Editor of *Anaesthesia News* continues to detail the many strategies that are being adopted by some insurance companies to try to induce consultants to charge fees which are in accordance with the maximum benefits which their schedules provide. These bear a close relationship with each other *(Anaesthesia News* 1995 No 90 et seq.). It is a sad scene.

BUPA formed a "Consensus Panel" for anaesthesia on which two nominees of the Council of the Association of Anaesthetists sit, but there are "concerns about its function".[491] There was some light at the end of the tunnel however. The Office of Fair Trading announced its intention to investigate the health insurance business! There is concern that the public is not getting value for money for the very large premiums which are currently being charged; bearing in mind that professional fees have been restrained in recent times there must be other causes for the current situation![493]

Medical Defence Society subscriptions. Responsibility for the settlement of legal claims against medical practitioners working in NHS hospitals was assumed by the Department of Health in 1988 as a temporary measure,[494] and made permanent in 1989.[478] Indemnity is, of course, still required for private practice. The Defence Societies began to introduce differential subscriptions based on the varying perceived risks of the individual specialties and the amount of private practice undertaken; but, by 1995 the subscriptions had risen very steeply and the possibility arose of some mitigation being obtained by risk management strategies including employment of modern monitoring techniques. Measures of this kind have been successful in reducing malpractice insurance premiums for anesthesiologists in the United States.[420] This was the subject of the 1993 BOC Health Care Lecture by professor Clayton Petty (Utah).[495]

The Chairmanship of the Committee is certainly no sinecure! It requires toughness, tact, and tenacity, as well as the wisdom of Solomon and the patience of Job, and it attracts a great deal of correspondence from Members of the Association which has to be answered. The Association has been fortunate in having the services of exceptional Chairmen during the eighties and nineties:- Michael Inman (1983-1989), Robin Weller (1990-1992), Anna-Maria Rollin (1993-1997) and R E Atkinson (1997 *et seq*).

Assistance for Anaesthetists

The Council of the Association of Anaesthetists and individual Members of the Association have been concerned over many years to ensure that, in the interests of safety and efficiency, practising anaesthetists are provided with adequate assistance at all times. They have also consistently tried to ensure that those who assist anaesthetists (particularly Operating Department Assistants (ODAs), but also nurses) have just and fair terms and conditions of service and proper remuneration commensurate with their skills (Chapters 7 and 8). The attempt to secure these objectives has been an uphill struggle.

This is re-emphasised by the reports of successive Linkman Conferences and in other documents placed in the archives of the Association of Anaesthetists in the nineteen eighties and nineties.[343,344,478,479,490,494,496-504]

The concept that anaesthetists required skilled assistance at all times was gradually accepted by the Department of Health and local administrators during the eighties. There was however a reluctance to provide funds for this objective to be properly realised, especially after the 1984 reorganisation when managers were under instructions to work within budgets and to pursue a policy of reducing costs as their primary aim. Anaesthetists in many hospitals had however achieved reasonable levels of assistance by the mid eighties by insistence, which often sadly had to be confrontational, on the standards which were deemed to be essential by the Association of Anaesthetists and the Faculty of Anaesthetists. There were still however, outlying areas, particularly in obstetric units, where assistance was unsatisfactory or non-existent.[496, 497]

The personnel who provided the assistance were a mixture of Operating Department Assistants (ODA), a few (all too few) trained Anaesthetic Nurses, and State Registered nurses (SRN) and State Enrolled Nurses (SEN) trained "on the job", many of whom were part-time and/or married. There was however no properly defined structure or career ladder for a service dedicated to providing assistance for anaesthetists, and many senior nurses, surgeons, and consultants of other disciplines continued to regard such provision as an unnecessary luxury; in addition a considerable number of theatre nurses were still suspicious of, or even hostile to, attempts to improve the status and training of ODAs because they saw such activities as a possible challenge to the traditional role of the operating theatre nurse of providing direct assistance for the surgeon, as was originally envisaged in the Lewin Report (Chapter 8).

Operating Department Assistants (ODAs) were still very poorly paid during the nineteen eighties; often, even when greatly experienced. Their take home pay was below that of the lowest grade of nurse appointed alongside them to assist the anaesthetist,[498] and they had no career structure beyond the single step to Senior Operating Department Assistant (SODA), the advantage of which was minimal in terms of remuneration.

The ODAs were transferred to the "Professional and Technical B Grade" by the Department of Health in 1984. This move could theoretically have brought better terms and conditions of employment, including regulated hours, and proper overtime payment for out of hours duties, instead of trivial "stand by" payments; however the reluctance of Health Authorities to implement the transfer properly in the absence of additional funding, or to pay overtime rates, actually often resulted in a reduction of the hours of availability of ODAs and in their take home pay.[342,343] There followed a period in the late eighties when many ODAs left official employment in the NHS and joined agencies in order that they could lease their services back to the same hospitals where they were previously employed. This system brought immediately increased remuneration for the ODAs and improved assistance for anaesthetists but, of course, NHS pension rights were not accumulated. It was immediately expensive for Health Authorities, but many of the new style General Managers preferred the flexibility and lack of career responsibility for agency personnel, to being committed to established employees, and especially to paying them for overtime.[498,499] Most of the ODAs who joined agencies in order to maintain a reasonable standard of living would have much preferred to have permanent employment if they could have achieved an appropriate salary, if necessary with a certain amount of fully rewarded overtime.[498,499] A situation developed in some hospitals in which almost the entire ODA staff were agency based, though working continuously in the same location (personal recollection).

Maurice Burrows (President 1988-1990) chaired a working party which produced an excellent but pragmatic Association of Anaesthetists document on *Assistance for Anaesthetists* in 1988 at a time when there was great difficulty in recruiting ODAs due to the low remuneration.[498] The introduction to this publication summed up the situation in 1988 as follows:-

> *"After seventeen years the changes introduced to implement them, the Lewin proposals [Chapter 8] have clearly failed to achieve their objective. The concept of a pluri-potent, non-nursing staff grade has not come about: nurses are still overwhelmingly assisting surgeons while anaesthetists are being assisted by a mixture of staff, predominantly non-nursing and ill-paid. Our assistants may be better educated and trained than twenty years ago but there is little change*

in the acknowledgement of their expertise and contribution..........

It is tempting, therefore, to suggest that we scrap the current system and start again. In terms of practical politics however, this is not likely to be achievable just because one professional organisation demands it, however good the arguments it develops .... we have to work with what exists and try to mould developments to achieve the objects of the Association [of Anaesthetists]."[498]

The objective of the Association of Anaesthetists as expressed in the document was simply stated, it was:-

"to ensure that patients have a safe and efficient service and that therefore every anaesthetist has adequate assistance at all times, and that the person providing the assistance is adequately skilled and adequately rewarded." [498]

The recommendations for realising this objective were defined in detail and were practical; in broad terms they were that a corps of ODAs and/or nurses should be created within the operating theatre organisation, dedicated to providing assistance for anaesthetists with a dedicated manager of either discipline as appropriate, and that "Anaesthetic Department Assistants" and "Anaesthetic Department Nurses" should have comparable remuneration according to experience.[498]

The document on "Assistance for Anaesthetists" was followed by, and complimentary to, an Association publication on the "Efficiency of Theatre Services" produced by a working party chaired by Michael Rosen (President 1986-1988) in 1989.[499] Both documents clearly had an influence on the report of a Department of Health Steering Group chaired by Professor Peter G Bevan (former Vice President of the Royal College of Surgeons of England) on a "Study of the management and utilisation of operating theatres" which was published in 1990.[505]

The ODAs were transferred to the new NHS grades of Medical Technical Officers (MTO) in 1989. There are five levels of MTO grades ranging from MTO 1 (£6,751 rising to £7,897 in five increments) to MTO 5 (rising to £21,895 after 8 years). Local individual assessments and regrading by District

Health Authorities were undertaken. This was similar to the notorious exercise instituted for nurses. Consultant Anaesthetists familiar with the system felt that the grade of MTO 3 would have been reasonable and, despite local managerial resistance and some injustices, some minimal enhancement of salaries for ODAs was achieved.[500] This regrading resulted in many ODAs leaving the agencies and returning to NHS employment; unfortunately by 1996 there was evidence that, due to the erosion of relative NHS pay levels for ODAs, many of them are beginning to feel the need to return to the agencies (personal communication John Ballance, Consultant Anaesthetist at Hereford and President of the British Association of Operating Department Assistants - BAODA).

The training of ODAs. The National Council for Vocational Qualifications (NCVQ) was set up by the Government in 1986 to develop a national framework of qualifications in a wide range of occupations based on in-house competence and assessment in the workplace.[506] This system has been accepted by the NHS Training Authority (NHSTA) as a replacement for the City and Guilds Examination so far as the training and assessment of ODAs is concerned.[478,479,494,498,502-504,506,507] The scheme offers a means of providing a qualification for the advancement of ODAs to the new grade of Operating Department Practitioner (ODP), in parallel with the Nurse Practitioner status which the nursing profession is seeking to promote in accordance with the aims of the Project 2000. Margaret Heath (Vice President 1991-1993), a member of the NHSTA working group on ODA training, was very active in coordinating the introduction of the NCVQ training scheme for ODAs and formed a "Communication Circle" of interested parties with the objective of keeping all concerned informed of the changes; since 1993 the Circle has been coordinated by Ann Naylor (Basildon, Essex).[478, 479,504,507]

Registration of ODAs. The objective of achieving registration for trained ODAs and ODPs, so that they may be regulated under an appropriate professional disciplinary code by an approved organisation, has been a long term objective of the British Association of Operating Department Assistants (BAODA) and the smaller organisation (the National Association of Professional and Technical Theatre Personnel) which has been renamed Theatre Personnel Nationwide (TPN). The proposed registration of ODAs and ODPs is supported by the Association of Anaesthetists. Registration would improve the professional status of these valuable members of the theatre operating team and enable their role to be extended (perhaps, for example in the matter for responsibility for controlled drugs which are required by the anaesthetists during an operating list; the 1995 document on controlled drugs published by the Association of Anaesthetists suggests how this might be achieved by amendments to the Misuse of Drugs Regulations published in 1985). It would incidentally, enhance their bargaining power so far as remuneration is concerned. It would also enable misconduct to be dealt with adequately; for example it would prevent an ODA or ODP "dismissed from a post for gross moral turpitude one day [being] re-employed in another Health Authority the next" as is at present possible.[507]

A high level meeting between the then President (W R MacRae) and Officers of the Association of Anaesthetists and representatives of BAODA and the Royal College of Nursing was held at 9 Bedford Square in 1993 with the objective of exploring the way forward with regard to registration.[507] Professor P G Bevan (the former Vice President of the Royal College of Surgeons of England) was also present; he had chaired the Department of Health Steering Group which had prepared the Authoritative report of the 1990 "Study of the Management of Operating Departments"[505] and was President of the National Association of Theatre Nurses (NATN). Several important facts emerged. The NATN were no longer opposed to the registration of ODPs, especially if their duties were to be concentrated on providing assistance for anaesthetists.[508] The United Kingdom Central Council for Nurses, Midwives and Health Visitors (UKCC) had been approached as a possible registering authority for ODAs, but it was considered that this would not be appropriate. The most likely registering body might be the Council for Professions Supplementary to Medicine (CPSM) under the Privy Council; this already included organisations representing such professionals as physiotherapists and chiropodists. BAODA met many of the qualifications of the CPSM guidelines for registration, but the absence of an educational qualification for entry to training as an ODA, and of an exit exam for the NCVQ Qualification, might present difficulties. It was decided to press for action through the various channels open to the individuals who attended the meeting.[507] Progress has been slow however. The Government is believed to be reconsidering the overall position of registration of professions supplementary to medicine, but so far little advance seems to have been accomplished in the matter of registration of ODAs and ODPs.

Anaesthetic Nurses. Those (unfortunately relatively few) anaesthetists who have worked with a properly organised service of anaesthetic nurses who have completed the six month ENB (English Nursing Board) 182 course have greatly appreciated their expert services.[509] They are registered professionals and as such can undertake responsibilities not usually undertaken by ODAs in relation to the custody and administration of drugs, as well as preparing the patient by, for example, setting up intravenous infusions. How far assistance to the anaesthetist could be extended, for instance to monitoring the anaesthetised patient during short absences of the medical anaesthetist from individual operating theatres but within the operating theatre suite, is a matter for debate, and certainly any thought of anything other than the one to one medical supervision of a patient under anaesthesia, or the independent administration by nurses in the operating theatre of drugs not directly and individually prescribed by the physician anaesthetist, is contrary to British practice. The development of anaesthetic nursing services during the eighties based on the ENB 182 course was however very limited. The 1988 Association report could only identify three ENB courses in the whole of the United Kingdom. The report also pointed out the managerial difficulties of organising mixed anaesthetic assistant services composed of nurses and ODAs.[498] Those nurses who completed the ENB 182 courses were also often disappointed to find that there were few career opportunities open to them other than in those few hospitals which themselves ran training courses. Theatre nursing superintendents also sometimes overtly made it very plain that they considered that an "anaesthetic sister" was an unnecessary luxury at a time when they were short of staff to assist the surgeons (personal experience)!

The concept of the nurse assisting the doctor rather than being an independent practitioner is also contrary to the philosophy of the nursing hierarchy in the nineteen nineties, but the idea of an extended role for the nurses as Nurse Practitioners in Anaesthetics, with wide responsibilities in the perioperative period including preoperative preparation as well as in the recovery period, is being actively canvassed.[510] Anaesthetists would welcome a skilled, well trained and cooperative nursing colleague in the operating suite.[511,512] Preoperative visiting by nurses has its dangers however; unless there is very close relationship with the anaesthetist the practice has led to real difficulties when the advice given is contrary to the views of the anaesthetist.

Some nurses in the nineties contemplate the possible further step to nurse anaesthesia in the United Kingdom, but it is doubtful whether the implications of this are fully understood.[510,511] Alex Crampton Smith (Emeritus Professor, Oxford), who has wide experience of working with nurse anaesthetists in Scandinavia and the USA, cautions against exporting systems for the delivery of anaesthetic care from one country to another, although he would welcome an enhanced status for the anaesthetic nurse in the United Kingdom.[512] It is doubtful, however, if the wider use of the trained anaesthetic nurses will be a practical proposition in the United Kingdom in the future. The new style Project 2000 student nurses are given little opportunity to undertake work experience in operating theatres, and it is likely that the absence of exposure during training will result in the diminution in the recruitment of personnel who have not had the opportunity to be attracted to work in this field. The future, so far as assistance for the anaesthetist is concerned would seem, in general, to lie in the hands of the ODP, properly trained, registered and organised, and adequately financed, so that he or she has attractive career prospects; only in this way will be most suitable candidates be recruited. The Association of Anaesthetists must try to ensure that progress towards these objectives is maintained.

The Educational Programme of the Association 1983-1995

It has already been noted that the move to 9 Bedford Square in 1985 was followed by a very considerable expansion in the educational programme of the Association. Development was further facilitated by the appointment of an Educational Coordinator in 1986. This post was generously funded by the Medical Division of the British Oxygen Company (later renamed Ohmeda Healthcare). The post was held by Mrs Catherine Goff from 1986 to 1988, when she was succeeded by Mrs Lesley Ogg, who became Administrative Manager in 1996, and was in turn succeeded by Mrs Louise Watts. This appointment, together with modest increases in the secretariat at 9 Bedford Square, computerisation, and the advent of desk-top publishing, has enabled the educational programme to be extended and conducted with increasing professionalism, but the continued inclusion of the wives of some of the executive officers in the registration teams at larger meetings still maintains a greatly appreciated link with the Association "family" atmosphere of the past.

The two original major meetings of the year (the Annual General, Scientific and Linkman meeting each September, and the Annual Meeting of the Group of Anaesthetists in Training in late March) continue to be increasingly well attended, but have been challenged in popularity by the Winter Scientific Meeting and Dinner held each January in London since the event was inaugurated in 1988. There is, in addition, the very successful seminar programme, and the Annual Continuing Medical Education Day (formerly Postgraduate Study Day) which has been run in conjunction with the Royal College (formerly Faculty) of Anaesthetists in October since 1982. The Association of Anaesthetists of Great Britain and Ireland also sponsored several other meetings during this period either on its own or jointly with other bodies.

Annual Scientific and General Meetings and Linkman Conferences 1983-1992 and the Annual Winter Meetings 1988-1992.

Year	Meeting	Location	Attendance
1983	Annual	Gosforth Park Hotel, Newcastle upon Tyne[331]	270
1984	Annual	University of Exeter[341]	c500
1985	Annual	Leicester Polytechnic[369]	450
1986	Annual	City University, London[356]	520
1987	Annual	University of Sheffield[362]	380
1988	Winter	Royal College of Surgeons of England, London[362,371]	400
	Annual	University of Southampton[363,513]	524
1989	Winter	Royal College of Surgeons of England, London[363,372]	379
	Annual	University College, Swansea[364,514]	521
1990	Winter	Royal College of Surgeons of England, London[364,373]	282
	Annual	Manchester Institute of Science and Technology[365,515]	481

1991	Winter	Queen Elizabeth II Conference, Centre, London[365,374]	218
	Annual	Harrogate International Congress Centre[325,516]	450
1992	Winter	Queen Elizabeth II Conference Centre, London. Diamond Jubilee Meeting [325,375]	300
	Annual	Bournemouth International Centre[391,517]	503

Meeting Venues. The very successful meetings and celebrations in Golden Jubilee year 1982, included the hosting by the Association of Anaesthetists of the 6th European Congress of Anaesthesiology (Chapter 8), were followed by the period from 1983 to 1990 when the increasingly popular Annual Scientific, General and Linkmen meetings continued to be held in University Centres outside London each September, with the local Departments of Anaesthesia responsible for the organisation for the scientific programme in concert with the Education and Research Committee. The only exception was in 1986 when the academic buildings of the City of London University were utilised[356] because it was felt that, after several years of holding Annual Meetings outside London, it was time that a meeting was held in the capital city. The increase in the number of registrants year by year began to strain the capacity of various University buildings, particularly in respect of the lecture theatres for plenary sessions and the space required for the number of exhibitors who wished to book in for the Trade Exhibition (personal recollection). The accommodation at the City of London University in 1986 was particularly cramped (the seating capacity of the auditorium was only 450 and there were over 500 registrants),[356] but fortunately the facilities at Sheffield 1987,[362] Southampton 1988[363,513] Swansea 1989[364,514] and Manchester 1990[365,515] proved to be adequate if rather crowded. The Officers and Council, prompted by the Education and Research Committee, therefore decided that the time had come to make use of the excellent Congress Centres which were opening up throughout the United Kingdom at that time; this despite the inevitable considerable increase in the cost of running the meetings. The Scientific Programme would be organised by one or other of the University Departments of Anaesthesia (not necessarily from the particular area) in collaboration with the Education and Research Committee and the social programme would be the responsibility of local anaesthetists.[502]

This arrangement has proved to be very satisfactory, and those concerned are to be congratulated on the very high standard achieved. Professor Alan Aitkenhead (Nottingham) was chairman of the Education and Research Committee from 1991 to 1995 and contributed a great deal to the development of the new arrangements for the Annual Meetings.

The first of the series was at the Harrogate International Congress Centre in September 1991 and effectively demonstrated the advantages of the new departure. The Leeds University Department (Professor J Gareth Jones) in conjunction with the Education and Research Committee originated the Scientific Programme and the stimulating social programme was organised by a team of Yorkshire anaesthetists.[325,516] Professor John Utting and his colleagues from Liverpool organised the scientific programme of the 1992 Annual Meeting in Bournemouth[392,517]

The policy of using the Congress Centres has been more than justified. The large number of registrants at the superb Birmingham International Centre in 1995 foreshadowed the future, now that the compulsory Royal College of Anaesthetists Postgraduate Medical Education programme which puts a premium on the attendance at scientific meetings has been initiated.

The Winter Scientific meetings each January, which were introduced in 1988 also continue to be popular. It was decided that the venue for the Diamond Jubilee celebrations of the Association of Anaesthetists in 1992 should rightly be in London where the organisation was founded, and the new Queen Elizabeth II Conference Centre in Westminster was therefore booked for a trial run in January 1991 as well as for the Jubilee meeting itself in January 1992. The pattern of holding the Winter Meeting at the Queen Elizabeth II Conference Centre in January each year, and the Annual Scientific, General and Linkman meeting in September at a major Congress Centre outside London subsequently became well established.

Joint meetings at home and abroad. The practice of inviting the national societies of other nations to participate jointly in the Scientific and Social programme of some of the Annual Scientific Meetings, which was begun in the seventies, and Members of the Association being invited to attend reciprocal meetings abroad, has continued in the eighties and nineties. A successful joint meeting held in Bonn in 1985 attracted some 300 Germans and over 100 British anaesthetists and was in return for the German visit to the Annual Scientific Meeting at Wembley Conference Centre in 1978. Seventy five British and Irish anaesthetists and "accompanying persons" were royally entertained at a 700 strong meeting of the Canadian Society in Ottawa in June 1989 during which a magnificent carving of a loon was presented to the Association of Anaesthetists of Great Britain and Ireland. This bird reappeared on the platform at the return meeting at the Scottish Exhibition Centre in Glasgow in 1993, somewhat to the astonishment of those British anaesthetists who had not attended the Ottawa meeting when they caught sight of it through a haze of whisky fumes.[366,518,524]

Association of Anaesthetists meetings and seminars on NHS management. The Officers and Council of the Association of Anaesthetists, from the start of the various reorganisations of the NHS in the eighties were concerned that, in their patients and their own interests, anaesthetists should play their full part in NHS management. Margaret Heath (Lewisham) suggested at the Linkman Conference in 1983 that the Association should follow the Regional lead given by Departments of Anaesthesia in Cardiff and the Trent Region, and hold a national meeting or course on management.[496] Meetings on management, which were well attended, were subsequently held in January 1985 and January 1987 at the Royal College of Surgeons in Lincoln's Inn Fields.[341,362] A considerable number of seminars at 9 Bedford Square have been subsequently devoted to management, and some have been provided for NHS managers. Working parties of the Association of Anaesthetists have also produced many informative pamphlets for the guidance of members and NHS managers over the years.

Sponsored meetings

The Association of Anaesthetists has often joined with other interested bodies in organising occasional meetings to mark important events and to underwrite special meetings.

The Second International Symposium on the History of Anaesthesia took place between 20 and 23 July 1984 at the Royal College of Surgeons of England.[525,526] The Symposium was under the patronage of Her Royal Highness Princess Alexandra who graced, with her charming presence, the Opening Ceremony presided over by Aileen Adams (Dean of the Faculty of

Anaesthetists 1985-1988), and the Reception in the Great Hall of Lincoln's Inn. The Organising Committee was chiefly composed of past and present Officers and Council Members of the Association of Anaesthetists. It was chaired by Tom Boulton (President 1984-1986) with Peter Baskett (later President 1990-1992) as Secretary General. The event attracted over 300 delegates from 25 countries who contributed many erudite papers which were later published as a Proceedings volume.[525] Full use was also made of the historic buildings in London for the social programme including the Banqueting House in Whitehall for the ceremonial banquet.[525,526]

A Tribute to Professor Sir Robert Macintosh on his 90th Birthday. A meeting was arranged to honour this occasion. It was organised jointly by the Section of Anaesthetics of the Royal Society of Medicine, the Association of Anaesthetists, and the Faculty (now Royal College) of Anaesthetists. The meeting was held at the RSM on 2 October 1987 and took the form of a symposium detailing aspects of Sir Robert's eventful life followed by a reception.[362] A souvenir volume was edited by W Dennis Smith (Leeds, President of the Anaesthetic Section of the RSM 1987-1988) and Gordon Paterson (Oxford).[527]

The Sir Ivan Magill Centenary Meeting was also organised jointly by the Section of Anaesthetics of the RSM, the Association of Anaesthetists and the Faculty (now Royal College) of Anaesthetists to celebrate the hundredth anniversary of the birth of the great pioneer, on 23 July 1888. Over 200 registrants attended a symposium based on the special interests of Sir Ivan. A Commemorative Dinner was held at which the first Sir Ivan Magill Gold Medal for Innovation in Anaesthesia was presented to John Nunn by the President Michael Rosen (1986-1988).[362]

The First Open Meeting of the European Academy of Anaesthesiology (Chapter 6) took place in London at the Royal College of Surgeons of England from 13-15 July 1989. It was organised by the Association of Anaesthetists and included a Refresher Course of 14 lectures. A prize of £1,000 (1996: £1,300), which had been presented by the European Section of the World Federation of Societies of Anaesthesiologists, was awarded to Colin S Goodchild (then of Leeds and now in Australia) for his paper on "The mechanism by which benzodiazepines spinally mediate analgesia".[363]

The First International Conference on Anaesthesia and Critical care in Disasters and War 18-21 July 1990. This very high level meeting at the Royal College of Surgeons of England in which many civil and military physicians from North America and a number of European Countries participated, was organised by Air Commodore Colin McLaren. It was under the patronage of the Surgeon General of the Armed Forces, the President of the Association of Anaesthetists (Maurice Burrows), and the President of the College of Anaesthetists (Michael Rosen).[364]

Technical Exhibitions and the Association Stand and Shop

The Technical Exhibitions are important features of all scientific meetings of the Association of Anaesthetists; year by year the equipment manufacturers and pharmaceutical firms show their support for the specialty of anaesthesia by their considerable financial contribution, and by exhibiting and demonstrating their products and answering the questions of the delegates. The Members of the Association are grateful to them for their interest and unfailing courtesy. Council endeavours to make their attendance at the Association meetings as congenial as possible. Ralph Vaughan from Cardiff was appointed by Council as Technical Exhibition Coordinator in 1985 (Council Minutes 1.2.1985).[27] His unfailing cheerfulness, personal knowledge and happy relationship with the exhibitors did much to promote mutual cooperation. He was awarded a Pask Certificate in 1990,[364,529] after which he shared the responsibility with Frederick Roberts (Exeter)[365] who took over sole charge in 1994.[366] The scope and standard of the Technical Exhibition facilities were greatly improved and expanded after the Association of Anaesthetists began to hold its Annual and Winter meetings in purpose built congress centres.

The Association of Anaesthetists demonstration stand and shop was formalised during 1986 when Wendy Scott (Milton Keynes) was invited to undertake the responsibility. A year or two previously a portable stand illustrating the activities of the Association and the Junior Anaesthetists' Group had been prepared for display at scientific meetings to demonstrate the varied activities of the Association to registrants. The only items identifiable as being connected with the Association, which were available for sale at the Association meetings up to the early eighties, were neck ties and wall shields bearing the coat of arms of the Association. These could be easily handled by the registration desk. A number of souvenir items were produced for the souvenir shop for the 1982 European Congress and some surplus stock remained;[324] by 1986 the "shopping list" of marketable goods had expanded considerably to include, besides a variety of ties, the increasing number of "glossy" information booklets, the reprinted Bryn Thomas historical apparatus book, and several slide sets, cuff-links, tie pins, golf umbrellas, and other presentation items bearing the coat of arms of the Association of Anaesthetists. Wendy Scott was awarded a Pask Certificate of Honour in 1990.[364,529] She was succeeded by Rachel Jane Chestnut (Kilmarnock),[365] and she in turn handed over this important responsibility to Hilary Aitken (Redditch) in 1994.[366]

An additional popular feature of the Association stand at meetings has been the display of selected items from the unique collection of historic audio video tapes built up by Ian McLellan (Leicester).

The Diamond Jubilee celebrations of the Association of Anaesthetists of Great Britain and Ireland, 9-11 January 1992

The decision to celebrate the 60th Anniversary of the foundation of the Association of Anaesthetists at the time of the Winter Scientific Meeting in London in January 1992 was wise.[365,530-533] It enabled the reigning President (Peter Baskett) to mastermind the entire proceedings as a unity, rather than having a change of President half way through the celebratory meeting, as would have been the case if the Annual General and Scientific meeting in September 1992 had been selected. A Working Party charged with planning the Diamond Jubilee celebrations was set up in 1990 under the Chairmanship of Peter Baskett as President Elect.[364,365] The Diamond Jubilee meeting was held at the Queen Elizabeth Conference Centre close to Westminster Abbey and the Houses of Parliament. This had already been used as a "trial run" for the Winter meeting the year before in 1991.[365]

The Opening Ceremony of the Diamond Jubilee Winter Scientific Meeting took place on Thursday 10 January 1992 in the Benjamin Britten Hall of the Queen Elizabeth Centre on the evening before the start of the scientific programme. It was a splendid occasion graced by the presence of the Patron of the Association of Anaesthetists, Her Royal Highness, The Princess Margaret, Countess of Snowdon.[325,531,532] The President, Peter Baskett, first invited the Princess to open the meeting in an erudite and witty speech. He recalled with pleasure his first "meeting" with the Princess as a Cadet No 516766 when she inspected his School Officers Training Corps in 1950 in the company of Queen Elizabeth the Queen Mother. He also thanked her for her patronage and interest in the Association of Anaesthetists and for her work for many charities.[533] Peter Baskett's speech also served as a citation for the election and admission of Princess Margaret as an Honorary Member of the Association of Anaesthetists, after which she was presented with her Certificate of Honorary Membership and a fine pair of sharp scissors for which she had asked. The Princess then opened the meeting and made a delightfully amusing, but nonetheless well informed, reply to Peter Baskett, and in doing so paid tribute to the achievements of the Association over the sixty years of its existence.[325,532] Next came a pause for a formal reception in the Rutherford Room where the Princess was introduced to Officers and elected and coopted Council Members and their wives and husbands.[325,531]

A visit to the extensive Trade Exhibition organised by Fred Roberts (Exeter) followed. Princess Margaret showed great interest in the items on display and talked vivaciously to the exhibitors.[325,531]

The Scientific Programme which was held on Friday and Saturday 11 and 12 January 1992, was organised by Tony Wildsmith of Edinburgh (later Professor of Anaesthesia, University of Dundee). There were six sessions. The first session was chaired by the reigning President and each of the others by a former President. Each session represented a chronological decade and each began with an historical overview of the decade or a relevant event within it. E T (Eddie) Mathews of Birmingham presented a particularly lively account and personal reminiscence of the colourful life of Henry Featherstone, the Founder President of the Association of Anaesthetists (Appendix A). Other papers included accounts of the introduction of revolutionary agents and techniques. The last session (1982-1992) brought the audience right up to date.[531,532]

The British Oxygen Company Health Care Lecture on "Clinical measurement and clinical care" was delivered by Professor Sir Keith Sykes (Oxford) in his usual stimulating and thought-provoking style.[325,531,532]

Honorary Membership was conferred on the President of the British Cardiac Society Douglas Chamberlain, CBE, MD, FRCP (Brighton) during the course of the scientific programme. He has had much to do with anaesthesia during his career, both in relation to the preoperative care of patients with heart disease, and particularly with the promotion of schemes of emergency management of circulatory arrest outside the hospital.

The Diamond Jubilee Dinner was held in the Banqueting Hall of the New Connaught Rooms in Covent Garden. Over three hundred diners enjoyed an excellent meal. There was a prestigious guest list including presidents and representatives of the Royal Medical Colleges and Specialist Associations, the British Medical Association, the Department of Health and the Armed Forces. The toast of "the guests" was proposed by the President and Professor Alastair Spence, CBE, President of the College of Anaesthetists responded.[325,531,533]

The Diamond Jubilee celebrations were superlatively successful and demonstrated the strength of the achievements of the Association over its sixty years of existence as a medicopolitical academic and social organisation.[325,531]

The Association and the World Federation of Societies of Anaesthesiologists (WFSA)

World Congresses of Anaesthesiologists and European Congresses of Anaesthesiology 1983-1992

8th World	1984	Manila, Philippines
7th European	1986	Vienna, Austria
9th World	1988	Washington DC, USA
8th European	1990	Warsaw, Poland
10th World	1992	The Hague, Netherlands

British anaesthetists continued to be prominent in the affairs of the WFSA. John Zorab (Bristol) was elected for a second term as Secretary General of the WFSA at the World Congress of Anaesthesiologists in 1984 and became its President (for 1988-1992) in 1988 at the World Congress in Washington DC.[325,363] Peter Baskett was Chairman of the European Section of the WFSA and of the European Resuscitation Council, and W Leslie Baird (Honorary Treasurer of the Association 1992 et seq) was elected Honorary Secretary of the European Section in 1991.[365] The elections at the 10th World Congress in the Hague, Netherlands in 1992 resulted in Michael Vickers (President of the Association 1982-1984) becoming Secretary General of the WFSA (and he was subsequently elected President 1996), Michael Rosen (President of the Association 1996-1998) being elected Treasurer, W R (Bill) MacRae (President of the Association 1992-1994) being elected to the Finance Committee, and Trevor Thomas (Bristol) appointed to chair the Obstetric Committee, while Roger Eltringham (Cheltenham) continued as a member of the Education Committee.[325]

A presentation of a Badge of Office for the President of the Polish Society of Anaesthetists was made on behalf of the Association of Anaesthetists of Great Britain and Ireland during the 8th European Congress in Warsaw in 1990 (Council Minutes 19.10.1990).[441]

The Creation of the College of Anaesthetists at the Royal College of Surgeons of England in 1988

The granting of a Supplementary Charter to the Charter of the Royal College of Surgeons of England. Michael Vickers was elected President of the Association of Anaesthetists in September 1982. He was the first President for over a decade to sit concurrently as an elected Member of the Board of Faculty of Anaesthetists of the Royal College of Surgeons of England, except for a few months at the start of Cyril Scurr's Presidency. The next two Presidents were also elected Members of the Board of Faculty; thus the Association view in favour of an independent College of Anaesthetists was strongly represented on the Board of Faculty in the years which led up to the establishment first of a College of Anaesthetists within the Royal College of Surgeons of England (RCS England) in 1988, and, ultimately, to the foundation by Royal Charter of an independent Royal College of Anaesthetists on 16 March 1992. Other elections to the Board of Faculty also represented a shift of opinion within the Board in favour of collegiate status for anaesthetists, and this reflected in turn a growing body of opinion within the electorate of the Faculty in favour of an independent College.

The desire for change in the constitution of the Faculty had of course already been expressed in the historic resolutions of the Board passed during John Nunn's Presidency in 1980 (Chapter 8), following which a new working party was set up to discuss matters with the Council of the RCS England. Sir Alan Parks, who was President of the RCS England from the middle of 1980 until his untimely death in November 1982, had showed considerable sympathy for constitutional reforms in favour of anaesthetists.

The next six years were a period of particularly felicitous relationships between the Presidents of the RCS England (Sir Geoffrey Slaney, 1982-1986 and Sir Ian Todd, 1986-1989) and the Deans of the Faculty of Anaesthetists (Professor (Sir) Donald Campbell, CBE, 1982-1985 and Aileen Adams, CBE, 1985-1988), but progress towards constitutional reform may be perceived as having been very slow. The records show that the joint Working Party charged with constitutional review met formally on average once each year, but much informal discussion between the Officers of the surgeons' College and the Officers of the Faculty took place and, in fact, real progress was made. It must also be remembered that the solution which emerged involved lengthy deliberation by the Privy Council.[535,541]

The Faculty held its first independent Diploma Ceremony in 1983[534,535] and the process of severance of its financial affairs from those of the surgeons' College as a whole, which had begun under the Presidency of Sir Alan Parks was completed:[535,537] these changes, together with the delegation of the control of the examinations and the award of diplomas, and other measures previously instituted (Chapter 8),[542-543] meant that for practical purposes the Faculty of anaesthetists was independent, except in name[541-543] and because, by statute, the Faculty of Anaesthetists was still subject to the Council of the Royal College of Surgeons of England.

The solution recommended by the Constitutional Working Party was one which had been dismissed *ex cathedra* as not being acceptable to the Privy Council by a former President of the RCS England in 1976 (Chapter 8)! It was simply to seek a Supplemental Charter to that of the RCS England giving it power to substitute the designation "College" for "Faculty" under separate Presidents.[536,537,541] This concept was fully supported by the Council of the Association of Anaesthetists which passed a resolution in 1983 "congratulating the Faculty and College (RCS England) on their achievements and pressed them to move forward to the formation of a College of Anaesthetists".[424]

The "College within a College" solution was viewed pragmatically by those who looked upon it as a generally acceptable step towards "the most stable end-point.... a College of Anaesthetists quite separate from the College of Surgeons".[542,543] It was also acceptable to those who were dedicated to maintaining the unity of the RCS England and its two Faculties (this included the senior officer of the RCS England Secretariat).[544] It also met the need of others who greatly valued the link of remaining joined to the prestigious RCS England, and satisfied those who enjoyed the ambience of the fine buildings in Lincoln's Inn Fields and those who viewed the difficulties and expense of equipping and administering a separate building with alarm; as Aileen Adams (Dean of the Faculty 1985-1988), who had been closely concerned with the negotiations, wrote in 1989:-

"The advantages of remaining physically within the Royal College of Surgeons are obvious, though if necessary they could have been dispensed with. More autonomy was not needed, because the Faculty had total control of its own affairs in a not inconsiderable way as well as contributing to the Affairs of the College [RCS England] as a whole, and to those of the profession through the Conference [of the Royal Medical Colleges and their Faculties]. What was needed was solely the status and prestige of the title of College and President."[541]

An attempt was made by the Secretariat of the RCS England to substitute the title "Master" for "President" for the senior professional officer of the proposed subsidiary college. This was on the grounds that there could not be two Presidents within the same organisation. This view was untenable however; it was pointed out that the Royal Society of Medicine as a whole has a President as also does each of its Sections (personal recollection).

The legal process of implementing the somewhat novel change to a "College within a College" was lengthy. It involved petitioning the Privy Council to advise Her Majesty the Queen to grant the Supplementary Charter to the Charter of the RCS England, and revision of the Ordinances of the surgeons' College.

The Creation of the College of Anaesthetists at the Royal College of Surgeons of England in 1988

The Supplemental Charter and revised Ordinances were signed by the Queen in July 1988 and the Great Seal was affixed on 14 October 1988.[538,539] The Council of the RCS England and the Faculty of Anaesthetists then passed the necessary orders and the "College of Anaesthetists at the Royal College of Surgeons of England" came into being by resolution on 19 October 1988 in the presence of a phalanx of former Deans of the Faculty[539,541] Professor Michael Rosen, who had succeeded Aileen Adams as Dean in June 1988 became the first President of the College of Anaesthetists. The President of the RCS England, (Sir) Ian Todd struck the College gong to usher in the new College; he then welcomed the partnership between the two Colleges and wished the College of Anaesthetists every success in the future.[539,540]

The Council of the Association noted the founding of the College of Anaesthetists "with great satisfaction" and congratulated its Immediate Past President, Michael Rosen on becoming the first President of the new College.[363] This circumstance echoed the precedent set in 1948 when Archibald Marsden the Immediate Past President of the Association of Anaesthetists became the first Dean of the Faculty of Anaesthetists, and earlier in 1932 when Featherstone, the Immediate Past President of the Section of Anaesthetics of the Royal Society of Medicine became the first President of the Association of Anaesthetists.

The College of Anaesthetists at the Royal College of Surgeons of England under its energetic President Michael Rosen lost no time in expanding its activities and influence in the dedicated pursuit of excellence in the practice of the specialty. The Standing Committees of the Faculty concerned with the education, examinations, hospital recognition for training, supervision of individual programmes leading to specialist accreditation, and Scottish affairs were taken over and revitalised; in addition new principal committees concerned with quality of practice (audit) and competence to practice, manpower, and the training of overseas doctors and fund raising were inaugurated and, by 1992 there were at least nine other internal committees and working parties concerned with the particular problems of the day.[545,546]

It was estimated in October 1989 (College of Anaesthetists Newsletter No 2) that it was represented on some 63 intercollegiate, governmental and other joint bodies.[545] These included the Department of Health Joint Consultants' Committee (JCC), and the Councils of the General Medical Council (GMC) and the RCS England, as well as the Association of Anaesthetists. An important and pleasing development was the cooption of the new President of the Association of Anaesthetists, Maurice Burrows, who was not an elected member of the College Council, to the important Council-in-Committee.[542,545]

The College of Anaesthetists collaborated with the RCS England in the production in 1990 of an important report on pain after surgery by a Working Party of the Commission on Surgical Services chaired by Alastair Spence[547] and in 1991 in the production of a revised document on the Workload of Consultant Anaesthetists in conjunction with the Association of Anaesthetists. It also produced its own document on the role and purpose of undergraduate education in anaesthesia.[548]

The College had to ensure that its views were heard in regard to the effects on training and standards of major Government initiatives in its early years under its first President Michael Rosen and his successor Alastair Spence (1991-1994), who was destined to preside over its transformation into the independent Royal College of Anaesthetists in 1992. These schemes included "Achieving a balance", which unfortunately concerned itself with reducing the number of Registrars rather than expanding the number of Senior Registrars and Consultants to absorb the excess, and despite the agreement to reduce the hours of junior doctors, the new regulation relating to the training of foreign postgraduates, and the controversial White Paper "Working for Patients" presaging the draconian reorganisation of the NHS which was to follow in 1992.

The Joint College and Association of Anaesthetists Senior Lectureship in intensive care. This was an imaginative and innovative collaboration in 1989 between the College and the Association. The annual cost, shared equally between the Association and the College, was £60,000 (1996: £80,000) per year for five years. The award was to a Department of Anaesthesia rather than an individual appointed solely jointly by the College and the Association; from a short list of three Departments, that of the University of Birmingham (Professor Peter Hutton) was selected.[363]

The Princess Royal, Princess Anne was admitted to Honorary Fellowship of the College at a ceremonial Extraordinary Meeting of the College Council on 21 November 1990 in the presence of 130 Fellows and guests.[545]

Staff and premises. All these activities necessitated a considerable increase in the Secretariat of the College (by February 1991 the number of staff had risen from 5 in 1988 to 12). One important development was the establishment in 1991 of an Examinations Department independent of the Department of the RCS England. The accommodation allocated to the Faculty on the ground floor of the surgeons' College had been extended during the nineteen eighties but it soon became apparent that more space was necessary. Additional accommodation was generously provided on the 6th floor of the Nuffield College building adjacent to the surgeons' College.[545]

The British Journal of Anaesthesia **(BJA)** became the "Official Journal of the College of Anaesthetists" from the January 1990 number onwards, but retained a great deal of its independence.[549,550] The President and one of the two Vice Presidents of the College of Anaesthetists sit *ex officio* on the Board of the BJA. The College is responsible for "ratifying" the appointment of Members of the Board but the Board acts independently to elect its Editor and Assistant Editors, and "the editorial independence of the Board is totally preserved in the new arrangement". The *BJA* remains primarily a high quality scientific journal; College news and information for Fellows is disseminated by the entirely separate *Royal College of Anaesthetists Newsletter* first published in February 1989.[540] Fellows of the College receive the *BJA* and the *Newsletter* as a privilege of Fellowship. The circulation of the *BJA* was increased considerably by the arrangement with the College, particularly in the United Kingdom; it now enjoys "a higher circulation within the United Kingdom and Europe than any other anaesthetic journal".[549, 550]

A grant of arms for the College of Anaesthetists. Application to the Sovereign through the College of Arms for a grant of a separate coat of arms for the College of Anaesthetists was made very soon after the new College was inaugurated. The Officers of the College of Arms (the Earl Marshall and the Heralds) were at first reluctant to recommend to the Queen the granting of the right to bear arms to an organisation which was a subsidiary of another body. A pragmatic solution to the problem was found however! The Letters Patent dated 1 March 1991 make the grant to the Royal College of Surgeons of England for the use of the College of Anaesthetists, but there is provision in the Letters Patent for the right to the use of the arms to pass absolutely to the College of Anaesthetists should it become completely independent at any time, which in due course it did in 1992.[551-553]

The arms though quite distinct, follow a tradition for corporate arms by adopting a format and charges derived from the arms of the institutions from which the College was derived, that is the Royal Society of Medicine, the Association of Anaesthetists of Great Britain and Ireland, and the Royal College of Surgeons of England (the Faculty of Anaesthetists was not, of course, an armigerous body). The two golden poppy heads "in chief" on a red field from the Arms of Association (Appendix B) are included. The supporters are the British pioneer specialist anaesthetists Snow and Clover and the unique motto is "Divinum sedare dolorem" ("It is divine (or praiseworthy) to alleviate pain"). The crest on the helmet includes floral emblems for England and Wales (the Tudor rose), Scotland (the thistle), and Ireland (the shamrock) thus denoting jurisdiction over all the constituent parts of the United Kingdom (there are separate surgical Colleges for England, Scotland and Ireland).[551,552]

The question of the bestowal of the Royal accolade and the petition for an independent Royal College of Anaesthetists

It is quite probable that, had the "College of Anaesthetists within the Royal College of Surgeons of England" been granted the status conferred by the Royal prefix, and become itself the Royal College of Anaesthetists (albeit "within the Royal College of Surgeons of England"), the position conferred under the Supplementary Charter would have been considered to be acceptable by most anaesthetists. The "Royal" College of Anaesthetists would then doubtless have remained attached to the Royal College of Surgeons of England, and within its portals in accommodation generously provided by the surgeons but, which was nonetheless, structurally divided and inadequate for its expanding role. The fact that the Royal College of Anaesthetists was a subsidiary college of the Royal College of Surgeons of England would probably have been actually or conveniently forgotten, and the "Royal" College of Anaesthetists would have sat comfortably alongside other medical

Royal Colleges in such bodies as the Conference of Royal Medical Colleges and their Faculties, the GMC and the JCC, and been recognised as equal by the Government and Civil Service.[554]

It is clear also that at first the Senior Officers of both the Association of Anaesthetists and the College of Anaesthetists considered that the "College-within-a-College" solution was satisfactory, and that only a short time would elapse before the essential Royal prefix was conferred to put a seal on the arrangement.[542,556]

It was not altogether surprising with hindsight however that, when one body which advises on the exercise of the Royal prerogative (the College of Arms) was unwilling to do so wholeheartedly for a subsidiary College, that another such body (the Privy Council) would decline to recommend the granting of the Royal prefix. It became certain, however, after six months consultation by "top professionals" that this would indeed be the case; as Alastair Spence (then Vice President of the College of Anaesthetists) wrote at the time:-

> *"The formula of a "College-within-a-College" was an innovative and much admired step that many considered to mark the end of fractionation of the institutes of medicine [which] other important groups were poised to follow."*[554]

The prospect of not being able to obtain the Royal accolade altered the position of the College of Anaesthetists and the attitude of the Councils of both the College and the Association;[365,556,557] as Alastair Spence also wrote in June 1990:-

> *"A Royal College is regarded.... in Britain as on a plane higher than a "non-royal" college or faculty. This has quite fundamental implications for the ease of access to Government and the likelihood of being included in discussions on important issues in the first place. The system is essentially British and therefore not quite logical but we [the College of Anaesthetists] can only thrive by playing to the rules."*[554]

The Council of the College of Anaesthetist took the unanimous decision to become an entirely independent College in June 1989 and informed the

The question of the bestowal of the Royal accolade and the petition for an independent Royal College of Anaesthetists

President and Council of the RCS England of its intention to do so.[556,557] The surgeons' College under its new President (Sir) Terence English accepted the decision with sadness but as an inevitable development and with kindly consideration.[556,557] The necessary mechanism for obtaining a new and independent Charter was the preparation of a petition from the President and Council of the Royal College of Surgeons of England, as the parent body, for separation of its subsidiary College of Anaesthetists.[558] The Council of the surgeons' College generously allowed the College of Anaesthetists three years to find separate premises from the prospective granting of its Royal Charter.[558]

The President of the College of Anaesthetists and members of the College Council toured the country during the second half of 1989 and the early months of 1990 to promote the concept of an independent College. They also emphasised that it would be necessary to acquire property to house the institution, and that there was consequently a need to raise funds.[556,557]

The Council of the Association of Anaesthetists of Great Britain and Ireland were supportive and passed the following resolution on 8 December 1989:-[364,441,559]

> *"Council of the Association of Anaesthetists recognises the need for the College of Anaesthetists to extend its development by seeking legal identity through a separate Charter, by seeking Royal Status and the acquisition of independent premises. Council of the Association is unanimous in expressing its strong support to the College of Anaesthetists in pursuing these aims."*[441,559]

Michael Rosen as President of the College of Anaesthetists, addressed the registrants at the 1990 Winter Scientific Meeting of the Association of Anaesthetists at the house of the Royal College of Surgeons of England in Lincoln's Inn Fields. He had recently been appointed Commander of the Order of the British Empire (CBE) and elected to the appointment of Honorary Professor in the University of Wales, and he received the acclamation of the audience for these honours. He then gave an account of the aspirations of the College and invited support for the College appeal for funds. The above Resolution of the Council of the Association of Anaesthetists was unanimously endorsed with acclamation.[364,559]

The Council of the College of Anaesthetists felt that the degree of support they were receiving made the need to hold a referendum amongst its Fellows unnecessary and this conclusion was accepted by the Privy Council; even so, at one time, the question of a possible need for a referendum to all Fellows of the Royal College (including surgical Fellows and those of the Faculty of Dental Surgery) was seriously considered (personal recollection).

Fund raising for the College of Anaesthetists began in earnest in June 1990, after the decision to seek the status of an independent College had been made and the requirement for separate premises became a necessity; however a personal appeal from the President to Council Members and Senior Fellows had already resulted in some £0.5 million being covenanted.[556]

The College Council Members responsible for fund raising were W R MacRae and Peter Morris. The Appeal was based on the Anaesthetists Academic Foundation which the Association of Anaesthetists had carefully husbanded and £172,287 was handed over to the College at the time of its foundation.[554,560,561] This sum consisted of the aggregate of all the donations made to the Academic Foundation with interest less the grant of £15,000 made when the Seminar Programme at 9 Bedford Square was inaugurated in 1986.

It would be neither pertinent nor appropriate to describe in detail the progress and development of the "Foundation Appeal" of the College of Anaesthetists in this history of the Association of Anaesthetists. It will suffice to record that several leading industrialists and other eminent people joined the Appeals Committee, under the Chairmanship of Sir Peter Gadsden (a former Lord Mayor of London, a distinguished professional engineer and a prominent businessman with a multitude of charitable, public, and professional interests and appointments).[562] The Appeal was pursued with great vigour by the Committee and the Officers and Members of Council of the College of Anaesthetists as is recorded in successive (Royal) College of Anaesthetists Newsletters.[545] The Association began by covenanting £10,000 each year over a five year period (Accounts of the Association of Anaesthetists Education and Research Trust 1989-1993) and later provided an unsecured loan and donation for the purchase of the College building. Industry responded magnificently. Contributions from individual Fellows of the College at first came somewhat slowly but later quickened;[545] by March 1992 £2,855,000 of the target £5,000,000 had been donated,[563] and by March 1994 over four million pounds, to which total over 1000 individual Fellows out of just over 5000 had contributed.[564]

The purchase of 48-49 Russell Square by the College of Anaesthetists. The College in its search for a suitable building first made an offer for Number 8 Bedford Square, next door to the Association of Anaesthetists at Number 9, and the legal process for its purchase was begun. This house, though already elegantly restored, would not have been large enough for all the administrative and social activities of the College and provisional arrangements were made to continue to rent the sixth floor of the Nuffield College in Lincoln's Inn Fields. This arrangement, necessitating operating on two sites, would not have been entirely satisfactory.[565,566] It was, therefore, a blessing in disguise that "a complicated legal issue" not involving the College or its advisers, "threatened the deal" within a realistic time-scale, and the offer was withdrawn.[566]

A larger and much more suitable property which would house the whole of the activities of the College except for plenary gatherings of Fellows was found in the adjoining Square to Bedford Square at 48-49 Russell Square. A deal was struck for a 105 year lease at a time when market conditions were highly favourable to buyers due to a depression in property prices. The College of Anaesthetists certainly got a bargain![567] The College of Anaesthetists' Secretariat moved into the new building on 22 August 1992 despite the fact that workmen on site had not completed the necessary alterations and decorations.[568]

The Contribution of the Association of Anaesthetists to the purchase of the College Building. The Council of the Association of Anaesthetists resolved to offer aid to the College of Anaesthetists to enable them to purchase a property during 1991 before Number 8 Bedford Square became available. When Number 8 did come on the market the College indicated that they wished to accept a loan. The Association initially offered an interest-free loan of £500,000 which would be repaid over a number of years subject to certain conditions being met. Advisory Committee, on behalf of Council, felt it would be advantageous if the Association's loan was expressed as a percentage of the equity, "this would avoid the need for repayments by the

College, and would be an elegant fulfilment of one of the original aims of the Association for the foundation of an independent body for [academic] anaesthesia".[365] The College of Anaesthetists did not agree to this proposition but, after further discussion, accepted the Association's offer of an unsecured loan of 0.5 million pounds from the Education and Research Trust to be divided into two equal tranches; £250,000 interest free, to be repaid in 10 equal instalments, the first of which was to be payable on the anniversary of the loan, and £250,000 interest free for the first two years and thereafter at interest based on the Midland Bank's base rate; repayment of this tranche was to be made in 10 equal instalments with the first of these payable on the first anniversary of the loan. The loan was, in the event, taken out and applied to the purchase of 48-49 Russell Square on 18 February 1992;[325,365,569] in fact, so successful was the (by then) Royal College of Anaesthetists Appeal that the loan was paid in full during 1994.[366] The Association of Anaesthetists then underlined its support for the Royal College by contributing the accrued interest on the loan, amounting to approximately £4,500, to the College Appeal Fund.[570]

The Inauguration of the Royal College of Anaesthetists

Her Majesty the Queen granted the Charter to the Royal College of Anaesthetists on 16 March 1992 even before the move to 48-49 Russell Square. Celebrations marking both the granting of the Charter and the move to 48-49 Russell Square took place later in 1992, and were crowned by the visit of Her Majesty the Queen on Thursday 8 July 1993.

The Lord Mayor of London, Sir Brian Jenkins, honoured the Royal College with a visit on Tuesday 15 September 1992 and viewed the almost completed building works.[568]

The Conference of Internationally Reciprocating Examining Boards in Anaesthesia held their periodic meeting at the new Royal College premises on 3 October 1992. This body was composed of the Presidents and Deans or Presiding Officers of the Examining Boards of Australasia, Canada, Ireland, South Africa, New Zealand and the United States.[568] It is sad, but inevitable considering their different system of Board Certification, that the American Board of Anesthesiology subsequently began a process of graduated withdrawal from the reciprocal arrangements in 1993.[572]

An ecumenical service of thanksgiving and dedication was held at St Clement Danes Church in the Strand on the morning of Monday 5 October 1992. This was the first of several ceremonial events celebrating the birth of the Royal College of Anaesthetists which took place on that day. The Archbishop of Westminster, His Eminence Cardinal Basil Hume OSB preached a moving and memorable sermon.[568,573]

The presentation of the College Medal to Professor Pradit Chareonthaitawee, President to the Royal College of Anaesthetists of Thailand took place later in the morning at a ceremony at the Guildhall, in the City of London prior to the Diplomate Ceremony. It surprised many that the (United Kingdom) Royal College was not the first Royal College of Anaesthetists, but the King of Thailand had, in fact, conferred the Royal prefix on the Thai College shortly before Her Majesty granted the Charter to the United Kingdom College.[574] It pleases the writer, however (as a committed nationalist and monarchist) that the designation "Royal", without a territorial designation, is invariably internationally accepted as referring to a British organisation, for example, besides the Royal Medical Colleges, the Royal Navy and the Royal Army Medical Corps!

The Ceremony of Presentation of Diplomates later in the morning of 5 October 1992 at the Guildhall was addressed by Virginia Bottomley JP, MP, Secretary of State for Health with a characteristic speech.[568,575]

The Symposium on continuing medical education (CME) was held at the Guildhall in the afternoon of 5 October 1992. It was masterminded by Professor A P (Tony) Adams of Guy's Hospital, London. The subject was, of course, well chosen as the Report of the Chief Medical Officers' Working Party was expected early in 1993. Speakers including distinguished representatives from Australasia, Canada, the United States and the United Kingdom, and Sir Robert Kilpatrick, then President of the General Medical Council, discussed various approaches to the provision of Continuing Medical Education (CME).[568,576,577]

An Open House and a Celebratory Party were held in the afternoon and evening of 5 October 1992. The College building at 48-49 Russell Square was open to inspection for Fellows and their families, donors and well-wishers to admire in the afternoon.

A celebratory party ended the day at the Hotel Russell across the Square. This was enjoyed to the full in the manner for which anaesthetists as a specialty are renowned. An excellent buffet supper was provided and a lively band for dancing was on hand.

It had been a truly memorable day marking an achievement for which many, including the members of the Association of Anaesthetists of Great Britain and Ireland, had waited and striven for so long.[568,577]

The use of postnominal letters for the diplomas of Fellowship, so customary in British practice, was the cause of some confusion amongst Fellows when the Faculty of Anaesthetists of the Royal College of Surgeons (FARCS) became in turn the College of Anaesthetists (CAnaes) and then the Royal College of Anaesthetists (RCA). The Fellowship could not use the postnominal "FCA" in the "College of Anaesthetists" phase because that was already generally used by the accountants (Fellow of (the Institute) of Chartered Accountants). Anaesthetists had therefore to settle for the rather ungainly "FC Anaes". There was some confusion when the Royal prefix was added as to whether "FRCA." should be used, but the Privy Council ruled that FRCA was acceptable.[577]

Who's Who (1995) lists the Royal College of Art as another body entitled to use the postnominal FRCA for its Fellowship, indeed it could be regarded as having precedence, but it is understood that, unlike FCA, this designation is rarely used. The Council of the Royal College of Anaesthetists ruled on 1 May 1992 that they wished the postnominal FRCA, and FRCA alone, to be employed irrespective of whether the individual Fellow received his Diploma of Fellowship in the FFARCS, FC Anaes, or FRCA eras.[577]

Stanley Neville Alan, LLB, Secretary successively to the Faculty, the College, and the Royal College of Anaesthetists, having faithfully served and organised the Secretariat of the developing institution for over 21 years, and seen it safely into its new home, retired in February 1993.[577,578] He will be remembered as one who had an encyclopaedic knowledge of the affairs of the organisation, and not least also for his good humour, ready welcome and sound counsel for all, however senior or junior, who visited the somewhat cramped offices in Lincoln's Inn Fields; nor should his ability to smooth over such difficulties as arose from time to time with the Association of

Anaesthetists and the parent surgeons' College be forgotten. His last official public duty was to oversee the ceremony of the Presentation of Diplomates at the Guildhall on 5 October 1992 with his accustomed faultless precision; this task is never easy as it is highly desirable that the less familiar names of some diplomates have to be pronounced with accuracy!

Sir Geoffrey de Deney, KCVO, MA, BCL, became Chief Executive of the Royal College of Anaesthetists at the beginning of 1993. He was formerly a civil servant of very considerable distinction and, latterly immediately before retirement from the Civil Service, Clerk to the Privy Council, in which post he was coincidentally concerned in the negotiations which led to the granting of the Charter of the College of Anaesthetists.[577,579]

Tangible gifts from the Association of Anaesthetists to the Royal College. The College itself earmarked a portion of the money gifted to the Association of Anaesthetists for the purchase of regalia for the President and Vice Presidents of the College, but the Council of the Association of Anaesthetists considered that it was appropriate to mark the granting of the Royal Charter with "a gift in keeping with the elegance of the new headquarters". An antique mahogany long case clock made by Nathaniel Newman about 1720 was selected for the Fellows (North American) Room. It was presented to the Council of the College at a ceremony on 16 March 1993.[580,581]

The Official Opening of the Royal College of Anaesthetists by Her Majesty the Queen took place on Thursday 8 July 1993. The Royal College was *en fête* for the President Professor Alastair Spence, CBE to receive Her Majesty on the fine sunny afternoon on a proud day for the discipline of anaesthesia.[582,583] The Bedford Estates had given permission for the erection of a large marquee in the gardens at the rear of the College adjoining its own small recently laid out garden with its bust of the pioneer John Snow. This bust had been sculpted by Mrs Jane Burgess and was the gift of the Obstetric Anaesthetists Association.[584]

Almost everyone associated with anaesthesia was present at the opening ceremony. The company included the newly elected Honorary Fellow of the Royal College, John Nunn (Head of the Division of Anaesthesia of the Medical Research Council, Research Centre, Northwick Park (1968-1991), Dean of the Faculty of Anaesthetists (1979-1982), Vice President (1988-1990) and first Magill Gold Medallist of the Association of Anaesthetists in 1988), as well as younger Fellows who had received their diplomas that morning at the ceremony at the University of London Senate House, and representatives of charitable foundations, industry, and other benefactors. There were many demonstrations, both historic and contemporary, and of a number of organisations and firms connected with anaesthesia, including the medical branches of the Defence Forces.[582,583]

Australian parallels

Historically, there has been a close relation between the Australian and the United Kingdom anaesthesia and in particular in the formation of its institutions.

The Australian Society of Anaesthetists celebrated its fiftieth anniversary in 1984, two years after the Association of Anaesthetists of Great Britain and Ireland. This was marked by the donation of a Presidential Medallion by the Association of Anaesthetists to the Australian Association. This Medallion was taken to Australia by John Nunn, who was the Australian Association's Official visitor in 1984. It was presented by him to the Australian Association on behalf of the Association of Anaesthetists of Great Britain and Ireland during the Golden Jubilee Celebrations in Adelaide in October 1984.[341,585]

The metamorphosis of the Faculty of Anaesthetists of the Royal Australasian College of Surgeons into the independent Australian and New Zealand College of Anaesthetists (ANZCA) occurred in 1992. The writer has a personal recollection that there was much interest in Australia in the latter half of 1989 in the formation of the College of Anaesthetists in London, but that interest was considerably diminished when it was explained to the Australians and New Zealanders that the move did not signify absolute independence from the Royal College of Surgeons of England at that stage. The Australasian Faculty became an independent College (ANZCA) by incorporation under Australian law on 7 February 1992 about one month before the Queen signed the independent Royal Charter of the Royal College of Anaesthetists.[586] It is known that there had been some discussion amongst rank and file Fellows of the Australasian Faculty (though not in the Australian Board of Faculty) as to whether New Zealand should be included with the new College. It is probably unlikely in the present political climate that the new College will seek to be granted the Royal prefix, but there is a rumour that some New Zealanders are keener on this than their Australian colleagues (personal communication)!

In memoriam 1983-1995

The decade which included the Diamond Jubilee year of the Association in 1992, and the two or three years which followed saw the deaths of no less than nine pioneers whose names figure prominently in the history of the Association of Anaesthetists of Great Britain and Ireland; taken together their careers provide a panorama of the development of the specialty of anaesthesia in the United Kingdom. Three of them were knighted (an all too rare honour for anaesthetists). One of them had been a Founder Member of the Association of Anaesthetists in 1932, all were Honorary Members of the Association, all had been officers, and seven of them had been Members of the Board of the Faculty of Anaesthetists of the Royal College of Surgeons of England (four being Founder Members). Two were nonagenarians, one died in his ninetieth year, four in their eighties and two in their late seventies, and the one remaining had achieved the allotted span of three score year and ten. This is possibly a hopeful precedent for British anaesthetists, but one does just wonder whether longevity could be attributed to the vast amounts of that wonderfully safe and effective agent ether, which all must have legitimately inhaled in the course of their practice in the specialty in earlier years before the development of scavenging!

Sir Ivan Whiteside Magill, KCVO (1888-1986) Northern Irishman; Member of Council (1933-1934) and Vice President (1948-1950); graduate of the Queens University, Belfast (1913), survivor of the trenches of the 1914-1918 War; originator of wide bore endotracheal anaesthesia; Consultant to the Brompton Hospital for Chest Diseases and Westminster Hospital; acknowledged foremost clinical anaesthetist in London from the nineteen twenties to the nineteen forties; originator of the Diploma in Anaesthetics in 1935.[587-589]

Christopher Langton Hewer (1897-1986); Member of Council 1935-1937, Vice President 1966-1968, Founder Editor of *Anaesthesia* (1946-1966); graduate (1918) and Member of the Consultant staff of St Bartholomew's

Hospital, London; author and later editor of 14 editions of *Recent Advances in Anaesthesia* (1932-1982).[590,591]

Professor Sir Robert Reynolds Macintosh (1897-1989); New Zealander; Member of Council 1937-1939, Vice President 1955-1957; fighter pilot in the Royal Flying Corps in the 1914-1918 War; graduate of Guy's Hospital, London (1924); first Nuffield Professor of Anaesthetics at the University of Oxford (1937-1965): this was the first departmental chair outside North America and, arguably the first independent University chair in the World); Air Commodore and organiser at the training of anaesthetists for the armed services in the 1939-1945 War; designer of the universally used Macintosh laryngoscope and the EMO graduated ether-air vaporiser for difficult environments; promoter of the use of spinal anaesthesia and other local anaesthesia techniques, and peripatetic lecturer and demonstrator in developing countries.[527,592,593]

Professor Sir Geoffrey Stephen William Organe (1908-1989). Born in Madras of English parents; Member of Council (1950-1958), President (1953-1956); graduate of the University of Cambridge and Westminster Medical School; Consultant 1939 and later Professor of Anaesthesia, Westminster Hospital, University of London (1966-1975); Dean of the Faculty of Anaesthetists (1958-1961); Founder Secretary Treasurer of the World Federation of Societies of Anaesthesiologists (1955-1964) and President (1964-1968); pioneer in the study of traumatic shock and muscle relaxants, and world-wide traveller and lecturer in the promotion of modern anaesthesia.[594]

John Alfred Lee (1906-1989) born in Liverpool; Member of Council (1969-1971); President (1971-1973, graduate of the Durham College of Medicine at Newcastle upon Tyne (1927); general practitioner and anaesthetist at Southend-on-Sea (1931-1940); Anaesthetist in the civilian Emergency Medical Service in the Second World War (1939-1947); Consultant Anaesthetist Southend-on-Sea (1947-1971). Author of the *Synopsis of Anaesthesia* (10 editions between 1947 and 1987 and translated into seven foreign languages); pioneer in departmental organisation for training, anaesthetic outpatient clinics (1948) and recovery wards and promoter of the use of spinal, epidural and other local anaesthetic techniques.[595]

John Warry Dundee, OBE (1921-1992); Northern Ireland; Member of Council (1980-1982); Vice President (1982-1984); graduate of Queens University, Belfast (1946); Consultant at Belfast 1958 (first Professor 1964-1988); Head of a remarkable Department of Anaesthesia, he supervised 50 theses for higher degrees); internationally recognised researcher, particularly for a lifetime study of the effects of intravenous drugs used in anaesthesia; he could as well have been a professor of pharmacology as of anaesthesia but he took his full share of clinical commitments. Founder Member and later Dean of the Faculty of Anaesthetics of the Royal College of Surgeons in Ireland and Board Member of the Faculty of Anaesthetics of the Royal College of Surgeons of England. Leading figure and educator in Northern Ireland, author of some 500 research papers, and presenter of innumerable communications to societies throughout the world.[596]

Professor William Woolf Mushin, CBE (1910-1993) born and educated in the East End of London and Essex, the son of a headmaster of Lithuanian origin; Member of Council (1968-1970); Vice President (1970-1972); qualified from the London Hospital 1933. First Assistant to Professor Macintosh at Oxford 1943-1947; Director (1947) and later Professor (1953) of the newly independent Department of anaesthesia at the University of Wales in Cardiff; his Department was initially modelled on Professor Macintosh's Department at Oxford and he made it a centre for Postgraduate Medical Education (PME) in Wales at a time when PME in the United Kingdom was at an elementary stage. Mushin was an expert clinician and an impressive lecturer and teacher; he had great administrative ability; he was a pioneer in record keeping and audit; he became Vice Provost of the Welsh National School of Medicine and Dean of the Faculty of Anaesthetists of the Royal College of Surgeons of England and was in demand as a member of many national and governmental committees.[597,598]

Arthur John Wells Beard (1908-1993); a Londoner; Member of Council (1964-1972), Honorary Treasurer (1966-1970), President (1969-1971); qualified from St Bartholomew's Hospital, London in 1931. He can be regarded as having been one of the last, if not the last of the General Practitioner Consultant Anaesthetists. He was a GP with an interest in anaesthesia before the Second World War; he continued as a GP throughout the 1939-1945 War while he was an anaesthetist in the Emergency Medical

Service, and remained a GP throughout his time as a Consultant in the National Health Service at the Royal Postgraduate Medical school and the National Heart Hospital (1948-1973), when he was amongst the leaders of the postwar development of the specialty, and afterwards until within a few weeks of his death in 1993. He was an outstanding and innovative clinician and a kindly and dedicated instructor. He became President of the Association of Anaesthetists and Postgraduate Dean at the National Heart Hospital.[599]

Philip John Helliwell (1915-1994) was a Yorkshireman; Member of Council (1964-1977), Honorary Secretary (1966-1968), President (1973-1976); he qualified at the University of Edinburgh in 1938; he was one of those young specialists who trained as a military anaesthetist during the Second World War 1939-1945, in his case in the Army in the Far East; he was the first Research Fellow of the Association of Anaesthetists (1947) and later the architect of the dramatic development of the Association of Anaesthetists as an organisation of great influence in the sixties and seventies; he was the only President since 1965 to be elected to serve a three year term; he promoted the concept of an independent College of Anaesthetists with single minded vigour and dedication. He later became the principal reference of the Help for the Sick Doctor scheme of the Association of Anaesthetists. His other great sphere of influence was at Guy's Hospital, London, where he became Consultant Anaesthetist in 1948 and Director of the Department in 1956; he then turned his talents as an administrator to the rebuilding and reorganisation of Guy's Hospital as Chairman of the project team and finally in the unique position as the last Superintendent of Guy's Hospital in 1966-1974; his career was central to the post-war development of both the specialty of anaesthesia in the United Kingdom and of Guy's Hospital; he lived to see in retirement the establishment in 1992 of the Royal College of Anaesthetists which he so much desired but, sadly the demise of the renowned and rebuilt Guy's Hospital as an independent institution after the iconoclastic reorganisation of the National Health Service in 1992.[600]

Oswald Peter Dinnick (1917-1995); Member of Council (1961-1969), Honorary Secretary (1963-1966), Vice President (1966-1968); he qualified from the Middlesex Hospital, London in 1939 and almost immediately joined the Royal Air Force Medical Branch on the outbreak of the Second World War 1939-1945; he trained as an anaesthetist in the wartime RAF and saw active service in the North African and Italian campaigns; he was elected to honorary staff of the Middlesex on his return in 1946, became a Consultant in the NHS in 1948 and Senior Anaesthetist at the Middlesex in 1959; he was Honorary Secretary of the Association of Anaesthetists from 1963-1966 at a time when the educational activities of the Association of Anaesthetists were being developed and the embryo Junior Anaesthetists' group was being formed; his greatest contribution to anaesthesia however was in his pursuit of safe practice, and his associated lengthy service as a member and Chairman of the British and International Standards Commissions on Anaesthetic Equipment; he was also a pioneer in the audit of deaths under anaesthesia; he was a career long "Association man" devoted to its objectives and a ready source of inside information about its postwar history and of amusing anecdotes about those who contributed to its development.[601]

1983-1992. A decade culminating in joyous celebrations tinged with some future uncertainties

The Council and the Members of the Association of Anaesthetists of Great Britain and Ireland could look with satisfaction at the achievements of the decade following the Golden Jubilee in 1982 as they celebrated the Diamond Jubilee in 1992. The membership of the Association had increased significantly, the finances had prospered, and the organisation had ceased to be a tenant organisation and now occupied its own prestigious headquarters at 9 Bedford Square. This move enabled a very considerable increase in the educational, medicopolitical and social activities of the Association to take place.

British anaesthetists had evaluated and introduced new agents and techniques and the Association had actively influenced the safe development of many aspects of clinical practice. These included prehospital emergency care, monitoring, day and minimal invasive surgery, the prevention of postoperative pain, recovery, high dependency, and intensive care, and along with the rest of the medical profession, the alleviation of the formidable consequences of acquired immune deficiency syndrome (AIDS).

The establishment of the independent Royal College of Anaesthetists in its own building was the fulfilment of a long time goal of the Association of Anaesthetists, and the Council and members had not been slow to express its support and to give considerable financial assistance.

The Association of Anaesthetists had also played its part in encouraging anaesthetists to participate in the new management structure of the British National Health Service which had resulted, for better or for worse, from the various medicopolitical reorganisations which took place during the decade. Many anaesthetists had in the process become amongst the most successful of the Clinical Directors.

The consequences of the 1991 reorganisation were not, however, fully apparent at the time the Association of Anaesthetists celebrated its Diamond Jubilee in January 1992, and the Chief Medical Officer's Working Group on specialist training, which was destined to initiate fundamental changes in training and postgraduate and continuing medical education had yet to report.[602] It was clear to the Officers and Council that the Association of Anaesthetists of Great Britain and Ireland would have much to do in both its active and its watchdog roles as the nineteen nineties progressed towards the third millennium.

10

Today, Yesterday and Tomorrow

1 January 1993 to 30 June 1997 *

"Hear the voice of the Bard
Who present, past and future sees"

William Blake (1757-1827) *Songs of Experience*

Executive Officers

Presidents:- W R MacRae (1992-1994)
S Morrell Lyons (1994-1996)
W L M Baird (1996-1998)

Honorary Treasurers:- W L M Baird (1992-1996)
D A Saunders (1996-1998)

Honorary Secretaries:- R S Vaughan (1992-1994)
D A Saunders (1994-1996)
D J Wilkinson (1996-1998)

Editor:- M Morgan (1991-1998)

Chairmen of the Group of Anaesthetists in Training: Elizabeth M Spencer (1990-1993), Susan M Geddes (1993-1995), J B Luntley (1995-1997), Claire Mallinson (1997 et seq)

The original objective of relating in context the history of the Association of Anaesthetists of Great Britain and Ireland from its foundation in 1932 to its Diamond Jubilee in 1992 was achieved by the completion of Chapter 9. This last chapter is by way of being a postscript. It records some of the political, medicopolitical, and medical developments which have occurred between the Diamond Jubilee year of 1992, and the change of government following the general election of 1 May 1997. The chapter goes on to consider the present

* Compiled by Anna-Maria Rollin from material supplied by T.B.B.

preoccupations of the Council and members of the Association of Anaesthetists up until the middle of 1997 and finally, and somewhat hesitantly, looks into the future.

The domestic scene in the United Kingdom (1993-1997)

The rate of technological development has accelerated through the 1990s, with *inter alia,* the opening of the Channel Tunnel, the ubiquitous mobile telephone and the astonishing impact of the Internet.[1,2]

The years 1993-1997 were not politically tranquil. The Conservative Government continued its policy of decentralisation, financial restriction and adherence to the dogma of market forces. Many public services and utilities were privatised, with deregulation often leading to anomalies and deterioration of services. Litigation, (after the American model) was on the increase. An attempt to 'curb' the professions brought with it the devaluation of experienced and dedicated staff, and this application of market forces resulted in job insecurity within the public services resulting in lowered morale.

The United Kingdom and the European Union (UK)

It is highly probable that most ordinary citizens of the United Kingdom thought the country was simply joining a free trade organisation when the government of Prime Minister Edward Heath acceded to the Treaty of Rome and the UK joined the European Economic Community (EEC) on 1 January 1973; however in the subsequent years the European Commission in Brussels has dictated many of the ways in which the UK conducts its internal affairs.[2-5] Not least of these, of course, is the fact that European regulations have altered fundamentally the way in which medical specialists are trained and accredited in the United Kingdom (see below).

Physician anaesthetists and medical practice in the mid-1990s

Certain medical, surgical and anaesthetic developments of the 1980s and early 1990s were considered in some detail in the last chapter. So far as surgical anaesthesia in the operating theatre is concerned, it is reasonable to predict further expansion of the use of pollution free total intravenous anaesthetic techniques (TIVA) at the expense of inhalation anaesthesia as better delivery and monitoring systems are developed. There are, however, several clinical issues which have come to the fore in the 1990s which have not been considered earlier. Some of them directly affect the practice of physician anaesthetists, particularly in the Intensive Care Unit; others are of more general interest.

Ethical considerations. The rise in consumerism, not just in medicine, but in all areas of life, has led to the growth of patient power, and a radical change in the doctor-patient relationship. The patient now expects to be involved in decisions about all aspects of his or her care, including those involving the anaesthetist.

Obstetrics can present many ethical problems for anaesthetists, especially since the practice of obstetrics involves a multidisciplinary team with midwives as independent practitioners and increasing emphasis on patient choice (Chapter 7).[6-8]

Intensive Care is an area in which British physician anaesthetists play an important part, both in treatment and as clinical directors (Chapters 7, 8 and 9). They are thus involved in many ethical dilemmas, including the selection (and rejection) of patients for admission to intensive care, the implementation of "Do Not Resuscitate" policies, and the problem of withdrawal of treatment.[9-11]

Anaesthetists are participants in the major debates currently occupying doctors, politicians and the general public. These include the problems of limited resources and rationing, euthanasia, antibiotic resistance and developments made possible by increased knowledge of genetics and molecular biology.[9-50]

Stress in anaesthetic practice, as in other walks of life, is inevitable. Nevertheless, in the 1990's, the hazards of excessive stress, both for the anaesthetist and his or her patients, became a topic of discussion. In 1997, a working party of the Association of Anaesthetists, under the chairmanship of Dr S Morrell Lyons, produced a valuable booklet on stress and its management for anaesthetists.[51]

The British National Health Service 1993-1997

The NHS was subjected to yet another period of major change in 1996 as the government attempted once again "to get the organisation right".[52] The

English Regional Health Authorities which had already been reduced from 14 to 8 were abolished and replaced by NHS Management Executive offices.[53] Regional Professional Advisory Committees giving advice on issues such as education, training and research were also abolished,[54,55] although the government belatedly introduced an amendment to the enabling legislation, to the effect that health authorities are required to take advice from doctors and other professional staff when making decisions on the delivery of healthcare.[56] Public health doctors at the new branch NHS Executive offices have become civil servants subject to the Official Secrets Act.[54,57]

Providers. Most acute hospitals in the United Kingdom are now administered as NHS Trusts. The basic method of provision of acute healthcare is, therefore, standardised but fragmented. Collusion between Trusts was deprecated on commercial secrecy grounds,[58,59] and this left the way open both for duplication and for deficiencies and unevenness in provision.[60] An Audit Commission report in 1994 found that Trust performance has been very variable from a financial point of view.[58] Nearly half the first wave (1991) Trusts and 22% of the second wave (1992) had failed to meet the government's target of earning a real return on capital of at least 6%.[61] Many hospital doctors subscribe to the view that in a truly national health service, competition between providers is inappropriate and that "Trusts should be cooperating in the interests of patients rather than competing".[60]

Purchasers. The provider element in hospital care in the present system is almost completely unified into individual Hospital Trusts, but the situation is very different on the purchaser side. By April 1997 it was estimated that 56% of the population of the United Kingdom were served by fundholding general practitioners. Some of the general practitioner fundholders were included in a pilot scheme of up to 50 practices of "total" fundholders who "purchased" the full range of hospital and community health services.[62]

There, therefore, continued to be two types of "purchasers". Health authorities contract for a population on a demographic basis, while general practitioner fundholders are responsible to individual patient demand.[63] The Family Health Service Authorities (FHSAs) merged with the District Health Authorities (DHAs) in 1996.[52,53] It remained to be seen whether a clash of interests between the different approaches to fundholding would ensue. Little comparative research had been attempted by the NHS Executive.[64]

The problem of intensive care provision in the new NHS. During the period under review, with the closure of hospital beds and, indeed, whole hospitals in London and other parts of the country, it became clear to all concerned with the direct care of patients that there was a dearth of intensive care beds.

In addition, the shortfall in intensive care beds, particularly for trauma victims, is related to the need for a coordinated system of trauma care units, as recommended by the Royal College of Surgeons in 1988 (Chapter 9). It is difficult to believe, however, that the problem of provision of emergency intensive care beds is fully understood by politicians when one considers the statement made by a Junior Minister in the Department of Health, that, "It is no good hospitals establishing intensive care units for peaks of demand. Highly staffed beds then lie empty for the rest of the year".[65] Would the Minister criticise the policy of having firemen standing by but ready to go into action if required?[66]

It is certainly possible to argue, as it is in the case of trauma (Chapter 9), and especially in the provision of paediatric intensive care[67-70] that, in our geographically compact country, centralisation, even of the existing number of intensive care beds into larger units, would result in both adequate provision and more expert care.[68] Such a scheme would, however, necessitate a highly efficient centrally directed transport service including helicopters, with dedicated specialist personnel.[71-73]

A computerised national bed register for intensive care was announced in September 1996 to start in the following December. This was an extension of the emergency bed service covering 100 intensive care units in south east England set up in 1995. The Chairman of the British Medical Association Junior Doctors' Committee doubted whether this would solve the problem; "If the register shows there aren't any beds, how will that help?"[74]

The provision of more High Dependency Units (HDUs) would be a potential solution to the lack of intensive care beds for patients who are breathing spontaneously but would require a high level of medical and nursing care and supervision.[66,75-77] This is particularly the case if the HDU is situated close to the Intensive Care Unit (ICU) and policies of flexible interchange of staff and transfer of patients between the ICU and the HDU are maintained.

The electronic "digivote" audit system used at the September 1996 Linkman Conference of the Association of Anaesthetists indicated that 50% of those present did not have an HDU at their hospital and had no prospect of one in the future; only 20% felt that there was sufficient provision for ICU beds, and 50% were aware of one cancellation or transfer per week due to deficiency of ICU or HDU facilities. Most disturbing of all, in this day and age, 59% stated that there were no recovery facilities at night! The British NHS has a long way to go in ICU, HDU and even recovery ward provision.[78]

NHS management problems following the 1991 reorganisation. The 1991 reorganisation of the NHS with its internal market concept was conceived and initiated in haste with minimal consultation with the health professions in the face of an impending general election (Chapter 9). The details of the new system had to be developed on an *ad hoc* basis.

Patient dissatisfaction, expressed in terms of increasing number of complaints, has been partly fuelled by the deliberately engineered arousal of expectations by *ex cathedra* declarations such as the Patients' Charter.[79-82]

Professional dissatisfaction has arisen because of the realisation that all targets set cannot be met in the context of prevailing restrictions on NHS funding and the demands for "efficiency savings" despite long-term underfunding.[83-84]

The development of clinical audit has been one of the few initiatives both promoted and directly financed by the Department of Health. The medical profession has taken up the challenge and is using audit to improve its practices and correct its mistakes.

The crisis in British Nursing in 1997

By 1996, there was a serious shortfall of nurses in the NHS.[85] This was partly due to conditions and pay in the hospital service and preference of nurses for posts in general practice,[86] and in the private hospital sector.[85] The need to recruit and retain nurses in the NHS was at last acknowledged early in 1997 when the Department of Health initiated a £32M recruitment campaign.[87]

Paradoxically, at a time when there is a grave shortage of nurses, especially in operating theatres, paediatrics and intensive care, the possibility of the introduction of nurse anaesthesia into the NHS has once again been raised (see below). The danger is that to substitute doctors by nurses could be regarded as a short or long-term response to medical staffing problems and could be seized on by politicians and management as a less expensive alternative.[88,89] There is fortunately considerable doubt as to whether there would be cost savings in such a doctor-to-nurse shift.[89]

The NHS in the Spring of 1997. Conditions in the acute hospital service in the winters which succeeded the 1991 reorganisation often did not seem to be markedly different to the practising clinician from those which preceded it, and which had, to some extent, precipitated the changes in the way NHS administration functioned (Chapter 9). The real problem was, and is (in June 1998), lack of funding in the face of ever increasing demand.[90]

The general election of 1 May 1997 and the NHS

By the run up to the general election scheduled for 1 May 1997, the Labour Party had become convinced of the advantages of the purchaser-provider split introduced by the Conservatives in 1991, and of the value of the concept of a primary care led service. In their election manifesto[91,92] Labour expressed its intention to "remove the disadvantages" of individual general practice fundholding. This was less draconian than earlier commitments to "abolish" fundholding.[93,94] They proposed to introduce local commissioning of hospital care by consortiums of 10 to 20 general practices which would negotiate a common budget with longer term (three to five years) agreements with hospitals for secondary care. They also expressed their intention of ending the internal market based on financial manipulation and its unfortunate consequences, such as competition rather than cooperation between Hospital Trusts, restriction of services for purely commercial reasons, and such mistaken economies as the introduction of mixed sex inpatient wards which are so disliked by the public.

Hospital Trusts were to be replaced by local health services with management boards meeting in public and more representative of local opinion.[92-94]

The Labour Party won the election by a landslide on 1 May 1997.[95] Tony Blair became Prime Minister and Frank Dobson was appointed Secretary of State for Health. The new administration, however, expressed a desire for caution now that it was in office! Frank Dobson has stated that it may take years for it to fulfil the Labour manifesto promise to replace the NHS internal market.[96]

The Calman Report and its implementation

The "Calman Report", more properly designated as *Hospital Doctors: Training for the Future. The Report of the Working Group on Specialist Medical Training, 1993,*[97] has result in the most major alterations in the training of medical specialists in the United Kingdom since the system was set up after the publication of the Todd Report in 1968 (Chapter 8). [97]

The events which led up to the Calman Working Group being formed in August 1992[99,100] have been outlined in previous chapters (Chapters 8 and 9). The terms of reference of the group were "to consider the present United Kingdom arrangements for post-graduate medical education, taking into account EC law", and to make proposals which would lead to harmonisation of the United Kingdom system of recognition of specialist status with that employed by other EU members.

The publication of the Calman Report in May 1993. The Report[97] recommended that there should be a single "Certificate of Completion of Specialist Training" (CCST) awarded by the General Medical Council on the advice of the relevant Royal College at the end of a satisfactorily completed, closely structured, specialist training programme of not more than seven years with a defined end point. The practitioner would then be regarded both as an independent specialist in EU terms and as an independent specialist ready for promotion to a consultant appointment in the British NHS. The T indicator of accreditation (Chapter 8) in the British *Medical Register* would be replaced by CT indicating the award of the CCST, and the holder of the certificate would apply to have his name included in a specialist register. The registrar and senior registrar grades would be amalgamated into a new "seamless" Specialist Registrar grade (SpR).[97,101-107]

The Royal Medical Colleges were charged with organising clearly defined curricula for training and the postgraduate deans with ensuring that the training was delivered.[97] This proposal consolidated the relationship and respective responsibilities of the Royal Medical Colleges and the Postgraduate Deans. The Royal Medical Colleges, represented regionally by the Regional Educational Advisors (REA), would determine and police the standards and curricula details of Postgraduate Medical Education (PGME). The Postgraduate Deans, through the network of district Clinical Tutors, would be responsible for ensuring that those responsible for the conditions and terms of employment, which would enable the standards to be met, fulfilled their obligations.[108,109] Just before publication of the Calman Report in May 1993, an "Executive Letter" of the Department of Health (EL (92) 63) became effective and the postgraduate deans were allocated the budget for 50% of the salaries (100% in Scotland) and 100% of the non-pay costs of all doctors in training. This has greatly enhanced the powers of the Postgraduate Deans in their dealings with NHS Hospital Trusts.

It was obvious from the start that "the only coherent solution" for ensuring the implementation of the recommendations of the Calman Report was an absolute expansion of the NHS consultant grade.[101] This was, firstly, because tightly structured training meant that both trainers and trainees would have less time for service work; secondly, because of the shorter and strictly time limited training more certified independent specialists would emerge and, therefore, more consultant posts would be required; thirdly, because patients and the NHS Executive expected more care to be delivered by fully trained specialists, and fourthly, because the implementation of the 1991 "New Deal" on junior doctors' working hours would reduce the time available for service commitments.[101] The vision of a consultant provided service has existed since the start of the NHS, but the corollary of consultant expansion, had only been half-heartedly applied.

The response of the Council of the Association of Anaesthetists to the Calman Report was orchestrated by the President (1994-1996) W R (Bill) MacRae.[105,110] The publication of the report brought a landslide of correspondence from concerned members.[111] The prospect of the reduction of the service commitment of the trainee grades and the fear that this would result in catastrophic changes in the nature of the work of consultants caused very grave concern.[101,110-117] After all, the percentage of trainees in the specialist pool (trainees plus certified specialists) in the United Kingdom was near to

50% compared with, for example, 8% in France and 9% in Italy.[113] The apprehension about dilatory authorisation of consultant increases or, even more important, funding of them, proved to some extent to be justified.[118,119] Anaesthesia in the United Kingdom, though a popular specialty with trainees, was a shortage specialty due to previous misplaced manpower controls.[110,111,113,119-125]

Council of the Association, in the document prepared by its working party which was chaired by MacRae and published in May 1994,[110] welcomed "in principle":

> "reduction in the duration of specialist training with more structured and intensive training programmes, the introduction of a unified training grade and a clear definition of a finishing point of specialist training marked by the award of a Certificate of Completion of Training."[110]

The document, however, after a detailed and exceptionally well researched analysis, continued:

> *"The Association of Anaesthetists of Great Britain and Ireland is of the opinion that, without significant financial investment in anaesthetic staff, primarily at consultant level, but also, for an interim period, in the training grades, implementation of the proposals in the Calman Report and an attempt to move anaesthetic services in the UK "into line" with Europe cannot succeed. Furthermore, even if sufficient new posts to support the existing service are funded, implementation of the Calman proposals will have to be gradual to ensure that enough, anaesthetists can be trained to the necessary standards."[110]*

The document pointed out *inter alia* that there were 10 to 12 trained specialist anaesthetists per 100,000 population in many countries in the European Union, whereas in the United Kingdom and Ireland there were only 4 to 5 consultant anaesthetists per 100,000. It was also emphasised that due to the fragmentation of the NHS in the latest (1991) reorganisation, Hospital Trusts had the "flexibility" to move away from centrally directed staffing policies and this might negate medical staffing expansion as it had done in the past.[110]

The Royal College of Anaesthetists' document on *Specialist Training in Anaesthesia, Supervision and Assessment* was published in May 1994,[126] well in advance of the deadline of July 1994 required by the Calman Report. The Council of the College had, in fact, been considering changes in specialist training since 1991.[103]

The College document described in detail a finite six year modular programme leading to the attainment of the CCST.[126] The first two years were to be basic specialist training as a senior house officer culminating in the passing of a newly structured examination for membership of the Royal College of Anaesthetists (MRCA). This was to be an essential step before sitting the examination for the FRCA during the first year of Higher Specialist Training (HST). The first year of HST (that is the third year of specialist training) would only be embarked upon after success in the MRCA examination and a selective interview with a statutory, properly constituted selection committee for promotion to the "unified training grade" (later designated as specialist registrar (SpR) grade).[126-128] The seventeen modules for the first three years of training (two of BST and one SpR) were defined in considerable detail and strict conditions of supervision and assessment were laid down. It was recognised that few hospitals could provide the complete training and therefore hospital departments would be expected to form "schools of anaesthesia".[126]

The College proposals, in their initial form, received "a less than rapturous welcome from the tutors".[129] The tutors declared 'with almost total unanimity that they [the proposals] were unrealistic and completely unworkable'.[106]

Following the response of consultants in the specialty, Professor Richard Ellis (Vice President of the RCA) and Professor John Norman (Member of Council of the RCA) headed a group which included College Tutors from district general hospitals, which produced a new trading guide, *Specialist Training for Senior House Officers in Anaesthesia* (1995).[130] This divided the training of SHOs into two parts (the "introductory six months" and the "next eighteen months"). The approach was much more flexible and a log book was introduced. There was, probably rightly, no concession to the requirements for close supervision, especially during the first six months of training.[130]

The examinations leading to the granting of the diploma of Fellowship of the Royal College of Anaesthetists underwent the first major changes since 1985 (Chapter 5).[131] They have been modified into a two-part format to conform with progress in the stages of the new six year training programme.[130-133] The passing of the "Primary" examination was one of the conditions to be met by the trainee before assessment for promotion to the new Specialist Registrar (SpR) grade, and the "Final" was to be taken towards the end of the first year of SpR training.

The original proposal of awarding the MRCA to those who passed the new primary FRCA examination was abandoned in 1995 (Annual Report of the Council of the RCA, 1995/1996). The postnominals of MRCA and FRCA would have been confusing and even perhaps exploited by employing authorities. The decision not to grant a Diploma in Anaesthetics (DA) at the same PGME stage is less easy to understand. The demise of the DA, awarded in recent years after passing Part 1 of the old examination (equivalent to the new Primary) is regretted by many, especially by trainers and trainees concerned to provide a practical workforce for developing countries.

The introduction of the new specialist registrar grade began on 1 December 1995 for general surgery and clinical radiology, and for other specialties, including anaesthesia, on 1 April 1996.[134,135] A period of intense activity for the Royal Colleges and Postgraduate Deans followed during the transitional phase, which was completed for anaesthesia in May 1996 just over a month after the starting date. Most senior registrars opted to continue with their own contracts but a large number of previous career grade registrars were transferred to the new grade. Anaesthesia was allocated 196 new SpR posts but only 60% of these were funded by December 1996.

The European Medical Specialist Qualifications Order in Council came into force on 12 January 1996. This order brought into being the Specialist Training Authority of the Medical Royal Colleges (STA) as the (British) "competent authority" for awarding the CCST under the European Regulations, and it ordered the creation of the new unitary Specialist Register for the (United Kingdom) General Medical Council (GMC). The former list of European specialists was discontinued.[128,136] Those eligible for inclusion in the all important GMC Specialist Register during the transition phase were:-

current and past United Kingdom Consultants, Senior Registrars awarded the old accreditation by their respective Royal Colleges who were not yet Consultants, those who were awarded the United Kingdom CCST during the transition phase, those holding European Economic Area (EEA) Specialist Certificates, and those in academic or research medicine "who have not followed a conventional (United Kingdom or EEA) training path, but whose expertise is assessed equivalent to CCST standards".

This latter group had (and have now since the end of the transitional phase) to apply to the STA and be assessed by the appropriate Royal College.

The importance of acceptance onto the Specialist Register of the GMC is that such registration, and not actually the possession of the CCST, has been a legal requirement for appointment to an established consultant post in the National Health Service in the United Kingdom since 1 January 1997.[136]

Many anaesthetists who had received part, or all, of their training overseas, outside the European Economic Area, applied for recognition of "equivalence" of training during 1996. The criteria applied by the Royal College of Anaesthetists were explicit, fair and unambiguous. Those anaesthetists in the official NHS nontraining, nonconsultant career grades of the NHS (Associate Specialists, Staff Grade doctors, Hospital Practitioners and Clinical Assistants)[137] did not qualify for the Specialist Registrar Grade unless, very unusually, they had been accredited before taking up such appointments; neither did those appointed by the independent NHS Trusts to peculiar grades of their own or those who had made a career as perpetual locums (unless, of course, they were accredited or could genuinely demonstrate equivalence to UK training). The RCA resisted the possibility of individuals gaining specialist registration by inappropriate promotion to consultant status in the transitional period.[136]

Continuing Medical Education (CME), as now understood, can be defined as the process of facilitating the maintenance and extension of the level of knowledge and the standards of practice reached at the end of specialist training throughout the career of the specialist (that is, for example, after appointment to consultant or other permanent grade in the NHS).

The Royal College of Anaesthetists (RCA), after a short pilot programme, began operating its CME scheme in April 1995 for all staff not in training grades, including consultants. Varying numbers of "credits" are awarded for attendance at RCA educational meetings, other national, regional, and local meetings, attendance at hospital case conferences, audit meetings, journal clubs and formal lectures delivered locally. So far as "self-learning" is concerned, visits to another centre, preparation of a lecture, publications and preparation of theses for higher degrees are all eligible for "credits", but personal study of journals and text books is excluded from the RCA scheme as being impractical, even though it has been successfully included in other countries, for example in the USA and Australia; this is a pity.[138,139]

The business of the Association 1992-1997

Many of the important items of business in this period have already been discussed by extension in Chapter 9 and earlier in this chapter.

Cooperation between the Association of Anaesthetists of Great Britain and Ireland and the Royal College of Anaesthetists. The polarised responsibilities of the Association of Anaesthetists (concern for the conditions in which anaesthetists work), and of the Royal College of Anaesthetists (concern for the maintenance of standards of practice of anaesthetists and their effect on patient care) are clearly defined and complementary. The areas of postgraduate and continuing education in which both bodies participate are of common concern.

A pleasing feature in recent years has been the increasing collaboration between the Presidents of the two bodies and the development of cross-representation between their two Councils. Apart from a few months at the beginning of Cyril Scurr's Presidency (1976-1978), Michael Vickers (1982-1984) was the first President of the Association of Anaesthetists to serve concurrently as an elected member of the Board of the Faculty (now Council of the Royal College) of Anaesthetists since J Alfred Lee (1971-1973). This circumstance may reflect the coolness between the two bodies over the "College issue" in the 70s (Chapter 8). However, the Dean of the Board of Faculty remained officially a coopted member of the Association Council and Advisory Committee during that period, although there was no official cross-representation on the Board.

There was, however, increasing unofficial cross-representation by members who were elected to both the Board of Faculty and the Council of the Association of Anaesthetists. Four of the seven Presidents of the Association since 1982 have been contemporaneously elected members of the Board of Faculty (since 1988 the College Council) and, happily, Maurice Burrows (1988-1990) was coopted to the Board in Committee of the College. Morrell Lyons (1994-1996), who was particularly instrumental in fostering a close relationship between the two bodies,[140] and his successors Leslie Baird and Maldwyn Morgan have been coopted as Members of the College Council. The President of the College is coopted both to the Council of the Association of Anaesthetists and the Advisory Committee. There is also an exchange of minutes between the organisations.[140-144] The elevation of the two coopted members of the committee of the Association's Group of Anaesthetists in Training to full membership of the Council of the Royal College of Anaesthetists is a pleasing demonstration of the close cooperation of the two bodies (Royal College of Anaesthetists' Annual Report 1995-1996).

Liaison with the Department of Health. Several meetings took place in 1994 and 1996 between the President of the Association of Anaesthetists (Morrell Lyons), the President of the Royal College of Anaesthetists (Cedric Prys-Roberts), and the Minister of Health (Gerald Malone) and officials of the NHS Executive. The purpose was to discuss matters of mutual concern to anaesthetists and the Department.[140-144] Topics which were discussed included: the service implications of the Calman Report, stress and suicide amongst anaesthetists, the effects of the constraints of funding, "rationalisation" and inefficiently managed competition on new developments, the perceived concerns of the Health and Safety Executive over pollution due to anaesthetic gases and vapours, the effect of the new management structure on teaching and research, the increasing incidence of consultant anaesthetists taking early retirement, the General Medical Council initiatives on poor performance amongst doctors, the need for High Dependency Units, and the reorganisation of the blood transfusion service.[140,142]

Nurse and non-physician anaesthesia again! It is not surprising that at a time of shortage of physician anaesthetists, some hard pressed consultant anaesthetists, and more particularly NHS managers, should be tempted to contemplate turning to nurses and other non-medically qualified anaesthetists for the administration of anaesthesia.[145]

The Association established a working party under the chairmanship of its President, Morrell Lyons, to re-examine and report on the issues. This it did early in 1996, in a booklet entitled *"Anaesthesia in Great Britain and Ireland: A Physician Only Service"*. This "made a clear statement about the paramount position of the medical anaesthetist in Great Britain and Ireland in the provision of an anaesthetic service."[146]

The report of Charles Reilly, Professor of Anaesthesia, Sheffield, (*Professional Roles in Anaesthetics: a Scoping Study*) was presented to the NHS Executive in March 1996.[142,148-150] The report drew attention to the fact that the United States was the only English speaking country in the world to allow nurses to work as independent anaesthesia providers. It concluded that there was no support from any national medical or nursing body for the introduction of nurse anaesthetists. There was support, however, for defining and developing the roles of anaesthetists' assistants, whether nurses or operating room assistants or practitioners, and there was a need to explore the framework of an ideal anaesthetic team. Such sentiments are, of course, very welcome to the Association of Anaesthetists which has long advocated adequate and properly organised and registered assistants for anaesthetists (Chapters 8 and 9).

The Reilly Report also advocated the setting up of a mechanism for a national overview of the development of anaesthetic services. The NHS Executive responded by setting up a steering group to evaluate further "professional roles in anaesthesia". Both the Association of Anaesthetists and the Royal College of Anaesthetists were strongly represented on the group and focused its efforts towards preoperative screening of patients, resuscitation, acute pain management and intensive care, rather than the use of nurses to deliver general anaesthesia.[147] A report of a working party of the Association of Anaesthetists entitled *"The Anaesthetic Team"* making recommendations in this direction has been published in 1998.

The Audit Commission also began evaluating anaesthetic services, including acute and chronic pain relief, in 1997, for one of their "value for money" investigations.[141] The President of the Association of Anaesthetists and the President of the Royal College of Anaesthetists were members of the "Advisory Group" of the Commission which generally supported the views of the Association of Anaesthetists in its report.[151]

The composition of the Advisory Committee had remained much the same since the Committee was reorganised in 1973 and 1974. It consisted of the President and Executive Officers of the Association of Anaesthetists, including the President-Elect if there was one, the Chairman of the Junior Anaesthetists' Group (later Group of Anaesthetists in Training), the Dean of the Faculty (later President of the Royal College of Anaesthetists) and the Chairman of the BMA Anaesthetic Subcommittee (if not an Executive Officer of the Association) plus three elected members of Council selected by the Council itself by ballot (Chapter 8). The function of the Advisory Committee remained, on paper, much as defined by Philip Helliwell at his first Council meeting as President in November 1973: that of giving "careful consideration to the Agenda for Council, presenting matters for discussion in a form that would ensure full consideration of the alternatives available". However, in later years, Advisory, having discussed a topic, tended sometimes to present a proposal to Council as a fait accompli rather than with alternatives. Morrell Lyons as President (1994-1996) was of the opinion that the full potential of elected members was not being utilised, that they lacked a forum, and that election to Advisory was divisive. Lyons proposed that all elected members should serve on Advisory in their second and subsequent years on Council, and that the agenda of Advisory should be tailored to allow longer discussion on specific topics. (Council Minutes 3.2.1995). These proposals received general approval and were accepted.[141]

The list of committees and working parties of the Association bears testimony to the large number of commitments of the Association of Anaesthetists in 1998. There are, first, the six major divisions, the Council and the Advisory Committee, the Group of Anaesthetists in Training, the Editorial Board of *Anaesthesia*, the Management Committee of *Anaesthesia News,* and the Standing Committee in Ireland of the Association of Anaesthetists of Great Britain and Ireland; then, the permanent standing committees, Finance, Safety, Standards, International Relations, Independent Practice, Museum, Library and Archives, Specialist Societies and the new Management and Working Practice Committee.

Finally, there are the working parties, the majority of which are preparing or revising reports and the now well known "glossy" booklets on specific topics relating to anaesthesia (in 1997 HIV and blood borne viruses, risk management, stress, the anaesthesia team, the provision of pain services, anaesthetic services for obstetrics (in conjunction with the Obstetric Anaesthetists' Association), and the checklist for anaesthetic equipment).[151]

The Journals of the Association of Anaesthetists of Great Britain and Ireland in the 1990s

The journal *Anaesthesia* under the editorship of Maldwyn Morgan of the Royal Postgraduate Medical School, London, with the assistance of a talented team of Assistant Editors produced its fiftieth annual volume in 1995. Mal Morgan wrote a perceptive and sympathetic editorial in the January 1995 issue detailing the history of the journal and its present policies.[152] Two pleasing aspects are that the present Editor continues to put emphasis on papers of obvious clinical relevance, because that is what interests most of his readers, and the continuance of a lively correspondence section.[152]

The fiftieth volume printed, in each of its twelve issues, a paper from a past year which was of significant importance at the time that it was published. The Editor and his immediate predecessor John Lunn (1982-1990), selected the articles; interestingly, all the twelve papers chosen were published between 1960 and 1969.

There have only been five Editors of *Anaesthesia*, Christopher Langton Hewer (1946-1966), Roger Bryce-Smith (1967-1972), Tom Boulton (1973-1982), John Lunn (1982-1990), and Maldwyn Morgan (1990-1998). Langton Hewer, the Founder Editor, died in 1986 in his ninetieth year.[153] The other four are alive and well at the time of writing. Three of them attended a luncheon hosted by the President of the Association and received presentations during the Golden Jubilee Year.[142] Professor Michael Harmer of Cardiff takes over the Editorship in 1999 after Maldwyn Morgan has become President of the Association of Anaesthetists.

The contract for the publication of *Anaesthesia* from January 1997 was awarded once again to Blackwell Science of Oxford who, as Blackwell Scientific Publications, had previously published Anaesthesia on behalf of the Association of Anaesthetists from 1973 to 1981 (Chapter 8). The parting with W B Saunders (previously Academic Press) was made amicably and with regret on a purely commercial basis.[142]

***Anaesthesia News*,** that lively and often humorous newsletter, which had taken over "the news and views" functions of *Anaesthesia* in 1987, also had cause for celebration in 1995 when it published its 100th issue in November.[154] *Anaesthesia News* was originally conceived by John Lunn, then Editor of *Anaesthesia*, as a separate publication to accommodate calendars of events and other nonscientific items, and thus to free up additional space in the parent journal for scientific material. *Anaesthesia News*, originally managed by the Editorial Board of *Anaesthesia*, achieved independent status within the Association of Anaesthetists with its own Management Board in 1990.

The 100th issue contained revealing articles by its two Editors (John Horton of Cardiff 1987-1992 and Ed (J E) Charlton of Newcastle upon Tyne, who was appointed in 1993), and many reminiscences and photographs of the events which the newsletter had covered during its existence.[154] *Anaesthesia News* now has its own unique place in the hearts of members of the Association for information, interest and amusement, and as a special forum for their own medicopolitical and clinical views, as well as those of the very perceptive Deefer Dog!

The Association of Anaesthetists' web site. The Association of Anaesthetists' home page was inaugurated officially in 1996, and was the first UK medical web site maintaining the Association's reputation for innovation. Ed Charlton and Roger Hayes had maintained an Association presence on the Internet for some time beforehand, and the Association web site was given to their care.[142,143]

The sesquicentennial (150th anniversary) celebrations of Morton's first public demonstration of ether anaesthesia in 1846

A meeting was held at the Queen Elizabeth II Conference Centre, Westminster on 16 January 1997 to celebrate the 150th anniversary of Morton's first successful public demonstration of anaesthesia by the inhalation of ether on 16 October 1846.[143,155]

The meeting was organised jointly by the Association of Anaesthetists of Great Britain and Ireland, the History of Anaesthesia Society, and the Sections of Anaesthesia and History of Medicine of the Royal Society of Medicine. A celebration dinner was held at the Dorchester, Park Lane the following day (17 January 1997), as had been the case fifty years before, for the centenary of Morton's demonstration (Chapter 5). The sponsorship of the meeting by Intavent, Zeneca and Abbott Laboratories, and of the dinner by Intavent, was greatly appreciated.[143,155]

Summary: The Association of Anaesthetists of Great Britain and Ireland, 1932-1997

This volume has traced the development and achievements of the Association of Anaesthetists of Great Britain and Ireland from its foundation in 1932 to the present, through over sixty years of dramatic sociological, political, scientific and medical change.

British anaesthesia 1932-1948. Developments in anaesthesia certainly occurred in the major teaching and specialist hospitals in the 30s, but elsewhere, anaesthesia remained a "rag and bottle" General Practitioner procedure. There is, therefore, no doubt that Harry Featherstone founded the Association of Anaesthetists of Great Britain and Ireland in 1932 primarily as an elite organisation, in order to better the conditions under which university anaesthetists worked; in addition, he had the vision to see that a specialist diploma in anaesthetics would greatly enhance their status. The new Association of Anaesthetists was, however, prepared to give kindly paternalistic advice to all those who practised anaesthesia but did not qualify for membership (Chapter 3).

The major achievement of the Association of Anaesthetists during the 1930s was in fact the establishment of the Diploma of Anaesthetics by the Conjoint Board, which they managed to have awarded without examination to members of the Association with suitable seniority (Chapter 4).

Paradoxically, it was the Second World War (1939-1945) which raised the status of anaesthesia, both clinically and professionally. The amalgamation of the civilian hospital services, both voluntary and municipal, into the Emergency Medical Service (EMS) at the beginning of the war brought with it a demand for salaried anaesthetists in the EMS. The great expansion of the medical branches of the British armed services (particularly the army) brought with it the need for young medical practitioners to administer anaesthesia in field surgical teams and military hospitals around the world. The senior members of the Association of Anaesthetists of Great Britain and Ireland, the only body representing anaesthetists in the United Kingdom at the time, were closely involved in the training of members of the expanding specialty and saw to it that the possession of the Diploma of Anaesthetics was a passport to higher military rank. There were, coincidentally, major medical developments which intimately concerned anaesthesia. These included the organisation of a first-class blood transfusion service and the discovery of penicillin. The performance of anaesthetists in preoperative resuscitation, in the operating theatre itself, and in the perioperative period resulted in added respect from their surgical colleagues (Chapter 5).

Anaesthesia in the post war period and in the British National Health Service. The end of the Second World War and demobilisation released a body of young, qualified and experienced anaesthetists ready and willing to staff the new United Kingdom National Health Service. The upgrading of the Diploma in Anaesthetics and the foundation of the Faculty of Anaesthetists (promoted by the Association of Anaesthetists with the backing of the Royal College of Surgeons) and the conversion of the upgraded Diploma into a Fellowship in Anaesthesia, led, after some considerable negotiation to the acceptance of anaesthetists as Consultants of equal rank with other specialties in the new NHS (Chapter 5).

The 1950s were a period of considerable development in techniques of clinical anaesthesia. The introduction of the muscle relaxants and the revolutionary new inhalation agent halothane, coupled with the use of controlled ventilation, was one of the great turning points in the practice of anaesthesia, in which British anaesthetists took the lead. The way was then open for the development of thoracic, cardiac and neurosurgical anaesthesia, and great improvements in techniques for abdominal surgery. The introduction of new and more effective local anaesthetic agents and the development of the epidural technique led, in the same period, to a revolution in obstetric anaesthesia. Administratively it was in the 1950s that the Association of Anaesthetists overcame its reluctance to enter into educational activities and began to have scientific programmes at its meetings. The 1960s were a decade in which many new drugs were introduced, particularly intravenous agents. Much more importantly, however, British and Irish physician anaesthetists began to develop services outside the operating theatre, which were, in many instances, unconnected with the actual administration of anaesthesia. These developments included managing and teaching the new techniques of cardiopulmonary resuscitation, the establishment of postoperative recovery rooms and subsequent development into the care of patients in intensive care units (ICU); so much so that anaesthesia became the dominant specialty in the ICUs of the United Kingdom.

It was also in the 1960s that the educational programme for registrars in the Association of Anaesthetists evolved into the foundation of the Junior Anaesthetists' Group (now the Group of Anaesthetists in Training) which has been a major success story for the specialty (Chapter 7).

The stable administrative structure based on the old voluntary hospital system had been very successful in promoting clinical development in the NHS in the first twenty years of its existence. The nineteen seventies were to be different. The cost of running the NHS, fuelled by very successful but unforeseen medical developments, far exceeded the original estimates. It was an unhappy time in the NHS with pay freezes and considerable industrial unrest. Paradoxically, the Association of Anaesthetists flourished in the seventies. It moved to its own suite of offices in BMA House, greatly improved its financial management, considerably enhanced its educational and research activities and initiated medical audit into perioperative deaths (Chapter 8).

In the 1980s and early 1990s a series of politically motivated reorganisations took place in the NHS (Chapter 9). The Association of Anaesthetists prospered and grew in stature during these difficult years, however, particularly after the acquisition of its own free-standing home, the elegant Georgian house at 9 Bedford Square, in 1985. The educational and research activities of the Association expanded, and the very successful seminar programme was introduced. The Association also played its part in preparing and encouraging its members to participate in the new management structure of the NHS and its Hospital Trusts (Chapter 9).

Summary: The Association of Anaesthetists of Great Britain and Ireland, 1932-1997

The Association celebrated its Diamond Jubilee in style in 1992 and, in the same year, the dream of the foundation of a Royal College of Anaesthetists, so long promoted by the Association of Anaesthetists, became reality, and the Royal College acquired its own premises close at hand in Russell Square with the financial support of the Association (Chapter 9).

Calman and its consequences 1993-1997. The government's Calman Working Group was originally formed to bring specialist training into line with the directives of the European Union, but the opportunity has been taken to reorganise completely the structure of postgraduate medical education and, to a large extent, to place a defined limit on the length of specialist training. The lead in the mid-1990s in these developments has rightly been taken by the new Royal College of Anaesthetists but the Association of Anaesthetists has played a very important part in influencing the process (Chapter 10).

The future of the Association of Anaesthetists of Great Britain and Ireland. Officers of the Association of Anaesthetists are often asked why the specialty of anaesthesia needs two powerful professional bodies (the Association and the Royal College of Anaesthetists) to represent its interests. The basic position is discussed at length in Chapter 8. The Royal College of Anaesthetists is a body which operates under a Royal Charter and ordinances sanctioned by the Privy Council, with the objective of regulating the professional conduct of its members and maintaining the professional standards of the specialty, including examining its trainees and assessing their competence to practise as independent specialists. A medical Royal College is allowed charitable status only by reason of the fact that it exists to protect the public and does not act in the pecuniary interests of its members. It can only be concerned with the conditions in which its members work if adverse circumstances prevent them practising their specialty to the standards which they have laid down. The Association of Anaesthetists, on the other hand, does not have a Royal Charter, has made its own rules and can support the legitimate interests of its members, and has widened its remit out of all recognition since its foundation in 1932.

What are the major preoccupations of the Association of Anaesthetists in 1998? The principal formal activities are over issues regarding terms and conditions of service, independent practice, etc., which cannot be undertaken by the Royal College of Anaesthetists because of its charitable status. These are illustrated by the long list of standing committees and working parties. This is only part of the story, however. Day by day, individual requests from members of the Association for information, guidance and support flood in to 9 Bedford Square. Such requests have greatly increased since the reorganisation of the 1990s and the introduction of structured and shortened training initiated by the Calman Report.

There are thus, in 1999, two organisations, the Association and the College of Anaesthetists, each with its own clearly defined responsibility, linked by a common interest in Postgraduate Medical Education (PGME). There are some PGME activities administered jointly by the two bodies, but there are generally differences in the nature and content of the educational meetings. This has been especially the case in recent years as the Association has paid particular attention to the continuing medical education (CME) of established anaesthetists in their consultant years including the demands of management.

Could the two organisations be brought together under the same roof? This would probably be possible since the Association of Anaesthetists has demonstrated that, for taxation purposes, it is possible for a charitable body (the Education and Research Trust) to coexist in the same building with one that does not have charitable status to the mutual benefit of both (Chapters 8 and 9). It would have to be a large building however, as probably the only directorates that could be organised jointly would be PGME and Finance.

Could the two bodies have a common Council? This is very doubtful as the two Councils differ considerably. The electorates are different for a start. Association rules permit only ordinary and trainee members from the United Kingdom and the Republic of Ireland to vote in elections. This is because a great deal of its business is, and always has been, connected with the terms and conditions of service relating to clinical practice in Great Britain and Ireland. All Fellows, however, both from the home countries and from overseas, vote to elect members of the Royal College Council. This difference, and the perceived function of the two institutions, result in a differing membership of the two Councils. By and large, academics and those from university hospitals are naturally elected to the College Council,[156] whereas the majority of members of the Association Council come from the rank and file of those employed by the British and Irish health services. The history of the corporate organisation of anaesthesia in Great Britain and Ireland related in this volume has surely demonstrated that there are considerable advantages in having two constitutionally differing bodies looking at those problems which are of mutual concern from different angles.

A conclusion

If Henry (Harry) Walter Featherstone looks down on the world in 1998, he is probably saddened by some of the social changes which have taken place, but he will be amazed and delighted at the enormous progress made in the practice of medicine and anaesthesia.

There is little doubt that Featherstone would approve of the present comprehensive nature of the Association (Chapter 5), representing as it does, the overwhelming majority (over 6,000) of the anaesthetists in the United Kingdom and the Republic of Ireland, both the fully qualified and those in training, as well as nearly 600 overseas members.

The Association of Anaesthetists of Great Britain and Ireland is a unique institution which, because of its independence, flexibility and informality, since its foundation in 1932 has been able to influence every major change in the corporate identity and practice of specialist anaesthesia in the United Kingdom and Ireland. It has also taken the lead in many developments in the international field. The Association has by good husbandry increased its assets so that it was able to disburse research and educational grants of £164,715 in the year April 1996 to March 1997.

Leslie Baird, the 26th successor to Harry Featherstone as President of the Association of Anaesthetists of Great Britain and Ireland has, however, emphasised the essential central commitment of the Association to individuals, in his message to its members in the 1997 Annual Report.[143]

> *"The Association acts as a "sounding board" for its members, reflecting their concerns, aspirations and endeavours. I and your Council look to you to help us maintain and develop communications between 9 Bedford Square and the membership so that our specialty can continue to take its rightful place in the forefront of medicine."*[143]

Harry Featherstone would have said "Amen" to that!

References

Note: in order to avoid needless repetition, single references are made under each chapter heading to the relevant minute books of the Association of Anaesthetists of Great Britain and Ireland (e.g. 16. *AAGBI Minute Book No 1: 1939-1947*; 1-195). Dates of individual meetings are provided in the text to facilitate easy reference.

The Annual Reports of Council from 1932 to 1944 were included in the Minute Books; from 1945 to 1977, the Reports were published. in separate pamphlets; from 1978 to 1995 the Annual Reports were included. in the journal *Anaesthesia* and numbered references are provided; from 1996 onwards the greatly enhanced reports will be kept at the headquarters of the Association separate from *Anaesthesia*.

Chapter 1 - Introductory

1. A new association of anaesthetists. *British Journal of Anaesthesia* 1931-2; **9**: 178.
2. Featherstone H W. The Association of Anaesthetists of Great Britain and Ireland. Its inception and purpose. *Anaesthesia* 1946; **1**: 5-9.
3. Helliwell P J. Editorial. *Anaesthesia* 1982; **37**: 392-7.
4. Obituary. H W Featherstone. *Anaesthesia* 1967; **22**: 532-3.
5. Department of Health. Distinction awards: analysis by type and award, specialty and percentage distribution at 31 December 1992 - England and Wales. *Health Trends* 1993; **25**: 152.
6. Helliwell P J. The Association of Anaesthetists of Great Britain and Ireland. Fifty years of service to the specialty of anaesthesia. *Anaesthesia* 1982; **37**: 913-23.
7. Editorial. Anaesthetic emergency work. *British Journal of Anaesthesia* 1930-31; **8**: 1-2.
8. Gray T C. Editorial 'Forward together'. *Anaesthesia* 1992; **47**: 369-70.

Chapter 2 - Whys and Wherefores

1. Correspondent. Fourth of the series of pioneers of modern anaesthesia. J Frederick William Silk, MD. *British Journal of Anaesthesia* 1926-27; **4**: 178-81.
2. Dinnick O P. The first anaesthetic society. In: Boulton T B, Bryce-Smith R, Sykes M K, Gillett G B, Revell A L. *Progress in Anaesthesiology. Proceedings of the Fourth World Congress of Anaesthesiologists*. 1968. Amsterdam. Excerpta Medica 1970; 181-6.
3. The Sections. Brief summary of proceedings. *British Medical Journal* 1912; **2**: 193.
4. Editorial. In memoriam. Dudley Wilmot Buxton, MD, MRCP. Consulting Anaesthetist University College Hospital. *British Journal of Anaesthesia* 1930-31; **8**: 129-31.
5. Cohen H M. Foreword. *British Journal of Anaesthesia* 1923-1924; **1**: 1-3.
6. Gray T C. Early history of the *British Journal of Anaesthesia*. In Rupreht J, Van Lieburg

M J, Lee J A, Erdmann W, eds. *Anaesthesia: Essays on its History*, 1985. Berlin: Springer-Verlag, 1985: 297-300.
7. Spence A A. The *British Journal of Anaesthesia*. Its evolution to the present position. In Rupreht J, Van Lieburg M J, Lee J A, Erdmann W, eds. *Anaesthesia. Essays on its History.* Berlin: Springer-Verlag, 1985: 301.
8. Power D A. Obituary. H M Cohen. *British Journal of Anaesthesia* 1929-30; **8**: 99.4951.
9. Evans F T. Obituary. H E G Boyle, *British Journal of Anaesthesia* 1942-43; 18: 43-4.
10. Mennell Z. Joseph Blomfield, *Anaesthesia* 1949; **4**: 89-93.
11. Betcher A M, Ciliberti B J, Wood P M, Wright L H. The Jubilee Year of organised anesthesia. *Anesthesiology* 1956; **17**: 226-64.
12. Ranney O. Francis Hoeffer McMechan. A brief sketch of his life and work. *Current Researches in Anesthesia and Analgesia* 1939; **18** (special supplement to No 6): 1-17.
13. Cohen H M. International contacts and publications. *British Journal of Anaesthesia* 1927-28; **5**: 21-3.
14. Editorial. Anaesthetists' worries. *British Journal of Anaesthesia* 1931-32; **9**: 57-8.
15. Editorial. *British Journal of Anaesthesia* 1931-32; **9**: 141.
16. A new Association of Anaesthetists. *British Journal of Anaesthesia* 1931-32; **9**: 178.
17. Ross J S. *The National Health Service in Great Britain. An Historical and Descriptive Survey*. Oxford: University Press, 1952.
18. Honigsbaum F. *The Division in British Medicine. A Short History of the Separation of General Practice from Hospital Care 1911-1968*. London: Kohan Page, 1979.
19. Waddy F F. Correspondence. *British Journal of Anaesthesia* 1930-31; **8**: 172.
20. Editorial. Our hospital emoluments. *British Journal of Anaesthesia* 1927-28; **5**: 107-8.
21 Jones W H. Anaesthetists in the unit system. *Lancet* 1931; **2**: 1156.
22. Annotation. Anaesthetists to surgical units. *Lancet* 1931; **2**: 1141-2.
23. Mortis R H. Anaesthetists in the unit system. *Lancet* 1931; **2**: 1211.
24. Webber H N. Anaesthetists in the unit system. *Lancet* 1931; **2**: 1211-2.
25. Clausen R C. Anaesthetists in the unit system. *Lancet* 1931; **2**: 1268.
26. Obituary. William Howard Jones, Surgeon Anaesthetist Charing Cross. *British Journal of Anaesthesia* 1935-36; **13**: 39-40.
27. Editorial. *British Journal of Anaesthesia* 1935-36; **13**: 1-2.
28. Edwards G. Emergency anaesthetics in hospitals. *British Journal of Anaesthesia* 1930-31; **8:** 15-18.
29. Editorial. Anaesthetic emergency work. *British Journal of Anaesthesia* 1930-31; **8**: 1-2.
30. Moir E. Correspondence. *British Journal of Anaesthesia* 1930-31; **8**: 79.
31. Ross J S, Fairlie H P. *Handbook of Anaesthetics*. Edinburgh: Livingstone, 1929.
32. Hewer C L. *Recent Advances in Anaesthesia and Analgesia*. London: Churchill, 1932.
33. Reviews. Recent Advances in Anaesthesia and Analgesia. *British Journal of Anaesthesia* 1932-33; **10**: 46.
34. Hornabrook R W. Correspondence. *British Journal of Anaesthesia* 1930-31; **8**: 125-8.
35. Editorial. Machines and men. *British Journal of Anaesthesia* 1929-30; **7**: 97-8.
36. "Robot". Correspondence. *British Journal of Anaesthesia* 1929-30; **7**: 184.
37. Hornabrook R W. A protest against the indulgence in the mechanical forms of anaesthetic administration. *British Journal of Anaesthesia* 1930-31; **8**: 36-9.
38. Boyle H E G. The anaesthetic equipment for the new surgical block of St Bartholomew's

Hospital. *British Journal of Anaesthesia* 1929-30; **7**: 130-4.
39. Finisterer F. The choice of anaesthetic for abdominal surgery. *British Journal of Anaesthesia* 1931-32; **7**: 143-61.
40. Mackenzie J R. Modern anaesthetics. The teaching of the undergraduate. *British Journal of Anaesthesia* 1931-32; **9**: 175-7.
41. Hadfield C F. Modern aids to anaesthesia. *British Journal of Anaesthesia* 1932-33; **10**: 62-73.
42. Clausen R J. Section of Anaesthetics Royal Society of Medicine. *British Journal of Anaesthesia* 1929-30; **7**: 180-1.
43. Jarman F S. General anaesthetics applicable to dental operations. *British Journal of Anaesthesia* 1929-30; **7**: 28-33.
44. De Caux F P. A system of anaesthesia for the dental anaesthetist. *British Journal of Anaesthesia* 1931-32; **9**: 22-40.
45. Mennell Z. Some difficulties which may occur in the administration of anaesthesia for cerebral operations. *British Journal of Anaesthesia* 1929-30; **7**: 52-8.
46. Mackenzie J R. Notes on anaesthesia for thoracic surgery. *British Journal of Anaesthesia* 1932-33; **10**: 19-24.
47. Jones W W. Spinal analgesia. A new drug. Percaine. *British Journal of Anaesthesia* 1929-30; **7**: 99-113.
48. Hall E F. Spinal anaesthesia. Spinocain and Duracain. *British Journal of Anaesthesia* 1930-31; **8**: 132-50.
49. Rowbotham S. Premedication. *British Journal of Anaesthesia* 1931-32; **9**: 41-55.
50. Crile G W, Lower W E. *Surgical Shock and the Shockless Operation through Anoci-association*. Philadelphia: Saunders, 1920.
51. Shipway F E. Resuscitation during anaesthesia and the newly born. *British Journal of Anaesthesia* 1931-32; **9**: 69-79.
52. Editorial. What of the future? *British Journal of Anaesthesia* 1926-27; **4**: 113-5.
53. Buxton D W. The teaching of anaesthetics in medical schools. *British Journal of Anaesthesia* 1926-27; **4**: 124-31.
54. Obituary. J R Mackenzie. *Anaesthesia* 1964; **19**: 153.

Chapter 3 - The Foundation, January to July 1932

1. Obituary. H W Featherstone. *Anaesthesia* 1967; **22**: 532-3.
2. Helliwell P J. Editorial. *Anaesthesia* 1982; **37**: 394-7.
3. Obituary. Henry Walter Featherstone. *Lancet* 1967; **1**: 1012-3.
4. APT. Obituary Notices. H W Featherstone. *British Medical Journal* 1967; **2**: 380.
5. Featherstone H W. President's Address. A visit to some of the hospitals in Canada and to the Mayo Clinic. *Proceedings of the Royal Society of Medicine* 1930-31; **24**: 103-6.
6. Section of Anaesthetics. *British Journal of Anaesthesia* 1930-31; **8**: 74.
7. Featherstone H W. The Association of Anaesthetists of Great Britain and Ireland. Its inception and purpose. *Anaesthesia* 1946; **1**: 5-9.
8. Featherstone H W. *Memorandum to the Association of Anaesthetists of Great Britain and Ireland* 1946. An unpublished document in the Archives of the Association of Anaesthetists of Great Britain and Ireland.
9. Obituary. William Howard Jones, Surgeon Anaesthetist, Charing Cross. *British Journal of*

Anaesthesia 1935-36; **13**: 39-40.
10. Boulton T B. Sir Geoffrey Marshall, Shock and nitrous oxide. *Survey of Anesthesiology* 1992; **36:** 40-5.
11. FTE Obituary. H E G Boyle *British Journal of Anaesthesia* 943; **18**: 43-4.
12. Hadfield C F. Eminent anaesthetists. H Edmund G Boyle. *British Journal of Anaesthesia* 1950; **22**: 107-17.
13. Obituary. Zebulon Mennell. *Anaesthesia* 1959; **4**: 210-12.
14. Mennell Z. The second Embley Memorial Lecture delivered at Melbourne University. *British Journal of Anaesthesia* 1935-36; **13**: 3-24.
15. H M. Obituary. Dr C W Morris. *Anaesthesia* 1969; **24**: 295-6.
16. *AAGBI Minute Book No 1: 1932-47*; pp 1-195.
17. W S McC. Obituary. Sir Francis Shipway, KCVO *Anaesthesia* 1969; **24**: 296.
18. A new Association of Anaesthetists. *British Journal of Anaesthesia* 1931-32; **9**: 178.
19. Editorial. *British Journal of Anaesthesia* 1931-32; **9**: 141-2.
20. Mennell Z. Obituary. Joseph Blomfield. *Anaesthesia* 1949; **4**: 89-93.
21. A R H. Obituary. E F Hill. *British Medical Journal* 1974; **3**: 746.
22. Obituary. Ashley Skeffington Daly. *Anaesthesia* 1959; **14**: 210-20.
23. Z M. John Henry Chaldecolt. A*naesthesia* 1950; **5**: 160.
24. Cohen H M. Foreword. *British Journal of Anaesthesia* 1923-24; **1**: 1-3.

Chapter 4 - The Prewar years, 2 July 1932 to 3 September 1939

1. Obituary. H W Featherstone. *Anaesthesia* 1967; **22**: 532-3.
2. Mennell Z. Obituary. Joseph Blomfield. *Anaesthesia* 1949; **4**: 89-93.
3. Obituary. Zebulon Mennell. *Anaesthesia* 1959; **14**: 210-12.
4. Obituary. H S Sington. *Anaesthesia* 1956; **11**: 185.
5. Obituary. William Howard Jones, Surgeon Anaesthetist Charing Cross. *British Journal of Anaesthesia* 1935-36; **13**: 39-40.
6. Ross J S. *The National Health Service in Great Britain. An Historical and Descriptive survey*. Oxford: University Press; 1952.
7. Owen D. Back to a two-tier health service. *St Thomas' Hospital Gazette* 1989; **81**: 189-94.
8. Honigsbaum F. *The Division in British Medicine. A History of the Separation of General Practice and Hospital Care*. 1911-1968. London: Kogan Page, 1979.
9. Dodd H G. Anaesthesia and the Law. *British Journal of Anaesthesia* 1938-39; **16**: 16-21.
10. Sykes W S. Anaesthesia, its present and future. *British Journal of Anaesthesia* 1935-36; **13**: 28-32 and 41-53.
11. Singer C, Underwood E A. *A Short History of Medicine*. Oxford: University Press, 1962: 693-7.
12. Rhodes P. *An Outline History of Medicine*. London: Butterworths, 1985: 142-5.
13. Woollam C H M. The development of apparatus for intermittent negative pressure respiration. In: Atkinson R S, Boulton T B. *History of Anaesthesia. International Congress Series* 134. London: Royal Society of Medicine, 1989: 393-401.
14. Mushin W W. Editorial. Professor Emeritus Sir Robert Reynolds Macintosh: 17 October 1897 - 28 August 1989. *Anaesthesia* 1989; **44**: 951.
15. Beinart J. *A History of the Nuffield Department of Anaesthetics Oxford 1937-1987*. Oxford: University Press, 1987.

16. Mackenzie J R. Modern Anaesthetics. The teaching of the undergraduate. *British Journal of Anaesthesia* 1931-32; **9**: 175-7.
17. Ross J S, Fairlie H P. *Handbook of Anaesthetics*. 4th edition. Edinburgh: Livingstone, 1935.
18. Minnitt R J. *Handbook of Anaesthetics. Formerly Ross and Fairlie, 5th edition*. Edinburgh: Livingstone, 1940.
19. Ayre P. The student anaesthetist. *British Journal of Anaesthesia* 1938-39; **16**: 10-15.
20. Elam J. The teaching of anaesthetic methods for use in general practice. *British Journal of Anaesthetics* 1939-41; **17**: 57-60.
21. Obituary. W S Sykes. *British Medical Journal* 1961; **1**: 1258-9.
22. Waters R M, Schmidt E R. Cyclopropane anaesthesia. *Journal of the American Medical Association* 1934; **103**: 975-83.
23. Griffith H R. Cyclopropane: a revolutionary anaesthetic agent. *Canadian Medical Association Journal* 1937; **35**: 496-500.
24. Rowbotham E S, Charter A, Jarman R, Phillips G R, Vaile T B. Cyclopropane anaesthesia: a report based on 250 cases. *Lancet* 1935; **2**: 1110-3.
25. Casual comments. *British Journal of Anaesthesia* 1933-34; **11**: 122-3.
26. Casual comments. Cyclopropane. *British Journal of Anaesthesia* 1933-34; **11**: 157.
27. Guedel A E. Cyclopropane anaesthesia. *Anesthesiology* 1940; **1**: 13-25.
28. Nosworthy M D. Anaesthesia in chest surgery with special reference to controlled respiration with cyclopropane. *Proceedings of the Royal Society of Medicine* 1941; **34**: 479-505.
29. Weese H, Scharpff W. Evipan, ein neuortiges Einsch lat mittel. *Deutsche Medizin ische Wochenschrift* 1932; **58**: 1205-7.
30. Lundy J S, Tovell R M. Intravenous anaesthesia. Preliminary report of the use of two new thiobarbiturates. *Proceedings of the Staff Meetings of the Mayo Clinic* 1935; **10**: 536-43.
31. Pratt T W, Tatum A L, Hathaway H R, Waters R M. Sodium ethyl (e-methyl butyl) thiobarbiturate. Preliminary experimental and clinical study. *American Journal of Surgery* 1936; **31**: 464-6.
32. Jarman R, Abel L. Evipan, an intravenous anaesthetic agent. *Lancet* 1933; **2**: 18-20.
33. Jarman R, Abel L. Intravenous anaesthesia with pentothal sodium. *Lancet* 1936; **1**: 422-3.
34. Anaesthetics Committee Medical Research Council and Royal Society of Medicine. A report on the clinical value of "Evipan". *British Journal of Anaesthesia* 1933-34; **11**: 23-8.
35. Bourne W Analgesia and anaesthesia in obstetrics. Pentothal sodium, cyclopropane and vinyl ether. *British Journal of Anaesthesia* 1937-38; **15**: 1-8.
36. Dixon C P. Some observations on pentothal sodium. *British Journal of Anaesthesia* 1937-38; **15**: 60-1.
37. Jarman R. The combination of intravenous with spinal anaesthesia, using pentothal and percaine. *British Journal of* Anaesthesia 1937-38; **15**: 20-4.
38. Marriott H L, Kekwick A. Continuous drip blood transfusion: with case records of very large transfusions. *Lancet* 1935; **1**: 977-81.
39. Laurie R D. New inventions. An apparatus for indicating the rate of flow of saline solution in subcutaneous and rectal administration. *Lancet* 1909; **1**: 248.
40. Helliwell P J. The Association of Anaesthetists of Great Britain and Ireland. Fifty years of service to the specialty. *Anaesthesia* 1982; **37**: 913-23.
41. Casual comments. *British Journal of Anaesthesia* 1932-33; **10**: 133-6.
42. *AAGBI Minute Book No 1. 1932-1947*. pp 1-195.

43. The Association of Anaesthetists. *British Journal of Anaesthesia* 1938-39; **16**: 71.
44. Featherstone H W. Association of Anaesthetists of Great Britain and Ireland. *British Medical Journal* 1932; **2**: 421-2.
45. Featherstone H W. Association of Anaesthetists of Great Britain and Ireland. *British Medical Journal* 1932; **2**: 539-40.
46. Annotation. An Association of Anaesthetists. *Lancet* 1932; **2**: 527.
47. The Association of Anaesthetists of Great Britain and Ireland. *British Journal of Anaesthesia* 1932-33; **10**: 38
48. Betcher A M, Gilberti B J, Wood P M, Wright L H. The Jubilee Year of organised anesthesia. *Anesthesiology* 1956; **17**: 226-64.
49. Chambers E J. The story of a journey in search of information. *British Journal of Anaesthesia* 1927-28; **5**: 158-67.
50. Dr Ralph M Waters' visit to London. *British Journal of Anaesthesia* 1936-37; **14**: 35-6.
51. FTE. Obituary. H E G Boyle. *British Journal of Anaesthesia* 1942-43; **18**: 42-3.
52. Foregger R. Gwathmey *Anesthesiology* 1944; **5**: 296-9.
53. Thomas K B. *The Development of Anaesthetic Apparatus. A History Based on the Charles King Collection of the Association of Anaesthetists of Great Britain and Ireland*. Oxford: Blackwell Scientific Publications, 1975.
54. Griffith H R. Obituary. Wesley Bourne 1886-1965. *Anaesthesia* 1965; **20**: 376-7.
55. Wilson G. *Fifty Years. The Australia Society of Anaesthetists 1934-1984*. Edge Cliff, Australian Society of Anaesthetists, 1987.
56. Mennell Z. The Second Embley Memorial Lecture delivered at the Melbourne University. *British Journal of Anaesthesia* 1935-36; **13**: 3-24.
57. Wilson G. Obituary. Geoffrey Kaye 1903-1986. *Anaesthesia and Intensive Care* 1987; **15**: 107-9.
58. Annual Report to Council 1935-1936 *British Medical Journal* 1936; **1**: Supplement p 215.
59. Annual Report of Council 1935-1936. *British Medical Journal* 1936; **1**: 207-8.
60. Annual Representative Meeting. *British Medical Journal* 1937; **2**: Supplement pp 56-8.
61. Annual Representative Meeting. *British Medical Journal* 1938; **2**: Supplement pp 74-75.
62. Annual Representative Meeting 1938. *British Medical Journal* 1938; **2**: Supplement 72-73.
63. Association of Anaesthetists of Great Britain and Ireland. Annual Report of Council 1989-1990. *Anaesthesia* 1991; **46**: 243-53.
64. Leading Article. A diploma in anaesthetics. *Lancet* 1935; **1**: 1451.
65. Edridge A W. Editorial. Sir Ivan Whiteside Magill. *Anaesthesia* 1987; **42**: 231-3.
66. Magill I W. An appraisal of progress in anaesthetics. Frederic Hewitt Lecture 1965. *Annals of the Royal College of Surgeons of England* 1966; **38**: 154-65.
67. C L H. Obituary. Charles Frederick Hadfield. *Anaesthesia* 1965; **20**: 514-5
68. Examining Board in England. Regulations for obtaining the Diploma in Anaesthetics. *British Journal of Anaesthesia* 1934-35; **12**: 184-7.
69. The Diploma in Anaesthetics. *British Journal of Anaesthesia* 1935-36; **13**: 33 & 54-55
70. The Diploma in Anaesthetics. *British Journal of Anaesthesia* 1936-37; **14**: 83-4 and 94.
71. The Diploma in Anaesthetics. *British Journal of Anaesthesia* 1937-38; **15**: 69-70 and 116.
72. The Diploma in Anaesthetics. *British Journal of Anaesthesia* 1938-39: **16**: 28, 109 and

141.
73. Editorial. The Diploma in Anaesthetics. *British Journal of Anaesthesia* 1938-39; **16**: 81-2.
74. Editorial. The Nuffield Professorship of Anaesthetics. *British Journal of Anaesthesia* 1936-37; **14**: 93-4.
75. Macintosh R R, Pratt F B. *Essentials of General Anaesthesia with Special Reference to Dentistry*. Oxford: Blackwell, 1940.
76. Casual comments. *British Journal of Anaesthesia* 1932-35; **10**: 133-6.
77. Association of Anaesthetists of Great Britain and Ireland. *British Journal of Anaesthesia* 1933-34; **11**: 84-6.
78. Editorial. Anaesthetics for midwifery. *British Journal of Anaesthesia* 1933-34; **11**: 1-2.
79. Casual comments. Confinements. *British Journal of Anaesthesia* 1933-34; **11**: 80-1.
80. Boulton T B. Anaesthesia and resuscitation in difficult environments. In: Hewer C L, ed. *Recent Advances in Anaesthesia and Analgesia* 11th edition. Edinburgh: Churchill Livingstone, 1972: 143-238.
81. T C G. Obituary. R J Minnitt. *British Medical Journal* 1974: **1**: 464.
82. Minnitt R J. Self-administered analgesia for midwifery in general practice. *Proceedings of the Royal Society of Medicine* 1934; **27**: 1313-18.
83. Minnitt R J. *Gas and Air Analgesia*. London: Bailliere, 1938.
84. Annotation. Coroners under review. *British Medical Journal* 1936; **1**: 318-9.
85. Casual comments. Coroners inquests. *British Journal of Anaesthesia* 1933-34; **11**: 157-8.
86. Coroners law and practice. The Departmental Committee Report. *British Medical Journal* 1936; **1**: 322-4.
87. Gordon-Taylor G. Obituary. Raymond Apperly. *Anaesthesia* 1960; **15**: 196-7.
88. Medical notes in Parliament. Coroners inquests: Committee of Inquiry. *British Medical Journal* 1935; **1**: 234-5.
89. Medical notes in Parliament. Coroners inquests. Personnel of Committee. *British Medical Journal* 1935; **1**: 509-10.
90. Featherstone H W. The Association of Anaesthetists of Great Britain and Ireland. Its inception and purpose. *Anaesthesia* 1946; **1**: 5-9.
91. Boulton T B. Editorial. C Langton Hewer. *Anaesthesia* 1986; **41**: 469.
92. HCC-D. Obituary. M D Nosworthy. 1980; 815.
93. Association news. *Anaesthesia* 1951; **6**: 124.
94. Association news. *Anaesthesia* 1952; **7**: 263.
95. Burns R. *To a mouse*. 1786.

Chapter 5 - War and Peace, 3 September 1939 to 31 December 1948

1. Obituary. Z Mennell. *Anaesthesia* 1959; **14**: 210-2.
2. Obituary. Ashley Skeffington Daly. *Anaesthesia*, 1978; **33**: 387-9.
3. W S M. Obituary. Archibald D Marston. *Anaesthesia* 1962; **17**: 260-1.
4. Helliwell P J, Pinkerton H H. Obituary. John Gillies. President of the Association of Anaesthetists of Great Britain and Ireland 1947-1950. *Anaesthesia,* 1976; **31**: 1311-13.
5. Obituary. H S Sington. *Anaesthesia* 1956; **11**: 185.
6. O P D. Obituary. Bernard Johnson. *Anaesthesia* 1959; **14**: 419-21.
7. Z M. Obituary. Joseph Blomfield. *Anaesthesia* 1949; **4**: 89-93.

8. R B W, W D W. Obituary. W A Low. *Anaesthesia* 1970; **25**: 587.
9. Pallister W K. Editorial. Sir Geoffrey Stephen William Organe. *Anaesthesia* 1989; **44**: 461-2.
10. Boulton T B. Editorial. C Langton Hewer. *Anaesthesia* 1986; **41**: 469.
11. Ross J S. *The National Health Service in Great Britain. An Historic Descriptive Survey.* Oxford: University Press, 1952.
12. Honigsbaum F. *The Division in British Medicine. A History of the Separation of General Practice from Hospital Care.* London: Kogan Page, 1979.
13. Edwards B. *The National Health Service. A Manager's Tale 1946-1992.* London: Nuffield Provincial Hospitals Trust, 1993.
14. Blair J S G. Mitchmer Lecturer 1994. *Journal of the Royal Army Medical Corps* 1995; **141**: 7-14.
15. Harris J. Beveridge, William Henry, Baron Beveridge (1879-1963). In: Williams E T and Nicholls C S, eds. *The Dictionary of National Biography*, 1961-1970. Oxford: University Press, 1981: 102-8.
16. Dunn C L. *The Emergency Medical Services.* London: Her Majesty's Stationery Office, 1952.
17. Mansfield R. Reminiscences of anaesthesia during the blitz and 10 happy years in India. In: Rupreht J, Lieburg M J V, Lee J A, Erdmann W, eds. *Anaesthesia. Essays on its History.* Berlin: Springer-Verlag, 1985: 228-33.
18. Lee J A, Lunn J N. Editorial. John Alfred Lee (1906-1989). *Anaesthesia* 1989; **44**: 631.
19. Atkinson R S, Rushman G B, Davies N J H. *Lee's Synopsis of Anaesthesia.* 11th edition. Oxford: Butterworth-Heinemann, 1993.
20. *AAGBI Minute Book No 1.* 1932-1947, pp 1-402.
21. Daly A S. Anaesthesia in the army. In: Cope Z, ed. *Surgery*. London: Her Majesty's Stationery Office, 1953: pp 220-3.
22. Featherstone H W. *The Association of Anaesthetists of Great Britain and Ireland. Notes on its Inception and Purpose.* An unpublished document in the archives of the Association of Anaesthetists. 1946.
23. Whitby L. The transfusion of blood and other fluids (i) Blood transfusion. In: Cope Z, ed. *Surgery.* London: Her Majesty's Stationery Office 1953: 46-57.
24. Macintosh R R. Anaesthesia in the Royal Air Force. In: Cope Z, ed.. *Surgery.* London: Her Majesty's Stationery Office, 1953: 223-33.
25. Association News. *Anaesthesia* 1952; **7**: 60.
26. M K S Obituary. Robert Reynolds Macintosh. *Lancet* 1989; **2**: 816.
27. Hall V *Reminiscences and Anaesthesia in India 1939-1946,* Published privately 1998. (Available at the Association of Anaesthetists of Great Britain and Ireland).
28. Obituary H K Ashworth. *Anaesthesia* 1979; **34**: 108.
29. P J H, D M C. Obituary. W S McConnell. *British Medical Journal* 1982; **285**: 67.
30. McConnell W S. Obituary. Thomas Alexander Britten Harris. *Anaesthesia* 1957; **12**: 240-1.
31. W J P. Obituary. R E Pleasance. *Anaesthesia* 1970; **25**: 439.
32. Mitchell J V. Burma revisited. *Anaesthesia* 1979; **34**: 811-21.
33. Laycock J D. Discussion on anaesthesia for major disasters. *Proceedings of the Royal Society of Medicine* 1959; **52**: 245-6.

34. Boulton T B. Nurse anaesthesia in South Vietnam. *Anaesthesia* 1970; **25**: 469-72.
35. Boulton T B. Anaesthesia and resuscitation in difficult environments. In: Hewer C L, ed. *Recent Advances in Anaesthesia and Analgesia*. 11th edition Edinburgh: Churchill Livingstone, 1972, 143-238.
36. Anonymous. The nurse-anaesthetist controversy. *British Journal of Anaesthesia* 1939-41; **17**: 108-11.
37. Woolmer R F. Anaesthetics in the Royal Navy. In: Cope Z, ed.. *Surgery*. London: Her Majesty's Stationery Office, 1953.
38. R W C. Obituary. Professor Ronald Woolmer. *Anaesthesia* 1963; **18**: 248-50.
39. Woolmer R F. *Anaesthetics Afloat*. London: Lewis, 1942.
40. Gillies D M M. Wynands J E. Obituary. Dr Harold Griffith. *Canadian Anaesthetists Society Journal* 1985; **32**: 370-2.
41. Griffith H R, Johnson G E. The use of curare in general anaesthesia. *Anesthesiology* 1942; **3**: 418-20.
42. Wilkinson D J. Dr F P de Caux: the first user of curare for anaesthesia in England 1928. *Anaesthesia* 1991; **46**; 49-51.
43. Keys T E. *The History of Surgical Anesthesia*. New York: Krieger, 1945.
44. Gray T C, Halton J. A milestone in anaesthesia (d-tubocurarine chloride). *Proceedings of the Royal Society of Medicine* 1945-46; **39**: 400-10.
45. Gray T C. Modern anaesthesia. *Transactions of the Medical Society of London* 1949; **65**: 80-7.
46. Prescott F, Organe G, Rowbotham S. Tubocurarine chloride as an adjunct to anaesthesia. Report on 180 cases. *Lancet* 1946; **2**: 80-4.
47. Simmons H J A. Preliminary investigation of the use of curare in anaesthetic practice and the treatment of spastic paralysis. *British Journal of Anaesthesia* 1946-47; **20**: 34-8.
48. Mallinson F B. Curarisation compared with other methods of securing relaxation in anaesthesia. *Anaesthesia* 1946; **1**: 17-21.
49. Boulton T B. T Cecil Gray and the "Disintegration of the nervous system". *Survey of Anesthesiology* 1994, **38**: 239-252.
50. Gray T C. Disintegration of the nervous system. Joseph Clover Lecture. *Annals of the Royal College of Surgeons of England* 1954; **15**: 402-19.
51. Editorial. *British Journal of Anaesthesia* 1938-39; **16**: 125-7.
52. Chivers E M, Evans W E F. Anaesthesia in surgical shock. *British Journal of Anaesthesia* 1939-41; **17**: 92-3.
53. Pask E A. General anaesthesia in traumatic shock. Some theoretical considerations. *British Journal of Anaesthesia* 1939-41; **17**: 129-66.
54. Cope Z. Shock and Resuscitation. In: Cope Z, ed.. *Surgery*. London: Her Majesty's Stationery Office, 1953: 90-216.
55. Mallinson F B. Casualty anaesthesia in the EMS. *British Journal of Anaesthesia* 1939-41; **17**: 107.
56. Bennetts F E. Thopectone anaesthesia at Pearl Harbor. *British Journal of Anaesthesia* 1995; **75**: 366-8..
57. Adams R C, Gray H K. Intravenous anesthesia with pentothal sodium in the case of gunshot wound associated with severe traumatic shock and loss of blood. Report of a case. *Anesthesiology* 1943; **4**: 70-3.

58. Editorial. The question of intravenous anesthesia in war surgery. *Anesthesiology* 1943; **4**: 74-7.
59. Presman D, Schotz S. A critical analysis of the use of intravenous morphine. *Anesthesiology* 1943; **4**: 53-66.
60. Beinart J. *The History of the Nuffield Department of Anaesthetics, Oxford 1937-1987*. Oxford: University Press, 1987.
61. Rushton M A. Oxford vaporiser for endotracheal anaesthesia. *Lancet* 1943; **2**: 509-10.
62. Boulton T B. Editorial. C Langton Hewer. *Anaesthesia* 1986; **41**: 469-71.
63. Hewer C L, Hadfield C F. Trichloroethylene as an inhalation anaesthetic. *British Medical Journal* 1941; **1**: 924-27.
64. Jowitt M D, Knight R J. Anaesthesia during the Falklands Campaign. The land battles. *Anaesthesia* 1983; **38**: 776-83.
65. Macintosh R. A new laryngoscope. *Lancet* 1943; **2**: 205.
66. R R M. Obituary. Professor E A Pask. *Anaesthesia* 1962; **21**: 437-38.
67. Macintosh R. Twenty years ago. *Anaesthesia* 1968; **23**: 282-4.
68. Editorial. *Anaesthesia* 1977; **32**: 843-5.
69. Editorial. *British Journal of Anaesthesia* 1939-41; **17**: 10
70. The Association of Anaesthetists of Great Britain and Ireland. *British Journal of Anaesthesia* 1939-41; **17**: 31-2.
71. A I P B. Obituary.. Dr John Challis. *Anaesthesia* 1939-41; **17**: 1.
72. Obituary. Dr William Sykes. *Anaesthesia* 1961; **16**: 383.
73. J S C. Obituary. Steel G C. *British Medical Journal* 1985; **290**: 475.
74. Association News. *Anaesthesia* 1948; **3**: 79-82.
75. Edridge A W. Sir Ivan Whiteside Magill. *Anaesthesia* 1987; **42**: 231-3.
76. Obituary. Rowbotham E S. *Anaesthesia* 1979; **34**: 709.
77. Obituary. R J Minnitt. *Anaesthesia* 1974; **29**: 382.
78. W S McC. Obituary. Sir Francis Shipway. *Anaesthesia* 1969; **24**: 269.
79. H B G. Obituary. Beverley Charles Leech. *Canadian Anaesthetists' Society Journal* 1960; **7**: 351-2.
80. F K B. Obituary. R M Tovell. *Anaesthesia* 1967; **22**: 362-3.
81. Obituary. John Frederick William Silk. *British Medical Journal* 1943; **2**: 731.
82. Obituary. Lord Webb-Johnson. *British Medical Journal* 1958; **1**: 1357-9.
83. Leading article. The nurse anaesthetist. *Lancet* 1940; **2**: 301.
84. Mennell Z, Blomfield J. Nurse anaesthetists. *British Medical Journal* 1940; **2**: 297-80.
85. Mennell Z, Blomfield J. Nurse anaesthetists. *Lancet* 1940; **2**: 307.
86. Anonymous. Casual comments. *British Journal of Anaesthesia* 1938-39; **16**: 142-4.
87. Special Article. Medicine and the Law. The nurse-anaesthetist. *Lancet* 1941; **1**: 223-4.
88. Gould R B. Nurse anaesthetists. *British Medical Journal* 1941; **1**: 419.
89. Notes, Comments and abstracts. Nurses' view of the nurse anaesthetist. *Lancet* 1940; **2**: 736.
90. Elam J. Nurse anaesthetists. *British Medical Journal* 940; **2**: 368.
91. Goode A F. Nurse anaesthetists. *British Medical Journal* 1940; **2**: 430.
92. Elam J. Nurse anaesthetists. *British Medical Journal* 1940; **2**: 430.
93. Elam J. Training in anaesthetics. *Lancet* 1940; **2**: 309.
94. Edwards G. Emergency anaesthetics in hospitals. *British Journal of Anaesthesia* 1930-31;

8: 15-18.
95. Loughnane F M. Nurse anaesthetists. *British Medical Journal* 1941; **2**: 463.
96. Rickards J F. The nurse anaesthetist. *Lancet* 1940; **2**: 405.
97. Parsons F B. Nurse anaesthetists. *British Medical Journal* 1940; **2**: 429.
98. Parsons F B. Nurse anaesthetists. *Lancet* 1940; **2**: 364.
99. Railton R, Barr M. *The Royal Berkshire Hospital 1839-1989. Reading: the Royal Berkshire Hospital 1989*: 137.
100. Obituary. Sir Frederic William Hewitt. *Lancet* 1916; **1**: 61.
101. Boulton T B, Cole P V. Anaesthesia in difficult situations. 9: Some solutions, new drugs and a conclusion. *Anaesthesia* 1968; **23**: 597-630.
102. Lawson J I M. Impressions of nurse anaesthesia in the United States. *Anaesthesia* 1970; **25**: 457-63.
103. Miller J S. Anaesthetic nurses in Sweden. *Anaesthesia* 1970; **25**: 464-8.
104. Macintosh R R. Training in anaesthetics. *Lancet* 1940; **2**: 345.
105. Macintosh R R. Supplementary anaesthetists. *Lancet* 1962; **1**: 157-8.
106. Toner J. Supplementary anaesthetists. *Lancet* 1961; **2**: 1452.
107. Organe G. Obituary. Ronald Jarman. *Anaesthesia* 1973; **28**: 127.
108. Grey-Turner E, Sutherland F M. *The History of the British Medical Association. Volume 2 1932-1981*. London: British Medical Association; 1982: 30-76.
109. Leading article. Social insurance and services. Medical parts of the Beveridge Plan. *British Medical Journal* 1942; **2**: 704-6.
110. Medical notes in Parliament. Health Service Bill. *British Medical Journal* 1946; **2**: 177-80.
111. Moran C, Webb Johnson A, Gilliatt W. National Health Service Act. Presidents of Royal Colleges and Mr. Bevan. *British Medical Journal* 1947; **1**: 66.
112. Bevan A. National Health Service. Mr. Bevan's reply. *British Medical Journal* 1947; **1**: 66-7.
113. Murley R. *Surgical Roots and Branches*. London: British Medical Association, 1990.
114. Obituary. Dr Gilbert Brown. *Anaesthesia,* 1960; **15**: 198.
115. Brown G. An address. *Medical Journal of Australia* 1935; **92**: 33-7.
116. Reconstruction. Staffing of County Hospitals. Posts and pay. *Lancet* 1945; **2**: 717-8.
117. AAGBI Minute Book No 2. 1947-1963.
118. Editorial. *British Journal of Anaesthesia*, 1950; **22**: 1-3.
119. Editorial. *British Journal of Anaesthesia*, 1951; **22**: 63-5.
120. Editorial. The next objective. *British Journal of Anaesthesia*, 1960; **32**: 395.
121. Association News. *Anaesthesia*, 1947; **2**: 122-3.
122. The Editor. Then and now. Anaesthesia thirty years ago (1947) Volume 2. *Anaesthesia,* 1977; **32**: 898-903.
123. Editorial. the struggle upward. *British Journal of Anaesthesia* 1939-41; **17**: 81-84.
124. Editorial. *Anaesthesia* 1948; **3**: 3.
125. Extracts from the regulations for obtaining the Diploma in Anaesthetics. *Anaesthesia*, 1948; **3**: 30-1.
126. The Examining Board in England. Diploma in Anaesthetics. *British Journal of Anaesthesia*, 1948-49; **21**: 158-9.
127. Boulton T B. Editorial. *Anaesthesia,* 1948; **3:** 3.

128. Association news. *Anaesthesia*, 1948; **3**: 79-82.
129. Obituary. George Edwards. *Anaesthesia*, 1990; **45**: 86.
130. Association news. *Anaesthesia*, 1948; **3**: 129.
131. Association news. The Annual General Meeting. *Anaesthesia*, 1948; **3**: 40-1.
132. Obituary notice. Katherine G Lloyd-Williams. *British Medical Journal*, 1973; **1**: 179.
133. Obituary. Ralph Blair Gould. *Anaesthesia* 1984; **39**: 1044.
134. Boulton T B. Editorial. *Anaesthesia* 1980; **35**: 1147.
135. Featherstone M W. The Association of Anaesthetists of Great Britain and Ireland. Its inception and purpose. *Anaesthesia*, 1946; **1**: 5-9.
136. The Editor. Then and now. Anaesthesia thirty years ago. *Anaesthesia*, 1976; **31**: 1103-7.
137. R J M. Obituary. Joseph Blomfield. *British Journal of Anaesthesia* 1948-49; **21**: 152-3.
138. ARH. Obituary. E F Hill. *British Medical Journal*, 1974; **3**: 746.
139. Editorial. *British Journal of Anaesthesia*, 1948-49; **21**: 105-6.
140. Spence A A. The British Journal of Anaesthesia. Its evolution and present position. In: Ruprecht J, Van Lieburg M J, Lee J A, Erdmann W, ed. Anaesthesia, *Essays on its History*. Berlin; Springer-Verlag 1985: 301-3.
141. Macintosh R R. Deaths under anaesthetics. *British Journal of Anaesthesia*, 1948-49; **21**: 107-36.
142. Gray T C. The early history of the *British Journal of Anaesthesia*. In: Ruprecht J, van Lieburg M J, Lee J A, Erdmann W, eds. *Anaesthesia. Essays on its History*. Berlin: Springer-Verlag, 1985: 297-300.
143. Editorial. *Anaesthesia*, 1951; **6**: 1.
144. Editorial. *British Journal of Anaesthesia*, 1951; **23**: 63-4.
145. Editorial. *The British Journal of Anaesthesia* and *Anaesthesia*. *British Journal of Anaesthesia*, 1959; **31**: 517.
146. Editorial. *Anaesthesia*, 1960; **15**: 1-20.
147. Smith G. Editorial I. Journal of the College of Anaesthetists. *British Journal of Anaesthesia*, 1990; **64**: 1-2.
148. P J H. Obituary. A M Hutton. *British Medical Journal* 1981; **282**: 160.
149. Helliwell P J, Hutton A M. Trichlorethylene anaesthesia. *Anaesthesia*, 1950; **5**: 4-13.
150. Helliwell P J, Hutton A M. Twenty years ago. *Anaesthesia*, 1968; **23**: 686-9.
151. Helliwell P J. The Association of Anaesthetists of Great Britain and Ireland. *Anaesthesia*, 1982; **37**: 913-23.
152. M W G. Obituary B L S Murtagh. *Anaesthesia*, 1970; **25**: 150-1.
153. Association news. *Anaesthesia*, 1947; **2**: 163.
154. Association news. *Anaesthesia*, 1946; **1**: 41.
155. Association news. *Anaesthesia*, 1947; **2**: 41.
156. Duncum B M. *The Development of Inhalation Anaesthesia: with Special Reference to the Years 1846-1900*. Oxford: University Press, 1947.
157. Photographs of the Presidential badge and the plaque unveiled at the Royal College of Surgeons. *Anaesthesia* 1947; **2**: 24-25.
158. Marston A D. Centenary of anaesthesia in Great Britain. *Anaesthesia*, 1946; **1**: 9-17.
159. Edinburgh centenary celebrations. *Anaesthesia*, 1948; **3**: 39.

Chapter 6 - Consolidation and Progress, 1 January 1949 to 31 December 1959

1. Helliwell P J. Obituary. John Gillies. *Anaesthesia* 1976; **31:** 1311-2.
2. R B W, W D W. Obituary. W A Low. *Anaesthesia* 1970; **25:** 587.
3. Pallister W K. Editorial. Sir Geoffrey Stephen William Organe 1908-1989. *Anaesthesia* 1989; **44:** 461-2.
4. Organe G S W. Obituary. Ronald Jarman. *Anaesthesia* 1973; **28:** 197.
5. O P D. Obituary. Dr Bernard Johnson. *Anaesthesia* 1959; **14:** 419-21.
6. Burn J M B. Obituary. Robert Patrick Webb Shackleton. *Anaesthesia* 1977; **32:** 819-21.
7. Lumley J. Editorial. Arthur John Wells Beard. *Anaesthesia* 1993; **48:** 483-4.
8. Boulton T B. Editorial. C Langton Hewer. *Anaesthesia* 1986; **41:** 469-70.
9. Royle T. *The Best Years of their Lives. The National Service Experience 1945-1963*. London: Michael Joseph, 1986.
10. Hutchinson J R H. Medical notes in Parliament. Army Medical Services. *British Medical Journal* 1952; **1:** 1212-13.
11. Clyne A J. Missile wounds in Malaya. *British Medical Journal* 1954; **2:** 10-16.
12. Lyons A S, Petrucelli R J. *Medicine. An Illustrated History*. New York; Abrams, 1987: 576-603.
13. Schatz A, Bugie E, Walksman S A. Streptomycin, a substance exhibiting antibiotic activity against gram positive and gram negative bacteria. *Proceedings of the Society of Experimental Biology and Medicine 1944*; **55:** 66-69.
14. Singer C, Underwood E A. *A Short History of Medicine*. 2nd edition. Oxford: University Press, 1962: 693-7.
15. Woodruff H B, Burg R W. The antibiotic explosion. In: Parnham M J, Bruinvels J. *Discoveries in Pharmacology*. Volume 3. Pharmacological Methods, Receptors and Chemotherapy. Amsterdam: Elsevier, 1986; 303-51.
16. Lassen H C A. A preliminary report on the 1952 epidemic of poliomyelitis in Copenhagen with special reference to the treatment of acute respiratory insufficiency. *Lancet* 1953; **1:** 37-41.
17. Salk J E. Vaccination against poliomyelitis; performance and prospect. *American Journal of Public Health* 1955; **45:** 576-96.
18. Public Health. Poliomyelitis in 1947. *British Medical Journal* 1948; **1:** 541.
19. Kolff W J. Modern therapy of uremia: especially peritoneal lavage and treatment with the artificial kidney (dialyser with large area). *Belgisch Tijdschrift Voor Geeneeshindig Documentate* 1946; **2:** 449-63.
20. Murray J E, Merrill J P, Harrison J H. Renal homotransplantation in identical twins. *Surgical Forum* 1955; 432-6.
21. Starzl T E. Personal reflections in transplantation. *Surgical Clinics of North America* 1978; **58:** 879-93.
22. Billingham R E, Krohn P L, Medawar P B. Effect of cortisone on survival of skin homografts in rabbits. *British Medical Journal* 1951; **1:** 1157-63.
23. Marriott H L. Water and salt depletion. *British Medical Journal* 1947; **1:** 245-50, 285-90 and 328-32.
24. LeQuesne L P. *Fluid Balance in Surgical Practice*. London: Lloyd Luke, 1955.

25. Jude J R. Origins and evolvement of cardiopulmonary resuscitation. In: Atkinson R S, Boulton T B. eds. *The History of Anaesthesia*. International Congress and Symposium Series 134. London: Royal Society of Medicine, 1989: 452-64.
26. Beck C S, Pritchard W H, Feil H S. Ventricular fibrillation of long duration abolished by electric shock. *Journal of the American Medical Association* 1947; **135**: 985-6.
27. Hewer C L, Lee J A. *Recent Advances in Anaesthesia and Analgesia (including oxygen therapy)* 8th edition. London: Churchill, 1957: 172-7.
28. Elam J. Rediscovery of expired air methods for emergency ventilation. In: Safar P, ed. *Advances in Cardiopulmonary Resuscitation*. New York: Springer-Verlag 1977: 263-5.
29. Kouwenhoven W B, Jude J R, Knickerbocker G G. Closed chest cardiac massage. *Journal of the American Medical Association* 1960; **173**: 1064.
30. Souttar H S. The surgical correction of mitral stenosis. *British Medical Journal* 1925; **2**: 603-6.
31. Ellis R H. The first transauricular mitral valvotomy. An account to mark the fiftieth anniversary of the operation. *Anaesthesia* 1975; **30**: 374-90.
32. Cutler E C, Levine S A, Beck C S. The surgical treatment of mitral stenosis. Experimental and clinical studies. *Archives of Surgery* 1924; **9**: 691-821.
33. Brock R C. Pulmonary valvulotomy for the relief of congenital pulmonary stenosis. Report of three cases. *British Medical Journal* 1948; **1**: 1121-32.
34. Bailey C P, Ramirez H P R, Larzelere H B. Surgical treatment of aortic stenosis. *Journal of the American Medical Association* 1952; **150**: 1647-52.
35. Gray T C, Riding J E. Anaesthesia for mitral valvotomy. The evolution of a technique. *Anaesthesia* 1957; **12**: 129-47.
36. Cooley D A. Perspectives of cardiac surgery with personal reflections. *Surgical Clinics of North America* 1978; **58**: 895-90.
37. Lewis F J, Taufic M. Closure of atrial septal defects with the aid of hypothermia. Experimental accomplishments and a report of one successful case. *Surgery* 1953; **33**: 52-9.
38. Gibbon J H. Artificial maintenance of circulation during experimental occlusion of the pulmonary artery. *Archives of Surgery* 1937; **34**: 1105-31.
39. Rendell-Baker L. History of thoracic anaesthesia. In: Mushin W W, ed. *Thoracic Anaesthesia*. Oxford: Blackwell Scientific Publications, 1963: 598-661.
40. Editorial. *Anaesthesia* 1947; **2**: 126.
41. Leading Article. Syringe sterilisation. *British Medical Journal* 1962; **1**: 1126-7.
42. Medical Research Council. *Memorandum 41* (Revision of War Memorandum 15). Her Majesty's Stationery Office, 1962.
43. The Nuffield Provincial Hospital Trust. *The Planning and Organisation of Central Syringe Services*. London: Nuffield Provincial Hospital Trust, 1957.
44. Bailey H. *Pye's Surgical Handicraft* 18th edition. Bristol: Wright, 1962: 60.
45. Parliament. *British Medical Journal* 1965; **1**: 394.
46. Pask E A. Committee on deaths associated with anaesthesia. Review of cases where postoperative care was inadequate to meet the circumstances which arose. *Anaesthesia* 1955; **10**: 4-8.
47. Gilston A. The management of respiratory distress after cardiothoracic surgery. *Thorax* 1962; **17**: 139-45.
48. Davies R M, Belcher J R, Boulton T B, Fraser A C, Gardner E, Lee J A, Pask E A. Discussion

on organisation for immediate postoperative recovery period. *Proceedings of the Royal Society of Medicine* 1958; **51**: 151-6.
49. Jolly C, Lee J A. Postoperative observation ward. *Anaesthesia* 1957; **12**: 49-56.
50. Gillies D M M, Wynards J E. The Contribution of Harold Randall Griffith (1896-1985) to Anaesthesia. In: Atkinson R S, Boulton T B. *The History of Anaesthesia*. International Congress and Symposium Series 134. London: Royal Society of Medicine, 1989: 614-7.
51. Scott D B. Inferior vena cava occlusion in late pregnancy and its importance in anaesthesia. *British Journal of Anaesthesia* 1968; 40: 120-8.
52. Cope R W. Woolley and Roe versus Ministry of Health and Others. *Anaesthesia* 1990; **45**: 859-64.
53. Hutter C D D. The Wooley and Roe Case. A reassessment. *Anaesthesia* 1990; **45**: 859-64.
54. Hingson R A, Edwards W B. Continuous caudal analgesia: analysis of the first ten thousand confinements thus managed with a report on the author's first thousand cases. *Journal of the American Medical Association* 1943; **123**: 538-46.
55. Galley A H. Continuous caudal analgesia in obstetrics. *Anaesthesia* 1949; **4**: 154-68.
56. Gray T C. A reassessment of the signs and levels of anaesthesia. *Irish Journal of Medical Science* 1960; 6th series **No 419**: 499-508.
57. Penfold J B. Postoperative changes in water and salt balance. *Anaesthesia* 1955; **10**: 9-17.
58. Jackson I. Arteriotomy in neurosurgery. *Anaesthesia* 1954; **9**: 13-6.
59. Wyman J B, Cox R, Gillies J. Discussion on hypotension during anaesthesia. *Proceedings of the Royal Society of Medicine* 1953; **46**: 605-12.
60. Griffiths H W C, Gillies J. thoracolumbar splenchinectomy and sympathectomy. Anaesthetic procedure. *Anaesthesia* 1948; **3**: 134-46.
61. Scurr C F. Reduction of hemorrhage in the operative field by the use of pentamethonium iodide: a preliminary report. *Anesthesiology* 1951; **12**: 253-4.
62. Enderby G E H, Pelmore J F. Controlled hypotension and postural ischaemia to reduce bleeding in surgery. *Lancet* 1951; **1**: 663-7.
63. Enderby G E H. Pentolinium tartrate in controlled hypotension. *Lancet* 1954; **2**: 1097-8.
64. Robertson J D, Armitage P. Comparison of two hypotensive agents. *Anaesthesia* 1959; **14**: 53-64.
65. Rovenstein E A, Batterman R I. The utility of demerol as a substitute for the opiates in preanesthetic medication. *Anesthesiology* 1943; **4**: 126-34.
66. Mushin W W, Rendell-Baker L. Pethidine as a supplement to nitrous oxide anaesthesia. *British Medical Journal* 1949; **2**: 472.
67. Pearce C. Intravenous pethidine in intravenous anaesthesia (a report of 330 cases). *British Journal of Anaesthesia* 1951; **23**: 205-13.
68. Ruben H, Andreassen A K. Pharmacological effects of pethidine on the larynx seen during intubation. *British Journal of Anaesthesia* 1951; **23**: 33-8.
69. Dundee J W. A review of chlorpromazine hydrochloride. *British Journal of Anaesthesia* 1954; **26**: 357-79.
70. Laborit H, Hugenard P. L'hibernation artificielle chez le grand choque. *Presse Medicale* 1951; **61**: 1029-30.
71. Editorial. *Anaesthesia* 1955; **10**: 3.
72. Bovet D, Depierre F, Lestrange Y. Propietes curarisantes des ethers phenoliques a fonctions ammonium quaternaires. *Comptes Rendus Hebdomadaires des Seances de l'Academie des*

Sciences 1947; **225**: 74-8.
73. Mushin W W, Wien R, Mason D J F, Langston G T. Curare-like actions of tri-(diethylaminoethoxy)-benzine triethyliodide. *Lancet* 1949; **1**: 726-8.
74. Organe G, Paton W D M, Zaimis E J. Preliminary trials of bistrimethyl ammonium decane and pentane di-iodide (C10 and C5) in man. *Lancet* 1949; **1**: 773-4.
75. Scurr C F. The introduction of depolarizing muscle-relaxants into clinical practice. In: Atkinson R S, Boulton T B, eds. *History of Anaesthetics*. International Congress and Symposium Series 134. London: Royal Society of Medicine, 1989: 9-12.
76. Scurr C F. A relaxant of very brief action. *British Medical Journal* 1951; **2**: 831-2.
77. Bevan D R, Bevan J C, Donati F. *Muscle Relaxants in Clinical Anaesthesia*. Chicago: Year Book Publishers, 1988: 247-77.
78. Suckling C W. Some chemical and physical factors in the development of Fluothane. *British Journal of Anaesthesia* 1957; **29**: 466.
79. Raventos J. The action of Fluothane. A new volatile anaesthetic. *British Journal of Pharmacology* 1956; **11**: 394-410.
80. Johnstone M. The human cardiovascular response to fluothane anaesthesia. *British Journal of Anaesthesia* 1956; **28**: 392-410.
81. Bryce-Smith R, O'Brien H D. Fluothane. A non-explosive volatile anaesthetic agent. *British Medical Journal* 1956; **2**: 969-72.
82. Virtue R W, Payne K W. Postoperative death after Fluothane. *Anesthesiology* 1958; **19**: 562.
83. Relton J E S, Britt B A, Seward D J. Malignant hyperpyrexia. *British Journal of Anaesthesia* 1973; **45**: 269-75.
84. Stoetling V K. The use of a new intravenous oxygen barbiturate 2598 for intravenous anaesthesia (a preliminary Report). *Anesthesia and Analgesia: Current Researches* 1957; **36**: (No 3) 49-57.
85. Dundee J W, Moore J. Thiopentone and Methohexital. A comparison as main agents for an operation. *Anaesthesia* 1961; **16**: 50-73.
86. Gordh T. Xylocain. A new local anaesthetic. *Anaesthesia* 1949; **4**: 4-9 and 21.
87. Braun H. Über einize neue orliche Anaesthetica (Stovain, Alypin, Novocaine). *Deutche Medizinische* Wochenschrift 1905; **31**: 1667-71.
88. Lunn J N. Editorial. William Woolf Mushin *Anaesthesia* 1993; **48**: 461-2.
89. R R M. Obituary. Professor E A Pask. *Anaesthesia* 1966; **21**: 437-8.
90. R W. Obituary. Professor Ronald Woolmer. *Anaesthesia* 1963; **18**: 248-50.
91. Obituary. Dundee J W. *Anaesthesia* 1992; **47**: 365.
92. G W B. Obituary. J Clutton-Brock. *British Medical Journal* 1986; **283**: 1381.
93. Murley R S. *Surgical Roots and Branches*. London: British Medical Association 1990: 189-201.
94. Rue E R. National Health Service in the U K: its structure. In: Walton J, Beeson P B, Scott R B. *The Oxford Companion to Medicine*. Oxford: University Press, 1986: 814-9.
95. Owen D. Back to a two tier health service. *St Thomas' Hospital Gazettee* 1989; **87**: 189-94.
96. Annotation. The nursing hierarchy. *Lancet* 1966; **1**: 1085-6.
97. Grey-Turner E, Sutherland F M. *History of the British Medical Association; Volume 2*, 1932-1981. London: British Medical Association, 1982: 101-64.

98. Report. Cost of the National Health Service. Report of the Guillebaud Committee. *British Medical Journal* 1956; **1**: (Supplement) 31-4.
99. Leading article. Trial by committee. *British Medical Journal* 1956; **1**: 279-80.
100. Critic. Young specialists in search of a job. *Lancet* 1948; **2**: 946-7.
101. Leading article. Medical staffing of hospitals. *British Medical Journal* 1961; **1**: 883-4.
102. Report. Surplus Senior Registrars. Minister's proposals. *British Medical Journal* 1953; **1**: (Supplement) 243.
103. Leading article. Emigration of British doctors. *British Medical Journal* 1962; **1**: 779-80.
104. Seale J. Medical emigration from Britain 1930-1961. *British Medical Journal* 1962; **1**: 782-7.
105. Davison R H. Medical emigration to North America. *British Medical Journal* 1962; **1**: 986-7.
106. Sykes M K. The American approach to anaesthesia. *British Medical Journal* 1956; **1**: 1148-50.
107. *AAGBI Minute Book No 2* 1947-1965: 25-271.
108. S R T H. Obituary. G Edwards. *British Medical Journal* 1989; **299**: 510.
109. Editorial. *Anaesthesia* 1957; **12**: 123.
110. Griffith H R. Obituary. Wesley Bourne 1886-1965. *Anaesthesia* 1965; **20**: 376-7.
111. Association and Faculty news. *Anaesthesia* 1949; **4**: 46-7.
112. Association news. *Anaesthesia* 1959; **14**: 104-7.
113. Association news. *Anaesthesia* 1951; **6**: 184-5.
114. Wishart H V, Holloway K B, Spence A A. Obituary. Henry Harvey Pinkerton. *Anaesthesia* 1982; **37**: 1143-5.
115. Faculty News. *Anaesthesia* 1953; **8**: 211-2.
116. Association news. *Anaesthesia* 1954; **9**: 222-4.
117. Association news. *Anaesthesia* 1950; **5**: 52-4.
118. Distinction awards. Analysis by type of award, specialty and percentage distribution. 31 December 1989. England and Wales. *Health Trends* 1990; **22**: 130.
119. Ely B. Medical and dental staffing prospects in the NHS in England and Wales in 1988. *Health Trends* 1989; **21**: 99-106.
120. Association news. *Anaesthesia* 1948; **3**: 40-1, 1949; **4**: 46-7, 1950; **5**: 52-4, 1951; **6**: 61-2, 1952; **7**: 60-2, 1953; **8**: 66-7, 1954; **9**: 61-2, 1955; **10**: 61-2.
121. Association news. *Anaesthesia* 1955; **10**: 321.
122. E A C. Obituary. M H A Davison. *British Medical Journal* 1970; **4**: 564.
123. Davison M H A. Ut non percipiatur dolor. *Anaesthesia* 1956; **11**: 118-34.
124. Association news. *Anaesthesia* 1957; **12**: 117-9.
125. R W C. Obituary. Professor Ronald Woolmer. *Anaesthesia* 1963; **18**: 248-50.
126. Obituary Notice. Katherine G Lloyd-Williams. *British Medical Journal* 1973; **1**: 179.
127. Association news. *Anaesthesia* 1957; **12**: 368.
128. Association news. *Anaesthesia* 1958; **13**: 105-6 and 245-8.
129. Editorial. Silver Jubilee 1932-1957. *Anaesthesia* 1958; **13**: 1-2.
130. Editorial. *Anaesthesia* 1958; **13**: 109-10.
131. Silver Jubilee Meeting. Summaries of Papers. *Anaesthesia* 1958; **13**: 179-222.
132. HCC-D. Obituary. M D Nosworthy. *British Medical Journal* 1980; **281**: 815.
133. Nosworthy M D. Pseudo-science and modern anaesthesia. *Anaesthesia* 1958; **13**: 111-23.

134. Association news. *Anaesthesia* 1958; **13**: 373-4.
135. Association news. *Anaesthesia* 1959; **14**: 104-7.
136. Edwards G. John Snow, MD. *Anaesthesia* 1959; **14**: 113-26.
137. Summaries of papers read at the Annual Meeting, Southport, 30 October-1 November 1958. *Anaesthesia* 1959; **14**: 76-83.
138. Davison M H A. Chloroform in modern anaesthesia. *Anaesthesia* 1959; **14**: 127-34.
139. E A C. Obituary. M H A Davison. *British Medical Journal* 1970; **4**: 564.
140. Galloon S. Controlled respiration in neurological anaesthesia. *Anaesthesia* 1959; **14**: 223-30.
141. Association News. *Anaesthesia* 1959; **14**: 305.
142. Association News. *Anaesthesia* 1960; **15**: 97-8.
143. Summaries of papers read at the Scientific Session of the Association of Anaesthetists, Stratford-upon-Avon. Friday 23 October 1959. *Anaesthesia* 1960; **15**: 65-74.
144. Benazon D. The experimental and clinical use of profound hypothermia. *Anaesthesia* 1960; **15**: 134-45.
145. R E L. Obituary. L F Wolfson. *British Medical Journal* 1980; **281**: 1646.
146. Sellick B A. Cricoid pressure to control regurgitation of stomach contents during induction of anaesthesia. *Lancet* 1961; **2**: 404-6.
147. P S L. Obituary. L F Wolfson. *British Medical Journal* 1981; **282**: 237.
148. Steinhaus J E. Anaesthesiology and pharmacology at Wisconsin in the 1930s. In: Ruprecht J, Van Lieburg M J, Lee J A, Erdmann W, eds. *Anaesthesia. Essays on its History*. Berlin; Springer-Verlag, 1985: 256-61.
149. Beecher H K, Todd D D. A study of the deaths associated with anaesthesia and surgery. Based on a study of 599, 548 anaesthetics in ten institutions 1948-1952 inclusive. *Annals of Surgery* 1954; **140**: 2-34.
150. Abstracts from current literature. The nurse anaesthetist by H K Beecher. *Anaesthesia* 1949; **4**: 201-2.
151. Beecher H K. The nurse anaesthetist. *Surgery Gynaecology and Obstetrics* 1948; **86**: 115-8.
152. Pask E A, Gillies J. The American approach to anaesthesia. *British Medical Journal* 1956; **1**: 1361.
153. Swarz W. Attempts to establish anaesthesiology as a specialty in German medicine. In: Atkinson R S, Boulton T B, eds. *The History of Anaesthesia*. International Symposium Series 134. London, Royal Society of Medicine, 1989: 170-5.
154. De Lange J J, Mauve M, Reeser L D J, Ruprecht J, Smalhout B, Bongertman-Diek J M, eds. *Van aether naar beter vertig jaar Nederlandse Vereninging voor Anesthesiologie 1943-1988*. Utrecht: Nederlandse Vereninging voor Anesthesiologie, 1987.
155. De Lange J J. Theodoor Hammes (1874-1951) the first professional anaesthetist (in Holland). In: Atkinson R S, Boulton T B, eds. *The History of Anaesthesia*. International Symposium Series *134*. London. Royal Society of Medicine, 1989: 89-92.
156. Organe G. An account of the development of the World Federation of Societies of Anaesthesiologists. In: Ruprecht J, Van Lieburg M J, Lee J A, Erdmann W, eds. *Anaesthesia. Essays on its History*. Berlin: Springer-Verlag, 1985: 311-313.
157. Soban D, Andonov V, Lalevic P, Ribaric L, Stagie A On the development of modern anaesthesia in Yugoslavia. In: Ruprecht J, Van Lieburg M J, Lee J A, Erdmann W, eds.

Anaesthesia. Essays on its History. Berlin: Springer-Verlag, 1985: 253-257.
158. Bennett J P. Obituary. R M Davies. *British Medical Journal* 1992; **304**: 569.
159. Vermeulen-Cranch. From open ether to open hearts. In: Ruprecht J, Van Lieburg M J, Lee J A, Erdmann W, eds. *Anaesthesia. Essays on its History*. Berlin: Springer-Verlag, 1985: 265-9.
160. Dworacek B, Keszler H. The development of anaesthesiology in Czechoslovakia. In: Ruprecht J, Van Lieburg M J, Lee J A, Erdmann W, eds. *Anaesthesia. Essays on its History*. Berlin: Springer-Verlag, 1985: 258-61.
161. Secher O. Anaesthesiology Centre Copenhagen. In: Ruprecht J, Van Lieburg M J, Lee J A, Erdmann W, eds. *Anaesthesia. Essays on its History*. Berlin: Springer-Verlag, 1985: 321-34.
162. Wilson G. *Fifty years. The Australian Society of Anaesthetists 1934-1984*. Edgecliff N S W: The Australian Society of Anaesthetists, 1987.
163. Betcher A M, Gliberti B J, Wood P M, Wright H H. The jubilee year of organised anaesthesia. *Anesthesiology* 1956; **17**: 226-64.
164. Wilson G. Obituary. Geoffrey Kaye 1903-1986. *Anaesthesia and Intensive Care* 1987; 15: 107-9.
165. 26th Annual Congress of Anaesthetists 1951. *Anesthesia and Analgesia. Current Researches*. 1951; **30**: 85-92.
166. Association News. *Anaesthesia* 1951; **6**: 184-5.
167. Association News. *Anaesthesia* 1952; **7**: 60-2.
168. International Congress of Anesthesiology. Paris, France, September 20, 21 and 22, 1951. *Anesthesia and Analgesia. Current Researches* 1951; **30**: 93-5.
169. Griffith H R. History of the World Federation of Anesthesiologists. *Anesthesia and Analgesia. Current Researches* 1963; **42**: 389-97.
170. Zorab J S M. Special article. The World Federation of Societies of Anaesthesiologists (WFSA). *Anaesthesia* 1976; **31**: 285-92.
171. Howat D D C. The World Federation of Societies of Anaesthesiologists 1968-1984. In: Ruprecht J, Van Lieburg M J, Lee J A, Erdmann W, eds. *Anaesthesia. Essays on its History*. Berlin: Springer-Verlag, 1985: 314-20.
172. Obituary Notice. Katherine G Lloyd-Williams. *British Medical Journal* 1973; **1**: 179.
173. Lawson J I M. Impressions of nurse anaesthesia in the United States. *Anaesthesia* 1970; **25**: 457-63.
174. Lund I. Reminiscences of the development of modern anaesthesia in Norway. In: Ruprecht J, Van Lieburg M J, Lee J A, Erdmann W, eds. *Anaesthesia. Essays on its History*. Berlin: Springer-Verlag, 1985: 291-2.
175. Gordh T. The influence of Ralph M Waters on the development of anaesthesiology in Sweden. In: Ruprecht J, Van Lieburg M J, Lee J A, Erdmann W, eds. *Anaesthesia. Essays on its History*. Berlin: Springer-Verlag, 1985: 36-41.
176. Miller J S. Anaesthetic nurses in Sweden. *Anaesthesia* 1970; **25**: 464-8.
177. Horner J. The nurse anaesthetist in Norway. In: Ruprecht J. Van Lieburg M J, Lee J A, Erdmann W, eds. *Anaesthesia. Essays on its History*. Berlin: Springer-Verlag, 1985: 366-8.
178. Association News. *Anaesthesia* 1952; **7**: 192-5.
179. Yamamura H. History of modern anaesthesia in Japan. In: Ruprecht J, Van Lieburg M J,

Lee J A, Erdmann W, eds. *Anaesthesia. Essays on its History.* Berlin: Springer-Verlag, 1985: 217-9.
180. Inamoto A. The influences of modern anaesthesia of other countries on the growth of anaesthesia in Japan. In: Ruprecht J, Van Lieburg M J, Lee J A, Erdmann W, eds. *Anaesthesia. Essays on its History.* Berlin: Springer-Verlag, 1985: 220-3.
181. Yung S. History of modern anaesthesia in China. In: Ruprecht J, Van Lieburg M J, Lee J A, Erdmann W, eds. *Anaesthesia. Essays on its History.* Berlin: Springer-Verlag, 1985:
182. W S M. Obituary. Dr Archibald D Marston. *Anaesthesia* 1962; **17**: 235-8.
183. Seldon T H. Special Article. Harold Randall Griffith. *Anesthesia and Analgesia* 1986; **65**: 1051-3.
184. Edridge A W. Editorial. Sir Ivan Whiteside Magill. *Anaesthesia* 1987; **42**: 231-3.
185. Association News. *Anaesthesia* 1952; **7**: 60-2.
186. Shackleton R P W. The World Congress of Anaesthesiologists 1955. Held at Scheveningen and The Hague, 5-10 September. *Anaesthesia* 1956; **11**: 112-3.
187. Howat D D C. The World Federation of Societies of Anaesthesiologists 1968-1984. In: Ruprecht J, Van Lieburg M J, Lee J A, Erdmann W, eds. *Anaesthesia. Essays on its History.* Berlin: Springer-Verlag, 1985: 314-20.
188. Bradbeer E G. Letter from Dr E G Bradbeer. *Anaesthesia* Points West 1968; **1**: 7.
189. A R H. The Manchester and District Society of Anaesthetists 1946-50. In: Elwood W J, Tuxford A F, eds. *Some Manchester Doctors. A biographical collection to mark the 150th Anniversary of the Manchester Medical Society 1834-1984.* Manchester: University Press, 1984.
190. Association News. *Anaesthesia* 1948; **3**: 79-82.
191. Helliwell P J, Hutton A M. Trichlorethylene anaesthesia. *Anaesthesia* 1950; **5**: 4-13.
192. Association News. *Anaesthesia* 1950; **5**: 105-7.
193. Association News. *Anaesthesia* 1952; **7**: 192-5.
194. Association News. *Anaesthesia* 1954; **9**: 222-4.
195. Thomas K B. The Development of Anaesthetic Apparatus. *A history based on the Charles King Collection of the Association of Anaesthetists of Great Britain and Ireland.* Oxford: Blackwell Scientific Publications, 1975.
196. Sykes W S. *Essays on the First Hundred years of Anaesthesia. Volume 3.* Ellis R H, ed. London: Churchill Livingstone, 1982: 185-267.
197. Association News. *Anaesthesia* 1949; **4**: 203-4.
198. Editorial. *Anaesthesia* 1949; **4**: 153.
199. Obituary. H J V Morton. *British Medical Journal* 1982; **284**: 988.
200. Association News. *Anaesthesia* 1951; **6**: 61-2.
201. Gould R B. Preventable anaesthetic deaths. Reflections on modern anaesthesia. *Anaesthesia* 1951; **6**: 100-9.
202. Editorial. *Anaesthesia* 1951; **6**: 189.
203. Association News. *Anaesthesia* 1951; **6**: 247-8.
204. Morton H J V, Wylie W D. Anaesthetic deaths due to regurgitation. *Anaesthesia* 1951; **6**: 190-201 and 205.
205. Committee on Deaths Associated with Anaesthesia. Report on 400 cases. *Anaesthesia* 1952; **7**: 200-5.
206. Edwards G, Morton H J V, Pask E A, Wylie W D. Deaths associated with anaesthesia. A

report on 1000 cases. *Anaesthesia* 1956; **11**: 194-220.
207. Committee on Deaths associated with Anaesthesia. Cases in which hypotension has been used. *Anaesthesia* 1953; **8**: 263-7.
208. Pask E A. Committee on Deaths Associated with Anaesthesia. Review of cases where post-operative care was inadequate to meet the circumstances which arose. *Anaesthesia* 1955; **10**: 4-8.
209. Editorial. *Anaesthesia* 1956; **11**: 193.
210. Leading Article. Anaesthetic Deaths. *British Medical Journal* 1956; **2**: 868-9.
211. J A L, G C S. Obituary Notices. C J Massey Dawkins. *British Medical Journal* 1975; **4**: 493.
212. Dawkins M, Elam J E. Anaesthetic deaths. *British Medical Journal* 1956; **2**: 995.
213. Murley R S. Anaesthetic Deaths. *British Medical Journal* 1956; **2**: 1173-4.
214. Obituaries. Hunter A R. *Anaesthesia* 1991; **46**: 604.
215. Hunter A R. Neostigmine-resistant curarisation. *British Medical Journal* 1956; **2**: 919-21.
216. Miles H N, Levin J, Boulton T B, Krigbaum E M. Neostigmine-resistant curarisation. *British Medical Journal* 1956; **2**: 1429-30.
217. Dinnick O P. Deaths associated with anaesthesia. Observations on 600 cases. *Anaesthesia* 1964; **12**: 536-56.
218. Lunn J N, Mushin W W. *Mortality Associated with Anaesthesia*. London: Nuffield Provincial Hospital Trust, 1982.
219. Campling E A, Devlin H B, Lunn J N. *The Reports of the National Confidential Enquiry into Perioperative Deaths*. London: Published independently, 1990, 1992 and 1993.
220. Leading Article. The banning of heroin. *British Medical Journal* 1953; **2**: 196.
221. Douthwaite A H. The ban on heroin. *British Medical Journal* 1953; **2**: 907-8.
222. Medical Notes in Parliament. Ban on heroin. *British Medical Journal* 1955; **1**: 1163.
223. Annual Representative Meeting, London 1955. The withdrawal of heroin. *British Medical Journal* 1955; **1**: Supplement 289-90.
224. Medical Notes in Parliament. *British Medical Journal* 1956; **1**: 298-9.
225. Bullingham R E S, McQuay H J, Moore R A. Extradural and intrathecal narcotics. In: Atkinson R S, Hewer C L, eds. *Recent Advances in Anaesthesia and Analgesia 14*. Edinburgh: Churchill Livingstone, 1982: 141-56.
226. Mushin W W, Gray T C, Wilson H B. The use of heroin by anaesthetists. *Anaesthesia* 1957; **12**: 125-8.
227. Editorial. *Anaesthesia* 1957; **12**: 247-8.
228. Low W A. President's address. *Proceedings of the Royal Society of Medicine* 1951; **44**: 219-24.
229. Editorial. *Anaesthesia* 1952; **7**: 133.
230. W S M. Obituary. Dr D Marston. *Anaesthesia* 1962; **17**: 260-1.
231. *Report of a Working Party on Anaesthetic Explosions including Safety Code for Equipment and Installations*. London: Her Majesty's Stationery Office, 1956.
232. Leading Article. Anaesthetic Explosions. *British Medical Journal* 1956; **2**: 1225-6.
233. Vickers M D. Explosion hazards. Recommendations of the Association of Anaesthetists of Great Britain and Ireland. *Anaesthesia* 1971; **26**: 155-7.
234. Obituary. A Charles King. *Anaesthesia* 1966; **21**: 439-40.
235. Wilkinson D J. A Charles King: a unique contribution to anaesthesia. *Journal of the Royal*

Society of Medicine 1987; 80: 510-4.
236. Wilkinson D J. Francis Percival de Caux. An anaesthetist at odds with social convention and the law. *Anaesthesia* 1991; **46**: 300-5.
237. Obituary. Robert James Minnitt. *Anaesthesia* 1974; **29**: 382.
238. R P W S. Mr A Charles King. *Anaesthesia* 1953; **8**: 138.
239. Obituary. Dr William Stanley Sykes. *Anaesthesia* 1961; **16**: 383.
240. *AAGBI Minute Book No 1 1932-1947*: 1-402.
241. Wilkinson D J, Eccles A. The BOC Museum (Charles King Collection of Historical Apparatus)-the evolution of a Collection into a Museum. *Journal of the History of Collections* 1992; **4**: 99-105.
242. Obituary. Kenneth Bryn Thomas. *Anaesthesia* 1979; **34**: 108.
243. Thomas K B. The A Charles King. Collection of early anaesthetic apparatus. *Anaesthesia* 1970; **25**: 548-564.
244. Mushin W W. Editorial. Professor Emeritus Sir Robert Reynolds Macintosh 17 October 1897 - 28 August 1989. *Anaesthesia* 1989; **44**: 951-2.
245. Thornton J L. John Snow: Pioneer specialist anaesthetist. *Anaesthesia* 1950; **5**: 129-34.
246. John Snow's Grave. *Anaesthesia* 1950; **5**: 48.
247. Association News. *Anaesthesia* 1952; **7**: 192-5.
248. Association News. *Anaesthesia* 1958; **13**: 481-2.

Chapter 7- Expansion and Extension, 1 January 1960 to 31 December 1969

1. Organe G S W. Obituary. Ronald Jarman. *Anaesthesia* 1973; **28**: 197.
2. Wishart H H, Holloway K B, Spence A A. Obituary. Henry Harry Pinkerton. *Anaesthesia* 1982; **37**: 1143-5.
3. Burn J M B, Zorab J S M. Obituary. Robert Patrick Webb Shackleton. *Anaesthesia* 1977; **32**: 819-21.
4. Lumley J. Editorial. Arthur John Wells Beard. *Anaesthesia* 1993; **48**: 483-4.
5. M H A D. Obituary. E A Pask. *British Medical Journal* 1966; **1**: 1486.
6. R I W B, W D W, R I B. Obituary. H J V Morton. *British Medical Journal* 1982; **284**: 988.
7. Zorab J S M. Editorial. Philip John Helliwell. *Anaesthesia* 1994; **49**: 659-60.
8. Boulton T B. Editorial. C Langton Hewer. *Anaesthesia* 1986; **41**: 469-70.
9. Cook C, ed. *Pears Cyclopaedia* 1889-90, 98th edition. Harmondsworth: Penguin Books, 1989.
10. Grey-Turner E, Sutherland F M. *History of the British* British Medical Association, 1982.
11. Notes and News. Oral contraceptives. *Lancet* 1961; **2**: 885-6.
12. Leathard A. *Health Care Provision. Past, present and future*. London: Chapman and Hall, 1990.
13. Leading Article. "Getting Married". *British Medical Journal* 1959; **1**: 705.
14. Turner G S, Piper G W, Hendry R P, Cockshut R W, Watson-Williams E, Pinniger R W, Cooper B S. Correspondence. "Getting Married". *British Medical Journal* 1959; **1**: 714-5.
15. Walton J, Baroness J A, Lock S, eds.. *The Oxford Companion to Medicine*. Oxford: University press, 1994.
16. Wilkinson D J. Francis Percival de Caux. An anaesthetist at odds with social convention and the law. *Anaesthesia* 1991; **46**: 300-5.

17. Leading Article. A deadly habit. *British Medical Journal* 1962; **1**: 696-7.
18. Williams G M. Status of renal transplantation today. *Surgical Clinics of North America* 1978; **58**: 273-84.
19. Starzl T E, Marchioro T L, Von Kaulla K N, Hermann G, Brittain M D, Waddell W R. Homotransplantation of the liver in humans. *Surgery, Gynecology and Obstetrics* 1963; **117**: 658-76.
20. Calne R Y, Williams R. Orthotopic liver transplantation: the first 60 patients. *British Medical Journal* 1977; **1**: 471-81.
21. Scott D L. Cardiac pacemakers as an anaesthetic problem. *Anaesthesia* 1970; **25**: 87-114.
22. Emmanuel R. Too ill for surgery? *British Medical Journal* 1968; **2**: 400-2.
23. Leading Article. Cardiac Transplantations. *British Medical Journal* 1967; **4**: 757-8.
24. Leading Article. First British cardiac transplantation. *British Medical Journal* 1968; **2**: 315-6.
25. Leading Article. Beyond the bounds. *British Medical Journal* 1968; **2**: 642.
26. Thomas F T. Heart transplantation - 1978. *Surgical Clinics of North America* 1978; **58**: 335-56.
27. Medical News. Cardiac Transplantation. *British Medical Journal* 1973; **1**: 431.
28. Knight P F. Anaesthesia for leaking abdominal aortic aneurysm. *Anaesthesia* 1963; **18**: 151-7.
29. Bowen R A. Anaesthesia in operations for the relief of portal hypertension. *Anaesthesia* 1960; **15**: 3-10.
30. Leading Article. total replacement of the hip. *British Medical Journal* 1972; **2**: 177-8.
31. Farman J V. Anaesthesia for transplant surgery. In: Hewer C L, Atkinson R S eds.. *Recent Advances in Anaesthesia and Analgesia*. 12th edition. Edinburgh: Churchill Livingstone, 1976: 92-119.
32. Rosborough D. Fat embolism in patients with fractured hips. *British Medical Journal* 1972; **2**: 528.
33. Ellis R H, Mulvein J. Total replacement of the hip. *British Medical Journal* 1972; **2**: 528.
34. Turner L. Too ill for surgery? *British Medical Journal* 1968; **2**: 558.
35. Manley R W. A new mechanical ventilator. *Anaesthesia* 1961; **16**: 317-23.
36. Editorial. *Anaesthesia* 1968; **23**: 163-4.
37. Hunter A R. Diallyl nortoxiferine. *British Journal of Anaesthesia* 1964; **36**: 406-20.
38. Baird W L M, Reid A M. The neuromuscular blocking properties of a new steroid compound, pancuronium bromide. A pilot study in man. *British Journal of Anaesthesia* 1967; **39**: 775-80.
39. Nilsson E. Editorial views. Origin and rationale of neuroleptanalgesia. *Anesthesiology* 1963; **24**: 267-8.
40. Stovner J, Endresen R. Diazepam in intravenous anaesthesia. *Lancet* 1965; **2**: 1298-9.
41. Cushman R P A. Diazepam in intravenous anaesthesia. *Lancet* 1966; **1**: 1042.
42. Dundee J W, Clarke R S J. Clinical studies of induction agents 9: a comparative study of a new Eugenol derivative, FBA 1420 with b29.505 and standard bartiburates. *British Journal of Anaesthesia* 1964; **36**: 100-5.
43. Scott J G. Propanidid. *Anaesthesia* 1984; **39**: 834.
44. Jarman R, Edghill H B. Methoxyflurane (Penthrane). *Anaesthesia* 1962; **18**: 265-78.
45. Richey J E, Smith R B. Renal failure after methoxyflurane anaesthesia. *Anaesthesia* 1972;

27: 9-13.
46. Jones P L, Molloy M J, Rosen M. the Cardiff penthrane inhaler. A vaporiser for the administration of Methoxyflurane in obstetric analgesia. *British Journal of Anaesthesia* 1971; **43**: 190-9.
47. Boivin P A, Hudon F, Jacques A. Properties of the fluothane-ether anaesthetic. *Canadian Anaesthetists' Society Journal* 1958; **5**: 409-413.
48. Howat D D C. A new azeotropic mixture. A comparison of halothane-methyl-n-propylether and halothane alone. *Anaesthesia* 1963; **18**: 446-461.
49. Rees G J, Gray T C. Methyl-n-propyl ether. *British Journal of Anaesthesia* 1950; **22**: 83-91.
50. Watt M J, Ross D M, Atkinson R S. A clinical trial of bupivacaine. A preliminary report on a new analgesic agent in extradural analgesia. *Anaesthesia* 1968; **23**: 2-13.
51. Davies D M. Clinical Forum. An extradural analgesia service in obstetrics. *Anaesthesia* 1971; **26**: 494-5.
52. Bryce-Smith R. Complications. In: Hewer C L, ed. *Recent Advances in Anaesthesia and Analgesia*. Edinburgh: Churchill Livingstone. 1972: 239-70.
53. Plumpton F S, Besser G M, Cole P V. Corticosteroid treatment and surgery. 1. An investigation of the indications for steroid cover. *Anaesthesia* 1969; **24**: 3-11.
54. Plumpton F S, Besser G M, Cole P V. Corticosteroid treatment and surgery. 2. The management of steroid cover. *Anaesthesia* 1969; **24**: 12-18.
55. Virtue R W, Payne K W. Postoperative death after fluothane. *Anesthesiology* 1958; **11**: 562-3.
56. Editorial. The National halothane study. *Journal of the American Medical Association* 1966; **197**: 811-2.
57. Neuberger J, Williams R. Occasional Review. Halothane anaesthesia and liver damage. *British Medical Journal* 1984; **289**: 1136-9.
58. Denborough M A, Lovell R R H. Anaesthetic deaths in a family. *Lancet* 1960; **2**: 45.
59. Ellis F R, Heffron J J A. Clinical and biochemical aspects of malignant hyperpyrexia. In: Atkinson R S, Adams A P, eds. *Recent Advances in Anaesthesia and Analgesia 15*. Edinburgh: Churchill Livingstone, 1985: 173-208.
60. Searle J F. Anaesthesia in sickle cell states. A review. *Anaesthesia* 1973; **28**: 48-58.
61. T B B. Editorial. *Anaesthesia* 1965; **20**: 1-2.
62. Smith W D A. Pollution and the anaesthetist. In: Hewer C L, Atkinson R S, eds. *Recent Advances in Anaesthesia and Analgesia 12*. Edinburgh: Churchill Livingstone, 1976: 131-73.
63. Editorial. *Anaesthesia* 1963; **18**: 133-4.
64. Hutchinson R. Awareness during surgery. A study of its incidence. *British Journal of Anaesthesia* 1961; **33**: 463-9.
65. Clutton-Brock J. Two cases of poisoning by contamination of nitrous oxide during anaesthesia. *British Journal of Anaesthesia* 1967; **39**: 388-920.
66. G W B. Obituary. J Clutton-Brock. *British Medical Journal* 1986; **283**: 1381.
67. Kouwenhoven W B, Jude J R, Knickerbocker G G. Closed chest cardiac massage. *Journal of the American Medical Association* 1960; **173**: 1064-7.
68. Editorial. *Anaesthesia* 1962; **17**: 1-2.
69. Milstein B B. Cardiac resuscitation. *British Journal of Anaesthesia* 1961; **33**: 498-515.
70. Marshall R D. A year of resuscitation. A report of a meeting of the North East Metropolitan

Regional Anaesthetists' Group. *Anaesthesia* 1966; 21: 86-91.
71. Sykes M K, Orr D S. Cardiopulmonary resuscitation. A report of two years experience. *Anaesthesia* 1966; **21**: 363-71.
72. Gilston A, Resnekov L. *Cardio-respiratory Resuscitation*. London: Heinemann, 1971.
73. R A B. Obituary. R A Binning. *British Medical Journal* 1989; **298**: 43.
74. Binning R. External cardiac compression. *British Medical Journal* 1962; **2**: 1753-4.
75. Gilston A. Intensive care in England and Wales. A survey of current practice, training and attitudes. *Anaesthesia* 1981; **36**: 188-93.
76. Rosen M (Chairman). *Report of a Working Party. Intensive Care Services - provision for the future*. London: Association of Anaesthetists of Great Britain and Ireland, 1988.
77. Editorial. *Anaesthesia* 1976; **31**: 371-3.
78. Campbell E M M. *British Medical Association Planning Unit Report. Intensive Care*. London: British Medical Association, 1968.
79. Mushin W W (President). Section of Anaesthetics. Discussion on intensive care units. *Proceedings of the Royal Society of Medicine* 1966; **59**: 1293-6.
80. Ibsen B. Intensive therapy: background and development. *International Anesthesiology Clinics* 1966; **4**: 277-94.
81. Bower A G, Bennett V R, Dillon J B, Axelrod B. Investigations on the care and treatment of poliomyelitis patients. *Annals of Western Medicine and Surgery* 1950; **4**: 561-582 and 686-716.
82. Secher O. The polio epidemic in Copenhagen 1952. In: Atkinson R S, Boulton T B, eds. *The History of Anaesthesia*. International Congress and Symposium Series 134. London: Royal Society of Medicine 1989: 425-32.
83. Ibsen B. The anaesthetist's viewpoint on the treatment of respiratory complications in poliomyelitis during the epidemic in Copenhagen 1952. *Proceedings of the Royal Society of Medicine* 1954; **48**: 72-4.
84. Beinart J. *A History of the Nuffield Department of Anaesthetics Oxford 1937-1987*. Oxford: University Press, 1987.
85. Spalding J M K, Smith A C. *Clinical Practice and Physiology of Artificial Respiration*. Oxford: Blackwell Scientific Publications 1963.
86. Salk J E. Vaccination against poliomyelitis: performance and prospect. *American Journal of Public Health 1955*; **45**: 576-96.
87. Lambert V F (Chairman). Discussion on the modern indications for tracheotomy with special reference to the management of those cases requiring artificial respiration. *Proceedings of the Royal Society of Medicine* 1955; **48**: 947-960.
88. Pearce D J. Experiences in a small respiratory unit of a general hospital with special reference to the treatment of tetanus. *Anaesthesia* 1961; **16**: 308-16.
89. Horton J A G. Major complications arising with treatment of tetanus. In: Boulton T B, Bryce-Smith R, Sykes M K, Gilbert G B, Revell A L, eds. *Progress in Anaesthesiology. Proceedings of the Fourth World Congress of Anaesthesiologists*. Amsterdam. Excerpta Medica 1970: 1104-9.
90. Smith A C. The treatment of severe tetanus by paralysing drugs and intermittent pressure respiration. *Proceedings of the Royal Society of Medicine* 1956; **51**: 1006-8.
91. Shackleton P. The treatment of tetanus. Role of the anaesthetist. *Lancet* 1954; **2**: 155-8.
92. Rushman G B, Richmond D J H, Miell R M, Boulton T B. The Intensive Care Unit. *St*

Bartholomew's Hospital Journal 1970; **74**: 242-4.
93. Cohen P J. Editorial Views. Critical care, critical times. *Anesthesiology* 1977; **47**: 81.
94. Jolly C, Lee J A. Postoperative observation ward. *Anaesthesia* 1957; **12**: 49-56.
95. Gardner E K. The recovery ward and intensive therapy unit. *Anaesthesia* 1964; **19**: 128-30.
96. Gilston A. The management of respiratory distress after cardiothoracic surgery. *Thorax* 1962; **17**: 139-45.
97. Gilston A. A. Facial signs of respiratory distress after cardiac surgery: a plea for the clinical approach to mechanical ventilation. *Anaesthesia* 1976; **31**: 385-7.
98. Spencer G T. Planning and Construction of Intensive Therapy Units. In: Boulton T B, Bryce-Smith R, Sykes M K, Gillett G B, Revell A L, eds. *Progress in Anaesthesiology. Proceedings of the Fourth World Congress of Anaesthesiology*. Amsterdam. Excerpta Medica, 1970: 479.
99. Partridge J F, Guedel J S. Cardiac arrest after myocardial infarction. *Lancet* 1961; **1**: 807-8.
100. Atkinson R S. Place of the anaesthetist in the intensive care unit. In: Hewer C L, ed. *Recent Advances in Anaesthesia and Analgesia*. 11th edition. Edinburgh: Churchill Livingstone 1972: 271-89.
101. Rees G J, Stead A L, Bush G H, Jones R S. Intensive therapy in paediatrics. *British Medical Journal* 1966; **2**: 1611-6.
102. Ministry of Health. Progressive Patient Care. Interim Report of a Departmental Working Group. *Monthly Bulletin of the Ministry of Health and the Public Health Laboratory Service* 1962; **21**: 218-23.
103. Boulton T B. Editorial. *Anaesthesia* 1982; **37**: 627-8.
104. Leading Article. Intensive care. *British Medical Journal* 1966; **2**: 1609-10.
105. Mushin W W, Lunn J N. The anaesthetist and intensive care. *British Medical Journal* 1969; **2**: 683-4.
106. Marshall R D. Intensive care and the anaesthetist. *British Medical Journal* 1969; **2**: 820.
107. Crockett G S. Intensive care and the anaesthetist. *British Medical Journal* 1969; **2**: 820.
108. Round the centres. St Bartholomew's Hospital. *Anaesthesia* 1968; **23**: 133-4.
109. Gilston A. Report of the First World Congress on Intensive Care, June 24-27, 1974. *European Journal of Intensive Care Medicine* 1975; **1**: 93-7.
110. Special correspondent. Monitoring in anaesthesia, present trends and future needs.. *British Medical Journal* 1970; **1**: 686-7.
111. M K S. Editorial. *Anaesthesia* 1970; **25**: 315-6.
112. Crul J S (Chairman). Symposium on Monitoring in Anaesthesia. In: Boulton T B, Bryce-Smith R, Sykes M K, Gillett G B, Revell A L, eds. *Progress in Anaesthesiology. Proceedings of the Fourth World Congress of Anaesthesiologists*. Amsterdam: Excerpta Medica 1970: 335-66.
113. Monks P S. Safe use of electro-medical equipment. *Anaesthesia* 1971; **26**: 264-80.
114. Hull C J. Electrocution hazards in the operating theatre. *British Journal of Anaesthesia* 1978; **50**: 647-57.
115. Csanky-Treels J C. Hazards of central venous pressure monitoring. *Anaesthesia* 1978; **33**: 172-7.
116. Adams A P, Morgan-Hughes J O, Sykes M K. pH and blood gas analysis. Methods of measurement and sources of error using electrode systems. Parts 1 and 2. *Anaesthesia*

1967; **22**: 575-97 and *Anaesthesia* 1968; **23**: 47-64.
117. Sykes M K. Venous pressure as a clinical indication of adequacy of transfusion. *Annals of the Royal College of Surgeons of England* 1963; **33**: 185-97.
118. Kelman G R. Interpretation of CVP measurements. *Anaesthesia* 1971; **26**: 209-15.
119. Editorial. The moment of death. *World Medicine Journal* 1967; **14**: 133-4.
120. Boulton T B. Definition of death. *St Bartholomew's Hospital Journal* 1969; **23**: 39-47.
121. Clinical Topics. Diagnosis of death. Statement issued by the Honorary Secretary of the Conference of Medical Royal Colleges and their Faculties in the United Kingdom. *British Medical Journal* 1976; **2**: 1187-8.
122. Leading Article. Invincible arrogance, and patients suffer. *British Medical Journal* 1980; **2**: 1509-10.
123. Leading Article. A television verdict on brain death. *Lancet* 1980: **2**: 841.
124. Searle J P. Editorial. *Anaesthesia* 1981; **36**: 253-5.
125. Belam O H, Dobney G H. Persistent pain. Treatment by nerve block (a preliminary report). *Anaesthesia* 1957; **12**: 345-51.
126. Editorial. *Anaesthesia* 1962; **17**: 267-8.
127. Swerdlow M. Four years pain clinic experience. *Anaesthesia* 1967; **22**: 568-74.
128. Lloyd J W. Use of anaesthesia. The anaesthetist and the pain clinic. *British Medical Journal* 1980; **281**: 432-4.
129. Lloyd J W. Pain relief clinics. *Journal of the Royal Society of Medicine* 1982; **75**: 151-2.
130. Bonica J J (Chairman). Symposium on pain. In: Boulton T B, Bryce-Smith R, Sykes M K, Gilbert G R, Revell A L, eds. *Progress in Anaesthesiology. Proceedings of the Fourth World Congress of Anaesthesiologists.* Amsterdam: Excerpta Medica 1970: 243-88.
131. Swerdlow M, Mehta M D, Lipton S. The role of the anaesthetist in chronic pain management. *Anaesthesia* 1978; **33**: 250-7.
132. Melzack R, Wall P D. Pain mechanisms. A new theory. *Science* 1965; **150**: 971-9.
133. Scott W E. The continuing problem of pain: a discussion paper. *Journal of the Royal Society of Medicine* 1982; **75**: 117-20.
134. Glyn C J. Domiciliary consultations within the pain relief service. *British Medical Journal* 1986; **292**: 222.
135. Mirkes P E. Teratology. In: Walton J. Beeson P B, Scott R B, eds. *The Oxford Companion to Medicine.* Oxford: University Press, 1986: 1374-8.
136. Hayman D J. Withdrawal of thalidomide (Distaval). *British Medical Journal* 1961; **2**: 1499.
137. Leading Article. Social Insurance and Services. Medical Parts of the Beveridge Plan. *British Medical Journal* 1942; **2**: 704-6.
138. Roberts F. The cost of the National Health Service. *British Medical Journal* 1949; **1**: 293-7.
139. Ministry of Health. *Hospital Plan for England and Wales.* London: HMSO, 1962.
140. Abel A L, Lewin W. Report on Hospital Buildings. *British Medical Journal* 1959; **1**: Supplement 109-14.
141. Leading Article. Royal Commission Report. *British Medical Journal* 1960; **1**: 556-7.
142. Beecham L. Review Body Reports. *British Medical Journal* 1992; **304**: 403.
143. Medicopolitical Digest. Review body Reports. *British Medical Journal* 1992; **304**: 449.
144. British Medical Association Third Report of Negotiations on Family Doctor Service *British Medical Journal* 1966; **1**: Supplement 135-45.

145. Leading Article. Hospital Medical Staff. *British Medical Journal* 1966; **2**: 1021-2.
146. BMA Working Party. "Charter" for Hospital Doctors. *British Medical Journal* 1966; **2**: Supplement 171-4.
147. Leading Article. Medical Staffing of Hospitals. *British Medical Journal* 1961; **1**: 883-4.
148. Editorial. *Anaesthesia* 1967; **22**: 1-2.
149. Blair J S G. Mitchiner Lecture 1994. *Journal of the Royal Army Medical Corps* 1995; **141**: 7-14.
150. Blair J S G. Mitchinner Lecture 1994. *Journal of the Royal Army Medical Corps* 1995; **141**: 7-14.
151. AAGBI. *Minute Book No 2*. 5.12.47-1.2.63.
152. A J S. Obituary. Lieutenant General Sir Alexander Drummond. *British Medical Journal* 1988; **297**: 1603.
153. Smith G, ed. Anaesthetic Research Society, Handbook of British Anaesthesia 1992-1993. London: *British Journal of Anaesthesia* 1992: 18.
154. Boulton T B, Bryce-Smith R, Sykes M K, Gillett G B, Revell A L, eds. *Progress in Anaesthesiology. Proceedings of the Fourth World Congress of Anaesthesiologists.* Amsterdam, Excerpta Medica Foundation Congress Series 200, 1970.
155. *AAGBI Minute Book No 3*. 5.4.63-6.7.73.
156. Pallister W K. Editorial. Sir Geoffrey William Organe 1908-1989. *Anaesthesia* 1989; **44**: 461-2.
157. Association News. *Anaesthesia* 1963; **18**: 124-6.
158. Annual Report to Council 1980-1981. *Anaesthesia* 1982; **37**: 228-35.
159. Obituary. Robert Reynolds Macintosh. *Lancet* 1989; **2**: 816.
160. Obituary. Michael Denis Nosworthy. *Anaesthesia* 1981; **36**: 98.
161. Obituary. Edgar Stanley Rowbotham. *Anaesthesia* 1979; **34**: 709.
162. Obituary. Harry James Shields. *Canadian Anaesthetists' Society Journal* 1974; **21**: 258-60.
163. Obituary. Edward Falkner Hill. *Anaesthesia* 1974; **29**: 768.
164. Obituary. Robert James Minnitt. *Anaesthesia* 1974; **29**: 382.
165. Obituary Notices. Katherine G Lloyd-Williams. *British Medical Journal* 1973; **1**: 179.
166. Obituary. Frankis Tilney Evans. *Anaesthesia* 1974; **29**: 768
167. R R M. Obituary. Professor E A Pask. *Anaesthesia* 1966; **27**: 437-9.
168. Editorial. *Anaesthesia* 1977; **32**: 843-5.
169. Obituary. Henry Evelyn Pooler. *Anaesthesia* 1977; **32**: 401.
170. Association News. Miss Joan Paternoster. *Anaesthesia* 1962; **17**: 127.
171. Obituary. Ralph Blair Gould. *Anaesthesia* 1984; **39**: 1044.
172. Lee J A, Lunn J N. Editorial. John Alfred Lee. *Anaesthesia* 1989; **44**: 631.
173. Editorial. *Anaesthesia* 1960; **15**: 103.
174. Editorial. *Anaesthesia* 1966; **21**: 323-4.
175. Hewer C L. Dr R P B Shackleton and *Anaesthesia*. *Anaesthesia* 1977; **32**: 1038-90.
176. Hewer C L. Editorial. *Anaesthesia* 1976; **31**: 1023-4.
177. Association News. *Anaesthesia* 1966; **21**: 313.
178. Obituary. A R Hunter. *Anaesthesia* 1991; **46**: 604.
179. P J H. Obituary. A M Hutton. *British Medical Journal* 1981; **282**: 160.
180. Spencer E M. *The History of the Group of Anaesthetists in Training.* London: Association

of Anaesthetists of Great Britain and Ireland, 1992.
181. Association News . Steering Committee of Associates in Training. *Anaesthesia* 1967; **22**: 191-2.
182. Association News. Registrars Meeting at Bristol. *Anaesthesia* 1968; **23**: 484-5.
183. G W B. Obituary. J Clutton-Brock. *British Medical Journal* 1986; **283**: 1381.
184. Platt R (Chairman). Medical Staffing in the Hospital Service. Report of a Joint Working Party. *British Medical Journal* 1961; **1**: Supplement 99-102.
185. Leading Article. Medical Staffing of Hospitals. *British Medical Journal* 1961; **91**: 883-4.
186. Strachan C I (Chairman). Revised Report of a subcommittee on hospital Medical staffing. *British Medical Journal* 1955; **1**: Supplement 177-81.
187. Sellors T. Hospital Medical Staffing. *British Medical Journal* 1964; **2**: 816.
188. Porritt A (Chairman). Report of Medical Services Review Committee. Summary of Conclusions and Recommendations. *British Medical Journal* 1962; **2**: 1178-86.
189. Leading Article. Porritt Report on the NHS. *British Medical Journal* 1962; **2**: 1171-3.
190. Ministry of Health Statement. Medical Staffing and Structure in Hospitals. *British Medical Journal* 1964; **2**: 438-40.
191. Summary of Ministry Circular HM(64)94. Hospital Medical Staffing. New Arrangements. *British Medical Journal* 1964; **2**: Supplement 193-4.
192. Leading Article. Hospital Medical Staffing. *British Medical Journal* 1964; **2**: 398-9.
193. Leading Article. Hospital Practitioner grade. *British Medical Journal* 1976; **2**: 1277.
194. Association News and Notices. Hospital Practitioner Grade. *Anaesthesia* 1976; **31**: 1319.
195. Scurr C F. Editorial. *Anaesthesia* 1977; **32**: 515-6.
196. Woodyard C. Hospital Practitioner Grade. *British Medical Journal* 1976; **2**: 1277.
197. Scurr C F. The Hospital Practitioner Grade. A reply from Dr Scurr. *Anaesthesia* 1978; **33**: 64.
198. Association News . *Anaesthesia* 1958; **13**: 105 and 373.
199. Spence A A. Tape-recorded lectures for anaesthetists. *British Journal of Anaesthesia* 1968; **40**: 1003-5.
200. Ellis F R, Spence A A. Clinical trials of metoclopramide (Moxolon) as an antiemetic in anaesthesia. *Anaesthesia* 1970; **25**: 368-71.
201. Spence A A, Smith G, Harris R. The influence of postoperative analgesia and operative procedures on postoperative lung function. A comparison of morphine with extradural nerve block. *Anaesthesia* 1970; **25**: 126.
202. Bushman J A, Collis J M. The estimation of gas losses in ventilator tubing. *Anaesthesia* 1967; **22**: 664-7.
203. Robinson J S, Cox L A, Bushman J, Inglis T. A pressure-cycled ventilator with multiple functional behaviour. *British Journal of Anaesthesia* 1969; **41**: 455-64.
204. R W C. Obituary. Professor Ronald Woolmer. *Anaesthesia* 1963; **18**: 248-50.
205. Association News. Essay Prize. *Anaesthesia* 1960; **15**: 97-8.
206. Association News. *Anaesthesia* 1965; **20**: 38.
207. Junior Anaesthetists' Group News. *Anaesthesia* 1974; **29**: 386-8.
208. Junior Anaesthetists' Group News. *Anaesthesia* 1973; **28**: 354-5.
209. Obituary. John Vernon Farman. *Anaesthesia* 1989; **44**: 92.
210. Faculty News. Adviser in Postgraduate Studies. *Anaesthesia* 1959; **14**: 306.
211. Farman J V. Anaesthetic problems facing developing countries. *Anaesthesia* 1967; **22**: 714-5.

212. Hingson R A. The World Federation of Societies of Anaesthesiologists extends education and emergency relief across the continents. In: Boulton T B, Bryce-Smith R, Sykes M K, Gillett G B, Revell A L, eds. *Progress in Anaesthesiology. Proceedings of the Fourth World Congress of Anaesthesiologists.* Amsterdam: Excerpta Medica Foundation Congress Series 200, 1970: 1115-20.
213. Zorab J S M. The World Federation of Societies of Anaesthesiologists (WFSA). *Anaesthesia* 1976; **31**: 285-92.
214. Wilson G. *Fifty Years. The Australian Society of Anaesthetists 1934-1984*. Edgecliff NSW: Australian Society of Anaesthetists, 1987: 439.
215. Adams A K (Chairman). Report on aid to developing Countries: Britain's contribution. *Anaesthesia* 1967; **22**: 281.
216. OPD. Obituary. Bernard Johnson. *Anaesthesia* 1959; **14**: 419-21.
217. Faculty News. Bernard Johnson Memorial Fund. *Anaesthesia* 1961; **16**: 517.
218. Commonwealth Medical Conference. *British Medical Journal* 1965; **2**: 993-4.
219. Boulton T B, Bryce-Smith R, Sykes M K, Gillett G B, Revell A L, eds. *Progress in Anaesthesiology. Proceedings of the Fourth World Congress of Anaesthesiologists.* Amsterdam: Excerpta Medica Foundation International Congress Series No 200, 1970.
220. Oduntan S A. Chloroform anaesthesia. A clinical comparison of chloroform and halothane administered from precision vaporisers. *Anaesthesia* 1978; **23**: 552-7.
221. Clinical Forum. *Anaesthesia* 1973; **28**: 679-95.
222. Wise C C, Robinson J S, Heath M J, Tomlin P J. Physiological response to intermittent methohexitone for conservative dentistry. *British Medical Journal.* 1969; **2**: 540-3.
223. Leading Article. Discontinuance of a libel case. *British Medical Journal* 1972; **4**: 254.
224. Our legal Correspondent. Defamation and medical Journals. *British Medical Journal* 1975; **2**: 46.
225. P S. Obituary. Stanley Lithgow Drumond-Jackson. *British Dental Journal* 1976; **140**: 73-4.
226. Vandam L D. The introduction of modern anaesthesia in the USA and the spread of the good news to the United Kingdom. In: Atkinson R S, Boulton T B, eds. *The History of Anaesthesia*. International Congress and Symposium Series 134. London: Royal Society of Medicine 1989: 64-9.
227. Ellis R H. *James Robinson and the Inhalation of Ether Vapour*. Eastbourne: Bailliere Tindall, 1983.
228. Boulton T B. Editorial. *Anaesthesia* 1979; **34**: 523-4.
229. Gray D J P. *Training for General Practice*. Plymouth: Macdonald and Evans, 1982: 161.
230. Report of a BDA Committee. The position of general anaesthesia in dentistry. *British Dental Journal* 1966; **120**: 89-91.
231. Dinsdale R C W, Dixon R A. Anaesthesia services to dental patients: England and Wales 1976. *British Dental Journal* 1978; **144**: 271-9.
232. Thornton J A. General anaesthesia and sedation for dentistry. In: Hewer C L, Atkinson R S, eds. . *Recent Advances in Anesthesia and Analgesia Number 13*. Edinburgh: Churchill Livingstone 1979: 117-37.
233. Tinkler S. The uses of hypnosis in dental surgery. In: Hartland J. *Medical and Dental Hypnosis and its Clinical Applications*. London: Bailliere Tindall and Cassell, 1966: 324-35.

234. Purves-Stewart J, Willcox W H. Poisoning by barbitone and allied drugs. *Lancet* 1934; **1**: 6-7.
235. Macintosh R R. Battle of the barbiturates. *Lancet* 1934; **1**: 154.
236. Holden G G P. Anaesthetics - a dentist's point of view. *Anaesthesia* 1981; **36**: 112-3.
237. Drummond-Jackson S L. A dental-anaesthetic death. *Lancet* 1966; **1**: 925.
238. Bourne J G. Safer dental anaesthesia. *British Medical Journal* 1967; **3**: 616-7.
239. T B B. The Salisbury meeting on dental anaesthesia. *Anaesthesia* 1968; **23**: 488-9.
240. Leading Article. Anaesthesia for dental extractions. *British Medical Journal* 1967; **1**: 447-8.
241. Bourne J G. A dental anaesthetic death. *Lancet* 1966; **1**: 879-80.
242. Bourne J G. Deaths with dental anaesthesia. *Anaesthesia* 1970; **25**: 473-81.
243. Pownall R H. A dental anaesthetic death. *Lancet* 1966; **1**: 879.
244. Coplans M P, Curson I. Deaths associated with dentistry. *British Dental Journal* 1982; **153**: 357-62 .
245. Bourne J G. Operator anaesthetists in dentistry. *Lancet* 1973; **2**: 611-2.
246. Bourne J G. Anaesthetics: time to delegate? *Lancet* 1970; **1** : 38
247. Boulton T B. Symposiun on the teaching of general anaesthesia for dental surgery. *Anaesthesia* 1964; **19**: 445-9.
248. Leading article. Safer dental anaesthesia. *British Medical Journal* 1967; **3**: 64-5.
249. Swiss R G (Chairman). *Report of a Joint Sub- Committee of the Minister of Health Standing Medical and Dental Advisory Committees of the Central Health Services Council*. London: Her Majesty's Stationery Office, 1967.
250. Editorial. *Anaesthesia* 1961; **16**: 123-4.
251. Yorkshire Society of Anaesthetists. Training in dental anaesthesia. *Anaesthesia* 1961; **15**: 125-8.
252. Annotation. *Lancet* 1964; **1**: 804-5.
253. BDA Committee. Report on the position of anaesthesia in dentistry. *British Dental Journal* 1966; **120**: 89-91.
254. M G. Obituary. A H Galley. *British Medical Journal* 1988; **297**: 737.
255. Parliamentary News. Dentists (anaesthetics). *British Dental Journal* 1966; **120**: 97.
256. Paper by the British Dental Association. General anaesthesia in dentistry. *British Dental Journal* 1967; **122**: 509-10.
257. GB. Summaries of Annual Conference Papers, Birmingham July 1967. Coplans M P. General anaesthesia for conservative dentistry. *British Dental Journal* 1967; **123**: 543-4.
258. Association News. Dental anaesthetics. *Anaesthesia* 1968; **23**: 311.
259. Galley A H. Reporting of Association and Faculty News. *Anaesthesia* 1969; **24**: 286-7.
260. MacRae W R, Vickers M D. New General Dental Council Guidance on general anaesthesia and sedation. *Anaesthesia* 1983; **38**: 804-5.
261. British Dental Association. Conference on general anaesthesia in dentistry. *British Dental Journal* 1967; **122**: Supplement 2-15.
262. Lawson J I M, Main D M G. The use of intravenous anaesthesia by dentists. *British Dental Journal* 1967; **122**: 21-3.
263. Hudson M W P. Safer dental anaesthesia. *British Medical Journal* 1967; **3**: 436.
264. Drummond-Jackson S L. Safer dental anaesthesia. *British Medical Journal* 1967; **3**: 436.
265. Annotation. Anaesthesia for dental surgery. *Lancet* 1967; **1**: 991-2.

266. Windeyer B (Chairman). General Anaesthesia for Dental Surgery. Report of the Windeyer Committee. *British Dental Journal* 1970; **128**: 295-6.
267. Parsons J D. The Windeyer Report. *British Dental Journal* 1970;**128**: 314.
268. Brown P R H, Main D N G, Lawson J I M. Diazepam in dentistry. Report on 108 patients. *British Dental Journal* 1968; **125**: 498-501.
269. Langa H. *Relative Analgesia in Dental Patients*. Philadelphia: Saunders, 1968.
270. Wylie W D (Chairman). *Report of the Working Party on Training in Anaesthesia*. London: Faculty of Dental Surgery and Faculty of Anaesthetists, 1978.
271. Hutton A M, Wedley J R, Seed R F. The teaching of anaesthesia to dentists. *British Dental Journal* 1978; **144**: 35-9.
272. News and Announcements. Intravenous anaesthesia for conservative treatment. Private fees pennissable in the NHS. *British Dental Journal* 1967; **123**: 189-90.
273. Howat D D C. Frederic Hewitt Lecture 1977. Anaesthesia as a career. *Anaesthesia* 1977 ; **32**: 979-95.
274. Scurr C. *NHS Dental Anaesthetics in General Dental Practice*. Pamphlet circulated to members in the Archives of the Association of Anaesthetists of Great Britain and Ireland), 1978.
275. Briefing. Dental Anaesthetics. GMSC recommends withdrawal of service. *British Medical Journal* 1977; **2**: 1434.
276. Annual Report of Council 1991-1992. Private Practice Committee. *Anaesthesia* 1993; **48**: 546-56.
277. Organe G S W, Beard A J W, Dinnick O P. *Report of a Subcommittee on Private Fees*. Archives of the Association of Anaesthetists of Great Britain and Ireland, 1964.
278. British Medical Association. *Private Consultant Work. BMA Guidelines 1990*. London: British Medical Association, 1990.
279. Annual Report to Council 1993-1994. *Anaesthesia* 1995; **50**: 272-282.
280. Higgs R H. The Institute of Operating Theatre Technicians. The staffing of operating theatres. In: Boulton T B, Bryce-Smith R, Sykes M K, Gillett G B , Revell A L, eds. *Progress in Anaesthesiology. Proceedings of the Fourth World Congress of Anaesthesiology*. Amsterdam: Excerpta Medica Congress Series No 200, 1970: 884-6.
281. Pamphlet. *Assistance for the Anaesthetist*. London: Association of Anaesthetists of Great Britain and Ireland, 1988.
282. Annual Report to Council 1990-1991. *Anaesthesia* 1992; **17**: 181-92.
283. Edridge A W. Editorial. Sir Ivan Whiteside Magill. *Anaesthesia* 1987; **42**: 231-3.
284. Lewin W (Chairman). *The Organisation of Staffing of Operating Theatres. A Report of a Joint Sub-Committee of the Standing Medical Advisory Committee and the Standing Nursing Advisory Committee of the Ministry of Health*. London: Her Majesty's Stationery Office, 1970.
285. Summaries of papers read at the Annual Meeting of the Association of Anaesthetists of Great Britain and Ireland, Dublin 1961. *Anaesthesia* 1962; **17**: 75-91.
286. Association News. The Annual Meeting. *Anaesthesia* 1962; **17**: 124-5.
287. Faculty News. The Royal College of Surgeons in Ireland. *Anaesthesia* 1960; **15**: 207.
288. Loder R E. The "Harrogate" anaesthetic room. An investigation into anaesthetists' requirements. *Anaesthesia* 1964; **19**: 557-61.
289. Association News. *Anaesthesia* 1966; **21**: 146-7.
290. Boulton T B. Report on the symposium on recovery wards. *Anaesthesia* 1966; **21**: 104-7.

291. Obituary. J W Dundee. *Anaesthesia* 1992; **47**: 365.
292. Wilkinson D J. A Charles King: a unique contribution to anaesthesia. *Journal of the Royal Society of Medicine* 1987; **80**: 510-4.
293. Galley A H. Association News. John Snow Medal. *Anaesthesia* 1970; **25**: 153-4.
294. Association News. The Annual Meeting 1962. *Anaesthesia* 1963; **18**: 124-6.
295. Association News . The Annual Meeting 1963. *Anaesthesia* 1964; **19**: 157-8.
296. Association News . The Annual Meeting 1964. *Anaesthesia* 1965; **20**: 111.
297. Association News. The Annual Meeting 1965. *Anaesthesia* 1966; **21**: 191.
298. Association News. The Annual Meeting of the Association, London 1970. *Anaesthesia* 1971; **26**: 117-8.
299. Association News. The thirty fifth Annual Meeting of the Association of Anaesthetists of Great Britain and Ireland 1967. *Anaesthesia* 1968; **23**: 156-8.
300. Association News. The Annual Meeting of the Association, Manchester 1969. *Anaesthesia* 1970; **25**: 153-6.
301. Howat D D C. The European Scene. The European Economic Community (EEC). *Anaesthesia* 1974; **29**: 211-21.
302. Second World Congress of Anaesthesiologists. *Anaesthesia* 1960; **15**: 452.
303. Shackleton R P W. Commonwealth and Foreign News. Report on the World Congress in Sao Paulo 1964. *Anaesthesia* 1965 ; **20**: 116-8.
304. Lee J A. Commonwealth and Foreign News. First European Congress of Anaesthesiology Vierma 1962. *Anaesthesia* 1963; **18**: 128-31.
305. Seward E H. Commonwealth and Foreign News. The Second European Congress of Anaesthesiology. *Anaesthesia* 1966; **21**: 610-2.
306. Shackleton R P W. Speech by the President of the Congress. In: Boulton T B, Bryce-Smith R, Sykes M K, Gillett G B, Revell A L, eds. *Progress in* Anaesthesiology. *Proceedings of the Fourth World Congress of Anaesthesiologists*. Amsterdam: Excerpta Medica Foundation Congress Series 200, 1970: x-xi.
307. Obituary. Cledwyn Bebb Lewis. *Anaesthesia* 1980; **35**: 729.
308. Obituary. F G Wood-Smith. *Anaesthesia* 1990; **45**: 905.
309. Wright R B. Congress retrospect. *Anaesthesia* 1969; **24**: 65-8.
310. Faculty of Anaesthetists of the Royal College of Surgeons of England. Admission of HRH Princess Alexandra to the Honorary Fellowship of the Faculty. *Anaesthesia* 1967; **22**: 537.
311. TBB. Overseas News. The Third European Congress of Anaesthesiology, Prague 1970. *Anaesthesia* 1971; **26**: 121-4.
312. Medicolegal. Death Certification and Coroners. *British Medical Journal* 1971; **4**: 498-500.
313. Association of Anaesthetists of Great Britain and Ireland. *Newsletter September 1970*. Association Archives.
314. The Secretariat, Advisory Committee on Distinction Awards. Analysis by type of award, specialty and percentage distribution at 31 December 1992 - England and Wales. *Health Trends* 1993; **25**: 152.
315. W J G. Obituary. Margaret Hawksley. *British Medical Journal* 1985; **291**: 680.
316. Association News. Association Tie, Anaesthesia 1963; **18**: 551.

Chapter 8 - Turbulent Years, 1 January 1970 - 31 December 1982

1. Lumley J. Editorial. Arthur John Wells Beard. *Anaesthesia* 1993; **48**: 843-4.
2. Lee J A, Lunn J N. Editorial. John Alfred Lee (1906-1989) *Anaesthesia* 1989; **44**: 631.
3. Zorab J S M. Editorial. Philip John Helliwell. *Anaesthesia* 1994; 49: 659-60.
4. Cook C, ed. *Pears Cyclopaedia*. London: Penguin Group, 1992: A2-A60 and G2-G78.
5. Hager K. *The Illustrated History of Surgery*. London: Starke, 1988.
6. Schwartz S I, ed. *The Year Book of Surgery*. Chicago: Year Book Medical Publishers, 1982: 127-57
7. Breckenridge A. Which Beta Blocker? *British Medical Journal* 1983; **286**: 1085-6.
8. Clarke R S J. The place of some newer nonanaesthetic drugs in anaesthetic practice. In: Hewer C L, ed. *Recent Advances in Anaesthesia and Analgesia*. 11th edition. Edinburgh: Churchill Livingstone, 1972: 15-40.
9. Jones R M. Calcium antagonists. In: Atkinson R S, Adams A P, eds.. *Recent Advances in Anaesthesia and Analgesia*, 15. Edinburgh: Churchill Livingstone, 1985: 89-106.
10. Gilston A. Techniques and complications of cardiac surgery. In: Hewer C L, Atkinson R S, eds. *Recent Advances in Anaesthesia and Analgesia*, 13. Edinburgh: Churchill Livingstone, 1979: 57-94.
11. Grunzig A R, Senning A, Siegenthaler W E. Nonoperative dilation of coronary artery stenosis. Percutaneous transluminal coronary angioplasty. *New England Journal of Medicine* 1979; **301**: 61-8.
12. Ikeda S, Yanai N, Ishikawa S. Flexible Bronchofiberscope. *Keio Journal of Medicine* 1968; **17**: 1-18.
13. Stiles C M, Stiles Q R, Denson T S. A flexible fibreoptic laryngoscope. *Journal of the American Medical Association* 1972; **221**: 1246-7.
14. Whitehouse W M, ed. *The Year Book of Diagnostic Radiology*. Chicago: Year Book Publishers, 1982: 11-84.
15. Blackwood W S, Maudgal D P, Pickard R G, Lawrence D, Northfield T C. Cimetidine in duodenal ulcer. Controlled trial. *Lancet* 1976; **2**: 174-6.
16. Wylie J H, Clark C G, Alexander-Williams J, Bell P R F, Kennedy T L, Kirk R M, MacKay C. Effect of Cimetidine on surgery for duodenal ulcer. *Lancet* 1981; **1**: 1307-8.
17. Ritchie J W K, Thompson W. A critical review of amniocentesis in clinical practice. In: Bonnar J, ed. *Recent advances in Obstetrics and Gynaecology*, 14. Edinburgh: Churchill Livingstone, 1982: 47-70.
18. Leading Article. Fertilisation in vitro. *British Medical Journal* 1979; **1**: 362.
19. Loder R E. The anaesthetist and the day-stay unit. *Anaesthesia* 1982; **37**: 1037-9.
20. Ogg T W. Assessment of pre-operative cases. *British Medical Journal* 1976; **1**: 82-3.
21. Burn J M B. A blueprint for day surgery. *Anaesthesia* 1979; **34**: 790-805.
22. Atkinson R S. Anaesthesia for day-care surgery. In: Atkinson R S, Hewer C L, eds. *Recent Advances in Anaesthesia and Analgesia*, 14. Edinburgh: Churchill Livingstone, 1982: 81-8.
23. Black G W. Metabolism and toxicity of volatile anaesthetic agents. In: Atkinson R S, Hewer C L, eds. *Recent Advances in Anaesthesia and Analgesia*, 14. Edinburgh: Churchill Livingstone, 1982: 31-44.
24. Hall R M, Boulton T B. Editorial. *Anaesthesia* 1979; **34**: 755-7.

25. Levy W J. Clinical anaesthesia with isoflurane. A review of the multicentre study. *British Journal of Anaesthesia* 1984; **56**: Supplement 101-112.
26. Nunn J F. Chairman's introduction. *British Journal of Anaesthesia* 1984; **56**: Supplement 1-2.
27. White P F, Way W L, Trevor H J. Ketamine. Its pharmacology and therapeutic uses. *Anesthesiology* 1982; **56**: 119-36.
28. Boulton T B. The clinical uses of ketamine with special reference to use in difficult environments. In Boulton T B, ed. *Lectures in Anaesthesiology* 1985; **Supplement 1**: 25-45.
29. Clarke R S J. Biotransformation of intravenous anaesthetic agents. In: Atkinson R S, Hewer C L, eds. *Recent Advances in Anaesthesia*.
30. Dundee J W, Clarke R S J. Clinical studies of induction agents 9. A comparative study of a eugenol derivative FBA 1420 with G 29.505 and standard barbiturates. *British Journal of Anaesthesia* 1964; **36**: 100-5.
31. Campbell D, Forrester A C, Miller D C, Hutton I, Kennedy J A, Lawrie T D V, Lorimer A R, McCall D A. A preliminary clinical study of CT1341 - a steroid anaesthetic agent. *British Journal of Anaesthesia* 1971; **43**: 14-24.
32. Morgan M, Whitwam J G. Editorial. Althesin. *Anaesthesia* 1985; 121-3.
33. Scott J G. Propanidid. *Anaesthesia* 1984; **39**: 834-5.
34. Editorial. Etomidate. *British Journal of Anaesthesia* 1976; **48**: 16.
35. Owen H, Spence A A. Editorial. Etomidate. *British Journal of Anaesthesia* 1984; **56**: 555-7.
36. Rogers K M, Dewar K M S, McCubbin T D, Spence A A. Preliminary experience with ICI 35868 as an i.v. induction agent. Comparison with Althesin. *British Journal of Anaesthesia* 1980; **52**: 807-10.
37. Cummings C, Dixon J, Kay N H, Windsor J P W, Major E, Morgan M, Sear J W, Spence A A, Stephenson D K. Dose requirements of ICI 35868 (propofol, "Diprivan") in a new formulation for induction of anaesthesia. *Anaesthesia* 1984; **39**: 1168-71.
38. Cole P. Sodium nitroprusside. In: Hewer C L, Atkinson R S, eds. *Recent Advances in Anaesthesia and Analgesia*, 13. Edinburgh: Churchill Livingstone, 1979: 139-49.
39. Behar M, Magora F, Olshwang D, Davidson J T. Epidural Morphine in treatment of pain. *Lancet*. 1979; **1**: 257-8.
40. Wang J K, Nauss I A, Thomas J E. Pain relief by intrathecally applied morphine in man. *Anesthesiology* 1979; **50**: 149-51.
41. Billingham R E S, McQuary H J, Moore R A. Extradural and intrathecal narcotics. In: Atkinson R S, Hewer C L, eds. *Recent Advances in Anaesthesia*, 14. Edinburgh: Churchill Livingstone, 1982: 141-56.
42. Graham J L, King R, McGaughey W. Postoperative pain relief using epidural morphine. *Anaesthesia* 1980; **35**: 158-60.
43. Franklin C B. Monitoring. In: Hewer C L, Atkinson R S, eds. *Recent Advances in Anaesthesia and Analgesia*, 13. Edinburgh: Churchill Livingstone, 1979: 167-83.
44. Editorial. *Anaesthesia* 1973; **28**: 597-8.
45. Mehta M. Chronic pain. In: Atkinson R S, Hewer C L, eds. *Recent Advances in Anaesthesia and Analgesia*, 14. Edinburgh: Churchill Livingstone, 1982: 157-77.
46. Lipton S. Pain relief. In: Hewer C L, Atkinson R S, eds. *Recent Advances in Anaesthesia*,

12. Edinburgh: Churchill Livingstone, 1982: 224-260.
47. Mason A A. Surgery under hypnosis. *Anaesthesia* 1955; **10**: 295-9.
48. Spence A A, Wall R A, Nunn J F. Environmental safety and the anaesthetist. In: Nunn J F, Utting J E, Brown B R, eds. *General Anaesthesia*, 5th edition. London: Butterworths, 1989: 595-608.
49. Vessey M P. Epidemiological studies of the occupational hazards of anaesthesia. A review. *Anaesthesia* 1978; **33**: 430-8.
50. Vickers M D. Pollution of the atmosphere of operating theatres. Advice to members from the Council of the Association of Anaesthetists of Great Britain and Ireland. *Anaesthesia* 1975; **30**: 697-9.
51. Department of Health. *Pollution in operating theatres etc by anaesthetic gases. HC(76)38 and SHHD/DS 76/65*. London: Department of Health, 1976.
52. Godber G. Chairman. *First report of a joint working party on the organisation of medical work in hospitals*. London: Her Majesty's Stationery Office, 1967.
53. Owen D. *Our NHS*. London: Pan Books, 1988.
54. Leathard A. *Health Care Provision. Past, Present and Future*. London: Chapman and Hall, 1990.
55. Edwards B. The National Health Service. *A Manager's Tale 1946-1992*. London: Nuffield Provisional Hospitals Trust, 1993.
56. Salmon B L. Chairman. *Report of the Committee on Senior Nurse Staffing Structure*. London: Her Majesty's Stationery Office, 1966.
57. *Evidence to the Royal Commission on the National Health Service*. A pamphlet in the Archives of the Association of Anaesthetists of Great Britain and Ireland, 1977.
58. Anonymous. NHS Reorganisation. *British Medical Journal* 1973; **2**: Supplement 158.
59. Grey-Turner E, Sutherland F M. *History of the British Medical Association. Volume 2, 1932-1981*. London: British Medical Association, 1982.
60. Anonymous. Hospital Disputes. Advice to consultants. *British Medical Journal* 1978; **2**: 1244.
61. Leading Article. Industrial anarchy in the NHS. *British Medical Journal* 1979; **1**: 364.
62. Leading Article. NHS Disputes. Effects on doctors and patients. *British Medical Journal* 1979; **1**: 426.
63. Supplement. BMA's evidence to the Review Body. Training grades in the service (Part 2). *British Medical Journal* 1975; **3**: 779-82.
64. Supplement. Review Body prices juniors' new contract. Two tier supplements for duties above 44 hours. *British Medical Journal* 1975; **3**: 782-5.
65. Leading Article. Hospital junior staff ballot. *British Medical Journal* 1975; **4**: 248.
66. Leading Article. Towards a better service. *British Medical Journal* 1975; **4**: 309-10.
67. Leading Article. Proposed new contracts for hospital junior staff. *British Medical Journal* 1973; **4**: Supplement 31-3.
68. Leading Article. Junior's viewpoint. Interview with the Group Council's Chairman. *British Medical Journal* 1973; **4**: Supplement 34-7.
69. Medical News. Juniors vote for industrial action. *British Medical Journal* 1975; **4**: 476.
70. Leading Article. Industrial action by doctors. *British Medical Journal* 1975; **4**: 544.
71. Supplement. Hospital Junior Staffs Committee. *British Medical Journal* 1975; 4: 600.
72. Supplement. Hospital Junior Staffs Committee. Committee recommends suspension of

sanctions. *British Medical Journal* 1975; **4**: 110.
73. Leading Article. Political facts of life. *British Medical Journal* 1976; **1**: 418.
74. Merrison A (Chairman). *Report of the Royal Commission on the National Health Service*. London: Her Majesty's Stationery Office, 1979.
75. Supplement. Hospital dispute. Royal Colleges statement. *British Medical Journal* 1975; **4**: 601-2.
76. Short D, Aldis A S, Cook C M, Jackson D M, Scorer C G, Walker R S. Should doctors strike again? *British Medical Journal* 1976; **1**: 1214.
77. Tasker P ("and nineteen other doctors from hospitals widely distributed throughout the country"). Junior hospital staff contract. *British Medical Journal* 1976; **1**: 45-6.
78. Leading Article. Consultant contract improvements. *British Medical Journal* 1979; **2**: 887.
79. Merrison A W. (Chairman). *Report of the Committee of inquiry into the regulation of the Medical profession*. London: Her Majesty's Stationery Office, 1975.
80. Leading Article. A good report. *British Medical Journal* 1975; **2**: 155-6.
81. *AAGBI Minute Book No. 4* (20.9.1973-2.8.1979).
82. General Medical Council. Appointed and nominated members. *British Medical Journal* 1979; **2**: 618.
83. Briefing. The Royal Commission on the NHS. The background. *British Medical Journal* 1979; **2**: 288-90.
84. Medical News. Royal Commission on the NHS. *British Medical Journal* 1976; **1**: 1221.
85. Rosen M, Vickers M D. *Evidence to the Royal Commission on the National Health Service*. A document in the Archives of the Association of Anaesthetists of Great Britain and Ireland 1977.
86. Merrison A W. (Chairman). *Royal Commission on the National Health Service*. London: Her Majesty's Stationery Office 1979.
87. Supplement. Royal Commission on the NHS. *British Medical Journal* 1979; **2**: 284-7.
88. Leading Article. Much to praise, not a little to criticise. *British Medical Journal* 1979; **2**: 227-8.
89. Supplement. "Patients First". Government proposals for the NHS. *British Medical Journal* 1979; **2**: 1605.
90. Riding J E. Annual Meeting of Fellows and Members 1978. Address by Dr J E Riding, Dean of the Faculty of Anaesthetists. *Annals of the Royal College of Surgeons of England* 1979; **61**: 77-78.
91. Nunn J F. Faculty of Anaesthetists Annual Meeting 18th March 1981. Address by the Dean, Dr J F Nunn. *Annals of the Royal College of Surgeons of England* 1981; **63**: 299-301.
92. Howat D D C. Editorial. *Anaesthesia* 1980; **35**: 1051-2.
93. Campbell D. Faculty of Anaesthetists Annual Meeting 16th March 1983. Address by the Dean, Professor Donald Campbell. College and Faculty Bulletin. *Supplement to Annals of the Royal College of Surgeons of England* 1983; **65** (No.4): 6-7.
94. Spencer E M. *The History of the Group of Anaesthetists in Training*. London: Association of Anaesthetists of Great Britain and Ireland 1992.
95. Howat D D C. The European Scene. The European Economic Community (EEC) *Anaesthesia* 1974; **29**: 211-21.
96. *AAGBI Minute Book No 3* (5.4.1963 - 6.7.1973).
97. *AAGBI Minute Book No 5* (2.8.1979 - 29.7.1983).

98. News and Notices. The Annual General Meeting of the Association of Anaesthetists of Great Britain and Ireland, 1977. *Anaesthesia* 1978; **33**: 88-9.
99. News and Notices. Miss Joyce Baxter. *Anaesthesia* 1974; **29**: 114-5.
100. Memorandum and Articles of the Association of Anaesthetists of Great Britain and Ireland No 1888799. 1985.
101. Financial Adviser. *Anaesthesia News* 1993; **No 70**: 3.
102. Smith R. Syme Oration 1977. Privileges and reform abilities of Royal Colleges. *Annals of the Royal College of Surgeons of England* 1977; **59**: 449-55.
103. Spence A A, Norman J. Editorial. Continuing controversy about a College of Anaesthetists. *British Journal of Anaesthesia* 1978; **50**: 313-5.
104. Murley R S. *Surgical roots and branches*. London. British Medical Association, 1990.
105. Helliwell P J (President). *From Council (to Members of the Association)*. Document in the Archives of the Association of Anaesthetists of Great Britain and Ireland, September 1976.
106. Boulton T B. Editorial. *Anaesthesia* 1979; **34**: 1-2.
107. Vickers M D. Editorial. *Anaesthesia* 1982; **37**: 1071-2.
108. Campbell D, Rees J, Gray T C, Robertson J D, Lee J A, Robson J G G, Lewis E B, Sellick B, Macintosh R, Utting J. College of Anaesthetists. *British Medical Journal* 1978; **1**: 574.
109. Beard J. *From the President*. Document in the Archives of the Association of Anaesthetists of Great Britain and Ireland, 1970.
110. MDV (Vickers M D). Editorial. *Anaesthesia* 1973; **28**: 233-4.
111. Baron D W, Baskett, P F, Bowes J, Davys R, Ellis T T, Kaufman L, Lunn J N, Mushin W W, Rosen M, Robinson J S, Tunstall M E, Woodcock J A. College of Anaesthetists. *British Medical Journal* 1972; **3**: 468-9.
112. Association News. Annual General Meeting of the Association. *Anaesthesia* 1972; **27**: 110-1.
113. The College's New Charter. *Annals of the Royal College of Surgeons of England* 1978; **60**: 152-5.
114. Shakespeare W. *Macbeth* 1606. I:vii.
115. Boulton T B. Editorial. *Anaesthesia* 1978; **33**: 1-2.
116. *Trust Deed of the Anaesthetists Academic Foundation*. Document in the Archives of the Association of Anaesthetists of Great Britain and Ireland. 1977.
117. Howat D D C. A College of Anaesthetists? *Anaesthesia* 1978; **33**: 300.
118. Gilston A. A College of Anaesthetists? A question. *Anaesthesia* 1978; **33**: 757.
119. Correspondence relating to Anaesthetists Academic Foundation. Copies in the Archives of the Association of Anaesthetists of Great Britain and Ireland. 1989.
120. Boulton T B. A College of Anaesthetists? The Editor replies. *Anaesthesia* 1978; **33**: 300-1.
121. Vickers M D. The Unity of the College of Surgeons. *Anaesthesia* 1978;
122. Boulton T B. College of Anaesthetists. *British Medical Journal* 1978; **1**: 648.
123. Baskett P, Zorab J, Hurdley J, Burn J M B. College of Anaesthetists. *British Medical Journal* 1978; **1**: 716-7.
124. Coplans M P. College of Anaesthetists. *British Medical Journal* 1978; **1**: 784.
125. Duncan J. College of Anaesthetists. *British Medical Journal* 1978; **1**: 987-8.
126. Hall V F. A College of Anaesthetists? *Anaesthesia* 1978; **33**: 635-6.
127. Hunter A R. A College of Anaesthetists? *Anaesthesia* 1978; **33**: 636-7.

128. Smith W D A. A College of Anaesthetists. Pros and Cons. *Anaesthesia* 1978; **33**: 754-6.
129. Vickers M D A. The Immediate Past Honorary Secretary replies. *Anaesthesia* 1978; **33**: 756-7.
130. Riding J E. Address by the Dean of the Faculty. *Annals of the Royal College of Surgeons of England* 1979; **61**: 241-3.
131. Nunn J F. Faculty of Anaesthetists; 32nd Anniversary 19 March 1980. Address by the Dean. *Annals of the Royal College of Surgeons of* 1980; **62**: 319-20.
132. Future of the Faculty of Anaesthetists. *Anaesthesia* 1980; **35**: 1221.
133. Nunn J F. Faculty of Anaesthetists Annual Meeting 18 March 1981. Address by the Dean. *Annals of the Royal College of Surgeons of England* 1981; **63**: 299-301.
134. Lord P H. Obituary. Sir Alan Parks. *College and Faculty Bulletin, Supplement to the Annals of the Royal College of Surgeons of England*, 1983; **65** (2): 4-5.
135. News and Notices. Annual General Meeting of the Association of Anaesthetists of Great Britain and Ireland 1980. *Anaesthesia* 1981; **36**: 98-9.
136. Boulton T B. Editorial. *Anaesthesia* 1980; **35**: 1147.
137. Nunn J F. Faculty of Anaesthetists Annual Meeting 17 March 1982. Address by the Dean. *Annals of the Royal College of Surgeons of England* 1982; **64**: 209-12.
138. College and Faculty News. Meeting of the Board of Faculty of Anaesthetists 20 October 1982. *College and Faculty Bulletin, Supplement to the Annals of the Royal College of Surgeons of England*, 1983; **65** (No 1): 1.
139. Vickers M D A. Editorial. What Next? *Anaesthesia* 1983; **38**: 929-30.
140. Burn J M B, Zorab J S M. Obituary. Robert Patrick Webb Shackleton. *Anaesthesia* 1977; **32**: 819-21.
141. Pallister W K. Editorial. Sir Geoffrey Stephen William Organe 1908-1989. *Anaesthesia* 1989; **44**: 461-2.
142. Lunn J N. Editorial. William Woolf Mushin. *Anaesthesia* 1993; **48**: 461-2.
143. Finch P, Nancekievill D G. The role of hospital medical teams at a major accident. *Anaesthesia* 1975; **30**: 666-76.
144. News and Notices. The Annual General Meeting of the Association of Anaesthetists of Great Britain and Ireland 1976. *Anaesthesia* 1977; **32**: 401-2.
145. Editorial. *Anaesthesia* 1977; **32**: 843-5.
146. Obituary. T P Ayre. *Anaesthesia* 1980; **35**: 104.
147. Boulton T B. Classical File. Pediatric anesthesia and the Jackson Rees Modification of Ayres' T-piece. *Survey of Anesthesiology* 1985; **29**: 139-148.
148. News and Notices. Obituaries. C J Massey Dawkins. *Anaesthesia* 1975; **30**: 842.
149. News and Notices. Obituaries. Thomas James Gilmartin. *Anaesthesia* 1987; **30**: 105.
150. Todd A (Chairman) *Report of the Royal Commission on Medical Education. London*: Her Majesty's Stationery Office 1968.
151. Middle article. Royal Commission on Medical Education. *British Medical Journal* 1968; **2**: 109-11.
152. Editorial. *Anaesthesia* 1972; **27**: 247-8.
153. Department of Health. Hospital Doctors. Training for the future. *The report of a working group on specialist Medical training*. London: Department of Health 1993.
154. Leading Article. Specialist Medical Training and the Calman report. Deserves and requires imaginative professional and managerial support. *British Medical Journal* 1993; **306**: 1281-2.

155. News. Specialist training may be overhauled. *British Medical Journal* 1993; **306**: 1287-8.
156. News and Notices. Visitor to the Association. *Anaesthesia News* 1993; **No 74**: 8.
157. News and Notices. The Linkman Conference 1976. *Anaesthesia* 1977; **32**: 402.
158. Editorial. *Anaesthesia* 1973; **28**: 1.
159. Boulton T B, Lunn J N. Editorial. *Anaesthesia* 1981; **36**: 1075.
160. Editorial. *Anaesthesia* 1976; **31**: 1.
161. Mapleson W W, Lunn J N. Editorial. *Anaesthesia* 1975; **30**: 601-3.
162. Anaesthesia and the Système International (SI). *Anaesthesia* 1975; **30**: 604-8.
163. Boulton T B. Editorial. *Anaesthesia* 1978; **33**: 303-6.
164. Christie R W, Marall O. Occasional Notes. Experiences with conversion to système international units. *New England Journal of Medicine* 1990; **323**: 1075-7.
165. Leading Article. Declaration of Vancouver. *British Medical Journal* 1978; **1**: 1302-3.
166. International Steering Committee of Medical Editors. Uniform requirements of manuscripts for biomedical journals. *British Medical Journal* 19? ; **1**: 1334-5.
167. Boulton T B. Editorial. *Anaesthesia* 1978; **33**: 303-6.
168. Boulton T B. Editorial. *Anaesthesia* 1982; **37**: 1155.
169. Boulton T B. Miss Dorothy F Atkins. Librarian Extraordinary. *Anaesthesia* 1982; **37**: 1145.
170. Lunn J N. Editorial. *Anaesthesia* 1983; **38**: 1.
171. Blake D, compiler. *Anaesthesia. Cumulative Index 1946-1975.* London: Academic Press, 1982.
172. News and Notices. Junior Anaesthetists Group. *Anaesthesia* 1978; **33**: 664-7.
173. News and Notices. Junior Anaesthetists Group. *Anaesthesia* 1975; **30**: 570-5.
174. Association News. Junior Anaesthetists Group News. *Anaesthesia* 1973; **28**: 354-5.
175. Wishart H H, Holloway K B, Spence A A. Obituary. Henry Harry Pinkerton. *Anaesthesia* 1982; **37**: 1143-50.
176. Scott D B. Editorial. Death Associated with Anaesthesia. *British Journal of Anaesthesia* 1977; **49**: 95-6.
177. Tomkinson J (Chairman). *Report on confidential enquiries into maternal deaths.* Department of Health and Social Security Report on Health and Social Subjects 26, 1976-1978. London: Her Majesty's Stationery Office, 1982.
178. Lunn J N. Editorial. *Anaesthesia* 1979; **34**: 229-30.
179. Nunn J F. Editorial. *Anaesthesia* 1982; **37**: 795-6.
180. Lunn J N, Mushin W W. *Mortality Associated with Anaesthesia.* London: Nuffield Provincial Hospitals Trust, 1982.
181. Lunn J N, Mushin W W. Special Communication. Mortality associated with anaesthesia. *Anaesthesia* 1982; **37**: 856.
182. Open forum. The Annual Conference of Linkmen of the Association of Anaesthetists of Great Britain and Ireland 1982. *Anaesthesia* 1983; **38**: 415-8.
183. Anonymous. Anaesthesia could cost 900 lives each year. *The Times* 1982; August 16: 2.
184. Leading Article. Deaths and Anaesthesia. *British Medical Journal* 1982; **285**: 530.
185. Leading Article. Six days to die. *Lancet* 1982; **2**: 424.
186. Manners J M. Deaths and Anaesthesia. *British Medical Journal* 1982; **285**: 731.
187. Scott P V. Deaths and Anaesthesia. *British Medical Journal* 1982; **285**: 731.
188. Wildsmith J A W. Deaths and Anaesthesia. *British Medical Journal* 1982; **285**: 731.

189. Vallance-Owen A J. Internal Medical Audit. *British Medical Journal* 1982; **285**: 896.
190. Buck N, Devlin H B, Lunn J N. *The Report of a Confidential Enquiry into Perioperative Deaths*. London: Nuffield Provincial Hospitals Trust and King Edward's Hospital's Fund for London. 1987.
191. Campling E A, Devlin H B, Hoile R W, Lunn J N. *The Report of the National Confidential Enquiry into Perioperative Deaths* 1989. London, 1990.
192. Campling E A, Devlin H B, Hoile R W, Lunn J N. *The Report of the National Confidential Enquiry into Perioperative Deaths* 1991/1992. London, 1993.
193. Boulton T B. Deaths and anaesthesia. *British Medical Journal* 1982; **285**: 730.
194. Charters P. Deaths and anaesthesia. *British Medical Journal* 1982; **285**: 1048.
195. Lunn J N. Editorial. Recovery from anaesthesia. Specially designated recovery areas are essential. *British Medical Journal* 1994; **308**: 804.
196. Lamb A S T. Deaths and anaesthesia. *British Medical Journal* 1982; **285**: 1048.
197. Lawler P G. Deaths and anaesthesia. *British Medical Journal* 1982; **285**: 1277-8.
198. Norcross K. Death from the anaesthetic. *Lancet* 1982; **2**: 612.
199. Lunn J N, Hunter A R, Scott D B. Anaesthesia related surgical mortality. *Anaesthesia* 1983; **38**: 1090-6.
200. Alment E A J (Chairman). *Competence to Practice. The report of a committee of enquiry set up for the medical profession in the United Kingdom*. London: Independently published ISBN 0/9505287/0/6, 1976.
201. Leading Article. Do sick doctors need more than the GMC? *British Medical Journal* 1981; **282**: 1-2.
202. Kessel N. Obituary. K Rawnsley. *British Medical Journal* 1992; **305**: 111.
203. Helliwell P J. The Association of Anaesthetists of Great Britain and Ireland 1932-1982. Fifty years of service to the specialty. *Anaesthesia* 1982; **37**: 913-23.
204. Supplement. Suspension for ill health. GMC Health Committee. *British Medical Journal* 1980; **281**: 1368.
205. Roy D. How to do it. Deal with problem colleagues. *British Medical Journal* 1987; **295**: 1190-2.
206. News and Notices. The Third Annual Conference of Linkmen of the Association of Anaesthetists of Great Britain and Ireland, 29 November 1978 at Wembley Conference Centre, London. *Anaesthesia* 1979; **34**: 404-8.
207. Baskett P J. Help for the sick doctor. *Anaesthesia* 1979; **34**: 288-9.
208. Association News and Notices. Competence to practice. *Anaesthesia* 1979; **34**: 710.
209. Mushin W W. Editorial. Professor Emeritus Sir Robert Reynolds Macintosh 17 October 1897-28 August 1989. *Anaesthesia* 1989; **44**: 951.
210. Association of Anaesthetists of Great Britain and Ireland. Annual Report of Council 1978-1979. *Anaesthesia* 1980; **35**: 526-35.
211. Association of Anaesthetists of Great Britain and Ireland. Annual Report to Council 1981-1982. *Anaesthesia* 1983; **38**: 188-98.
212. Zorab J S M. Special Article. Anaesthetists and the Common Market. *Anaesthesia* 1977; **32**: 252-6.
213. News and Notices. Linguistic competence of doctors from other EEC countries. *Anaesthesia* 1978; **33**: 97.
214. Brearley S. Medicine in Europe. Medical Education. *British Medical Journal* 1992; **304**: 41-4.

215. Howat D D C. Special Article. The European Scene. The European Economic Community. *Anaesthesia* 1974; **29**: 211-21.
216. Lister J. Editorial. Accreditation: who needs it? *British Journal of Hospital Medicine* 1985; **34**: 323.
217. Akle C A. Accreditation after Goldstein. *British Medical Journal* 1992; **304**: 840.
218. Beecham L. News. Trying to satisfy the directives on specialisation. *British Medical Journal* 1992; **305**: 332.
219. Brahams D. Medicine and the Law. Specialist training and accreditation. *Lancet* 1991; **338**: 1585-6.
220. Dyer C. Goldstein loses case in High Court. *British Medical Journal* 1993; **306**: 950-1.
221. Brearley S. Leading Article. Accreditation after Goldstein. Time for higher training committees to reconsider their procedures. *British Medical Journal* 1992; **304**: 518-9.
222. News. Junior doctors want single tier of specialist. *British Medical Journal* 1992; **304**: 1651-2.
223. Medicopolitical Digest. The week in Nottingham. Accreditation and certification. *British Medical Journal* 1992; **305**: 194.
224. Brearley S. Leading Article. Specialist medical training and the European Community. *British Medical Journal* 1992; **305**: 661-2.
225. Hunter S, McLaren P. Editorial. Specialist medical training and the Calman Report. Deserves and requires imaginative professional and managerial support. *British Medical Journal* 1993; **306**: 1281-2.
226. Beecham L. News. Specialist training may be overhauled. *British Medical Journal* 1993; **306**: 1287-8.
227. MacRae W R. Representation of the specialty in the European Union. *Anaesthesia News* (Newsletter of the Association of Anaesthetists of Great Britain and Ireland) 1994; **No 82**: 1-2.
228. Zorab J S M. International News. The European Academy of Anaesthesiology. *Anaesthesia* 1979; **34**: 126-7.
229. Lassner J. Editorial. The European Academy of Anaesthesiology. *Anaesthesia* 1984; **39**: 1-2.
230. News and Notices. European Academy of Anaesthesiology. *Anaesthesia* 1980; **35**: 132.
231. Gilston A, Lassner J. The European Academy of Anaesthesiology. *Anaesthesia* 1984; **39**: 502.
232. Association of Anaesthetists of Great Britain and Ireland. Annual Report of Council 1978-79. *Anaesthesia* 1980; **35**: 526-35.
233. Association of Anaesthetists of Great Britain and Ireland. Annual Report of Council 1979-80. *Anaesthesia* 1981; **36**: 90-7.
234. Association of Anaesthetists of Great Britain and Ireland. Annual Report of Council 1980-81. *Anaesthesia* 1982; **37**: 228-35.
235. Association of Anaesthetists of Great Britain and Ireland. Annual Report of Council 1981-82. *Anaesthesia* 1983; **38**: 188-98.
236. Association of Anaesthetists of Great Britain and Ireland. Annual Report of Council 1983-84. *Anaesthesia* 1985; **40**: 111-120.
237. Boulton T B. Editorial. *Anaesthesia* 1979; **34**: 523-4.
238. Hutton A M, Wedley J R, Seed R F. Teaching anaesthesia to dentists. *British Dental Journal*

1978; **144**: 35-9.
239. Dinsdale R C W, Dixon R A. Anaesthetic dental services to dental patients: England and Wales 1976. *British Dental Journal* 1978; **144**: 271-9.
240. Coplans M P, Curson I. Deaths associated with dentistry. *British Dental Journal* 1982; **153**: 357-62.
241. Editorial. *Anaesthesia* 1976; **31**: 167-9.
242. Wylie W D (Chairman). *Report of the Working Party on Training in Dental Anaesthesia.* London: Royal College of Surgeons of England, 1978.
243. Contemporary Themes. Dental anaesthesia: two working parties. *British Medical Journal* 1981; **283**: 1529-30.
244. Lewis B. Safe dental anaesthesia. *British Medical Journal* 1981; **283**: 1495.
245. Seward G R (Chairman). *Report of the Inter-Faculty Working Party considering the Implementation of the Wylie Report.* London: Royal College of Surgeons of England, 1981.
246. Lewis B. Deaths and Dental Anaesthetics. *British Medical Journal* 1983; **286**: 3-4.
247. Boulton T B. Deaths and Dental Anaesthesia. *British Medical Journal* 1983; **286**: 303.
248. Editorial. General anaesthesia for dentistry. *British Dental Journal* 1981; **151**: 357.
249. Kember T, Macpherson G. *The NHS: a Kaleidoscope of Care: Conflicts of Service and Business Values.* London: Nuffield Provincial Hospital Trust, 1994.
250. From the GMS Committee. Dental Anaesthetics. *British Medical Journal* 1981; 282: 1170.
251. From the GMS Committee. Dental Anaesthesia. *British Medical Journal* 1981; **283**: 303.
252. From the GMS Committee. Training for dental anaesthetics. *British Medical Journal* 1983; **286**: 410-11.
253. Vickers M D. No objection to proper training. *British Medical Journal* 1983; **286**: 805-6.
254. Ball J G. No objection to proper training. *British Medical Journal* 1983; **286**: 1217.
255. Dental Education. The Report of a Committee of Inquiry appointed by the Nuffield Foundation: Paragraph 21. *British Dental Journal* 1980; 149: 342-3.
256. MacRae W R, Vickers M D. Special Article: New General Dental Council Guidance on general anaesthesia and sedation. *Anaesthesia* 1983; **38**: 804-5.
257. Association of Anaesthetists of Great Britain and Ireland. Annual Report of Council 1982-1983. *Anaesthesia* 1984; **39**: 89-98.
258. Editorial. Fluoride Supplementation. *British Dental Journal* 1981; **150**: 261.
259. McGimpsey J G, Kawar P, Gamble J A S, Browne E S, Dundee J W. Midazolam in dentistry. *British Dental Journal* 1983; **155**: 47-50.
260. Boulton T B. Presidential Address. The rise and fall of general anaesthesia in the dental chair. *SAAD Digest* 1980; **4**: 156-65.
261. Poswillo Report. Principal recommendations of the report. *British Dental Journal* 1991; **170**: 46.
262. Scurr C F. *NHS Dental Anaesthetics in General Dental Practice.* Document in the Archives of the Association of Anaesthetists of Great Britain and Ireland, 1976.
263. News and Notices. Anaesthetists Sub-committee of the Central Committee for Hospital Medical Services (CCHMS). Dental Anaesthetic Fees. *Anaesthesia* 1976; **31**: 840.
264. News and Notices. The Second Annual Conference of Linkmen of the Association of Anaesthetists of Great Britain and Ireland, 3 November 1977. *Anaesthesia* 1978; **33**: 282-90.
265. Supplement. Dental anaesthetic fees. Letter from BMA Chairman and the President of the

Association of Anaesthetists. *British Medical Journal* 1977; **2**: 1680.
266. Cameron J, Scurr C F. Lifting the ban on dental anaesthetics. *British Medical Journal* 1978; **2**: 1025.
267. Scurr C F. Dental anaesthetic fees. All is now clear. *British Medical Journal* 1978; **2**: 1302.
268. Smith W D A. Under the Influence. *A history of nitrous oxide and oxygen anaesthesia*. London: MacMillan, 1982.
269. Smith W D A. Perspective. *Proceedings of the Royal Society of Medicine* 1974; **67**: 987-9.
270. Wilkinson R T. Measuring the effects of environment upon performance. *Proceedings of the Royal Society of Medicine* 1974; **67**: 994-6.
271. Smith W D A. An approach to fatigue in the practice of anaesthesia. In: Gomez Q J, Egay L M, Craz-Odi M F, eds. *Anaesthesia: Safety for All: Proceedings of the 8th World Congress of Anaesthesiologists, Manila*. Amsterdam: Elsevier, 1984: 583-7.
272. WDAS. *Fatigue Working Party*. London: Documents in the Archives of the Association of Anaesthetists of Great Britain and Ireland, 1981.
273. Klein L. *The Role of the anaesthetist: an exploratory study*. London: Association of Anaesthetists of Great Britain and Ireland, 1980.
274. Reeve P E. Personality characteristics of a sample of anaesthetists. *Anaesthesia* 1980; **35**: 559-68.
275. Editorial. The Gasman goeth. *Lancet* 1980; **2**: 409.
276. T B B. The 1978 Annual Scientific Meeting. *Anaesthesia* 1979; **34**: 390-402.
277. Reeve P E, Vickers M D, Horton J N. Selecting Anaesthetists. The use of psychological tests and structured interviews. *Journal of the Royal Society of Medicine* 1993; **86**: 400-3.
278. Reeve P, Lunn J. Editorial. *Anaesthesia* 1981; **36**: 857-9.
279. Klein L. The role of the anaesthetist. A reply to the September 1981 Editorial. *Anaesthesia* 1981; **36**: 1142-3.
280. Lewin W (Chairman). *Report of a Joint Sub-committee of the Standing Medical Advisory Committee and the Standing Nursing Advisory Committee. The Organisation and Staffing of Operating Departments*. London: Her Majesty's Stationery Office, 1970.
281. Medical News. Operating theatres and staff. *British Medical Journal* 1971; **1**: 681.
282. Obituary. Walpole Lewin. *British Medical Journal* 1980; **280**: 323-4.
283. Horsey P J (Chairman). *Report on the Working Party on the Implementation of the Lewin Report on the Organisation of Operating Departments*. London: Association of Anaesthetists of Great Britain and Ireland, 1974.
284. Horsey P J (Chairman). *Operating Department Assistants. Development and current status*. Report of a Working Party of Council. London: Association of Anaesthetists of Great Britain and Ireland, 1975.
285. Editorial. *Anaesthesia* 1970; **25**: 455-6.
286. Inman M T (Chairman). *Report of a Working Party on Assistants for Anaesthetists*. London: Association of Anaesthetists of Great Britain and Ireland, 1982.
287. Hunter A R. Editorial. *Anaesthesia* 1978; **33**: 427-9.
288. Burrows M M (Chairman). *Report of a Working Party on Assistance for the Anaesthetist*. London: Association of Anaesthetists of Great Britain and Ireland, 1988.
289. *Criteria for Recognition of Hospital Posts under the FFARCS Regulations*. London: Faculty of Anaesthetists of the Royal College of Anaesthetists, 1980.
290. Heath M L. *Memorandum to the Communication Circle, assistance for anaesthetists, 5*

April 1993. London: Association of Anaesthetists of Great Britain and Ireland, 1993.
291. *Workload for the Consultant Anaesthetist.* London: Association of Anaesthetists of Great Britain and Ireland, 1983, 1984, 1990, 1991.
292. Rosen M. From the Honorary Secretary. Distinction unrewarded. *Anaesthesia* 1977; **32**: 936-7.
293. Loder R E. The anaesthetists and distinction awards. *Anaesthesia* 1982; **37**: 1126-9.
294. News and Notices. Distinction awards. Regional "C" Awards Committee for England and Wales. *Anaesthesia* 1977; **32**: 939- 42.
295. Association News and Notices. Region Higher Distinction Awards Committees for England and Wales. *Anaesthesia* 1978; **33**: 395-9.
296. Padfield A. Distinction and merit awards. *Today's Anaesthetist* 1994; **9**: 69.
297. Secretariat, Advisory Committee on Distinction Awards. Distinction Awards. Analysis by type of award, specialty and percentage distribution at 31 December 1992 - England and Wales. *Health Trends* 1993; **25**: 152.
298. News and Notices. The Second Annual Conference of Linkmen of the Association of Anaesthetists of Great Britain and Ireland. 3 November 1977. *Anaesthesia* 1978; **33**: 282-90.
299. News and Notices. The Third Annual Conference of the Linkmen of the Association of Anaesthetists of Great Britain and Ireland, 29 November 1978 at the Wembley Conference Centre, London. *Anaesthesia* 1979; **34**: 404-8.
300. Baskett P. From the Assistant Honorary Secretary. The Private Practice Committee. *Anaesthesia* 1978; **33**: 565-8.
301. News and Notices. The 1980 Annual Conference of Linkmen of the Association of Anaesthetists of Great Britain and Ireland. *Anaesthesia* 1981; **36**: 100-5.
302. News and Notices. The Annual Conference of Linkmen of the Association of Anaesthetists of Great Britain and Ireland 1981. *Anaesthesia* 1982; **37**: 237-44.
303. Editorial. Think again. *British Medical Journal* 1974; **1**: 211-2.
304. Hospital Medical Services: New Fees. Family Planning Services. *British Medical Journal* 1975; **3**: 185.
305. Family Planning Services. Hospital Fees. *British Medical Journal* 1975; **3**: 260.
306. Powell D E B, Douglas C P. Fees for Family Planning Services. *British Medical Journal* 1975; **3**: 437-8.
307. Parliament. Family Planning. *British Medical Journal* 1975; **4**: 656.
308. Baptiste C E and 12 others. Family planning for anaesthetists. *British Medical Journal* 1975; **4**: 105-6.
309. Association News and Notices. British Standards Institute new draft standards. *Anaesthesia* 1976; **31**: 978.
310. Memorandum from the Safety Committee on Safety in Anaesthesia of the Association of Anaesthetists of Great Britain and Ireland. Oxygen supply pressure failure warning and protection devices. *Anaesthesia* 1978; **31**: 316-8.
311. Editorial. Elective surgery and the pill. *British Medical Journal* 1976; **2**: 546.
312. RLH, AGD, RSA. Editorial. *Anaesthesia* 1974; **29**: 527-8.
313. Hargrove R L. The neurological complications of spinal and epidural analgesia. *Anaesthesia* 1981; **36**: 454-5.
314. Edmonds-Seal J, McNeilly R H. Special communication. Career opportunities for doctors with domestic commitments. A report of a working party. *Anaesthesia* 1981; **36**: 1040-3.

315. The Editor and Atkinson R S, Benyon D G, Birt R C, Cameron A, Lee J A, Rushman J B, Thorne T C, Watt M J, Prior F N. Requiem for trichloroethylene. *Anaesthesia* 1979; **34**: 903-4.
316. Heath M L. Deaths after intravenous regional anaesthesia. *British Medical Journal* 1982; **285**: 913-4.
317. Heath M. The hazards of intravenous regional anaesthesia (IVRA). *Anaesthesia* 1982; **38**: 417.
318. Reynolds F. Editorial. Bupivacaine and intravenous regional anaesthesia. *Anaesthesia* 1984; **39**: 105-7.
319. Bickford Smith P J. Junior anaesthetists and stress. *Anaesthesia* 1983; **38**: 417-8.
320. Association News and Notices. Annual Scientific Meeting of the Association 7-8 November 1974. Joint meeting with Dansk Anaesthesiologisk Selskab (Danish Society of Anaesthetists). *Anaesthesia* 1975; **30**: 264-72.
321. Atkinson R S. Joint meeting of the Association of Anaesthetists of Great Britain and Ireland and the Danish Society of Anaesthesiologists (Copenhagen 10-12 June 1976). *Anaesthesia* 1976; **31**: 1321-4.
322. Lassner J. Editorial. *Anaesthesia* 1977; **32**: 741-2.
323. Vickers M D. News and Notices. Joint meeting between the Société Francais d'Anesthésie et Réanimation and the Association of Anaesthetists of Great Britain and Ireland 14 June 1975. *Anaesthesia* 1975; **30**: 862-3.
324. News and Notices. The Annual Scientific Meeting of the Association of Anaesthetists of Great Britain and Ireland. *Anaesthesia* 1978; **33**: 89-95.
325. T B B. News and Notices. The 1978 Annual Scientific Meeting. *Anaesthesia* 1979; **34**: 390-402.
326. Association of Anaesthetists of Great Britain and Ireland. Annual Report of Council 1984-1985. *Anaesthesia* 1986; **41**: 120-7.
327. Association News and Notices. Congress Travel Arrangements. Annual Meeting of the Canadian Society of Anaesthetists 23-26 June 1975. *Anaesthesia* 1975; **30**: 111.
328. Padfield A. International News. The Canadian Anaesthetists Society Meeting (22-26 June 1975). *Anaesthesia* 1975; **30**: 863-4.
329. Association News and Notices. The Annual Meeting of the Association of Anaesthetists of Great Britain and Ireland, 24-25 September 1981 at Queens Medical Centre, Nottingham. *Anaesthesia* 1982; **37**: 365.
330. Association News and Notices. The Association of Anaesthetists of Great Britain and Ireland Anglo-American Meeting 10-11 September 1980. *Anaesthesia* 1981; **36**: 547-61.
331. Clothier C M. John Snow Memorial Lecture 1980. *Anaesthesia* 1981; **36**: 483-91.
332. Edridge A W. Editorial. Sir Ivan Whiteside Magill. *Anaesthesia* 1987; **42**: 231-3.
333. News and Notices. Anaesthetic Section of the Royal Society of Medicine. Sir Ivan Magill: 90th Birthday celebrations. *Anaesthesia* 1978; **33**: 866-8.
334. Scurr C. Editorial. *Anaesthesia* 1978; **33**: 577-80.
335. Menu. *Golden Jubilee Dinner 1982*. London: Archives of the Association of Anaesthetists of Great Britain and Ireland.
336. Spierdijk J, Rolly G, Feldman S A. The European Congress of Anaesthesiology. *Anaesthesia* 1978; **33**: 371.
337. News and Notices. The 6th World Congress of Anaesthesiology. *Anaesthesia* 1976; **31**: 983-93.

338. Atkinson R S. Sixth European Congress of Anaesthesiology. Report. *Anaesthesia* 1982; **37**; 1226-7.
339. Boulton T B, Atkinson, R S, eds. Sixth European Congress of Anaesthesiology 8-15 September 1982. Volume of Summaries. *Anaesthesia* 1982; **37**: supplement.
340. Postgraduate Course. Royal Festival Hall, London 8 September 1982. *Anaesthesia* 1982; **37**: 118 and 483.

Chapter 9 - The Sixth Decade, 1 January 1983 to 31 December 1992

1. Cook C, ed. *Pears Cyclopaedia* 1993-1994. London: Penguin Books, 1993.
2. Edwards B. *The National Health Service 1946-1992. A manager's tale*. London: Nuffield Provincial Hospitals Trust, 1993.
3. Kember T, Macpherson G. *The NHS. A kaleidoscope of care. Conflict of service and business values*. London: Nuffield Provincial Hospitals Trust, 1994.
4. Harrison S, Pollitt C. *Controlling the professionals. The future work and organisation of the National Health Service*. Buckingham: Open University Press, 1994.
5. Stocking B. Patients' Charter. New rights issue. *British Medical Journal* 1991; **303**: 1148-9.
6. Warden J. Patients first. *British Medical Journal* 1991; **303**: 1153.
7. Hart. The Week. *British Medical Journal* 1991; **303**: 1158.
8. Orwell G. *Animal Farm. A fairy story*. London: Secker and Warburg, 1945.
9. Goodman P, Hyslop L. The privatisation of PC. *Sunday Times* 1994; 14 August: 13.
10. Brown L, Editor. *The New Shorter English Dictionary on Historical Principles*: . Editor. *The Shorter Oxford Dictionary*. Oxford: Clarendon Press, 1993. 1680-1..
11. Gottlieb M S, Schanker H M, Fan P R, Saxon A, Weisman J D. Pneumocystis pneumonia - Los Angeles. *Morbid Mortal Weekly Report* 1981; **30**: 250-2.
12. Friedman-Kien A, Lanbenstein L, Marmor M. Karposi's sarcoma and pneumocystis pneumonia among homosexual men - New York City and California. *Morbid Mortal Weekly Report* 1981; **30**: 305-8.
13. Brennan R B, Durack D T. Gay compromise syndrome. *Lancet* 1981; **2**: 1338-9.
14. Waterson A P. Regular review. Acquired immune deficiency syndrome. *British Medical Journal* 1983; **286**: 743-6.
15. DuBois R M, Branthwaite M A, Mikhail J R, Batten J C. Primary Pneumocystis carinii and cytomegalovirus infections. *Lancet* 1981; **2**: 1339.
16. Barre-Sinoussi F, Chermann J C, Reg F. Isolation of a T-lymphotrophic retrovirus from a patient at risk for acquired immunodeficiency syndrome (AIDS). *Science* 1983; **220**: 868-70.
17. Gallo R C, Salahuddin S Z, Popovic M. Human T-lymphotrophic retrovirus HTLV-III isolated from AIDS patients and donors at risk for AIDS, *Science* 1984; **224**: 500-3.
18. Mortimer P P, Jesson W J, Vandervelde E M, Pereira M S. Prevalence of antibody to human T-lymphotrophic virus type III by risk group and area, United Kingdom 1978-1984. *British Medical Journal* 1985; **290**: 1176-8.
19. Editorial. The cause of AIDS? *Lancet* 1984; **1**: 1053-4.
20. Collier C. *The 20th century plague*. Tring: Lion Publishing, 1987.
21. DeCock K M. For debate. AIDS: an old disease in Africa? *British Medical Journal* 1984; **289**: 306-8.

22. McEvoy M, Tillett E. Some problems in the prediction of future numbers of cases of the acquired immunodeficiency syndrome in the United Kingdom. *Lancet* 1985; **2**: 541-2.
23. Moss A. *HIV and AIDS, Management by the primary care team*. Oxford: University Press, 1992.
24. Tillet H E, McEvoy M. Reassessment of predicted number of AIDS patients. *Lancet* 1986; **2**: 1104.
25. Notes and News. BMA statement on AIDS. *Lancet* 1985; **1**: 938.
26. Adler M W, Weller I V D. AIDS: sense not fear. *British Medical Journal* 1984; **288**: 1177-8.
27. *AAGBI Minute Book No 6* (22.9.1983 - 4.12.1987).
28. Searle J F (Chairman). *HIV and other blood borne viruses: guidance for anaesthetists*. London: Association of Anaesthetists of Great Britain and Ireland, 1992.
29. Lee K G, Soni N. AIDS and anaesthesia. *Anaesthesia* 1986; **41**: 1011-6.
30. Jeffries D J. Editorial. HIV and hepatitis: some way to go. *Anaesthesia* 1992; **47**: 921-2.
31. O'Donnell N G, Asbury A J. The occupational hazard of human immunodeficiency virus and hepatitis B infection. I: perceived and preventive measures adopted by anaesthetists: a postal survey. *Anaesthesia* 1991; **47**: 923-8.
32. O'Donnell N G, Asbury A J. The occupational hazard of human immunodeficiency virus and hepatitis B virus infection. II Effect of grade, age, sex and region of unemployment on perceived risks and preventive measures adopted by anaesthetists. *Anaesthesia* 1992; **47**: 929-35.
33. Jones J F. Recent changes in transfusion practice. In: Kaufman L, ed. *Anaesthesia Review 7*. Edinburgh: Churchill Livingstone, 1990: 177-91.
34. Leading Article. Blood transfusion, haemophilia and AIDS. *Lancet* 1984; **2**: 1433-5.
35. Jones P, Hamilton P J, Bird G, Fearn M, Oxley A, Tedder R, Cheinsong-Popov R, Codd A. AIDS and haemophilia: morbidity and mortality in a well defined population. *British Medical Journal* 1985; **291**: 695-9.
36. Weller I V D, Hindley D J, Adler M W, Meldrum J T. Gonorrhoea in homosexual men and media coverage of the acquired immunity deficiency syndrome in London 1982-3. *British Medical Journal* 1984; **289**: 1041.
37. Medical News. Don't aid AIDS: the Government's campaign. *British Medical Journal* 1986; **292**: 832.
38. News and Political Review. Headlines. Ten million infected with HIV. *British Medical Journal* 1991; **303**: 1494.
39. Adler W, ed. *ABC of AIDS*, 3rd ed. London: British Medical Journal Publishing, 1993.
40. News and Political Review. Headlines. No immediate vaccine for HIV. *British Medical Journal* 1991; **303**: 1494.
41. Stall R. How to lose the fight against AIDS among gay men. Declare victory and leave the field. *British Medical Journal* 1994; **309**: 685-6.
42. Johnson A M. Medicine and the media. Out of the shadows. *British Medical Journal* 1991; **303**: 1484.
43. Warden J. AIDS: rights versus responsibilities. *British Medical Journal* 1991; **303**: 540-1.
44. Mann J, Wilson M E. AIDS. Global lessons from a global epidemic. New international threats demand international responses. *British Medical Journal* 1993; **307**: 1574-5.

45. Tedder R S. Hepatitis B in hospitals. *British Journal of Hospital Medicine* 1980; **23**: 266-279.
46. Zuckerman A J. Who should be immunised against hepatitis B? *British Medical Journal* 1984; 289: 1243-4.
47. Blumberg B S, Alter H J, Visnich S. A "new" antigen in leukaemia. *Journal of the American Medical Association* 1965; **191**: 541-6.
48. Blumberg B S, Gertsley B J, Hungerford D A, London W T, Sutnick A I. A serum antigen (Australia antigen) in Down's syndrome, leukaemia, and hepatitis. *Annals of Internal Medicine* 1967; **66**: 924-31.
49. Tonks A. NHS adopts tougher measures against hepatitis B. *British Medical Journal* 1993; **307**: 522.
50. Evans T I. Regional anaesthesia for transutheral resection of the prostate. Which methods and which segments? *Anaesthesia and Intensive Care* 1974; **2**: 240-2.
51. Jacobaeus H C. Über die Moglichkeit die zystoskopie bei untersuchung seroser Hohlungen anzuwenden. *Munchener Medizinische Woehenschrift* 1910; **57**: 2090-2
52. Atkinson R S. Anaesthesia for endoscopy. In: Hewer C L, Atkinson R S, eds. *Recent Advances in Anaesthesia and Analgesia 12.* Edinburgh: Churchill Livingstone, 1976: 44-57.
53. Steptoe P C. *Laparoscopy in Gynaecology*. London: Livingstone, 1967.
54. Wickham J E A. Editorial. *Minimal Invasive Therapy* 1991; **1**: 1-5.
55. Wickham J E A. Minimal Invasive Surgery. Treatment of urinary tract stones. *British Medical Journal* 1993; **307**: 1414-7.
56. Russell R G. Minimal Invasive Surgery. General Surgery. *British Medical Journal* 1993; **307**: 1266-9.
57. Hamberg P, Gillquist J, Lysholm J. A comparison between arthroscopic menisectomy and modified open menisectomy. A prospective study with emphasis on postoperative rehabilitation. *Journal of Bone and Joint Surgery. British volume* 1984; **66-B**: 189-92.
58. Dubois F, Icard P, Berthelot G, Levard H. Coelioscopic cholecystectomy. Preliminary report of 36 cases. *Annals of surgery* 1990; **211**: 60-2.
59. Semm K. Endoscopic appendicectomy. *Endoscopy* 1983; **15**: 59-64.
60. Wastell C. Laporoscopic cholecystectomy. Better for patients and the Health Service. *British Medical Journal* 1991; **302**: 303-4.
61. Monson J R T. Minimal Invasive Surgery. Advanced techniques of abdominal surgery. *British Medical Journal* 1993; **307**: 1346-50.
62. Kerbl K, Clayman V, McDougall E M, Kavoussi L R. Minimal Invasive Surgery. Laparoscopic nephrectomy. *British Medical Journal* 1993; **307**: 1488-9.
63. Banta H D. Diffusion of Minimally Invasive Therapy in Europe. *Minimal Invasive Therapy* 1992; **1**: 189-95.
64. Banta H D. Minimal Invasive Surgery. Implication for hospitals, health workers and patients. *British Medical Journal* 1993; **307**: 1546-9.
65. Wickham J E A. Minimal Invasive Surgery. Future developments. *British Medical Journal* 1994; **308**: 193-6
66. Skinner A C. Minimal Invasive Surgery. More invasive than it looks. *British Medical Journal* 1994; **308**: 532-3.
67. Turner W H, Smith J C. Laparoscopic nephrectomy unproved in controlled trials. *British*

Medical Journal 1994; **308**: 533.
68. News Headlines. Training centres set up to teach keyhole surgery. *British Medical Journal* 1993; **307**: 754.
69. The Senate of the Royal Surgical Colleges of Great Britain and Ireland. *Quality Assurance: the role of training, certification, audit and continuing professional education in the maintenance of the highest possible standards of surgical practice.* London: Royal College of Surgeons of England, 1994.
70. Campbell W J, Moorefield R J. Junior surgeons lack practical experience. *British Medical Journal* 1993; **307**: 871-2.
71. McKibbin B, Irving M, Baskett, P J F, Murley R. *Saving Lives. The NHS Accident and Emergency Service and How to Improve it.* London: Institute of Economic Affairs, 1991.
72. Wyatt J P. Personal view. My accident was my fault. *British Medical Journal* 1993; **306**: 1009.
73. Snook R. Management of trauma. Deserves higher priority. *British Medical Journal* 1993; **306**: 1539.
74. Baskett P F J, Diamond A W, Cochrane D F. Urban mobile resuscitation. Training and service. *British Journal of Anaesthesia* 1976; **48**: 377-85.
75. R A B. Obituary. R A Binning. *British Medical Journal* 1962; **2**: 1753-4.
76. Binning R. External cardiac compression. *British Medical Journal* 1962; **2**: 1753-4.
77. Pantridge J F, Geddes J S. A mobile intensive care unit in the management of myocardial infarction. *Lancet* 1966; **1**: 807-8.
78. Pantridge J F. Editorial. Prehospital coronary care. *British Heart Journal* 1974; **36**: 233-7.
79. White N M, Parker W S, Binning R A, Kimber E R, Ead H W, Chamberlain D A. Mobile coronary care provided by ambulance personnel. *British Medical Journal* 1973; **3**: 618-22.
80. Briggs R S, Brown P M, Crabb M E, Cox T J, Ead H W, Hawkes R A, Jequier P W, Southall D P, Grainger R, Williams J H, Chamberlain D A. The Brighton resuscitation ambulances. A continuing experiment in prehospital care by ambulance staff. *British Medical Journal* 1976; **2**: 1161-5.
81. Mackintosh A F, Crabb M E, Grainger R, Williams J H, Chamberlain D A. The Brighton resuscitation ambulances. Review of forty consecutive survivors of out-of-hospital cardiac arrest. *British Medical Journal* 1978; **1**: 1115-8.
82. Baskett P. The organisation of immediate care. *Journal of the British Association of Immediate Care Schemes* 1978; **1** (No 2): 9-18.
83. Wilby J M. The British Ambulance Service. In: Baskett P J F, ed. *Immediate Prehospital Care. The Proceedings of the International Congress of Immediate Care 1980.* Chichester: Wiley, 1981. 23-9.
84. Goglen E. *Road Accidents.* Manchester: Geigy, 1965.
85. National Committee of Trauma and the Committee on Shock. *Accidental Death and Disability. The Neglected Disease of Modern Society.* Washington: National Academy of Sciences of the National Research Council, 1966.
86. Frey C F, Huelke D F, Bikas P W. Resuscitation and survival in motor vehicle accidents. *Journal of Trauma* 1969; **9**: 292-310.
87. Mackay G M. Aspects of emergency care. Some features of traffic accidents. *British Medical Journal* 1969; **4**: 799-801.

88. Snook R. Road accidents and the family doctor. Resuscitation at road accidents. *British Medical Journal* 1969; **4**: 348-50.
89. Easton K C. The General Practitioner and the rescue services. *Community Health* 1970; **2**: 81-7.
90. Irving M (Chairman). *Report of the Working Party on the Management of Patients with Major Injuries.* London: Commission on the Provision of Surgical Services of the Royal College of Surgeons of England, 1988.
91. Stewart R D. Prehospital Care. The American System. In: Baskett P J F, ed. *Immediate Prehospital Care. The Proceedings of the International Congress of Immediate Care 1980.* Chichester: Wiley, 1981: 45-54.
92. Collins J. Organisation and function of the accident flying squad. *British Medical Journal* 1966; **2**: 578-80.
93. Hall M H. The trapped motorist. *Lancet* 1965; **1**: 904-6.
94. Snook R. Accident flying squad. *British Medical Journal* 1972; **3**: 569-74.
95. Poulsen H, Lysgaard A. Emergency aid organisation. *Acta Anaesthesiologica Scandinavica* 1968; Supplement **29**: 283-92.
96. Zorab J S, Baskett P J F. *Immediate Care.* Eastbourne: Saunders, 1977.
97. Baskett P J F, Withnell A. The use of Entonox in the Ambulance Service. *British Medical Journal* 1970; **2**: 41-3.
98. *DHSS Health Notice HN(76) 204.* November 1976.
99. Baskett P J F, Boulton T B. Editorial. *Anaesthesia* 1979; **34**: 989-991
100. Baskett P J F. Special Communication. The need to disseminate knowledge of resuscitation into the community. *Anaesthesia* 1982; **37**: 74-6
101. The 1979 Annual Conference of Linkman of the Association of Anaesthetists of Great Britain and Ireland. *Anaesthesia* 1980; **35**: 107-11.
102. The Annual Conference on Linkman of the Association of Anaesthetists of Great Britain and Ireland, 1982. *Anaesthesia* 1983; **38**: 415-8.
103. Annual Conference of Linkman of the Association of Anaesthetists of Great Britain and Ireland, 1990. *Anaesthesia* 1991; **46**: 606-11.
104. Buck N, Devlin H B, Lunn J N. *The report of a Confidential Enquiry into Perioperative Deaths.* London: Nuffield Provincial Hospitals Trust and King Edward's Hospital's Fund for London, 1987.
105. Dooley A. Evaluation as a function of organisation. Projection of a model emergency service. In: Easton K, ed. *Rescue Emergency Care.* London: Heinemann, 1977: 459-73.
106. Driscoll PA. Trauma. Today's problems tomorrow's solutions. *Injury* 1992; **23**: 151-8.
107. Sparling R. Personal View. Flying doctor in London. *British Medical Journal* 1992; **304**: 647.
108. Hunt M. Personal View. Hanging on for dear life. *British Medical Journal* 1993; **307**: 452-3.
109. Bruce J (Chairman). *Report of a Joint Working Party.* London: Joint Consultants Committee, 1971.
110. Lewin W (Chairman). *Committee on Medical Staffing of Accident and Emergency Services.* London: British Medical Association, 1978.
111. O'Kelly T J, Westaby S. Trauma centres and the efficient use of financial resources. *British Journal of Surgery* 1990; **77**: 1142-4.

112. West J G, Trunkey D D, Lim R C. Systems of trauma care. A study of two counties. *Archives for Surgery* 1979; **114**: 455-60.
113. Trunkey D D. Society of University Surgeons. Presidential address. On the nature of things that go bang in the night. *Surgery* 1982; **92**: 123-32.
114. West J G, Williams M J, Trunkey D D, Wolferth C C. Concepts of emergency and critical care. Trauma systems. Current status - future challenges. *Journal of the American Medical Association* 1988; **259**: 3597-3600.
115. R E L. Obituary. Wolfson L J. *British Medical Journal* 1980; **281**: 1646.
116. Wolfson L J. *Anaesthesia for the Injured*. Oxford: Blackwell Scientific Publications 1962.
117. Skinner D V. Management of trauma. *British Medical Journal* 1993; **307**: 382.
118. Skinner D V. Editorial. Advanced trauma life support. *Injury* 1993; **24**: 147-8.
119. Rosen M (Chairman). *Report of a Working Party on the Efficiency of Theatre Services*. London: Association of Anaesthetists of Great Britain and Ireland (with the Association of Surgeons of Great Britain and Ireland and the British Orthopaedic Association) 1989.
120. Baskett P J F. (Chairman) *Report of a Working Party on the Role of the Anaesthetist in the Emergency Service*. London: Association of Anaesthetists of Great Britain and Ireland, 1991.
121. Annual Conference of Linkman of the Association of Anaesthetists of Great Britain and Ireland 1991. *Anaesthesia* 1992; **47**: 723-8.
122. Clark C. Improving the management of major trauma. *British Journal of Anaesthesia* 1990; **64**: 139-41.
123. Baskett P, Weller R, eds. *Medicine for Disasters*. London: Wright, 1988.
124. Walsh M, ed. *Disasters. Current Planning and Recent Experience*. London: Edward Arnold, 1989.
125. Morgan M, Lunn J, eds. Experiences with Propofol. Papers based on proceedings of an international symposium at the Royal College of Physicians in November 1987. *Anaesthesia* 1988; **.45**: *Supplement* 1-121.
126. Aitkenhead A R, Pepperman M L, Willats S M, Coates P D, Park G R, Bodenham A R, Collins C H, Smith M B, Ledingham I A, Wallace P G M. Comparison of propofol and midazolam for sedation in critically ill patients. *Lancet* 1989; **2**: 704-8.
127. Mackenzie S J, Kapida F, Grant I S. Propofol infusion for the control of status epilepticus. *Anaesthesia* 1990; **45**: 1043-5.
128. Eger E I, Johnson B H. Rates of awakening from anaesthesia with I-653, halothane, noflurane, and seroflurane. A test of the effect of anaesthetic concentration and duration in rats. *Anaesthesia and Analgesia* 1987; **66**: 977-82.
129. Jones R M. Desflurane and sevoflurane. Inhalation anaesthetics for this decade? *British Journal of Anaesthesia* 1990; **65**: 527-36.
130. Wrigley S R, Fairfield J E, Jones R M, Black A E. Induction and recovery characteristics of desflurane in day case patients. A comparison with propofol. *Anaesthesia* 1991; **46**: 615-22.
131. Adams A P, Hewitt P B. The new muscle relaxants atracurium and vecuronium. In: Atkinson R S, Adams A P, eds. *Recent Advances in Anaesthesia and Analgesia* 15. Edinburgh: Churchill Livingstone, 1985: 13-26.
132. Scott R P F, Norman J. Editorial III. Do we need more muscle relaxants? *British Journal*

of Anaesthesia 1988; **61**: 528-30.
133. Parkhouse J, Lambrechts E, Simpson B R J. The incidence of postoperative pain. *British Journal of Anaesthesia* 1961; **33**: 345-53.
134. Editorial. *Anaesthesia* 1975; **30**: 305-6.
135. Ferrante F M, Covino B G. Patient controlled analgesia. A historical perspective. In: Ferrante F M, Ostheimer G W, Covino B G, eds. *Patient Controlled Analgesia*. Oxford: Blackwell Scientific Publications, 1990: 3-9.
136. Boulton T B. Editorial. *Anaesthesia* 1982; **37**: 627-8.
137. Evans J M, Rosen M, MacCarthy J, Hogg I M. Apparatus for patient controlled administration of intravenous narcotics during labour. *Lancet* 1976; **1**: 17-8.
138. Black A M S, Alexander J I. Analgesia for postoperative pain. In: Atkinson R S, Adams A P. *Recent Advances in Anaesthesia and Analgesia* 17. Edinburgh: Churchill Livingstone, 1992: 119-35.
139. Spence A (Chairman). *Commission on the Provision of Surgical Services. Report of the Working Party on Pain after Surgery*. London: Royal College of Surgeons of England, 1990.
140. Morgan M. Editorial. *Anaesthesia* 1982; **37**: 527-8.
141. Crosby D L, Rees G A D, Gill J. The role of the high dependency unit in postoperative care. An update. *Annals of the Royal College of Surgeons of England* 1990; **72**: 309-12.
142. Ready B, Oden R Chadwick H S, Benedetti C, Rooke G A, Caplan R, Lorie M, Wild L M. Development of an Anesthesiology-based postoperative pain management service. *Anesthesiology* 1988; **68**: 100-6.
143. Adams A P. Safety in anaesthetic practice. In: Atkinson R S, Adams A P. eds.. *Recent Advances in Anaesthesia and Analgesia* 17. Edinburgh: Churchill Livingstone, 1992: 1-24.
144. Sykes M K. Essential Monitoring. British Journal of *Anaesthesia* 1987; **59**: 901-12.
145. *Recommendations for Standards of Monitoring and Recovery*. London: Association of Anaesthetists of Great Britain and Ireland, 1988 (revised 1994)
146. Eichorn J H, Cooper J B, Cullen D J, Maier W R, Philip J H, Seeman R G. Standards for patient monitoring during anaesthesia at the Harvard Medical School. *Journal of the American Medical Association* 1986; **256**: 1017-20.
147. Appendix 2. Royal College of Anaesthetists Guide to Basic Specialist Training. *British Journal of Anaesthesia. Handbook of British Anaesthesia*. London: Professional and Scientific Publications, 1994/5: 65.
148. Adams A P. Capnography and pulse oximetry. In: Atkinson S, Adams A P, eds. *Recent Advances in Anaesthesia and Analgesia* 16. Edinburgh: Churchill Livingstone, 1989: 155-75.
149. Jones J G. Editorial. Memory of intraoperative events. Patients remember more than we think. *British Medical Journal* 1994; **309**: 967-8.
150. Brain A I J. The laryngeal mask. A new concept in airway management. *British Journal of Anaesthesia* 1983; **55**: 801-5.
151. Brain A I J, McGhee T D, McAteer E J, Thomas A, Abu-Saad M A W, Barham J A. The laryngeal mask airway. Development and preliminary trials of a new type of airway. *Anaesthesia* 1985; **40**: 356-61.
152. Brodrick P M, Webster N R, Nunn J F. The laryngeal mask airway. A study of 100 patients

during spontaneous breathing. *Anaesthesia* 1989; 44: 238-41.
153. Magill I W. Endotracheal anaesthesia. *Proceedings of the Royal Society of Medicine* 1929; **22**: 83-87.
154. Verghese C, Smith T G C, Young E. Prospective survey of the use of the laryngeal mask airway in 2359 patients. *Anaesthesia* 1993; **48**: 58-60.
155. Payne J. The use of the fibreoptic laryngoscope to confirm the position of the laryngeal mask. *Anaesthesia* 1989; **44**: 865.
156. Chadwick I S, Vohra A. Anaesthesia for emergency Caesarean section using the Brain laryngeal airway. *Anaesthesia* 1989; **44**: 261-2.
157. Maltby J R, Loken R G, Watson N C. The laryngeal mask airway: clinical appraisal on 250 patients. *The Canadian Journal of Anaesthesia* 1990; **37**: 509-13.
158. Results of a multicentre trial. The use of the laryngeal mask airway by nurses during cardiopulmonary resuscitation. Results of a multicentre trial. *Anaesthesia* 1994; **49**: 3-7
159. McCrirrick A, Ramage D T O, Pracilio J A, Hickman J A. Experience with the laryngeal mask in 200 patients. *Anaesthesia and Intensive Care* 1991; **19**: 256-60.
160. Benumof J L. Management of the difficult adult airway; with special emphasis on awake tracheal intubations. *Anesthesiology* 1991; **75**: 1087-1110.
161. Pennant J H, White P F. *Anesthesiology*. The Laryngeal Mask Airway. Its uses in anesthesiology 1993; **79**: 144-163.
162. Association of Anaesthetists of Great Britain and Ireland. Annual Report of Council 1991-1992. *Anaesthesia* 1993; 48: 546-56.
163. Owen D. *Our NHS*. London: Pan Books, 1988.
164. Leathard A. *Health Care Provision*. London: Chapman and Hall, 1990.
165. Griffiths E R (Chairman). *NHS Management Inquiry*. London: Department of Health and Social Security, 1983.
166. Editorial. NHS Management Inquiry. Small, central management board recommended. *British Medical Journal* 1983; **287**: 1391-4.
167. Chantler C. How to do it. Be a manager. *British Medical Journal* 1989; **298**: 1505-8.
168. Dyson R. Personal perspective. In: Burrows M, Dyson R, Jackson P, Saxton H, eds. *Management for Hospital Doctors*. Oxford: Butterworth-Heinemann, 1944: 8-15.
169. Porritt A (Chairman). Report of the Medical Services Review Committee. Summary of conclusions of recommendations. *British Medical Journal* 1962; **2**: 1178-86.
170. Department of Health and Social Security. *Implementation of the NHS Management Inquiry HC 84 (13)*, 1984.
171. Department of Health and Social Security. *Patients First*. London: Her Majesty's Stationery Office, 1979.
172. Griffiths R. Introduction to general management. In: Burrows M, Dyson R, Jackson P, Saxton H, eds. *Management for Hospital Doctors*, 1994: 41-4.
173. Baker M R. The role of medical directors in trusts. In: Burrows M, Dyson R, Jackson P, Saxton H, eds. *Management for Hospital Doctors,* 1994: 50-4.
174. Stuart J. Pathology. In: Burrows M, Dyson R, Jackson P, Saxton H, eds. *Management for Hospital Doctors*, 1994: 300-2.
175. Chant A D B. Practising doctors should not manage. *Lancet* 1984; **1**: 1398.
176. Chalmers E, McLellan I, Naylor A, Shaw T. Editorial. Where now? The anaesthetist's development in management. *Anaesthesia* 1993; **48**: 279-80.

177. Jones B. Nursing: obstetrics and gynaecology. In: Burrows M, Dyson R, Jackson P, Saxton H, eds. *Management for Hospital Doctors*, 1994: 293-5.
178. Chantler C. Paediatrics. In: Burrows M, Dyson R, Jackson R, Saxton H, eds. *Management for Hospital Doctors*, 1994: 293-5.
179. Chantler C. The role of doctors in policy making. In: Burrows M, Dyson R, Jackson P, Saxton H, eds. *Management for Hospital Doctors*, 1994: 45-9.
180. Buckland R W. Anaesthesia. In: Burrows M, Dyson R, Jackson P, Saxton H, eds. *Management for Hospital Doctors*, 1994: 280-4.
181. Naylor A. Theatre. In: Burrows M, Dyson R, Jackson P, Saxton H, eds. *Management for Hospital Doctors*, 1994: 324-6.
182. Horton J N, Vickers M D. Administration in clinical units. Experiences in a Department of Anaesthetists. *Health Trends* 1984; **16**: 58-60.
183. Klein R. Lessons from the financial scandals in Wessex and the West Midlands. Health Authority members found wanting. *British Medical Journal* 1994; **308**: 215-6.
184. Warden J. The Ghost of Gladstone stirs. A whiff of scandal in the air. *British Medical Journal* 1994; **308**: 294.
185. Griffiths R. Seven years of progress. General management in the NHS. *Health Economics* 1992; **1**: 61-70.
186. Social Services Committee. *The Future of the National Health Service. Fifth Report: Session 1987-8.* London: Her Majesty's Stationery Office, 1988.
187. Smith T. New Year Message. *British Medical Journal* 1988; **296**: 1-2.
188. National Association of Health Authorities (NAHA). *The Autumn Survey 1987. Financial Position of District Health Authorities.* London: NAHA, 1987.
189. Delamothe T. The way we live now. Casualties. *British Medical Journal* 1987; **295**: 1628-33.
190. Smith R. Twenty steps towards a "closed society" on health. *British Medical Journal* 1987; **296**: 1633-4.
191. Lock S. NHS 1948-1988. Less ideology more humanity. *British Medical Journal* 1988; **297**: 1-3.
192. Hoffenburgh R, Todd I P, Pinker G. Crisis in the National Health Service. *British Medical Journal* 1987; **295**: 505.
193. Warden J. Letter from Westminster. A lesson in real politics. *British Medical Journal* 1988; **296**: 368.
194. Scrutator. The week. A personal view of medicopolitical events. *British Medical Journal* 1988; **296**: 367.
195. Day P, Klein R. NHS Review. The broad picture. Waiting for the small print. *British Medical Journal* 1989; **298**: 339-40.
196. Edwards B. The increasing power of the consumer. In: Owen AV, ed. *The Health Debate Live: 45 Interviews for "Leading for Health".* London: British Medical Association 1992: 129-35.
197. Enthoven A. *Reflections on the Management of the National Health Service.* London: Nuffield Provincial Hospital Trust, 1985.
198. British Medical Association. *Leading for Health: a BMA Agenda for Health.* London: BMA, 1992.
199. Chawner J. Consultants performance and counter productive incentives. In: Owen AV,

ed. *The Health Debate Live: 45 Interviews for "Leading for Health"*. London: British Medical Association, 1992: 76-80.
200. Medicopolitical Digest. Increase in NHS managers' pay. *British Medical Journal* 1993; **306**: 724.
201. Secretaries of State for Health, Wales, Northern Ireland and Scotland. *Working for Patients*. London: Her Majesty's Stationery Office, 1989.
202. Seaton A. Patients first; I wonder. *British Medical Journal* 1991; **302**: 1474.
203. Warden J. Letter from Westminster. Clarke's radical caution. *British Medical Journal* 1989; **298**: 351-2.
204. Lock S. Pride and prejudice. Time to recognise the weakness of the White Paper. *British Medical Journal* 1989; **298**: 1197.
205. Ham C. *The new National Health Service*. Oxford: Radcliffe Medical Press, 1991
206. Burrows M M. The Prime Minister's Review of the National Health Service. *Anaesthesia News* 1989; **No 23 (June): 1**.
207. The Annual Conference of Linkman of the Association of Anaesthetists of Great Britain and Ireland 1989. *Anaesthesia* 1990; **45**: 263-9
208. Smith R. Medicines core values. *British Medical Journal* 1994; **309**: 1247-8.
209. Shock M. Medicine at the centre of the nation's affairs. *British Medical Journal* 1994; **309**: 1730-3.
210. Light D W. Observation on the NHS reforms. An American perspective. *British Medical Journal* 1994; **309**: 568-70.
211. Scrutator. The week. Clarke's legacy of efficiency. *British Medical Journal* 1990; **301**: 1066.
212. News. New Secretary of State for Health. *British Medical Journal* 1990; **301**: 1062.
213. Roberts J. Kenneth Clarke: Hatchet man or remoulder? *British Medical Journal* 1990; **301**: 1382-3.
214. Warden J. The Bevan factor. *British Medical Journal* 1992; **304**: 338.
215. Hart. The week. *British Medical Journal* 1992; **304**: 338.
216. Maxwell R. Aneurin Bevan on the NHS. *British Medical Journal* 1992; **304**: 200.
217. Klein R. NHS reforms: the first six months. Judgement suspended. *British Medical Journal* 1992; **304**: 199-200.
218. Klein R. Labour's Health Policy. The conflict between the two main parties is now over means not ends. *British Medical Journal* 1992; **304**: 517-8.
219. Warden J. Britain's health manifestos. *British Medical Journal* 1992; **304**: 526.
220. Warden J. Letter from Westminster. The lib-lab solution. *British Medical Journal* 1992; **304**: 528.
221. Hart. The week. *British Medical Journal* 1992; **304**: 466.
222. Brearley S. Accreditation after Goldstein. Time for higher training committees to reconsider their procedures. *British Medical Journal* 1992; **304**: 518.
223. Beecham L. Junior doctors want single tier of specialist. *British Medical Journal* 1992; **304**: 1651-2.
224. Beecham L. Trying to satisfy EC directives on specialisation. *British Medical Journal* 1992; **305**: 332.
225. Department of Health. *Hospital Doctors Training for the Future. The Report of a Group on Specialist Medical Training*. London: Department of Health, 1993.

226. Hunter S, McLarren P. Specialist Medical training and the Calman report. Deserves and requires imaginative professional and managerial support. *British Medical Journal* 1993; **306**: 1281-2.
227. Ashton J. The Health of the nation. A new consensus emerges. *British Medical Journal* 1991; **302**: 1413-4.
228. Gabby J. The health of the nation. *British Medical Journal* 1992; **305**: 129-30.
229. Delamothe T. Towards a healthier England. *British Medical Journal* 1992; **305**: 135-6.
230. Warden J. Health trilogy. *British Medical Journal* 1992; **305**: 140.
231. Hart. The week. *British Medical Journal* 1991; **302**: 1424.
232. Warden J. Election battle cry. *British Medical Journal* 1991; **302**: 988
233. Warden J. Patients first. *British Medical Journal* 1991; **303**: 1153.
234. Stocking B. Patients' Charter. New rights issue. *British Medical Journal* 1991; **303**: 1148-9.
235. Warden J. First steps. *British Medical Journal* 1991; **302**: 810.
236. Warden J. Whipped to frenzy. *British Medical Journal* 1992; **305**: 139-40.
237. Warden J. The manager is king. *British Medical Journal* 1991; **302**: 1298.
238. Warden J. High and low NHS. *British Medical Journal* 1991; **302**: 1424.
239. Hart. The week. *British Medical Journal* 1991; **303**: 1018.
240. National Health Service Management Executive. *The NHS Reforms. The First Six Months.* London: Department of Health, 1992.
241. Klein R. NHS Reforms: the first six months. Judgement suspended. *British Medical Journal* 1992; **304**: 199-200.
242. Warden J. Reforms on course, say Government. *British Medical Journal* 1992: **304**: 204-5.
243. Radical Statistics Health Group. NHS Reforms: the first six months. Proof of progress or a statistical smokescreen? *British Medical Journal* 1992; **304**: 705-9.
244. Klein R. Society, health and the NHS. The BMA marshals the issues for debate. *British Medical Journal* 1991; **303**: 867-8.
245. News and Political Review. Photograph and caption. *British Medical Journal* 1992; **304**: 660.
246. Ford J. NAHAT Survey. *British Medical Journal* 1991; **303**: 1351-2.
247. Beecham L. Government upbeat on fundholding and waiting lists. *British Medical Journal* 1992; **304**: 661.
248. Paton C M. Problems with the NHS reforms. *British Medical Journal* 1992; **304**: 918.
249. Warden J. Reform begats reform. *British Medical Journal* 1992; **304**: 466.
250. Coulter A. Fundholding general practices. Early success - but will they last? *British Medical Journal* 1992; **304**: 397-8.
251. Sutherland V J, Cooper C L. Job stress, satisfaction, and mental health among general practitioners before and after the introduction of the new contract. *British Medical Journal* 1992; **304**: 1545-8.
252. Hart. The week. *British Medical Journal* 1992; **304**: 662.
253. Yates J. Lies damned lies and waiting lists; or lies, damned lies and politicians. *British Medical Journal* 1991; **303**: 802.
254. Medicopolitical digest. Two year waiting lists slashed. *British Medical Journal* 1992; **304**: 988.

255. Smith J. First Steps in fundholding. *British Medical Journal* 1992; **304**: 401-2.
256. Hart. The week. *British Medical Journal* 1992; **304**: 338.
257. Beecham L. Medicopolitical digest. Problems with extracontractural referrals continue. *British Medical Journal* 1992; **305**: 370.
258. Craft N. Secrecy in the NHS. *British Medical Journal* 1994; **309**: 1640-3.
259. Smith R. Twenty steps towards a "closed society" on health. *British Medical Journal* 1987; **295**: 1633-4.
260. Macdonald V. Put patients last. The Sunday Telegraph 1994; **No 1745 (13 Nov)**: 10.
261. Lock S. Realities and (some) visions. Not all gloom at Godber Symposium. *British Medical Journal* 1993; **307**: 280.
262. Timmins N. Audit and accountability in the NHS. In: Lock S, ed. *Eighty-five Not Out. Essays to Honour Sir George Godber.* London: King Edward's Hospital's Fund, 1993: 49-54.
263. Barley M G. The patient comes first. *Sunday Telegraph* 1994; **No 1746 (20 Nov)**: 10.
264. Anonymous. Personal view. No smoke without fire. *British Medical Journal* 1993; **307**: 1075.
265. Tomlin P J. Suspended doctors. *British Medical Journal* 1993; **307**: 1355.
266. Beecham L. NHS sackings. *British Medical Journal* 1992; **304**: 1588.
267. Simpson J, Smith R. "Macho" management in the NHS. may wreck everything. *British Medical Journal* 1992; **304**: 1598.
268. Hart. The week. The heart has its reasons. *British Medical Journal* 1992; **304**: 866.
269. Warden J. From Bevan to Bottomley. *British Medical Journal* 1992; **304**: 1004.
270. Warden J. New ministers. *British Medical Journal* 1992; **304**: 1136.
271. Beecham L. Medicopolitical digest. *British Medical Journal* 1992; **304**: 1183.
272. Beecham L. Medicopolitical digest. *British Medical Journal* 1992; **305**: 777-80.
273. Beecham L. Medicopolitical digest. *British Medical Journal* 1992; **305**: 894-5.
274. Dyer C. RHA told to reinstate "redundant" Helen Zeitlin. *British Medical Journal* 1992; **305**: 1177.
275. Harrison P. Doctors are vulnerable to managers. *British Medical Journal* 1993; **307**: 325-6.
276. Dyer O. Paediatrician wins complaints case. *British Medical Journal* 1994; **308**: 1258.
277. Birley J L T. Whistleblowing. The National Health Service as an open society. *Journal of the Royal Society of Medicine* 1996; **89**: 541-2.
278. Heys R F. Whistleblowing. *British Medical Journal* 1993; **306**: 210.
279. Smith R. Whistleblowing: a curse on ineffective organisations. Better management, not gagging is the answer. *British Medical Journal* 1992; **305**: 308-10.
280. Baddeley P G. Sympathy for the whistleblower. *British Medical Journal* 1992; 304: 1572.
281. Warden J. MPs slighted by advice to whistleblowers. *British Medical Journal* 1993; **307**: 345-60.
282. Beecham L. Whistleblowers may tell MPs. *British Medical Journal* 1993; **307**: 1216.
283. Villar R. Personal view. Praise will get more results. *British Medical Journal* 1993; **306**: 939.
284. Hart. NHS plc. *British Medical Journal* 1992; **305**: 1386.
285. Clarke A, McKee M. The Consultant episode. An unhelpful measure. Time to replace it

with a single episode of disease? *British Medical Journal* 1992; **305**: 1307-8
286. Bury B. Letter to Mrs Bottomley. *British Medical Journal* 1993; **306**: 702-3.
287. MacRae W R (Chairman). *NHS Management Changes. Implications for Anaesthetists.* London: The Association of Anaesthetists of Great Britain and Ireland, 1992.
288. Medical News. What nurses think. *British Medical Journal* 1988; **296**: 1474-5.
289. Scrutator. The week. A personal view of medicopolitical events. *British Medical Journal* 1988; **296**: 439.
290. Delamothe T. Nursing grievances. I: Voting with their feet. *British Medical Journal* 1988; **296**: 25-8.
291. Delamothe T. Nursing grievances. II: Pay. *British Medical Journal* 1988; 296: 120-5
292. Delamothe T. Nursing grievances. III: Conditions. *British Medical Journal* 1988; **296**: 183-5.
293. Delamothe T. Nursing grievances. IV: Not a profession, not a career. *British Medical Journal* 1988; **296**: 271-4.
294. Delamothe T. Nursing grievances. V: Women's work. *British Medical Journal* 1988; **296**: 406-8..
295. Delamothe T. Nursing grievances. VI: Other places, other solutions. *British Medical Journal* 1988; **296**: 406-8.
296. Delamothe T. Nurses: where do they go from here? *British Medical Journal* 1988; **296**: 449.
297. Mitchell J R A. Is nursing any business of doctors? A simple guide to the "nursing process". *British Medical Journal* 1984; *288*: 216-9.
298. Rowden R. Doctors can work with the nursing process. A reply to Professor Mitchell. *British Medical Journal* 1984; **288**: 219-21.
299. Currie C T. The nursing process. Revolutionary philosophy or a passing phase? *British Medical Journal* 1984; **289**: 1218-9.
300. Delamothe T. Nurses make the grade. *British Medical Journal* 1988; **296**: 1344.
301. Greenhalgh T. Skill mix. *British Medical Journal* 1993; **307**: 71.
302. Cohen P. Buying-out appeals. *Nursing Times* 1993; **89**: 18.
303. Briggs A (Chairman). *Report of the Committee on Nursing.* London: Her Majesty's Stationery Office, 1972.
304. United Kingdom Central Council for Nursing, Midwifery and Health Visiting (UKCC). *Project 2000. A New Preparation for Practice.* London: UKCC, 1986.
305. United Kingdom Central Council for Nursing, Midwifery and Health Visiting (UKCC). *Project 2000. The Only Option.* London: UKCC, 1986.
306. Fennell E. Lighting the way to higher standards. NCVQ. Supplement NCVQ. *The Times* 1995; **16 February: 3**.
307. Salvage J. Thumbs up from government for reform of nurse training. *British Medical Journal* 1988; **296**: 1553.
308. Mangan P. The new game in town. *Nursing Times* 1993; **89 (No 15)**: 52.
309. Lavelle M. Lessons for the teacher. *Nursing Times* 1993; **89 (No 15)**: 32-3.
310. Payne D. The bursary blues. *Nursing Times* 1994; **90 (No 48)**: 20-1.
311. Pennington S, Payne D. RCN warns of staffing crisis. *Nursing Times* 1994; **90 (No 49)**: 5.
312. Mangan P. Preparation for change. *Nursing Times* 1993; **89 (No 17)**: 58-60.

References: Chapter 9

313. Elkan R, Robinson J. Project 2000. Back to basics. *Nursing Times* 1993; **89 (No 4)**: 32-3.
314. Livesley B. Running out of staff for the NHS. Reductions in school leavers plus Project 2000 may bring the NHS to its knees. *British Medical Journal* 1989; **299**: 1-2.
315. Redfern L. Health care assistants. The challenge to nursing staff. *Nursing Times* 1994; **90 (No 48)**: 31-3.
316. Cole A. Disappearing act. *Nursing Times* 1995; **91 (No 1)**: 17.
317. Friend B. Under fire. *Nursing Times* 1993; **89 (No 17)**: 19.
318. David A. Worth their salt. *Nursing Times* 1994; **90 (No 51)**: 14.
319. Anonymous. P2K provides skills for change. *Nursing Times* 1994; *90 (No 51)*: 22.
320. Marsland L. Modern studies. *Nursing Times* 1993; *89 (No 15)*: 33-4.
321. Maynard A. Drunken sailor syndrome. *Health Service Journal* 1991; **101**: 17.
322. Vickers M. Lazy Sunday afternoon. *Health Service Journal* 1992; **102**: 1.
323. Vickers M D. Editorial. What manpower crisis?. *Today's Anaesthetist* 1995; **10**: 67.
324. Association of Anaesthetists of Great Britain and Ireland. Annual Report of Council 1981-1982. *Anaesthesia* 1983; **38**: 188-98.
325. Association of Anaesthetists of Great Britain and Ireland. Annual Report of Council 1991-1992. *Anaesthesia* 1993; **48**: 546-56.
326. Association of Anaesthetists of Great Britain and Ireland. *Minutes of the Annual General Meeting*, 1981.
327. Association of Anaesthetists of Great Britain and Ireland. *Minutes of the Annual General Meeting*, 1992.
328. Wylie W D. The search of 9 Bedford Square. *Anaesthesia News* 1987; **No 4 (October)**: 2.
329. Wylie W D. *Further note about the purchase of 9 Bedford Square.* Document in the Archives of the Association of Anaesthetists of Great Britain and Ireland, 1987.
330. Association of Anaesthetists of Great Britain and Ireland. *Minutes of the Annual General Meeting* 1984. London.
331. Association of Anaesthetists of Great Britain and Ireland. Annual Report of Council 1983-1984. *Anaesthesia* 1985; **40**: 111-20
332. Association of Anaesthetists of Great Britain and Ireland. *Minutes of the Annual General Meeting* 1984. London .
333. *The Director's Reports and Financial Statements of the Association of Anaesthetists of Great Britain and Ireland and the Education and Research Trust.* London: Association of Anaesthetists of Great Britain and Ireland, 1998.
334. Tite G. *Number Nine Bedford Square - An Illustrated History with Maps.* Sutton: Sussex Histories, 1986.
335. Fuge C A. Bedford Square. A connection with mesmerism. *Anaesthesia* 1986; **41**: 726-30.
336. Lee S. Editor. Wakley, Thomas (1795-1862). *Directory of National Biography.* **Volume 59**. London: Smith, Elder and Co., 1899: 4-8.
337. Thornton J L. The Medical College from its origins to the end of the nineteenth century. In: Medvei VC, Thornton J L, eds. *The Royal Hospital of Saint Bartholomew 1123-1973.* Ipswich: Cowell, 1974: 43-77.
338. Lee S. Editor. Scott, John, first Earl Eldon (1751-1838). *Dictionary of National Biography.* **Volume 51**. London: Smith, Elder and Co., 1897: 49-56.

339. Ellis R H, ed. *James Robinson on the Inhalation of the Vapour of Ether.* London: Bailliere Tindall, 1983.
340. Rosen G. Mesmerism and Surgery. A strange chapter in the history of anaesthesia. *Journal of the History of Medicine* 1946; **1**: 527-50.
341. Association of Anaesthetists of Great Britain and Ireland. Annual Report of Council 1984-1985. *Anaesthesia* 1986; **41**: 120-7.
342. Association of Anaesthetists of Great Britain and Ireland. Annual Conference of Linkmen, 1984. *Anaesthesia* 1985; **40**: 1263-6.
343. Association of Anaesthetists of Great Britain and Ireland. Annual Conference of Linkmen, 1985. *Anaesthesia* 1986; **41**: 464-8.
344. Association of Anaesthetists of Great Britain and Ireland. Annual Conference of Linkmen, 1986. *Anaesthesia* 1987; **42**: 459-64.
345. Edridge A W. Editorial. Sir Ivan Whiteside Magill. *Anaesthesia* 1987; **42**: 231-3.
346. Pallister W K. Editorial. Sir Stephen William Organe 1908-1989. *Anaesthesia* 1989; **44**: 461-2.
347. Obituary. Gilmartin T J. *Anaesthesia* 1987; **42**: 105.
348. Eastcott H H G. Obituary. Lord Porritt. *College and Faculty Bulletin. Supplement to the Annuals of the Royal College of Surgeons of England* 1994; 76: 80-2.
349. Lee S. Editor. Morton, John (1420-1500). *Dictionary of National Biography*. London: Smith, Elder and Co., 1894: 151-3.
350. Lunn J N. The opening ceremony. *Anaesthesia News* 1987; **No 4 (October)**: 2.
351. Horton J N. Editor. Association Benefactor honoured. *Anaesthesia News* 1988; **No 6 (January)**: 3.
352. Charlton J E. Editor. The loon hoots but the caravan moves on. *Anaesthesia News* 1993; **No 76 (November)**: 8.
353. Horton J N. Editor. Presentation of portrait of Dr Henry Featherstone. *Anaesthesia News* 1988. **No 11 (June)**: 3.
354. Souvenir programme. *Opening of 9 Bedford Square by Her Royal Highness, The Princess Margaret, Thursday 9 July 1987.* London: Association of Anaesthetists of Great Britain and Ireland, 1987.
355. Mushin W W. Editorial. Professor Emeritus Sir Robert Reynolds Macintosh. *Anaesthesia* 1989; **44**: 951-2.
356. Association of Anaesthetists of Great Britain and Ireland. Annual Report of Council, 1986-1987. *Anaesthesia* 1988; **43**: 83-9.
357. Tite G. Georgian Masterpiece. *Period Homes* 1987; **8**: 40-3.
358. Eccles A. Historical Resources at 9 Bedford Square, Part I: The BOC Museum (Charles King). *Anaesthesia News* 1991; **No 46 (May): 2-3.**
359. Wilkinson D J, Eccles A. The BOC Museum (The Charles King Collection of Historical Apparatus). The evolution of a collection into a museum. *Journal of the History of Collections* 1992; **4**: 99-105.
360. Boulton T B, Wilkinson J, Eccles A. The British Oxygen Company Museum and Charles King Collection of Historical Anaesthetic Apparatus at the Association of Anaesthetists of Great Britain and Ireland, 9 Bedford Square, London WC1. *Today's Anaesthetist* 1994; **9**: 33.
361. Eccles A. Historical resources at 9 Bedford Square. Part 2. Written and audiovisual

material. *Anaesthesia News* 1991; **No 47 (June)**: 2-3.
362. Association of Anaesthetists of Great Britain and Ireland. Annual Report of Council 1987-1988. *Anaesthesia* 1989; **44**: 280-9.
363. Association of Anaesthetists of Great Britain and Ireland. Annual Report of Council 1988-1989. *Anaesthesia* 1990; **45**: 92-100.
364. Association of Anaesthetists of Great Britain and Ireland. Annual Report of Council 1989-1990. *Anaesthesia* 1991; **46**: 243-53.
365. Association of Anaesthetists of Great Britain and Ireland. Annual Report of Council 1990-1991. *Anaesthesia* 1992; **47**: 181-192.
366. Association of Anaesthetists of Great Britain and Ireland. Annual Report of Council 1993-1994. *Anaesthesia* 1995; **50**: 272-82.
367. Association of Anaesthetists of Great Britain and Ireland. Annual Report of Council 1981-1982. *Anaesthesia* 1983; **38**: 188-98.
368. Horton J N. Editor. Seminars at 9 Bedford Square. *Anaesthesia News* 1987; **No 3 (August)**: 2.
369. Association of Anaesthetists of Great Britain and Ireland. Annual Report of Council 1985-1986. *Anaesthesia* 1987; **42**: 119-28.
370. Horton J N. Editor. Seminars at 9 Bedford Square. *Anaesthesia News* 1988; **No 13 (August)**: 2.
371. Horton J N. Editor. The Winter Scientific Meeting 1988. *Anaesthesia News* 1988; **No 9 (April)**: 1.
372. Horton J N. Editor. Association of Meeting at the College. *Anaesthesia News* 1989; **No 20 (March)**: 1.
373. Vaughan R S. Winter Scientific Meeting. *Anaesthesia News* 1990; **No 32 (March)**: 1.
374. Horton J N. Editor. Association Winter Meeting. *Anaesthesia News* 1991; **No 44 (March)**: 8.
375. Horton J N. Editor. Winter Meeting marks Jubilee Year. *Anaesthesia News* 1992; **No 56 (March)**: 1-3.
376. Charlton J E. Editor. Winter Scientific Meeting. *Anaesthesia News* 1995; **No 93 (April)**: 1-2.
377. Charlton J E. Editor. Ohmeda Health Lecture 1995. *Anaesthesia News* 1995; **No 92 (March)**: 3.
378. Charlton E. Editor. Penlon Garden opens. *Anaesthesia News* 1993; **No 13 (August)**: 1.
379. Editorial. House of Commons Social Services Committee Report. *British Medical Journal* 1981; **283**: 997-8.
380. Young G. Are isolated maternity units run by general practitioners dangerous? *British Medical Journal* 1987; **294**: 744-6.
381. Young G. Anaesthetic services in obstetrics. Association report warnings about small obstetric units. *Anaesthetic News* 1988; **No 10 (May)**: 1.
382. Perry J R. Some obstetric units can cope. *Anaesthesia News* 1988; **No 15 (October)**: 3.
383. Rosen M. A reply to Dr Young. *Anaesthesia News* 1988; **No 10 (May)**: 3.
384. Rosen M. The obstetric anaesthesia report. *Anaesthesia News* 1988; **No 16 (May)**: 1.
385. News and Political Review. Home truths about maternity services. *British Medical Journal* 1992; **304**: 657.
386. Charlton J E. Editor. New Government report on maternity services. *Anaesthesia News*

1993; **No 75 (October)**: 1.
387. Court C. Childbirth Trust calls for rights to home births. *British Medical Journal* 1995; **310**: 212.
388. Scott W E. Editorial. Ethics in obstetric anaesthesia. *Anaesthesia* 1996; **51**: 717-718.
389. Charlton J E. Editor. Association members meet in Bournemouth. *Anaesthesia News* 1992; **No 64 (November)**: 1.
390. Baskett P J F, Charlton J E. Association Administrator retires. *Anaesthesia News* 1992; **No 62 (September)**: 1.
391. Charlton J E. Citation: Miss Ann Muir. *Anaesthesia News* 1992; **No 65 (December)**: 7
392. Association of Anaesthetists of Great Britain and Ireland. Annual Report of Council 1992-1993. *Anaesthesia* 1994; **49**: 360-9.
393. Zorab J S M. Editorial. Philip John Helliwell. *Anaesthesia* 1994; **49**: 659-60.
394. Lunn J N. Editor. Obituary. Thomas James Gilmartin. *Anaesthesia* 1987; **42**: 105.
395. Lunn J N. Editorial. The evolution of Anaesthesia. *Anaesthesia* 1988; 43: 1.
396. Horton J N. Editor. Honorary Membership. *Anaesthesia News* 1992; **No 55 (February)**: 2.
397. Horton J N, Lunn J N. Editorial. *Anaesthesia News* 1987; **No 1 (April)**: 1.
398. Vickers M D. Unfinished business. 1. What's going on. *Anaesthesia News* 1988; **No 6 (January)**: 4.
399. Buck N. Is there anybody there? SOAP and the Linkmen: the facts. Can we contact your Linkman? *Anaesthesia News* 1988; **No 7 (February)**: 1.
400. Baird W L M, Lunn J N. *Survey of Anaesthetic Practice*. London: Association of Anaesthetists of Great Britain and Ireland, 1988.
401. Rollin A-M. The Linkman network. *Anaesthesia News* 1988; **No 10 (May)**: 3.
402. Cartwright D P. Do we need Linkmen? *Anaesthesia News* 1988; **No 14 (September)**: 3
403. Vickers M D. Unfinished business. 8. The Linkman Conference. Is it still worthwhile? *Anaesthesia News* 1988; **No 17 (December)**: 3.
404. Vickers M D. Unfinished business. 3. The Junior Anaesthetists' Group. *Association News* 1988. **No 8 (March)**: 4.
405. Spencer E M. *The History of the Group of Anaesthetists in Training*. London: Association of Anaesthetists of Great Britain and Ireland, 1992.
406. Goodwin A P L. Editor. *The Group of Anaesthetists in Training*. Yearbook 1993/4. London: Association of Anaesthetists of Great Britain and Ireland, 1993.
407. Berry C B. Editor. *The Group of Anaesthetists in Training Yearbook 1995*. London: Association of Anaesthetists of Great Britain and Ireland, 1995.
408. Allan L. Juniors' problems. *Anaesthesia News* 1988; **No 13 (August)**: 3.
409. *Handbook for Trainee Anaesthetists*, London: Association of Anaesthetists of Great Britain and Ireland, 1991.
410. Spencer L. Bristol hosts Trainee Silver Jubilee Meeting. *Anaesthesia News* 1992; **No 59 (June)**: 1-2.
411. Charlton J E. Editor. Winter meeting marks Jubilee Year. *Anaesthesia News* 1992; **No 56 (March)**: 1-3.
412. O'Flaherty D. Anaesthesia in the United Kingdom and Ireland. *Anaesthesia News* 1988; **No 13 (August)**: 1.
413. Horton J N. Editor. Ireland to have Standing Committee. Irish professional fees well

below UK levels. *Anaesthesia News* 1988; **No 16 (November)**: 4.
414. Fitzgerald P. Convenor. *Anaesthesia in Ireland. Provision of a Safe Service*. London: Association of Anaesthetists of Great Britain and Ireland, 1991.
415. Cahill J. Chairman. *Workload for Consultant Anaesthetists in Ireland*. London: Association of Anaesthetists of Great Britain and Ireland, 1991.
416. Cahill J. Chairman. Standing Committee. *Republic of Ireland National Manpower Survey*. London: Association of Anaesthetists of Great Britain and Ireland, 1994.
417. Cahill J, O'Toole D. Coordinators. *Irish National Survey of Intensive Care Units*. London: Association of Anaesthetists of Great Britain and Ireland, 1994.
418. Cahill J. Irish Standing Committee March 1994. *Anaesthesia News* 1994; **No 82 (May)**: 8.
419. Charlton J E. Editor. Association strength in Ireland grows. *Anaesthesia News* 1993; **No 66 (January)**: 1-2.
420. Association of Anaesthetists of Great Britain and Ireland. Annual Report of Council 1994-1995. *Anaesthesia* 1996; **51**: 295-305.
421. Cahill J. Fees Committee recommends acceptance of VHI offer. *Anaesthesia News* 1995; **No 92 (March)**: 1-2.
422. Association News and Notices. Register of Meeting dates. *Anaesthesia* 1975; **30**: 111
423. *AAGBI Minute Book No 5 (4.5.1979-29.7.1983)*.
424. Association of Anaesthetists of Great Britain and Ireland. Annual Report of Council 1982-1983. *Anaesthesia* 1984; **39**: 89-98.
425. Charlton J E. Association events. *Anaesthesia News* 1995; **No 99 (October)**: 1.
426. Horton J N. Editor. Golden handshake! *Anaesthesia News* 1988; **No 6 (January)**: 1.
427. Smith G. Editorial. Research in anaesthesia: the key to the future. *British Journal of Anaesthesia* 1995; **75**: 383-6.
428. *Educational Awards*. London: Association of Anaesthetists of Great Britain and Ireland, 1990.
429. Eltringham R J. Help needed overseas. Opportunities for service in the developing world. *Anaesthesia News* 1988; **No 8 (March)**: 1.
430. Carter M. Have exam, will travel...... again and again. *Association News* 1989; **No 25 (August)**: 1.
431. Obituary. Jeffrey Selwyn Crawford. *Anaesthesia* 1989; **44**: 373.
432. *Guidelines for Overseas Lecturers to Developing Countries*. London: Association of Anaesthetists of Great Britain and Ireland, 1993.
433. Charlton J E. Steel City hosts GAT. Another enormous success. *Anaesthesia News* 1993; **No 71 (June)**: 1-3.
434. Charlton J E. All change at GAT. *Anaesthesia News* 1995; **No 95 (June)**: 1-2.
435. Parbrook G D. Editorial. Death for anaesthesia in the general and community dental service. *British Journal of Anaesthesia* 1986; **58**: 369-70.
436. Hancocks S. Sixty proposals on dental anaesthesia. *British Medical Journal* 1990; **301**: 1351-2.
437. Coplans M P, Curson I. Deaths associated with dentistry. *British Dental Journal* 1982; **153**: 357-62.
438. Coplans M P, Curson I. Deaths associated with dentistry and dental disease 1980-1989. *Anaesthesia* 1993; **48**: 435-8.

439. Allen N A, Dinsdale R C W, Reilly C S. A survey of general anaesthesia and sedation in dental practice in two cities. *British Dental Journal* 1990; **169**: 168-72.
440. Seward M. Editor. Reprieve for dental general practice. *British Dental Journal* 1991; **170**: 43.
441. *AAGBI Minute Book No 7 (4.3.1988-3.2.1995).*
442. Poswillo D E. Chairman. *Report of an Expert Working Party. General Anaesthesia, Sedation and Resuscitation in Dentistry*. London: Standing Dental Advisory Committee Department of Health, 1990.
443. Seward M. Editor. Poswillo Report. Principal recommendations of the report. *British Dental Journal* 1991; **170**: 46.
444. Horton J N. Editor. Report sets high standards for dental anaesthesia and sedation. *Anaesthesia News* 1991; **No 43 (February)**: 1.
445. Sykes P. Editor. The Poswillo Report. *SAAD Digest* 1991; **8**: 26-32.
446. Mason D. Statement from the President of the GDC. *British Dental Journal* 1991; **170**: 47.
447. Padfield A. Proposals on dental anaesthesia. *British Medical Journal* 1991; **302**: 182.
448. Cartwright DP. "Reprieve for dental anaesthesia". *British Dental Journal* 1991; **170**: 129
449. James D W. A personal view. General anaesthesia, sedation and resuscitation in dentistry. *British Dental Journal* 1991; **171**: 344-7.
450. Seward M. Editor. Poswillo - the beginning of the end? *British Dental Journal* 1991; **171**: 339.
451. Robson J S. General anaesthesia and resuscitation in dentistry. *British Dental Journal* 1992; **172**: 134.
452. Seward M. Editor. Funding for Poswillo. *British Dental Journal* 1992; **172**: 83.
453. Sutherland DA. Funding for Poswillo. *British Dental Journal* 1992; **172**: 179.
454. Mason D. President's Address to the General Dental Council. *British Dental Journal* 1992; **172**: 361-3.
455. Boulton T B. Presidential Address. The rise and fall of general anaesthesia in the dental chair. *SAAD Digest*; 1980; **4**: 156-65.
456. Saeed N R. The establishment of dental anaesthetic clinics. *British Dental Journal* 1993; **175**: 308.
457. Hancocks S. Dentists vote to accept continuing care contract. *British Medical Journal* 1990; **301**: 77.
458. Hancocks S. How fares the dentists' contract? *British Medical Journal* 1990; **301**: 1352-3.
459. Strunin L. President's Statement. *Royal College of Anaesthetists Newsletter* 1999; **No 44 (January)**: 1-3..
460. Warden J. Dentistry in decay? *British Medical Journal* 1992; **305**: 1316.
461. Corson M A, Wilson M A. A survey of general anaesthesia and intravenous sedation within General Dental Practice in the City of Manchester 1991-1993. *SAAD Digest* 1995; **12**: 10-12.
462. Holt R D, Davenport E S, Fung D E. The use of general anaesthesia for tooth extraction in London: a multicentre trial. *British Dental Journal* 1992; **173**: 333-9.
463. Barnett P J, Skinner A C, Whelan E. Chair dental anaesthesia. A survey of current and intended practice in the Mersey Region. *Anaesthesia* 1994; **49**: 728-30.

464. Ross I D. Poswillo implementation. The non-consultant dental anaesthetists certification. *SAAD Digest* 1995; **12**: 16-7.
465. Spence A A. Dentistry and anaesthesia. *British Dental Journal* 1993; **175**: 135-8.
466. Whelan E, Skinner A. The anaesthetic fairy. *British Dental Journal* 1994; **177**: 87.
467. Mitchell J. A fundamental problem of consent. *British Medical Journal* 1995; **310**: 43-6
468. White G M J. Dental chair anaesthesia. "Unexpected hazard" defined by the High Court. *Today's Anaesthetist* 1996; **11**: 11-8.
469. Greenan J. New contract "rewards the cavalier anaesthetist". *British Dental Journal* 1991; **170**: 89.
470. Jack A. Judgement on unexpected hazard fee. *SAAD Digest* 1995; 12 (July): 23.
471. Lunn J N, Adams A P. What is not expected? *British Dental Journal* 1991; **171**: 353.
472. White G M J. "What is not expected". *British Dental Journal* 1992; **172**: 179-80.
473. Dillner L. Private medical fees investigated. *British Medical Journal* 1992; **305**: 667.
474. Charlton J E. Editor. Monopolies and private health. A sting in the tail. *Anaesthesia News* 1993; **No 68 (March)**: 8.
475. Charlton J E. Editor. Monopolies and private health. *Anaesthesia News* 1993; **No 69 (April)**: 1.
476. Beugg C. On your own, or in a company scheme? *Daily Telegraph* (Supplement: Managing Health Care) 1995; November 25: 15.
477. Pallot P. Just how much money is being wasted? *Daily Telegraph* (Supplement: Managing Health Care) 1995; November 25: 2.
478. Association of Anaesthetists of Great Britain and Ireland. The Annual Conference of Linkmen 1990. *Anaesthesia* 1991; **46**: 243-53.
479. Association of Anaesthetists of Great Britain and Ireland. The Annual Conference of Linkmen 1991. *Anaesthesia* 1992; **47**: 723-8.
480. Charlton J E. Editor. The dogs bark and the caravan moves on. *Anaesthesia News* 1993; **72 (July)**: 2.
481. Inman M T, Chairman Private Practice Committee. *Guidance on the Conduct of Private Practice*. London: Association of Anaesthetists of Great Britain and Ireland, 1988.
482. Charlton J E. Editor. Monopolies and private health. *Association News* 1993; **No 69 (April)**: 1.
483. Baskett P J F. Readers' points. *Anaesthesia News* 1994; **No 81 (April)**: 8.
484. Thelwall-Jones H. Readers' points. *Anaesthesia News* 1994; **No 83 (June)**: 7.
485. Charlton J E. Editor. The dogs bark and the caravan moves on. *Anaesthesia News* 1993; **No 70 (May)**: 3.
486. Beecham L. British Government bans BMA private fees guide. *British Medical Journal* 1994; **308**: 492-3.
487. Rollin A-M. Monopolies and Mergers Commission Report. *Anaesthesia News* 1994; **No 80 (March)**: 3.
488. Charlton J E. Editor. The dogs bark and the caravan moves on. *Anaesthesia News* 1994; **No 83 (June)**: 7.
489. Charlton J E. Editor. The dogs bark and the caravan moves on. *Anaesthesia News* 1995; **No 97 (August)**: 2
490. Charlton J E. Editor. The dogs bark and the caravan moves on. *Anaesthesia News* 1995; **No 98 (September)**: 2.

491. Association of Anaesthetists of Great Britain and Ireland. Annual Conference of Linkmen 1988. *Anaesthesia* 1989; **44**: 712-7.
492. Charlton J E. Editor. Winter Scientific Meeting. The BOC Health Care Lecture 1993. Professor Clayton Petty. *Anaesthesia News* 1993; **No 68 (March)**: 2-3.
493 Association of Anaesthetists of Great Britain and Ireland. Annual Conference of Linkmen 1983. *Anaesthesia* 1984; **39**: 397-400.
494. Heath M L. *Memorandum to the Communication Circle, Assistance for Anaesthetists*, 5 April 1993. London: Association of Anaesthetists of Great Britain and Ireland, 1993.
495. Charlton J E. Editor. Winter Scientific Meeting. The BOC Health Care Lecture 1993. Professor Clayton Petty. *Anaesthesia News* 1993; **No 63 (March)**: 2-3.
496. Association of Anaesthetists of Great Britain and Ireland. Annual Conference of Linkmen 1983. *Anaesthesia* 1984; **39**: 397-400.
497. Heath M L. *Memorandum to the Communication Circle, Assistance for Anaesthetists*, 5 April 1993, London: Association of Anaesthetists of Great Britain and Ireland, 1993.
498. Burrows M M, Chairman. *Report of a Working Party on Assistance for the Anaesthetist.* London: Association of Anaesthetists of Great Britain and Ireland, 1988.
499. Rosen M, Chairman. *Efficiency of Theatre Services. A Report of a Working Party of the Association of Anaesthetists, and the Association of Surgeons of Great Britain and Ireland.* London: Association of Anaesthetists of Great Britain and Ireland, 1989.
500. Birkinshaw K. The fate of ODAs. *Anaesthesia News* 1989; **No 29 (December)**: 3.
501. Association of Anaesthetists of Great Britain and Ireland. Annual Conference of Linkmen 1987. *Anaesthesia* 1988, **43**: 721-5.
502. Association of Anaesthetists of Great Britain and Ireland. Annual Linkman Conference 1989. *Anaesthesia* 1990; **45**: 263-9.
503. *Annual Conference of Linkmen 1992*. London: Association of Anaesthetists of Great Britain and Ireland, 1992. (Note: *not published in Anaesthesia*).
504. Association of Anaesthetists of Great Britain and Ireland. The 18th Annual Linkman Conference 1993. *Anaesthesia* 1994; **49**: 462-6.
505. Baird W L M. Government report on operating theatres in line with the Association's recommendations. *Anaesthesia News* 1990; **No 33 (April)**: 1.
506. Fennell E. Lighting the way for higher standards. NCVQ. *The Times* 1995; 16 February (Supplement on National Council of Vocational Qualifications): 3.
507. *Notes of a Meeting Held on 26 November 1993 at 9 Bedford Square to Consider the Registration of Operating Department Assistants (ODAs)*. London: Association of Anaesthetists of Great Britain and Ireland, 1993.
508. Charlton J E. Editor. News and Notices. Theatre personnel plan links. *Anaesthesia News* 1993; **No 75 (October)**: 8.
509. Lloyd J. Anaesthetic nurses. In: *A Tribute to Sir Robert Macintosh for his 90th Birthday.* London: Royal Society of Medicine, 1988: 30-2.
510. Bailey R, Alladi V. What's in a name? *Nursing Standard* 1995; **10 (No 8)**: 23-5.
511. Lyons M, Prys-Roberts C, Martin A J. Beware nurse anaesthetists say the medical bodies. *Nursing Times* 1995; **91 (No 45)**: 22-3.
512. Smith A C. Nurse anaesthetists - or anaesthetic nurses. *Anaesthetic News* 1990, **No 33 (April)**: 4.
513. Horton A N. Editor. Association meeting at Southampton. *Anaesthesia News* 1988; **No 16**

(November): 1 and 3.
514. Horton J N. Editor. Swansea hosts Association Scientific Meeting. *Anaesthesia News* 1989; **No 28 (November)**: 1.
515. Vaughan R S. Association members meet in Manchester. *Association News* 1990; **No 41 (December)**: 1 and 3.
516. Horton J N. Harrogate hosts the Association meeting. *Anaesthesia News* 1991; **No 52 (November)**: 1-3.
517. Horton J N. Association members meet in Bournemouth. *Association News* 1992; **No 64 (November)**: 1-3.
518. Charlton J E. Annual Scientific Meeting in Glasgow. *Anaesthesia News* 1993; **No 76 (November)**: 1-3.
519. Charlton J E. Association meeting in Brighton. *Anaesthesia News* 1994; **No 88 (November)**: 1-3.
520. Charlton J E. Winter Scientific Meeting. *Anaesthesia News* 1994; **No 80 (March)**: 1-2.
521. Atkinson R E. Winter Scientific Meeting 1995. *Anaesthesia News* 1995; **No 93 (April)**: 1-2.
522. Charlton J E. First Scientific Meeting at Birmingham ICC. *Anaesthesia News* 1996; **No 102 (January)**: 1-2.
523. Lunn J N. Successful Joint Canadian-British Meeting. *Anaesthesia News* 1990; **No 27 (October)**: 1.
524. Charlton J E. Editor. The loon hoots but the caravan moves on. *Anaesthesia News* 1993; **No 76 (November)**: 8.
525. Atkinson R S, Boulton T B, eds. *The History of Anaesthesia. International Symposium Series 134.* London: Royal Society of Medicine, 1989.
526. Baskett P J F. The Second International Symposium on the History of Anaesthesia. *Anaesthesia News* 1987; **No 5 (December)**: 3.
527. Smith W D A, Paterson G M C. *A Tribute to Sir Robert Macintosh for his 90th Birthday.* London: Royal Society of Medicine, 1988
528. Horton J N. Editor. The Sir Ivan Magill Centenary Meeting. *Anaesthesia News* 1988; **No 12 (July)**: 1.
529. Horton J N. Editor. Photograph and caption. *Anaesthesia News* 1991; **No 42 (January)**: 2.
530. Horton J N. Editor. 1992 will be our Diamond Jubilee. *Anaesthesia News* 1991; **No 45 (April)**: 1.
531. Horton J N. Editor. Winter Meeting marks Jubilee Year. *Anaesthesia News* 1992; **No 56 (March)**: 1-2.
532. *Diamond Jubilee Scientific Meeting 1992.* Programme in the Archives of the Association of Anaesthetists of Great Britain and Ireland. London.
533. Baskett P. *Speech on the Opening of the Diamond Jubilee Winter Meeting 1992.* Script in the Archives of the Association of Anaesthetists of Great Britain and Ireland, London.
534. Faculty of Anaesthetists. Ceremony of presentation of diplomates. *Annals of the Royal College of Surgeons of England* 1983; **65** *(Supplement 6)*: 6-7.
535. Campbell D. Faculty of Anaesthetists Annual Meeting 21 March 1984. Address by the Dean. *Annals of the Royal College of Surgeons of England* 1984; **66** *(Supplement 4)*: 5.
536. Campbell D. Faculty of Anaesthetists Annual Meeting 20 March 1985. Address by the Dean.

Annals of the Royal College of Surgeons of England 1985; **67** *(Supplement 4):* 5-6.
537. Adams A K. Chairman. Faculty of Anaesthetists Annual Meeting 1987. *Annals of the Royal College of Surgeons of England* 1987; **69** *(Supplement 4):* 8-10.
538. C J L. The Supplemental Charter of 1988. *Annals of the Royal College of Surgeons of England* 1989; **71** *(Supplement 1):* 15-7.
539. College of Anaesthetists. The Inaugural Meeting of the Council of the College 19 October 1988. *Annals of the Royal College of Surgeons of England* 1989; **71** *(Supplement 1):* 6-9.
540. RSA. College News. *College of Anaesthetists Newsletter* 1989; **1 (February)**: 2-5.
541. Adams A K. The evolution of the College of Anaesthetists. *Anaesthesia News* 1989; **No 22 (May)**: 3.
542. Burrows M M. One more step? *Anaesthesia* 1989; **44**: 803-4.
543. Vickers M D. Editorial. *Anaesthesia* 1982; **37**: 1071-2.
544. Vickers M D. Editorial. Transmogrified? Just so. *Today's Anaesthetist* 1995; **10**: 146-7.
545. *College of Anaesthetists Newsletters 2-11*; February 1990 to March 1992.
546. *Royal College of Anaesthetists Report and Accounts 1991/1992*.
547. Spence A A. Chairman. *Report of the Working Party of the Commission on the Provision of Surgical Services on Pain after Surgery*. London: Royal College of Surgeons of England, 1990.
548. Rosen M. Chairman. *Academic Departments of Anaesthesia in Undergraduate Education. An Undervalued Resource*. London: College of Anaesthetists, 1990.
549. Rosen M. From the President. *College of Anaesthetists Newsletter* 1989; **No 2 (October)**: 1-2.
550. Smith G. Editor. Editorial 1. Journal of the Royal College of Anaesthetists. *British Journal of Anaesthesia* 1990; **64**: 1-2.
551. Boulton T B. The Armorial Bearings of the College of Anaesthetists. *College of Anaesthetists Newsletter* 1990; **No 4 (June)**: 8-10.
552. Boulton T B. The Arms of the College of Anaesthetists. *Association News* 1991; **No 48 (July)**: 2.
553. Spence A A. From the President. *College of Anaesthetists Newsletter* 1992; **No 11 (June)**: 1.
554. Spence A A. Constitutional changes for the College of Anaesthetists. *College of Anaesthetists Newsletter* 1990; **No 4 (June)**: 2-3.
555. Rosen M. From the President. *College of Anaesthetists Newsletter* 1989; **No 1 (February)**: 1.
556. Rosen M. From the President. *College of Anaesthetists Newsletter* 1990; **No 3 (February)**: 1.
557. Rosen M. From the President. *College of Anaesthetists Newsletter* 1990; **No 4 (June)**: 1.
558. Rosen M. From the President. *College of Anaesthetists Newsletter* 1991; **No 7 (June)**: 1.
559. Lunn J N. One hundred per cent support. *Anaesthesia News* 1990; **No 32 (March)**: 1.
560. MacRae W R. Fund raising for your College. *College of Anaesthetists Newsletter* 1990; **No 4 (June)**: 4.
561. Morris P. Fund raising for our College. *College of Anaesthetists Newsletter* 1990; **No 5 (October)**: 2.
562. Browne D R G. Editor. The College of Anaesthetists appeal. *College of Anaesthetists Newsletter* 1992; **No 10 (March)**: 5.

563. Browne D R G. Editor. Fund raising update. *Royal College of Anaesthetists Newsletter* 1992; **No 11 (June)**: 2.
564. Rubin A P. Fund raising activities. *Royal College of Anaesthetists Newsletter* 1994; **No 17 (March)**: 16-7.
565. Spence A. From the President. *College of Anaesthetists Newsletter* 1991; **No 8 (September)**: 1.
566. Spence A. From the President. *College of Anaesthetists Newsletter* 1991; **No 9 (December)**: 1
567. Spence A. From the President. *College of Anaesthetists Newsletter* 1992; **No 10 (March)**: 1-2.
568. Browne D R G. Editor. An account of the activities at the Royal College of Anaesthetists, August to October 1992. *Royal College of Anaesthetists Newsletter* 1992: **No 12 (December)**: 3-6.
569. *Annual Accounts for the Year Ending 31 March 1993*. London: Association of Anaesthetists of Great Britain and Ireland, 1993: 20.
570 Charlton J E. Editor. Loan to the Royal College of Anaesthetists repaid. *Association News* 1994; **No 85 (August)**: 1.
571. Horton J N. Editor. The College's finest year. *Anaesthesia News* 1992; **No 58 (May)**: 1
572. Browne D R G. Editor. American Board of Anesthesiology. Recognition of qualifications. *Royal College of Anaesthetists Newsletter* 1993; **No 15 (Special issue, October)**: 9.
573. Hume B. Service of thanksgiving and dedication. *Royal College of Anaesthetists Newsletter* 1993; **No 13 (March)**: 2.
574. Browne D R G. Editor. College News. *Royal College of Anaesthetists Newsletter* 1992; **No 10 (March)**: 15.
575. Bottomley V. Ceremony of the presentation of diplomates. *Royal College of Anaesthetists Newsletter* 1993; **No 13 (March)**: 3.
576. Spence A. From the President. *Royal College of Anaesthetists Newsletter* 1992; **No 12 (December)**: 1-2.
577. Spence A. From the President. *Royal College of Anaesthetists Newsletter* 1993; **No 13 (March)**: 1.
578. Atkinson R S. Editor. Staff profile. *Royal College of Anaesthetists Newsletter* 1991; **No 6 (February)**: 5.
579. Browne D R G. Editor. Sir Geoffrey de Deney, KCVO. *Royal College of Anaesthetists Newsletter* 1993; **No 14 (June)**: 2.
580. Charlton J E. Editor. Association gift to the College. *Anaesthesia News* 1993; **No 70 (May)**: 1-2.
581. Browne D R G. Editor. The North American Room. *Royal College of Anaesthetists Newsletter* 1993; **No 14 (June)**: 14-16.
582. Spence A. From the President. *Royal College of Anaesthetists Newsletter* 1993; **Special issue No 15 (October)**: 1.
583. Browne D R G. Editor. The visit to the Royal College of Anaesthetists by Her Majesty Queen Elizabeth II. *Royal College of Anaesthetists Newsletter* 1993; **Special issue No 15 (October)**: 2-8.
584. Browne D R G. Editor. The donation of the bust of John Snow. *Royal College of Anaesthetists Newsletter* 1993; **No 16 (December)**: 8.

585. Barry B. Years of fulfilment 1962-84. In: Wilson G, ed. *Fifty Years. The Australian Society of Anaesthetists 1934-1984*. Edgecliff, NSW: Australian Society of Anaesthetists, 1987: 427-75.
586. Browne D R G. Editor. News. *Royal College of Anaesthetists Newsletter* 1992; **No 11 (June)**: 13.
587. Scurr C. Editorial. Sir Ivan Whiteside Magill, KCVQ. *Anaesthesia* 1978; **33**: 577-8.
588. Edridge A W. Sir Ivan Whiteside Magill, KCVQ. *Anaesthesia* 1987; **42**: 231-3.
589. Boulton T B. Classical file. Sir Ivan Whiteside Magill, KCVO (1888-1986) and anaesthesia for thoracic surgery. *Survey of Anesthesiology* 1988; **32**: 387-98.
590. Hewer C L. Forty years on. Frederic Hewitt Lecture. *Anaesthesia* 1959; **14**: 311-30.
591. Boulton T B. Editorial. C. Langton Hewer. *Anaesthesia* 1986; **41**: 469-71.
592. Mushin W W. Editorial. Professor Emeritus Sir Robert Reynolds Macintosh. *Anaesthesia* 1989; **44**: 951.
593. Boulton T B. Professor Sir Robert Macintosh, 1897-1989. Personal reflections on a remarkable man and his career. *Regional Anaesthesia* 1993; **18**: 145-54.
594. Pallister W A. Editorial. Sir Geoffrey Stephen William Organe. *Anaesthesia* 1989; **44**: 461-2.
595. Lee J A, Lunn J N. Editorial. J. Alfred Lee. *Anaesthesia* 1989; **44**: 631.
596. Clarke R S J. Obituary. J W Dundee. *British Medical Journal* 1992; **304**: 710.
597. Gray C. Obituary. W W Mushin. *British Medical Journal* 1993; **306**: 851-2.
598. Lunn J N. Editorial. William Woolf Mushin. *Anaesthesia* 1993; **48**: 461-2.
599. Lumley J. Editorial. Arthur John Wells Beard. *Anaesthesia* 1993; **48**: 843-4.
600. Zorab J S M. Editorial. Philip John Helliwell. *Anaesthesia* 1994; **49**: 659-60.
601. Bennett P J. Obituary. Oswald Peter Dinnick. *British Medical Journal* 1995; **311**: 1566.
602. Department of Health. *Hospital Doctors. Training for the Future. The Report of a Working Group on Specialist Medical Training*. London: Department of Health, 1993.

Chapter 10 - Today, Yesterday and Tomorrow, 1 January 1993-30 June 1997

1. Charlton J E. *Anaesthesia News* 1996-1997; **Nos 111-119** (October 1996-June 1997).
2. Cook C, Editor. *Pears Cyclopaedia* 1996-1997. 105th edition. London: Penguin Books, 1996.
3. Booker C, North R. *The Castle of Lies. Why Britain Must Get Out of Europe*. London: Duckworth, 1996.
4. Lamont N, Aims of those who took UK into EEC. *The Times* 1997; **26 January**: 21.
5. Redwood J. Tuesday Review. Exposed: the arrogant builders of Europe. *The Daily Telegraph* 1996: **19 November**: 17.
6. Scott W. Anaesthesia in pregnancy. In: Scott W E, Vickers M D, Draper H. Editors. *Ethical Issues in Anaesthesia*. London: Edward Arnold, 1995.
7. Scott W E. Editorial. Ethics in obstetric anaesthesia. *Anaesthesia* 1996; **51**: 717-8.
8. Naftalin N J. Ethics in obstetric anaesthesia. *Anaesthesia* 1997; **52**: 181.
9. Dyson R. Rational resource allocation. Management perspectives. In : Pace N, McLean S A M. Editors. *Ethics and the Law in Intensive Care*. Oxford: University Press, 1996: 158-66.
10. Pace N. Withholding and withdrawing medical treatment In: Pace N, McLean S A M. Editors. *Ethics and the Law in Intensive Care*. Oxford: University Press, 1996: 47-67.

11. Beddell S E, Pelle D, Maher P L, Cleary P D. Do-Not-Resuscitate orders for the critically ill. How are they used and what is their impact? *Journal of the American Medical Association* 1986; **256**: 233-7.
12. McTurk L. Rational resource allocation. In: Pace N, McLean S A M. Editors. *Ethics and the Law in Intensive Care.* Oxford: University Press, 1996:167-78.
13. McLean S A M. Advance directives. Legal and ethical considerations. In: Pace N, McLean S A M. Editors. *Ethics and the Law in Intensive Care.* Oxford: University Press, 1996:68-83.
14. Cranford R. Misdiagnosing the persistent vegetative state. An apparently high rate of misdiagnosis demands critical review and action. *British Medical Journal* 1996; **313**: 5-6.
15. Tinker J, Brown D R G, Sibbald W J. Editors. *Critical Care. Standards, Audit and Ethics.* London: Arnold, 1996.
16. Gibson R. Euthanasia, withholding life prolonging treatment, and moral differences between killing and letting die. *Journal of Medical Ethics* 1988; **14**: 115-7.
17. Hoffenburg R, Chairman. Resuscitation from cardiopulmonary arrest. Training and organisation. A Report of the Royal College of Physicians. *Journal of the Royal College of Physicians of London* 1987; **21**: 175-82.
18. Walsh M. Euthanasia. In Scott W E, Vickers M D, Draper H. Editors. *Ethical Issues in Anaesthesia.* Oxford: Butterworth-Heinemann, 1994: 129-39.
19. Walton J N (Lord). Dilemmas of Life and Death: parts 1 and 2. *Journal of the Royal Society of Medicine* 1995; **88**: 311-15 and 372-6.
20. Twycross R G. Euthanasia: going Dutch. *Journal of the Royal Society of Medicine* 1996; **89**: 320-30.
21. Editorial. Managing a comfortable death. *Lancet* 1996; **347**:1777.
22. Zinn C. Second Australian dies under euthanasia act. *British Medical Journal*, 1997; **314**: 92.
23. Fergusson A. Euthanasia. An update. *Journal of the Christian Medical Fellowship* 1997; **43**: 7-12.
24. Urwin J L, Knapp M B. Medicolegal aspects of Critical care. In Tinker J, Browne D R G, Sibbald W J. Editors. *Critical Care Standards, Audit and Ethics.* London: Arnold, 1966: 367-90.
25. Roberts J, Kiellsband C. Jack Kevorkian: A medical hero. Rare heroism to make us all feel uncomfortable. *British Medical Journal* 1996; **312**: 1434.
26. Quill T E, Cassell C K, Meier D. Care of the hopelessly ill. Proposed clinical criteria for physician assisted suicide. *New England Journal of Medicine* 1992; **327**: 1380-3.
27. Brody H. Assisted death. A compassionate response to medical failure. *New England Journal of Medicine* 1992; **327**: 1384-8.
28. Quill T E. Death and dignity. A case of individual decision making. *New England Journal of Medicine* 1991; **324**: 691-6.
29. Dyer C. GMC tempers justice with mercy in Cox case. *British Medical Journal* 1992; **305**: 1311.
30. Saunders C. Into the valley of the shadow of death. *A personal therapeutic journey.* British Medical Journal 1996; **313**: 1599-1601.
31. Benrubi G I. Euthanasia. The need for procedural safeguards. *New England Journal of Medicine* 1992; **326**: 197-8.

32. Hopkin P M, Ellis F R. Inherited disease affecting anaesthesia. In: Healy T E J, Cohen P J. Editors. *Wylie and Churchill-Davidson's a Practice of Anaesthesia.* London: Edward Arnold, 1995.
33. Kingston H M. *ABC of Clinical Genetics.* London: British Medical Association, 1989.
34. Morgan P G, Sedensky M M. A review of molecular genetics for the anaesthetist. *European Journal of Anaesthesiology* 1995; **12**: 221-47.
35. Weatherall D. Genetics and medical practice. In: Walton J, Barondess J A, Lock S. Editors. *The Oxford Medical Companion.* Oxford: University Press, 1994: 313-20.
36. Lachmann P J. Molecular biology in medicine. In: Walton J, Barondess J A, Lock S. Editors. *The Oxford Medical Companion.* Oxford; University Press, 1994: 604-7.
37. Kemietowicz Z. Health put at risk by insurers' demands for gene test results. *British Medical Journal* 1997: **314**: 625.
38. Sikora K. First five years of gene therapy for cancer. *Lancet* 1994; **344**: 1631-2.
39. Walton J, Barondess J A, Lock S. Editors. Genetic engineering. *The Oxford Medical Companion.* Oxford: University Press, 1994: 312-3.
40. Crocker J, Burnett D, Lowe D, Smith R. The clinical promise of molecular pathology and the birth of a new BMJ journal. *British Medical Journal* 1994; **309**: 624.
41. Cherfas J. "Naked" genes trial for melanoma sufferers. *British Medical Journal* 1992; **304**: 1202.
42. Hawkes N. At war over the field of genes. *The Times* 1996; **9 September**: 21.
43. Warden J. MPs seek more control over genetics. *British Medical Journal* 1996; **312**: 1119.
44. Travis J. Reviving the antibiotic miracle? *Science* 1994; **264**: 260.
45. Neutt H C. The crisis in antibiotic resistance. *Science* 1992; **257**: 1064-72.
46. Cohen M L. Epidemiology of drug resistance. Implications for a post antimicrobial era. *Science* 1992; **257**: 1050-5.
47. Goldman D A, Weinstein R A, Wenzel R P, Tablan O C, Dunn R J, Gaynes R P, Schlasser J, Martone W J. Strategies to prevent and control the emergence and spread of antimicrobial-resistance micro-organisms in hospitals. A challenge to hospital leadership. *Journal of the American Medical Association* 1996; **275**: 234-40.
48. Cookson B. Is it time to stop searching for MRSA? Screening is still important. *British Medical Journal* 1997; **314**: 664-5.
49. Bloom B R, Murray J L. Tuberculosis. Commentary on a reemergent killer. *Science* 1992; **257**: 1055-63.
50. Fox R. The post-antibiotic era beckons. *Journal of the Royal Society of Medicine* 1966; **89**; 601-2.
51. Lyons S M (Chairman) *Stress in Anaesthetists.* London: Association of Anaesthetists of Great Britain and Ireland, 1997.
52. Ham C. Where now for NHS reform? Making them up as they go along. *British Medical Journal* 1994; **309**: 351-2.
53. Warden J. New high command for the NHS. *British Medical Journal* 1993; **307**: 1091.
54. Smith J. Public Health gets a boost in NHS streamlining. *British Medical Journal* 1994; **309**: 357-8.
55. Beecham L. BMA raises concerns about NHS restructuring. *British Medical Journal* 1995; **310**: 334.
56. Headlines. UK Government agrees to statutory advice. *British Medical Journal* 1995;

310: 484.
57. Sheard S. Gagging public health doctors. *British Medical Journal* 1994; **309**: 1643-4.
58. Court C. Trust audit highlights variations in performance. *British Medical Journal* 1994; **308**: 997-8.
59. LeGrand J. Internal market rules OK. New rules take account of market behaviour. *British Medical Journal* 1994; **309**: 1596-7.
60. Bury B. Letter to Mrs Bottomley. *British Medical Journal* 1993; **306**; 702-3.
61. Headlines. NHS trusts fail to meet targets. *British Medical Journal* 1994; **308**: 998.
62. Beecham L. Tories extend general practice fundholding. *British Medical Journal* 1994; **309**; 1039.
63. Ham C. The future of purchasing. Tolerance of diversity will be necessary. *British Medical Journal* 1994; **309**: 1023-3.
64. Ham C, Shapiro J. The future of fundholding. Voluntary for general practitioners, compulsory for health authorities. *British Medical Journal* 1995; **310**: 1150-1.
65. Court C. Report highlights wide variations in intensive care. *British Medical Journal* 1995; **310**: 420.
66. Rosen M (Chairman) *Intensive Care Services. Provision for the Future.* London: Association of Anaesthetists of Great Britain and Ireland, 1988.
67. Hawkes N. Call to replace NHS casualty units with "trauma centres". *The Times* 1997; **9 January**: 8.
68. Tibby S, Hatherill M, Marsh M J, Murdoch I A. Paediatric intensive care beds: the problem is distribution rather than numbers. *British Medical Journal* 1996; **312**: 773.
69. Levene M. Neonatal intensive care and the NHS reforms. *British Medical Journal* 1992; **304**: 1694
70. Wilson C O. Nurse shortage deprives children of intensive care. *The Sunday Telegraph* 1996; **14 January**: 13.
71. Bull A R. Crisis reaction to shortages should be replaced by analysis of strategic services. *British Medical Journal* 1995; **310**: 110.
72. Bell B A. Neurosurgical intensive care in the south east. *British Medical Journal* 1995; **310**: 111.
73. Earbender. Everyone needs good neighbours. *Today's Anaesthetist* 1996; **11**: 41 (quoting) *Hospital Doctor* 1996; **8 February**: 12.
74. Warden J. Emergency bed register announced. *British Medical Journal* 1996; **313**: 575.
75. Bion J. Rationing intensive care. Preventing critical illness is better and cheaper than cure. *British Medical Journal* 1995; **310**: 682-3.
76. Ryan D W. Providing Intensive care High dependency units and bed registers will help, but not without more resources. *British Medical Journal* 1996; **312**: 654.
77. Ryan D W, Bayly P J M, Weldon C G W, Jingree M. A prospective two-month audit of the lack of provision of a high-dependency unit and its impact on intensive care. *Anaesthesia* 1997; **52**: 265-75.
78. Atkinson R E. 21st Annual Linkman Conference. *Anaesthesia News* 1996; **No. 113 (October)**: 1-2.
79. Department of Health. *The Patients' Charter.* London: Her Majesty's Stationery Officer 1991.
80. Beecham L. Revised Patients' Charter promises shorter waiting times *British Medical*

Journal 1995; **310**: 264.
81. Herd B, Herd A, Mathers N. The wizard and the gatekeeper of castles and contracts. *British Medical Journal* 1995; **310**: 1042-4
82. Harrison S, Pollit C. *Controlling the Professionals.* Buckingham: Open University Press, 1994.
83. Ham C. How go the NHS reforms? Despite some progress they have done little to compensate for long term underfunding. *British Medical Journal* 1993; **306**: 77-8.
84. Beecham L. Doctors continue to report funding problems. *British Medical Journal* 1997; **314**: 232.
85. Boulton A. Nursing shortfall hits Britain. *British Medical Journal* 1996; **312**: 139.
86. Venning P, Rowland M. New opportunities in practice nursing. Roles matter more than titles. *British Medical Journal* 1995; **311**: 3.
87. Beecham L. Government initiates a £32M nursing campaign. *British Medical Journal* 1997; **314**: 448.
88. Salvage J. What's happening to nursing? The traditional division of labour between doctors and nurses is changing. *British Medical Journal* 1995; **311**: 274-5.
89. Wilson S. Report queries savings with doctor-nurse shift. *British Medical Journal* 1995; **311**: 280.
90. Fletcher D. Health service facing worst cash crisis for 20 years claims BMA. *The Daily Telegraph* 1996: **18 October**: 11.
91. Warden J. Labour fudge on fundholding. *British Medical Journal* 1997; **314**: 1067.
92. Warden J. Spot the difference? *British Medical Journal* 1997; **314**: 1068-9.
93. Court C. Labour unveils its health reforms. *British Medical Journal* 1995; **311**: 79.
94. Warden J. At last: a political division on the NHS. *British Medical Journal* 1996; **313**: 1506.
95. Warden J. Labour finds power is heaven on earth. *British Medical Journal* 1997; **314**: 1438.
96. Hall C. NHS change will take years, says Dobson. *The Daily Telegraph* 1997; **20 May**: 60.
97. Calman K (Chairman). *Hospital Doctors: Training for the Future. The Report of a Working Group on Specialist Medical Education.* London: Department of Health, 1993.
98. Middle article. Royal Commission on Medical Education. *British Medical Journal* 1968; **2**: 109-11.
99. Beecham L. Working Party on specialist training starts work. *British Medical Journal* 1992; **305**: 603.
100. Beecham L. Trying to satisfy EC directives on specialisation. *British Medical Journal* 1992; **305**: 332.
101. Hunter S, McLaren P. Specialist medical training and the Calman Report: deserves and requires imaginative professional and managerial support. *British Medical Journal* 1993; **306**: 1281-2.
102. Brahms D. EC directives and specialists. *Lancet* 1993; **341**: 1017-8.
103. Geddes S. Specialist training in anaesthesia. What does the future hold? *Anaesthesia News* 1993; **No 77 (December)**: 1-2.
104. Beecham Linda. Junior doctors want single tier specialist. *British Medical Journal* 1992; **304**: 1651-2.

105. Editorial. Calman. *Anaesthesia News* 1994; **No 84 (July)**: 1.
106. Vickers M D. Don't panic, don't panic, Mr Mainwaring. *Today's Anaesthetist* 1994; **9**: 103.
107. Prys-Roberts C. From the President. *Royal College of Anaesthetists Newsletter* 1995; **No 22 (May)**: 1.
108. MacDonald R G. The evolving role of the Postgraduate Dean. *Royal College of Anaesthetists Newsletter* 1994; **No 19 (October)**: 2-4.
109. Biggs J. Postgraduate medical education in the NHS. Increasing effort and impact through 25 years. *Health Trends* 1994; **26**: 5-7.
110. Council of the Association of Anaesthetists (President MacRae W R). *Doctors: Training for the Future (the Calman Report). Implications for Anaesthetists.* London: Association of Anaesthetists of Great Britain and Ireland, 1994.
111. Charlton J E (Editor). Calman. *Anaesthesia News* 1994; **84 (July)**: 1.
112. Bailey J. Rethinking Consultants. Time for a change in working practices. *British Medical Journal* 1995; **310**: 788-90.
113. Smith J. Consultants of the future. Need to acknowledge organisational goals and play to their strengths. *British Medical Journal* 1995; **310**: 953-4.
114. Spence A. From the President. *Royal College of Anaesthetists Newsletter* 1994; **No 17 (March)**: 1-2.
115. Scotland A. Consultant oligarchy or workers cooperative. *British Journal of Hospital Medicine* 1990: **44**: 152.
116. Roberts J. Specialists in the United States. What lessons? *British Medical Journal* 1995; **310**: 724.
117. Rees J. Where medical science and human behaviour meet. *British Medical Journal* 1995; **310**: 724.
118. MacDonald V. Shortage of consultants sparks crisis in hospitals. *The Sunday Telegraph* 1995; **29 October**: 3.
119. MacRae W R (Chairman of Committee). Manpower. *The Royal College of Anaesthetists Report and Accounts* 1995-1996: 13 and 20.
120. Hull C J. Is there a manpower crisis and if there is when will it end? *Royal College of Anaesthetists Newsletter* 1995; **No 25 (December)**: 2-3.
121. Vickers M D. What manpower crisis? *Today's Anaesthetist* 1995; **10**: 67.
122. Smith J. The year that manpower controls finally crumbled. *British Medical Journal* 1994; **308**: 80.
123. MacRae W R. Implementation of the Calman Report. *Anaesthesia News* 1994; **No 80 (March)**: 80.
124. Brearley S. Medical Manpower. *British Medical Journal* 1991; **303**: 1534-6.
125. Newell J P, Herwick M J. Selecting Specialist Registrars. An appointment process. *Royal College of Anaesthetists Newsletter* 1997; **No 34 (May)**: 8-9.
126. Healy T E J (Chairman). *Specialist Training in Anaesthesia Supervision and Assessment.* London: Royal College of Anaesthetists, 1994.
127. Biggs J. New arrangements for specialist training in Britain. Guidance notes for implementing the specialist registrar grade. *British Medical Journal* 1995; **311**: 1242-3.
128. Norman J. "A Guide to Specialist Registrar Training". A Commentary. *Royal College of Anaesthetists Newsletter* 1996; **No 26 (March)**: 2-4.

129. Prys-Roberts C. From the President. *Royal College of Anaesthetists Newsletter* 1994; **No 19 (October)**: 1.
130. Ellis F R (Chairman). *Specialist Training for Senior House Officers in Anaesthesia. A College Guide for the First Two Years.* London: Royal College of Anaesthetists, 1995.
131. Hall C J. Examination update. *Royal College of Anaesthetists Newsletter* 1995; **No 22 (May)**: 2.
132. Royal College of Anaesthetists. *Specialist Registrars in Anaesthesia. A Training Guide.* London: Royal College of Anaesthetists, 1996: 1-23.
133. Royal College of Anaesthetists. *Primary and Final Examinations for the FRCA. Regulations.* Royal College of Anaesthetists, 1995: 1-16.
134. Beecham L. Specialist Registrar grade will start on 1 December. *British Medical Journal* 1995; **311**: 1233.
135. Biggs J. New arrangements for specialist training in Britain. Guidance notes for implementing the Specialist Registrar grade. *British Medical Journal* 1995; **311**: 1242-3.
136. Prys-Roberts C. President's statement and review of the year. *Royal College of Anaesthetists Annual report and Accounts* 1995-1996.
137. Morris P (Chairman). *Working Party on Non-Consultant Career Grade Anaesthetists.* London: Association of Anaesthetists of Great Britain and Ireland, 1993.
138. Hayes T M. Continuing Medical education: a personal view *British Medical Journal* 1995; **310**: 994-6.
139. Charlton J E. Demise of the cognate point. *Anaesthesia News* 1995; **No 97 (August)**: 8.
140. Lyon S M. State of Play. *Anaesthesia News* 1997; **No 115 (February)**: 1-2.
141. Association of Anaesthetists of Great Britain and Ireland. Annual Report 1994-1995. *Anaesthesia* 1996; **51**:295-306.
142. Association of Anaesthetists of Great Britain and Ireland. Annual Report 1995-1996. *Anaesthesia* 1997; **52**: 815-29.
143. Association of Anaesthetists of Great Britain and Ireland. *Annual Report* 1996-1997.
144. Prys-Roberts C. President's statement and review of the year. *Report and Accounts 1995-1996.* London: Royal College of Anaesthetists, 1997.
145. Charlton J E (Editor). Skill mix. *Anaesthesia News* 1994; **No 85 (August)**: 3.
146. Lyon S M (Chairman). *Anaesthesia in Great Britain and Ireland. A Physician Only Service.* London: Association of Anaesthetists of Great Britain and Ireland, 1996.
147. Charlton J E (Editor). Nurse anaesthesia and anaesthetic staffing. *Anaesthesia News* 1996; **No 103 (February)**: 1.
148. Reilly C, Barrett A, Challands A, Read S. *Professional Roles in Anaesthetics: A Scoping Study.* London: NHS Executive, 1996.
149. Norman J. Professional roles in anaesthetics. A scoping study. Professor C Reilly, Mrs A Barrett, Mr A Challands and Dr S Read. *Newsletter of the Royal College of Anaesthetists* 1997; **No 33 (March)**: 11.
150. Lyons S M. Professional roles in anaesthetics. A scoping study. *Anaesthesia News* 1997; **No 118 (May)**: 3.
151. Association of Anaesthetists of Great Britain and Ireland. *Annual Report* 1997-1998.
152. Morgan M. Editorial. *Anaesthesia* 50th year of publication. *Anaesthesia* 1995; **50**: 1-2.
153. Boulton T B. Editorial. C Langton Hewer. *Anaesthesia* 1986; **41**: 469-471.
154. Charlton J E (Editor). *Anaesthesia News* 100th issue. *Anaesthesia News* 1995; **No 100**

(November): 1-12.
155. Barr A M (Editor). *The History of Anaesthesia Society Proceedings*; **Volume 20**. Maidenhead: Abbott Laboratories, 1997.
156. Norman J. Editorial. *Royal College of Anaesthetists Newsletter* 1997; **No 32 (January)**: 1.

APPENDIX A

Henry Walter Featherstone
1894-1967
First President of the Association of Anaesthetists of Great Britain and Ireland

by

E T Mathews, MB, ChB, FRCA
Consultant Anaesthetist, Birmingham General Hospital

Henry (Harry) Featherstone was born in Erdington on 5 April 1894; Erdington became part of Birmingham in 1912. His father was a general practitioner and alderman. His mother was the eldest daughter of a successful businessman from Brooklyn, USA. She opened the Erdington Laundry in 1898, unknowingly providing a generation of medical students with material for jokes about anaesthetists washing surgeons' dirty linen.

Childhood and Education

As a child he spent long summer holidays in Brittany living with a French family and learning the language. He visited this family throughout his life and described their friendship as "one of the joys of my life".

Henry was educated at King Edward's School, Birmingham, Trinity College, Cambridge, and the Birmingham Medical School. He qualified during the Great War 1914-1918.

Service in the Great War 1914-1918

Featherstone joined the Royal Army Medical Corps (RAMC) and saw some of the terrible aspects of the 1914-1918 war. He was first medical officer to the 7th battalion Kings Royal Rifle Corps who lost 500 of their original strength of 530; later in the war he spent Christmas 1917 in the Advanced Dressing Station at Passchendale, a place where in 21 days his unit lost half of its effective strength. Later still he was gassed. He always described the incident as "slight", but he was unable to see for a time. After three weeks in hospital in France he was evacuated to England. His brother, who was in the Royal Artillery, was killed. Henry spoke and wrote about these events, and he subsequently revisited the scenes of his experience and maintained friendships with other survivors.

Medical Career

Featherstone returned to Birmingham after the war and took up resident medical posts at the General Hospital. These included that of Resident Medical Officer, which was then the accepted route to the post of Consultant Physician. Such a post had been his father's ambition, but, encouraged by Dr W J McCardie, who was probably the first full time provincial anaesthetist,[1] Henry took up anaesthetics and was appointed Assistant Anaesthetist in 1919 and Honorary Anaesthetist in 1926. Henry Featherstone had great admiration for McCardie, whose professional status at one time was such that he was consulted before the surgeon was selected and received fees equal to those of the surgeon.

Featherstone's contributions to the literature included some 27 items in journals and chapters in four books. They covered a wide range of subjects. An early paper described a combined mask and airway and the Featherstone gag for oral surgery is still used. It has jaws lined with soft gun-metal. His paper on the pulmonary complications of anaesthesia was well received and this topic was also the subject of his MD thesis. He also had a special interest in explosive vapours, both in anaesthesia and in industry, and in this context he worked closely with the Chief of the Birmingham Fire Brigade.

He was introduced into the Section of Anaesthetics of the Royal Society of Medicine (RSM) by McCardie who had been its President in 1907. Featherstone himself became President in 1930. He was also Vice President of the British Medical Association subgroup on anaesthesia and played a leading part in the local medical societies of Birmingham. He was at one time President of the Birmingham Medical Institute and also the Editor of the *Birmingham Medical Review*.

The foundation of the Association of Anaesthetists of Great Britain and Ireland

Featherstone made several visits to the leading centres in Canada and the United States, sometimes with fellow members of the Royal Society of Medicine. He discussed with them, and other colleagues, his concern about the lowly status of anaesthesia and he believed that anaesthetists needed an independent organisation. Others agreed, but it was Featherstone who took action. Philip Helliwell has summarised what Featherstone did - "Featherstone of Birmingham must be given credit for firstly conceiving, and then providing the impetus and organising ability, which led to the formation of the Association of Anaesthetists of Great Britain and Ireland".[2] Featherstone was elected its first President 1932-35, and then held the office of Honorary Secretary 1936-1939. His description of these events was the first paper in the first number of the journal *Anaesthesia*,[3] which was first published in 1946.

Service in the Second World War 1939-1945

Featherstone was in the Territorial Army Reserve. He was already in uniform and away at camp as the Administrative Officer of 14th General Hospital, when war was declared. This unit was sent to France on 1 April 1940 with orders to set up a 1000 bed tented hospital at Etaples across the estuary from Le Touquet. Le Touquet still had its colony of English residents; they included P G Woodhouse, the humorous novelist, and his wife who gave the unit much assistance. Their gifts included a radio which became the unit's only source of information when the blitzkrieg began. The hospital made ready for casualties, but, on 21 May 1940, they were ordered to evacuate immediately.

The convoy was dive bombed on the road to Boulogne and Henry and his colleagues had to take to the ditches, but the unit held together. They boarded the *Queen of the Channel*, a London-Southend Ferry, which was one of the armada which came to the rescue. She took them safely to Dover but she was sunk a few days later. The defence of the jetty at Boulogne lasted a further 48 hours.

Back in England he had a variety of postings. When the Americans arrived he was attached to the United States Army as chief anaesthetist to a thousand bedded hospital. With his American background he enjoyed this posting, except that the final meal of the day was at 5.30 p.m. He was used to dining much later and hunger woke him early each morning. His early rising impressed the American team.

In preparation for the D-Day landings he was posted to teach airborne medical officers the use of chloroform, the only agent they were permitted to take with them.

His own role for the D-Day landings was in command of a hospital ship (*Hospital Carrier 64*). In peacetime she was the *Amsterdam*, on the Harwich to Hook of Holland route. He trained his teams thoroughly; they loaded and unloaded 300 Canadian sailors as mock casualties in simulated disasters. From D-Day onwards he worked from the Normandy landing beaches. The ship was anchored close inshore as Casualty Clearing Station for Juno Beach where there were many French Canadians and, consequently, his command of the language was useful. Featherstone's son landed on the adjacent Sword Beach and was badly wounded. At 7 am on 7 August 1944, whilst sailing from Juno Beach to Southampton, the *Amsterdam* was shaken by two almost simultaneous explosions. The ship broke in two, and sank in less than a quarter of an hour. The training which the unit personnel had received was such that everyone behaved as if on another exercise. Over 200 of the 260 patients were saved; what loss of life there was, was caused almost entirely by the explosions. There was no rescue ship about and no signal could be sent, but eventually a naval launch came along and a cruiser was called up to rescue them. Henry was awarded the OBE for this exploit. His next posting was to the hospital ship *Empire Clyde*, sailing between the Mediterranean ports and the UK but ill health caught up with him and he was boarded out on the day after VE Day.

The postwar years

Henry resumed his post at Birmingham General Hospital. He had been away almost six years, but he was still only 51 years of age and, while he was on active service, others had taken over many of the roles he had played at local, regional and national level. Much of his private practice had gone; so too had his seat on the Council of the Association, though he became a Trustee.

He was still an enthusiastic teacher of medical students in his hospital practice and, although he was the most senior consultant he would regularly anaesthetise for the minor operations list done by the house surgeon. He taught the history of anaesthesia and demonstrated the use of historical apparatus including Hewitt's nitrous oxide apparatus. He rarely used trichloroethylene; he objected to its cost because he knew that it was supplied, without waxoline blue, for dry cleaning at a fraction of the medical price. He spoke highly of its use in dry cleaning. Featherstone was contracted for four sessions when the National Health Service was introduced in 1948. He also continued his overseas visits and was invited to present papers at prestigious conferences in Boston and Montreal.

The Association of Anaesthetists awarded him the first John Snow Medal in 1946, and in 1947 he received the honorary degree of Doctor of Laws from Edinburgh University as part of the Simpson chloroform centenary commemoration, and he was elected an Honorary Fellow of the Faculty of Anaesthetists of the Royal College of Surgeons of England in 1962.

Commercial, social and domestic interests

Henry Featherstone took an active interest in the management of the Erdington Laundry, which with its subsidiaries had become the leading laundry and dry-cleaning business in the Midlands, and he had other commercial interests too.

He went to live on his 700 acre (280 hectare) family estate which was some 30 miles from Birmingham. He lived first at The Knoll, in Barton under Needwood, and later at Yoxall Lodge, Newchurch. Barton under Needwood is mentioned in Denis (WDA) Smith's book *Under the Influence*, in connection with the first use of nitrous oxide anaesthesia in England;[4] surely an appropriate place for an anaesthetist to live. The location was also appropriate to his interest in explosions; just to the north of his estate the largest explosion in Britain took place in 1944. Bombs stored in a gypsum mine exploded. It was a wartime secret that was well kept; 46 years later in November 1990 a memorial was erected.

The estate was in good hunting country. Henry was a brave horseman; on one occasion when he was thrown from his horse and dislocated his shoulder he devised a method of self-reduction using a five bar gate. The gate also enabled him to remount without assistance and continue the chase. Featherstone fought against ill health for many years - he had several heart attacks and some serious gastrointestinal bleeds, and he had to undergo several major operations. He gave the writer this valuable advice about postoperative fluids after one operation: the patient should have a case of half bottles of champagne in his room; a half bottle being a suitable size to share with a close friend in the early postoperative period and later a suitable amount to have with a meal; whereas if whole bottles are opened the wrong type of people come to the room!

Henry was proud of his membership of the Octette, a select Midland Group based on the old eighteenth century scientific Lunar Society.[4] He was a Magistrate, a Commissioner of Taxes, Chairman of the YMCA, and a Trustee of the William Salt Library which houses the major collection of historical material relating to Staffordshire.

He loved the countryside and endeavoured to improve it by planting more trees on his estate. A few weeks before his death in 1967 he and his wife invited a hundred friends to lunch and a walk in their woods. He is buried in the churchyard at Newchurch where there is a commemorative plaque in the church. It records that he was the Founder and First President of the Association of Anaesthetists of Great Britain and Ireland.

He was indeed a remarkable man, who played an important part in the development of the specialty; he lived in interesting times and places, and he was, as he once described himself, "a dutiful old soldier".

References

1. Thomas K Bryn. *The Development of Anaesthetic Apparatus.* Oxford: Blackwell, 1975: 256.
2. Helliwell P J. Editorial. *Anaesthesia* 1982; **37**: 394-97.
3. Featherstone H W. The Association of Anaesthetists of Great Britain and Ireland. Its Inception and its Purpose. *Anaesthesia* 1946; **1**: 5-9.
4. Smith W D A. *Under the Influence - A History of Nitrous Oxide and Oxygen Anaesthesia.* London: Macmillan, 1982.

APPENDIX B

The Arms of the Association of Anaesthetists of Great Britain and Ireland

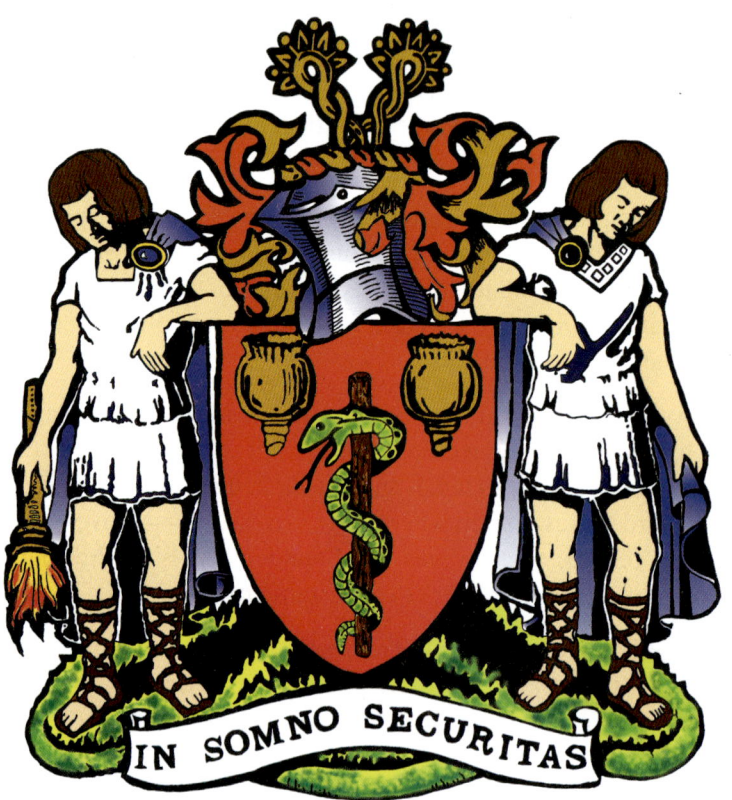

The grant of Arms of the Association of Anaesthetists

The grant of the right to bear heraldic arms by the Sovereign, acting through the College of Arms, is regarded in the United Kingdom as a significant step in the recognition in the status of a corporate body by the establishment. Any organisation or individual person can design and use a logo or register a trade mark, but the right to bear arms is an honour granted by the Monarch.[1-2]

The Association of Anaesthetists received its grant of arms at the behest of his late Majesty King George VI in Letters Patent. These were signed by the Garter Principal King of Arms and dated 12 February 1945 "in the 9th year of the King's reign". The imposing document now hangs in the Council Room of the Association of Anaesthetists at its headquarters at 9 Bedford Square, London.[2] The legal fees were donated by a benefactor, Mr Leslie Gamage (Chapter 5).

The Armorial Bearings of the Association of Anaesthetists

The shield or "escutcheon" is the primary component of a "coat of arms". It may be used alone, separately from the other elements which constitute the complete "achievement" of the arms, on documents or other items belonging to the organisation as a whole (for example as it is on the flag of the Association of Anaesthetists), or to its individual members (for example on cufflinks).

The escutcheon of the Association of Anaesthetists is "blazoned" (described) in heraldic terms as "gules a rod of Aesculapius proper, in chief two poppy heads or"; that is a shield with a red background with a rod of Aesculapius in its natural colours surmounted by two golden poppy heads.

It should be noted that the staff of Aesculapius (the god of healing) is correctly depicted as a single snake entwined round a rough staff cut from the branch of a tree, and not as the winged staff with two snakes (the caduceus) which is more correctly the emblem of the messenger god Mercury or Hermes (as depicted on the badge of the Royal Corps of Signals). This winged staff with two snakes is erroneously employed as a symbol of medicine by some medical organisations; although, the Royal Air Force has some excuse for using the winged staff for its medical branch![1,2]

The single snake Aesculapian staff on the Arms of the Association symbolises the status of British anaesthetists as physicians, which nowadays can be taken to include the functions of physician anaesthetists in the intensive care unit, in emergency medicine, and in the pain clinic.[1,2]

The two golden opium "poppy heads" or seed boxes represent morphia, one of the principal pain killing drugs used by the specialty of anaesthesia. The red ("gules") background or field is the traditional medical or surgical colour. Heraldic blazon makes no distinction of the shade of red but, in the British tradition, it is often painted as maroon or crimson on medical flags or coat of arms (as distinct from the scarlet of the military General Staff and the Guards regiments of the British Army). The flag of the Royal Army Medical Corps has horizontal, maroon, yellow and blue stripes, which are occasionally, rather irreverently, referred to as "blood, pus and cyanosis", conditions which are often sadly unavoidable in war.

The two golden poppy heads "in chief" on a red (or maroon) field have been incorporated into the escutcheon of the Royal College of Anaesthetists to signify the part which the Association of Anaesthetists played in its creation (Chapters 5, 8 and 9).[3,4]

The helmet allocated to the Association of Anaesthetists is that of an "esquire" or gentleman (it has a closed visor and is turned to one side). This is in accordance with the social and professional standing of physician anaesthetists.

The crest carried on the top of the helmet was originally intended as an additional means of identification of the wearer of the helmet in the heat of battle when the visor was closed. Sometimes the shield, or even the whole armorial achievement, is loosely referred to as "the crest" but this is not the correct usage of the term. The heraldic crest proper may, however, be used as a free standing device on its own (as is the crest consisting of the flowers of the herb Allheal of the Royal Society of Medicine on its ties). The Association crest has, however, not been used in this manner.

The crest of the Association of Anaesthetists consists of "two mandrakes in pile" (two mandrakes in the form of a wedge). This is a reminder that, in classical and medieval times, an extract of mandrake root was used as an anaesthetic and analgesic.

The mantling or lambrequin was originally a cloth cover to keep the sun off the helmet but, in heraldry it is often portrayed with symbolic and artistic licence. The colours of the lambrequin of the Association of Anaesthetists echo the predominant red and gold of the shield.

Supporters are normally reserved for Grants to peers in personal grants of arms; they are only granted to knights as a mark of special distinction, and hardly ever to individual esquires. Supporters are not granted to all institutions and, when they are, it is an additional honour.

The supporters of the shield of the Association of Anaesthetists are "on the dexter side" (that is on the right of the shield as held in front of the body) a representation of Somnus, the god of sleep, holding in his exterior hand a torch pointing downwards, and "on the sinister side" Morpheus, the son of Somnus, the god of pleasant dreams. These supporters can be regarded as representing effective, safe and pleasant anaesthesia. The reversed torch has been said to represent the diminished but surviving flame of life under general anaesthesia, as well as the educational functions of the Association of Anaesthetists.

It cannot be said that the supporters were well chosen by the College of Arms, or thoughtfully accepted by the 1945 Council of the Association. The symbolism is not obvious and the fact that both figures are depicted as asleep with heads bent has given rise to some embarrassment. Unkind detractors from other disciplines have described the two figures as sleeping, or even drunken, anaesthetists![1,3,5]

The motto was originally a battle cry, but nowadays, other than in the football stadium, it is normally a slogan of more peaceful import. The phrase *"in somno securitas"* was reasonably appropriate at the time that the grant of arms originated in 1945 when practically the only *raison d'etre* of British physician anaesthetists was the technical administration of general anaesthesia; even so it does not cover local anaesthetic techniques when the patient is awake but free from pain, nor, in the context of the present day, the activities of physician anaesthetists outside the operating theatre in intensive care, in pain management, or in emergency medicine.

Present day anaesthetists may also be concerned at the apparent equation of "sleep" with the very different state of pharmacological unconsciousness produced by general anaesthesia. Would not the much derided supporters be obstructed and cardiovascularly compromised if they were not asleep but anaesthetised in the upright position with flexed necks? Some knowledgeable scholars have even implied that the Latin of the motto might be translated to imply ambiguously that "all is well with the patient while the anaesthetist is peacefully asleep"! It may be that the Greek words *Katheudontas parateroumen* ("we watch closely those who sleep") which are used by the Canadian Society are rather more appropriate.[6]

Comment

These points made about the Arms of the Association of Anaesthetists were carefully taken into consideration when the design of the armorial bearings of the College of Anaesthetists was discussed with Heralds at the College of Arms in 1989.

The blazon of a coat of arms cannot be altered except by initiating an expensive new Grant from the Heralds at the College of Arms. Most individuals and organisations are content to accept and be proud of the historic arms as they were granted. Mr (later Professor) Peter Cull (Medical Artist at St Bartholomew's Hospital, London) redrew the coat of arms according to the original written blazon, when the Association of Anaesthetists was host to the 4th World Congress of Anaesthesiology in 1968 (Chapter 7). The new version was subsequently adopted for the cover of the journal *Anaesthesia* and for other publications of the Association of Anaesthetists.

References

1. Boulton T B. Arms and the Anaesthetist. A note from the Editor. *Anaesthesia* 1974; **29**: 627-8.
2. Boulton T B. The Arms of the Association of Anaesthetists of Great Britain and Ireland. *Anaesthesia News* 1991; **No 43 (February):** 2.
3. Boulton T B. The Armorial Bearings of the College of Anaesthetists. *College of Anaesthetists Newsletter 1990*; **No 4 (June):** 8-10.
4. *Anaesthesia News* 1991; **No 48 (July):** 2.
5. Thomas D V. Arms and the Anaesthetist. Un crie coeur. *Anaesthesia* 1974; **29**: 627.
6. Griffith HR. Obituary. Wesley Bourne. *Anaesthesia* 1965; **20**: 376-7.

APPENDIX C

Honours and Awards of the Association of Anaesthetists of Great Britain and Ireland

Honorary Members

Note: Honorary Membership is the Association of Anaesthetists oldest honour and dates from the Inaugural Meeting in 1932 (Chapter 3).

Honorary Members are nominated by the Officers and Council, and elected and admitted after a citation at an Annual General Meeting. Anaesthetists from the United Kingdom and Ireland have not normally been considered for Honorary Membership until after they retire. Honorary Members need not be anaesthetists or qualified in medicine.

1932

J F Silk

Honorary Anaesthetist to King's College Hospital, London Founder and President of the first Society of Anaesthetists in 1893.

R J Probyn-Williams
Honorary Anaesthetist to the London (now Royal London) Hospital.

C Carter Braine
Honorary Anaesthetist to Charing Cross Hospital, London.

R Gill
Honorary Anaesthetist to St Bartholomew's Hospital, London.

F H McMechan
Anaesthetist, New York, United States of America.
Founder of the National [USA] Anaesthesia Research Society 1919 (renamed the International Research Society in 1925). Founder Editor of *Current Researches in Anaesthesia* (1922-1949).

1936

The Right Honourable Viscount Nuffield, GBE, CH (William Morris).
Motor Manufacturer and Philanthropist.
Founder by endowment of the Nuffield Chair of Anaesthetics at the University of Oxford (1936).

R M Waters
Professor of Anaesthesia, Mayo Clinic, Rochester, Minnesota, USA. First Anaesthetist to be appointed as a Professor (1933-1949).
Hickman Medallist of the Royal Society of Medicine (1938).

1939

H E G Boyle, OBE
Honorary Anaesthetist, St Bartholomew's Hospital, London. Founder Member of Council (1932-1934).
One of the two original Examiners for the Diploma in Anaesthetics in 1935.

1942

Sir Francis Shipway, KCVO
Honorary Anaesthetist, Guy's Hospital, London.
Founder Member of Council (1932-1933) and Vice President (1935-1937).
Anaesthetist to several members of the Royal Family.

1943

H Bellamy Gardner
Honorary Anaesthetist, Charing Cross Hospital, London.

B C Leech
Professor of Anaesthesia, Regina, Saskatchewan, Canada.
Colonel Royal Canadian Army Medical Services.
Assistant Director of Medical Services, 2nd Canadian Division.

R M Tovell
Canadian born, Director of Anaesthetics, Hartford, Connecticut, USA.
Lieutenant Colonel, United States Army Medical Service. Adviser in Anaesthetics to the American Forces in Europe.

1945

Sir (later Lord) Alfred Webb-Johnson, Bt, KCVO, CBE, DSO.
Honorary Surgeon, The Middlesex Hospital, London.
President of the Royal College of Surgeons of England (1941-1949).
Supporter of the status of anaesthetists as consultants during the preparations for the British National Health Service and instigator of the inauguration of the Faculty of Anaesthetists of the Royal College of Surgeons of England (1948).

1953

H R Griffith
Professor of Anaesthesia, Montreal, Canada.
Pioneer of the use of curare in modern anaesthesia (1942).

1955

Wesley Bourne
Professor of Anaesthesia, McGill University, Canada.
First Hickman Medallist of the Royal Society of Medicine (1935). First Canadian Professor of Anaesthesia 1945.
The only expatriate to be President of the American Society of Anesthesiologists (1942).

1956

Ashley S Daly
Consultant Anaesthetist, the London (now Royal London) Hospital.
Founder Council Member (1932-35).
President of the Association of Anaesthetists (1941-1944).
Adviser in Anaesthesia to the British Army (Brigadier) 1939-1945.

Sir Ivan Magill, KCVO
Consultant Anaesthetist, Westminster Hospital, London.
Member of Council (1933-1948).
Pioneer of wide bore endotracheal anaesthesia.

1957

H W Featherstone, OBE
Honorary Anaesthetist, Birmingham (Appendix A).
Founder, First President and Honorary Secretary of the Association of Anaesthetists (1932-1942).

1959

John Gillies, MC, CVO
Consultant Anaesthetist, Edinburgh.
President of the Association of Anaesthetist (1947-1950).

Sir Robert Macintosh
Nuffield Professor of Anaesthetics Oxford (1937-1965).
First anaesthetist to be elected to an established University Chair in Anaesthetics.
Adviser in Anaesthetics to the Royal Air Force (Air Commodore) 1941-1945.
Member of Council of the Association of Anaesthetists 1944-1948 and 1953-1956.

A D Marston, CBE
Consultant Anaesthetist, Guy's Hospital, London.
Honorary Secretary and President Association of Anaesthetists (1941-1948).
First Dean of the Faculty of Anaesthetists (1948-1952).

1960

E S Rowbotham
Consultant Anaesthetist, Royal Free and Charing Cross Hospital, London.
Member of Council of the Association of Anaesthetists (1943-1944 and 1947-1950).
Pioneer of wide-bore endotracheal anaesthesia.

H J Shields
Professor of Anaesthesia, Toronto, Canada on the occasion of the 2nd World Congress of Anaesthesiologists in Toronto (1960).

1961

E Falkner Hill
Consultant Anaesthetist, Manchester.
Founder Council Member (1932-1934).
Editor, *British Journal of Anaesthesia* (1949-1962).

R J Minnitt
Consultant Anaesthetist, Liverpool
Founder Member (1932).
Member of Council (1941-1944).
Developer of Obstetric Analgesia with nitrous oxide and oxygen.

1962

G A Vandervell

A generous benefactor to the Research Funds of the Association of Anaesthetists.

1966

C Langton Hewer
Consultant Anaesthetist, St Bartholomew's Hospital, London. Editor of *Anaesthesia* 1946-1966.
Founder Member (1932).
Council Member and Vice President of the Association of Anaesthetists (1935-1936).

R Jarman, DSC
Consultant Anaesthetist, Royal Marsden (Cancer) Hospital, London.
President of the Association of Anaesthetists (1959-1962).
Founder Member (1932) and Member of Council (1943-1965).

1967

Katherine G Lloyd Williams, CBE
Consultant Anaesthetist and Dean of the Royal Free Medical School, London.
Council Member of the Association of Anaesthetists (1947-1950).

1968

Frankis T Evans
Consultant Anaesthetist, St Bartholomew's Hospital, London.
Dean of the Faculty of Anaesthetist (1955-1958).
Founder Member (1932) and Council Member of the Association of Anaesthetists (1938-1945).

M D Nosworthy
Consultant Anaesthetist, St Thomas Hospital, London.
Member of Council of the Association of Anaesthetist (1937-1938).
Pioneer of thoracic anaesthesia.

1969

Vernon F Hall, CBE, CVO
Consultant Anaesthetist, King's College Hospital, London.
President of the Association of Anaesthetists (1962-1965).
Member of Council, Honorary Treasurer and Vice President (1942-1945, 1948-1951 and 1955-1968).

1971

H H (Tony) Pinkerton
Consultant Anaesthetist, Glasgow.
President of the Association of Anaesthetists (1965-1967).
Member of Council and Vice President (1949-1952 and 1960-1969).

1972

T P Ayre
Consultant Paediatric Anaesthetist, Newcastle upon Tyne.

H J V Morton
Consultant Anaesthetist, Hillingdon.
Honorary Treasurer and Vice President of the Association of Anaesthetists (1960-1969).
Member of Council (1951-1954 and 1959-1969).

R P W Shackleton, CBE
Consultant Anaesthetist, Southampton.
President of the Association of Anaesthetists (1968-1970).
Member of Council, Honorary Secretary and Vice President (1949-1958 and 1960-1971).
First Regional Postgraduate Dean of Southampton Medical School.

1973

C J Massey Dawkins
Consultant Anaesthetist, University College Hospital, London.
Pioneer of Epidural Anaesthesia.

1974

A John W Beard
Consultant Anaesthetist, Royal Postgraduate Medical School (London) and General Practitioner.
President of the Association of Anaesthetists (1969-1971).
Member of Council, Honorary Secretary and Vice President (1953-1963 and 1966-1973).
Possibly the last Consultant Anaesthetist to continue to practice as a General Practitioner.

Sir Geoffrey Organe, CBE
Professor of Anaesthesia, University of London.
Consultant Anaesthetist, Westminster Hospital, London.
President of the Association of Anaesthetists (1953-1956).

Member of Council, Honorary Secretary and Vice President (1947-1959).
President of the World Federation of Societies of Anaesthesiology (1964-1968).
Dean of the Faculty of Anaesthetists (1958-1961).

1975

W W Mushin, CBE
Head of the Department of Anaesthetics, Cardiff (1947-1975).
First Professor of Anaesthetics, University of Wales (1953).
Member of Council and Vice President of the Association of Anaesthetists (1952-1959).
Dean of the Faculty of Anaesthetics (1961-1964).
Holder of numerous University and Government Advisory posts.

K F Stephens, CB, OBE
Major General, Army Medical Services.
Commandant Royal Army Medical College.
Army Advisor in Anaesthetics and Coopted Council Member (1961-1963).

1976

S Cullen
Professor, San Francisco, USA.

F F F Foldes
Professor of Anaesthesia, New York, USA.

T J Gilmartin
First Professor of Anaesthesia, Royal College of Surgeons in Ireland.
First Dean of the Irish Faculty of Anaesthetists (1960-1963).
Member of Council and Vice President of the Association of Anaesthetists (1958-1961, 1964-1967 and 1973-1975).

T Gordh
Professor of Anaesthesia, Stockholm, Sweden.

J Alfred Lee
Consultant Anaesthetist, Southend-on-Sea.
President of the Association of Anaesthetists (1971-1973).
Member of Council of the Association of Anaesthetists (1959-1962).

E M Papper
Professor of Anaesthesia, New York, USA.

1977

J J Bonica
Professor of Anaesthesia, Seattle, USA.

A C Forrester
First Professor of Anaesthesia, University of Glasgow.
Member of Council of the Association of Anaesthetists (1957-1960).

T Cecil Gray, CBE, KCSG, OSTJ
Professor of Anaesthesia, Liverpool.
President of the Association of Anaesthetists (1956-1959).
Member of Council, Honorary Treasurer and Vice President (1948-1962).
Dean of the Medical School of Liverpool University.
Dean of the Faculty of Anaesthetists (1964-1967).

J Lassner
Professor of Anaesthesia, Paris, France. First President of the European Academy of Anaesthesiology (1977).

1978

John Lundy
Professor of Anaesthesia, Mayo Clinic, Rochester, USA.
Pioneer of intravenous barbiturate anaesthesia.

Pritam Singh
Professor of Anaesthesia, Amritsar, India.

1979

P J Helliwell
Consultant Anaesthetist, and last Superintendent of Guy's Hospital, London (1967-1974).
President of the Association of Anaesthetists (1973-1976).
Member of Council, Honorary Secretary and Vice President (1951-1979).

1980

Rudolph Frey
Professor of Anaesthesia, Mainz, Germany.

Victor A Goldman
Consultant Anaesthetist, Eastman Dental Hospital, London.

A R Hunter
Professor of Anaesthesia, Manchester.
Council Member of the Association of Anaesthetists (1957-1960). Vice Dean of the Faculty of Anaesthetists (1968-1970).

M T Jenkins
Professor of Anaesthesia, Dallas, Texas, USA.

Sir William Paton, CBE, FRS.
Professor of Pharmacology, University of Oxford.
Adviser to the journal *Anaesthesia* (1966-1983).

1981

E Warburton
Financial Adviser to the Association of Anaesthetists (1974-1992). Chief Finance Officer, Guy's Hospital, London.

F G Wood-Smith
Consultant Anaesthetist, Royal Postgraduate Medical School, London.
Member of the Council of the Association of Anaesthetists (1957-1960).

1982

George Edwards
Consultant Anaesthetist, St George's Hospital, London.
First John Snow Lecturer (1958).
Member of Council of the Association of Anaesthetists (1945-1949).

Q J Gomez
Professor of Anaesthesia, Manila, Philippines.
President of the World Federation of Societies of Anaesthesiologists (1980-1984).

1983

H Lehmann
Professor of Biochemistry, University of Cambridge.
Adviser to the journal *Anaesthesia* (1974-1983).

Stanley A Mason
Consultant Anaesthetist, King's College Hospital, London.
President of the Association of Anaesthetists (1978-1980).
Member of Council and Honorary Treasurer (1969-1982).

Doreen Vermeulen-Cranch, CBE
Professor of Anaesthesia, Amsterdam, Holland. British born.

1984

W D Wylie
Consultant Anaesthetist and Dean of the Medical School, St Thomas' Hospital, London.
President of the Association of Anaesthetists (1980-1982).
Member of Council (1956-1959 and 1980-1984).

1985

G Jackson Rees
Consultant Anaesthetist, Alder Hey Children's Hospital, Liverpool.

1986

O P Dinnick
Consultant Anaesthetist, The Middlesex Hospital, London.
Member of Council, Honorary Secretary and Vice President (1961-1968 and 1973-1975).

D D C Howat
Consultant Anaesthetist, St George's Hospital, London.
Council Member, Honorary Treasurer and Vice President of the Association of Anaesthetists (1964-1967 and 1969-1981).
Vice Dean of the Faculty of Anaesthetists (1979-1981).

Sir Gordon Robson, CBE
Professor of Anaesthesia, Royal Postgraduate Medical School, London.
Dean of the Faculty of Anaesthetists (1973-1976).
Consultant Adviser to the Department of Health.

C F Scurr, CBE, LVO
Consultant Anaesthetist, Westminster Hospital, London.
President of the Association of Anaesthetists (1976-1978).
Member of Council (1956-1965 and 1973-1980).

1987

Sir Cecil Montacute Clothier, KCB, QC
Parliamentary Commissioner for Administration.
John Snow Lecturer (1982), and Chairman of the Association of Anaesthetists Appeal 1983-1984.

M H Holmdahl
Professor of Anaesthesia and Rector, University of Uppsala, Sweden.

K Rawnsley, CBE
Professor of Psychological Medicine, Welsh National School of Medicine.
Collaborator with the Association of Anaesthetists in establishing the "Help for the Sick Doctor" scheme 1978.

1988

Aileen K Adams, CBE
Consultant Anaesthetist, Cambridge.
Honorary Secretary of the Association of Anaesthetists (1969-1971).
Member of Council (1966-1973).
Dean of the Faculty of Anaesthetists (1985-1988).

J W Dundee, OBE
Professor of Anaesthetics, Queens University, Belfast.
Dean of the Irish Faculty of Anaesthetists (1971-1972).

The Right Honourable Lord Smith of Marlow, KBE
Consultant Surgeon to St George's Hospital, London.
President of the Royal College of Surgeons of England (1973-1977).

1989

M P Coplans
Consultant Anaesthetist, St George's Hospital, London.
Honorary Secretary of the Association of Anaesthetists (1970-1972).
Joint Secretary of the Association Fund Raising Committee (1983-1984).

M W Johnstone
Consultant Anaesthetist, Manchester.
Pioneer in the use of halothane in anaesthesia 1956.

Professor Carlos Parsloe
Sao Paulo, Brazil. President of the World Federation of Societies of Anaesthesiologists 1984-1988.

J P Payne
British Oxygen Professor of Anaesthesia, Royal College of Surgeons of England (1963-1987).
Vice President of the Association of Anaesthetists (1984-1986).

1990

T B Boulton, OBE
Consultant Anaesthetist, Oxford and Reading.
President of the Association of Anaesthetists (1984-1986).
Editor of *Anaesthesia* (1973-1982).
Member of Council and Vice President (1973-1988).

R J Maxwell, CBE
Secretary and Chief Executive, King Edward's Hospital Fund for London.

O K Mayrhofer
Professor of Anaesthesia, Vienna, Austria.
President of the World Federation of Societies of Anaesthesiology (1972-1978).

H Ruben
Professor of Anaesthesia, Copenhagen.
Pioneer in modern respiratory resuscitation and an inventive genius.

1991

M M Burrows
Consultant Anaesthetist, Wirral, Merseyside.
President of the Association of Anaesthetists (1988-1990).
Member of Council, Honorary Treasurer and Vice President (1978-1991).
Chairman and Member of important Government and British Medical Association Committees.

D A Chamberlain, CBE, KCSG
Consultant Cardiologist, Brighton.
President of the British Cardiac Society (1991-1992).

W W Mapleson
Professor of the Physics of Anaesthesia, University of Wales.

J F Nunn
Director of Anaesthesia, Medical Research Council, Medical Research Centre, Harrow.
Member of Council of the Association of Anaesthetists (1973-1976) and Vice President (1988-1990).
Dean of the Faculty of Anaesthetists (1979-1982).

1992

R S Atkinson, OBE
Consultant Anaesthetist, Southend-on-Sea.
Council Member of the Association of Anaesthetists (1979-1982) and Vice President (1987-1989).
Vice Dean of the Faculty of Anaesthetists.

Sir Keith Sykes
Nuffield Professor of Anaesthetics, University of Oxford (1980-1991).
Adviser in Anaesthesia to the Department of Health.
Vice President of the Association of Anaesthetists (1990-1992).

Ann Muir
Administrative Secretary, Association of Anaesthetists (1973-1992).

1993

Sir Donald Campbell, CBE
Professor of Anaesthetics, University of Glasgow.
Member of Council of the Association of Anaesthetists (1974), Vice President (1974-1980).
Dean of the Faculty of Anaesthetists (1982-1985).
President of the Royal College of Physicians and Surgeons of Glasgow (1992-1994).

A Doughty
Consultant Anaesthetist, Kingston-upon-Thames.
Pioneer in the use of epidural analgesia for obstetrics.
President of the Obstetric Anaesthetists Association Fellow *ab eundemn* of the Royal College of Obstetricians and Gynaecologists.

M Rosen, CBE
Consultant Anaesthetist and Honorary Professor of Anaesthesia, University Hospital of Wales.
President of the Association of Anaesthetists (1986-1988).
Member of Council, Honorary Secretary and Honorary Treasurer and Vice President (1972-1988).
Dean of the Faculty of Anaesthetists and First President of the (now Royal) College of Anaesthetists (1988-1990).
President of the Obstetric Anaesthetists Association.
Fellow *ab eundem* of the Royal College of Obstetricians and Gynaecologists.

Barbara M Q Weaver
Reader in Veterinary Anaesthesia, Bristol University.
President of the Association of Veterinary Anaesthetists.

1994

R S J Clarke
Professor of Anaesthesia, Queens University, Belfast.
Dean of the Faculty of Anaesthetists of the Royal College of Surgeons in Ireland (1991-1994).

J N Lunn
Reader in Anaesthetics, University of Wales.
Member of Council, Editor of *Anaesthesia* and Vice President of the Association of Anaesthetists (1982-1993).

M E Tunstall
Consultant Anaesthetist and Senior Lecturer, University of Aberdeen.
Member of Council of the Association of Anaesthetists (1978-1981).
President of the Obstetric Anaesthetists Association.
Pioneer in the use of premixed nitrous oxide and oxygen in obstetric analgesia.

1995

P Morris
Consultant Anaesthetist, Manchester.
Member of Council, Honorary Secretary and Vice President of the Association of Anaesthetists (1982-1991).
Vice President of the Royal College of Anaesthetists (1993-1995).
President of the Association of Paediatric Anaesthetists.

1996

M D A Vickers
Professor of Anaesthetics, University of Wales.
President of the Association of Anaesthetists (1982-1984).
Member of Council, Honorary Secretary and Vice President (1968-1986).
Elected President of the World Federation of Societies of Anaesthesiologists 1996.

Jean Horton
Consultant Anaesthetist, Cambridge.
Member of Council, Honorary Secretary and Vice President of the Association of Anaesthetists (1976-1987).

W S Wren
Consultant Anaesthetist, Dublin.
Member of Council and Vice President of the Association of Anaesthetists (1971-1978).

Dean of the Faculty of Anaesthetists of the Royal College of Anaesthetists in Ireland (1973-1976).

J S M Zorab
Consultant Anaesthetist, Bristol.
Member of Council, Honorary Secretary and Vice President of the Association of Anaesthetists (1968-1981).
President of the World Federation of Societies of Anaesthesiologists (1988-1992).

1997

W R MacRae
Consultant Anaesthetist, Edinburgh Royal Infirmary.
President of the Association of Anaesthetists 1992-1994.
Member of Council, Honorary Secretary, Vice President and Honorary Treasurer 1979-1998.

Margaret Branthwaite.
Barrister.
Consultant Anaesthetist and Physician, Royal Brompton Hospital 1969-1993.
John Snow Lecturer 1996.

1998

P J F Baskett
Consultant Anaesthetist, Bristol Royal Infirmary and Frenchay Hospital.
President of the Association of Anaesthetists 1990-1992.
Council Member, Honorary Secretary and Vice President 1976-1993.

J Cooper
Consultant Anaesthetist, Belfast.
Dean of the Faculty of Anaesthetists of the Royal College of Surgeons in Ireland.

P D Wall
Professor of Anatomy, University College London.
John Snow Lecturer 1993.

The Sir Ivan Magill Gold Medal

The Sir Ivan Magill Gold Medal "for innovation" was instituted in 1988 to commemorate the centenary of the birth of the pioneer anaesthetist Sir Ivan Magill, KCVO, who had died in his ninety eighth year in 1986. It is awarded for uniquely outstanding innovative contributions to the specialty of anaesthesia. It has been awarded three times between 1988 and 1998. The three recipients have certainly made unique innovations to the specialty in outstanding, but none-the-less interestingly different ways. The Medal is cast in gold. The obverse bears the relief portrait of Sir Ivan Magill. The name and date of the recipient is on the reverse and there is a bar on the ribbon bearing the inscription "For Innovation".

Candidates for the award of the Magill Gold Medal are nominated by Council and elected and presented with their award after a citation at an Annual General Meeting.

1988

John Francis Nunn (Head of the Division of Anaesthesia of the Medical Research Council, Research Centre, Harrow 1968-1991) has indisputably made unique contributions to the study of respiratory physiology and in particular, though not exclusively, to its application to the basic principles which underlie the practice of clinical anaesthesia. He has in addition been an innovative clinician and an able departmental and natural administrator (Chapter 7 and the above list of Honorary Members for 1991).

1993

Michael Rosen, CBE (Consultant and Honorary Professor, University of Wales) led the British specialty through the period which immediately preceded and finally achieved the establishment of the Royal College of Anaesthetists. He presided successively with single minded dedication and perseverance over the Association of Anaesthetists of Great Britain and Ireland (President 1986-1988), the Faculty of Anaesthetists of the Royal College of Surgeons of England (Dean 1988), and the (now Royal) College of Anaesthetists both before and after it achieved independence from the Royal College of Surgeons of England (President 1988-1991). See Chapters 8 and 9 and the above list of Honorary Members for 1993.

1995

Archibald Ian Jeremy Brain (Consultant Anaesthetist, Newham General Hospital, London 1983-1990 and later Honorary Consultant, Newham, Norwich Park, Harrow and the Royal Berkshire Hospital, Reading) is the inventor and developer of the laryngeal mask which revolutionised the delivery of inhalation anaesthesia and emergency air-way management with amazing rapidity in the United Kingdom and many other countries since its commercial release in 1989 (Chapter 9).

The John Snow Silver Medal

The John Snow Medal was cast in bronze from its introduction in 1946 until 1967 (Chapter 5) since when a silver medal has been presented. The change was made when a similar bronze medal for the John Snow Lecturer was introduced (Chapter 7). The John Snow Medal is cast in sterling silver and bears the arms of the Association on the obverse and the name of the recipient and the date on the reverse.

The medal has an interesting history. The medal originated after Professor (Sir) Robert Macintosh proposed to Council on 6 December 1945 that the three anaesthetist members of the armed forces who had been decorated for distinguished conduct during the Second World War (1939-1945) should be elected to Honorary Membership (or "Fellowship" as it was then designated). This was considered inappropriate but that "some other form of recognition should be explored". It was subsequently decided that a (bronze) medal should be struck and the medals were awarded "amidst great enthusiasm" to the three gallant recipients at the 1946 Annual General Meeting in October 1946 (Chapter 5).

The Council Minutes do not define the criteria laid down for future awards of the medal, and the 1946 Annual Report indicates simply that it had been "decided to establish the John Snow Medal to be awarded to anaesthetists for distinguished services", but implies that the awards to the three original recipients were not intended to be unique. Zebulon Mennell (President and Honorary Treasurer), who had been on Council since the foundation of the Association of Anaesthetists in 1932 and had looked after civilian anaesthesia so well during the Second World War (1939-1945), received the fourth John Snow Medal in 1947. No more awards were made until 1958 when four senior anaesthetists were honoured; three medals were awarded in the sixties and three in the seventies. An annual routine review of possible candidates for Association honours was instituted in the early eighties; eight medals were awarded in the eighties and six between 1990 and 1998; of the 29 recipients all have been from Great Britain and Ireland, 23 (including two of the original medallists) were Executive Officers of the Association of Anaesthetists, all except two had been members of Council at one time or another, and all except three were also elected to Honorary Membership.

Candidates for the award of the John Snow Medal are anaesthetists who are deemed to have made a major contribution to anaesthesia, particularly as Executive Officers of the Association but also outstandingly to the specialty in general. The nominations for the awards (usually nowadays at or after retirement from clinical practice) are made by Council and confirmed and presented at an Annual General Meeting.

*See also notes in the list of Honorary Members.

1946

*H W Featherstone, OBE
Lieutenant Colonel RAMC: President 1932-1935.

E A Pask, OBE
Squadron Leader RAF: Honorary Treasurer 1960-1966.

L G Morrison, MC
Major RAMC: Consultant Anaesthetist, Edinburgh.

1947

Z Mennell
President and Honorary Treasurer 1932-1947.

1958

*J Gillies, CVO, MC
President 1947-1950.

1966

*C Langton Hewer
Editor of *Anaesthesia* 1946-1966.

Appendix C: Honours and Awards of the AAGBI 733

1967

*Sir Robert Macintosh
Honorary Member.

*M D Nosworthy
St Thomas', Pioneer thoracic anaesthetist.

1969

*R Jarman, DFC
President 1959-1963.

1970

*R P Shackleton, CBE
President 1967-1969.

1972

*Sir Geoffrey Organe, CBE
President 1953-1956.

1974

*W W Mushin, CBE
Professor, University of Wales.

1982

*T Cecil Gray, KCSG, CBE
President 1956-1959.

1984

*C F Scurr, CBE, LVO
President 1976-1978.

1985

*T J Gilmartin
Professor, Dublin. Vice President of the Association of Anaesthetists 1973-1975.

1986

*Sir Gordon Robson, CBE
Professor, Royal Postgraduate Medical School.

1987

*P J Helliwell
President 1973-1976.

1988

*W D Wylie
President 1980-1982.

1992

*G Jackson Rees
Paediatric Anaesthetist, Liverpool.

*Sir Keith Sykes
Nuffield Professor of Anaesthesia, Oxford 1980-1991.

*J S M Zorab
Secretary General, World Federation of Societies of Anaesthesia.

1994

*T B Boulton, OBE
President 1984-1986.

*J N Lunn
Editor of *Anaesthesia* 1982-1991.

1996

*M D A Vickers
President 1982-1984.

1997

*W R MacRae
President 1992-1994.

1998

*P J F Baskett
President 1990-1992.

The Pask Certificate of Honour

The institution of the Pask award of honour arose out of the desire of Council to honour the gallantry of a Registrar Anaesthetist at the Moorgate Underground

Railway disaster in 1975. It was acknowledged that by custom the award of the John Snow Silver Medal had become unsuitable for the purpose (see the above section). Council, however, decided to institute an award with wider and more flexible terms of reference "to honour those who have rendered distinguished service, either with gallantry in the performance of their clinical duties, to the specialty of anaesthesia as a whole or to the Association itself, either in a single meritorious act, or consistently and faithfully over a long period" (Chapter 8).

The award is named after Professor E A Pask, OBE (1912-1966). Pask had a distinguished career in the Royal Air Force Medical Branch as an experimental physiologist in the Second World War (1939-1945). This included dangerous self experimentation requiring considerable personal courage. He then became the first Professor of Anaesthetics at Newcastle upon Tyne (*Anaesthesia* 1977; **32**: 843-5)

The Pask Certificate of Honour was designed by (Professor) Peter Cull, Medical Artist at St Bartholomew's Hospital, London. Peter Cull was himself awarded a Pask Certificate in 1986.

The award is made by resolution of the Council of the Association of Anaesthetists. It can therefore be made at any time in the year independently of the Annual General Meeting of the Association of Anaesthetists as a whole. It has, however become customary to present the Certificate at Annual General Meetings whenever possible.

An asterisk* indicates a professional anaesthetist. Locations listed are in the United Kingdom unless otherwise stated.

1977

Mrs Muriel Pask
Widow of the late Professor Edgar Alexander Pask, OBE, MD, FFARCS, in recognition of the outstanding services to anaesthesia of her late husband.

*P M Finch
St Bartholomew's Hospital, London, in recognition of his gallantry in the performance of his clinical duties at Moorgate on 28 February 1975.

*R Bryce-Smith
Oxford, in recognition of his distinguished service as Editor of *Anaesthesia*.

*O P Dinnick
Middlesex Hospital, London, former Honorary Secretary in recognition of his distinguished services to the Association of Anaesthetists of Great Britain and Ireland over many years.

*G H Ellis
St Bartholomew's Hospital, London, in recognition of his distinguished service to anaesthesia as Chairman of the Organising Committee of the 4th World Congress of Anaesthesiologists in London in 1968.

*E Jacobson
Denmark, in recognition of the hospitality of the Dansk Anaesthesiologisk Selskab to the Association under his Presidency, Copenhagen, June 1976.

Professor W W Mapleson
University of Wales, in recognition of his outstanding contribution to research on the physics of anaesthesia.

1978

*M P Coplans
St George's Hospital, London, in recognition of his distinguished services to the Association of Anaesthetists of Great Britain and Ireland over many years.

*B Haxholdt
Denmark, at the Joint Meeting with the Danish Society in London. President of the Dansk Anaesthesiologisk Selskab.

*Z Lett
Hong Kong, in recognition of his distinguished services to anaesthesia in Hong Kong.

*Karl H Weis
Federal German Republic, in recognition of the Joint Meeting with the German Society in London on 29 November to 1 December 1978.

1979

*Professor F N Prior
Ludhiana, in recognition of his work at The Christian Medical College, Ludhiana, Punjab, India over many years.

*K B Pinson,
Manchester, in recognition of his pioneer work in the design of ventilators and vaporisers.

*Professor J D Robertson, Edinburgh in recognition of his services to international anaesthesia.

R H Salt
Oxford, Chief Anaesthetic Technician, in recognition of his services to anaesthesia over many years as chief anaesthetic technician in Oxford.

*A Tindal
Glasgow,. in .recognition of his pioneer .work in hyperbaric. medicine.

1980

E K Hillard
Cardiff, Chief Anaesthetic Technician, in recognition of his distinguished service to anaesthesia through the Society of Anaesthetic Laboratory Technicians.

*J Moyers
United States, in recognition of his outstanding contribution to the Association's Anglo-American Meeting held in London in 1980.

1981

*J S Inkster
Newcastle upon Tyne, for distinguished service to paediatric anaesthesia and long service to the Association.

*M W Johnstone
Manchester, for his contribution to the introduction of halothane into clinical anaesthesia.

*P P Papworth
Kenya, for his contribution as anaesthetist to the Flying Doctor Service in Kenya.

1982

*D V Bateman
Epping, in appreciation of his long and distinguished service as Honorary Proof Reader of *Anaesthesia*.

*F F Waddy
Northampton, a Founder Member of the Association of Anaesthetists, and innovator of the concept of recovery wards.

1983

Pask Certificate of Honour awarded to the Defence Medical Services of the United Kingdom, in recognition of the services of anaesthetists in the Falklands Island Campaign 1982:

Lieutenant Colonel J Anderson, *Surgeon Lieutenant Commander D J Baker, *Major A K Banerjee, *Surgeon Commander P T Bull, *Surgeon Lieutenant Commander I F Geraghty, MBE, *Major M Jowitt, *Lieutenant Colonel R J Knight, *Surgeon Commander S B Merrill, *Surgeon Commander R A Moody, *Surgeon Lieutenant S J Squires, *Surgeon Lieutenant G J Stoot, *Surgeon Lieutenant S Q M Tighe, Surgeon Lieutenant Commander A Yates and Captain R Wagon.

1984

*Patricia Coyle
Australia, for services to anaesthesia in Uganda and elsewhere.

*H Grant-Whyte
South Africa, for services to anaesthesia in South Africa and internationally.

*W D A Smith, OBE
Leeds, for his contribution to research into nitrous oxide anaesthesia and the history of anaesthesia.

1985

*W M Brown
Belfast, for contribution to anaesthesia in Northern Ireland.

*Margaret L Heath
Lewisham, for her contribution to the work of the Association for many years.

C G Jones
Chief Anaesthetic Technician, East Grinstead, for his contribution to anaesthesia in peace and war.

*D F Kettler
German Federal Republic, President of the German Society of Anaesthetists.

*H O Stoeckel
German Federal Republic, Organiser of the joint meeting with the German Society in Bonn.

1986

P Cull
St Bartholomew's Hospital, London, for his contribution, as honorary artistic adviser, to the work of the Association.

*S Lipton, OBE
Liverpool, for his contribution to the development of the management of pain.

*Ruth E Mansfield, MBE
Christian Medical College, Vellore, India, for her contribution to anaesthesia in Vellore and the United Kingdom.

*A J Merrifield
Air Commodore, Royal Air Force, for his distinguished service to anaesthesia and aviation medicine.

1987

*Valerie Major
Christian Medical College, Vellore, India, for distinguished service to the teaching and practice of anaesthesia in India.

*P R Rayner
Chesterfield, for gallant action at the site of an air disaster near Donnington Park.

L Small
Department of Health and Social Security, for his contribution to anaesthesia as a member of the Scientific and Technical Branch DHSS.

1988

*J E Fairfield
Guy's Hospital, London, for gallant action at the King's Cross Underground station fire disaster.

M F Freeman
Chairman of the British Anaesthetic Respiratory Equipment Manufacturers Association, for his work with the Association in pursuit of the highest standards in the manufacture of equipment.

1989

*P Duncan
Canada, President of the Canadian Anaesthetists' Society, on the occasion of the joint meeting in Ottawa.

*J Cowan
Canada, Chairman of the Council of the Canadian Anaesthetists' Society, on the occasion of the joint meeting in Ottawa.

*P J Butler
Leicester, for gallant action at the site of the Kegworth air disaster.

*M J Mowbray
Nottingham, for gallant action at the site of the Kegworth air disaster.

*E Egan
Tanzania, for services for anaesthesia in Tanzania.

S Savage (deceased)
Glasgow, for his outstanding contribution to the knowledge of the chemistry of muscle relaxants.

1990

*L Kaufman
University College Hospital, London, in recognition of his work as collator of the Anaesthetic Literature section in *Anaesthesia*.

*Wendy E Scott
Milton Keynes, in recognition of her service as Association Exhibition Stand Co-ordinator.

B R Sugg
Secretary of the British Anaesthetic and Respiratory Equipment Manufacturers Association, in recognition of his contribution to anaesthesia and the Association.

*R S Vaughan
Cardiff, in recognition of his service to the Association as co-ordinator of technical exhibitions.

1991

*Ruth Hutchinson
Zimbabwe, in recognition of services to anaesthesia in Africa.

R Stratton
British Standards Institute, London, in recognition of his contribution to the safe practice of anaesthesia through his work with the British Standards Institute.

1992

*A I J Brain
Reading, in recognition of his development of the laryngeal mask airway.

*R Greenbaum
University College Hospital, London, in recognition of his work as Assistant Editor of *Anaesthesia* for many years.

*J N Horton
Cardiff, in recognition of his work as founding Editor of *Anaesthesia News*.

*P W Thompson, MBE
Cardiff, for his contribution to the development of British Standards for anaesthesia.

*I R Verner
The Middlesex Hospital, London, for his contribution as Press Officer to the Association's Diamond Jubilee celebration.

1994

*M Inman
Plymouth, for his contribution over many years to the development of links with Nepal.

1995

*R J Eltringham
Gloucester, in recognition of his outstanding contribution to the work of the Association and to education in anaesthesia in the Developing World.

*B Hayes
Birmingham, in recognition of his outstanding contribution to the promotion of safety standards in anaesthesia.

1996

*M Dobson
Oxford, in recognition of his contribution to education in anaesthesia particularly in developing countries.

1997

*N Burn
Newcastle upon Tyne, in recognition of his important contribution to the specialty as Chief Technician to Professor Pask and in particular in the design of ventilators and other anaesthetic equipment.

*J Cahill
Cork, in recognition of his invaluable work as Secretary and Chairman of the International Relations Committee.

*I McLellan
Leicester, in recognition of his invaluable work as the Association's Honorary Librarian.

*D J Wilkinson
London, in recognition of his invaluable work as Honorary Archivist and for his work in Chairing the Organising Committee of the Sesquicentennial Meeting.

* R G Walsh
Sydney, for his work in fostering the relationship between the Association and the Australian Society of Anaesthetists and for his outstanding contribution as President of the 11th World Congress in Sydney in 1996.

Appendix C: Honours and Awards of the AAGBI 743

* G Wotherspoon
Sydney, in recognition of his distinguished service to anaesthesia as President of the Australian Society of Anaesthetists and to the 11th World Congress in Sydney in 1996.

*I White
Winnipeg, in recognition of his invaluable work in promoting close cooperation between the Association and the Canadian Anaesthetists' Association.

1998

*J C Edwards
Southampton, for services to the Association of Anaesthetists of Great Britain and Ireland and his role as Curator of the Association's Art Competition.

*P Fenton
Malawi, in recognition of his invaluable work in establishing anaesthesia services in Malawi.

*D Zuck
London, for services to the Association of Anaesthetists of Great Britain and Ireland and his promotion of the history of the specialty.

Registrars' Prize and President's Medal

The Registrars' Prize for the best 10 minute presentation at the Annual Meeting for Anaesthetists in Training was inaugurated in 1974.

The prize has been accompanied by the award of the President's Medal since 1985. The gilt medal has the enamelled shield of the Association of Anaesthetists on the obverse and the recipients name on the reverse. Several of the winners of the Registrars' Prize have subsequently become leading academic anaesthetists.

1974   P Griffiths (Bristol)
"Thoracic epidural analgesia."

1975   J Asbury (Birmingham)
"Study of dreaming in short duration casualty anaesthetics."

1976 Margaret Berry (Stockton-on-Tees)
"Suxamethonium apnoea in patients undergoing ECT."

1977 Alan Aitkenhead (Glasgow)
"High spinal block for large bowel anastomosis."

1978 W S Nimmo (Edinburgh)
"Gastric emptying in the perioperative period."

1979 R B Young (Westminster Hospital, London)
"Suxamethonium for peritoneal closure."

1980 P S Sebel (The London Hospital)
"The effects of high dose fentanyl anaesthesia on the electroencephalogram."
and
A MacDonald (Glasgow)
"A new method for the central rewarming of hypothermic subjects."

1981 A Chambers (Edinburgh)
"Extradural morphine for postoperative pain."

1982 S G Greenbough (Manchester)
"Computerising data obtained with flow directed balloon filled pulmonary artery catheters."

1983 P R Layman (Oxford)
"Experience of transtracheal ventilation as the alternative to difficult intubation in oral surgery."

1984 B J M Bowles (Salford)
"Premedication in practice: efficacy and side effects."

1985 N C T Wilton (Southampton)
"Single breath induction using halothane, nitrous oxide and oxygen."

1986 A Allison (Edinburgh)
"Sciatic nerve blockade using a low power peripheral stimulator."

1987 E A Thornbury (Southampton)
"The effect of temperature on neuromuscular blockade."

1988 M S McKinnery (Northern Ireland)

Appendix C: Honours and Awards of the AAGBI 745

1989 A J Martin (Manchester)
      "A study of the effect of pH adjustment on discomfort caused by intradermal injection of lignocaine."

1990 S A Ridley (Glasgow)
      "Long time output from the intensive care unit."

1991 C Frerk (Manchester)
      "Assessment of the potentially difficult intubation."

1992 T Strang (Manchester)
      "Poestle laryngeal mask compromise cricoid pressure?"

1993 E McCoy (Belfast)
      "The levering larynoscope."

1994 J Isaac
      "A better spinal needle?"

1995 W E Jewell (Oxford)
      "Is the size of the laryngeal mask important?"

1996 T Cook (Bath)
      "Cricoid pressure: one hand or two?"

1997 D Buggy (Cork)
      "The prevention of hypotension with spinal anaesthesia."

1998 E Hammond (Poole)
      "Exam technique and performance in multiple choice question examinations."

APPENDIX D

Eponymous Lecturers of the Association of Anaesthetists of Great Britain and Ireland.

The John Snow Lecture

The eponymous John Snow Memorial Lecture was introduced in 1958 following a proposal by C Langton Hewer, the founder Editor of *Anaesthesia*. It marks the centenary of the death of John Snow (1813-1858) the first professional anaesthetist. The Lecturer was voted an emolument from the time of its introduction but, in 1967 a bronze medal similar in design to that of the John Snow Memorial Medal has been presented in addition: from then on the John Snow Memorial Medal has been struck in silver.

*only five anaesthetists have delivered this lecture.

1958 *George Edwards. Consultant Anaesthetist, St George's Hospital, London.
"John Snow MD."

1959 W Grey Walter. Scientific Consultant, Burden Neurological Institute, Bristol.
"The Control of Consciousness."

1960 Sir Ralph Stevenson, GCMG. Diplomat.
"From the Mediterranean to the Far East and back."

1961 Erskine Childers. Minister for Power and Transport for the Republic of Ireland. (later President of Ireland).
"The Irish Heritage."

1962 Lord Cohen of Birkenhead, CH. Professor of Medicine, University of Liverpool.
"John Snow and his Contemporaries."

1963 Lord James of Rusholm. Vice Chancellor of York University. Educationalist.
"The education of the scientist."

1964 *Professor W W Mushin, CBE. Professor of Anaesthesia, University of Wales.
"Craft and intellect."

Appendix D: Eponymous Lecturers of the AAGBI 747

1965 Sir Derrick Dunlop. Professor of Therapeutics and Clinical Medicine, University of Edinburgh.
"The evaluation of drugs."

1966 Sir John Wolfenden, CBE. Chairman, University Grants Commission. Educationalist.
"Some problems of medical education."

1967 Sir Ian Fraser, DSO, OBE. Senior Surgeon, Royal Victoria Hospital, Belfast.
"John Snow and his surgical friends."

1968 *There was no lecture in the year of the 4th World Congress of Anaesthesiologists in London.*

1969 *Sir Geoffrey Organe, CBE. Professor of Anaesthesia, Westminster Hospital, London.
"Anaesthesia 1939."

1970 Professor Henry Miller. Professor of Neurology and Vice Chancellor of the University of Newcastle upon Tyne.
"Medical education and medical research."

1971 Professor Sir Melville Arnott. Professor of Medicine, University of Birmingham.
"The pulmonary circulation."

1972 Lord Robens of Woldingham, PC. Chairman of the National Coal Board.
"The lesson of John Snow."

1973 Professor Dorothy Hodgkin, OM, FRS. Chancellor of the University of Bristol.
"Science, one subject."

1974 Sir William Armstrong, PC, CCB. Chairman of the Midland Bank. (Head of the Home Civil Service 1968-1974).
"The Civil Service and Medicine from John Snow to the present time."

1975 Sir Alec Merrison, FRS. Vice Chancellor of the University of Bristol.
"Doctor and patient, the regulation of the profession."

1976 Professor Sir Keith Simpson, CBE. Emeritus Professor of Forensic Medicine in the University of London.
"The Anaesthetist and the Law."

1977 Dr T K Whitaker. Chancellor of the National University of Ireland.
"Anaesthesia in the EEC."

1978 Lord Annan, OBE. Vice Chancellor, University of London.
"British Broadcasting."

1979 Lord Kearton of Whitchurch, OBE, FRS. Chairman of the National Oil Corporation.
"Energy and apathy."

1980 Sir Cecil Montacute Clothier, KCB, QC. Parliamentary Commissioner for Administration and the Health Service.
"The price of excellence."

1981 Professor Sir John Butterfield, OBE. Regius Professor of Physic, University of Cambridge.
"The modern epidemiology."

1982 *Professor M D A Vickers. Professor of Anaesthetics, University of Wales.
"In the public interest."

1983 Professor Sir John Walton. President of the General Medical Council.
"Training tomorrow's doctors."

1984 M O'Donnell. Medical writer and broadcaster.
"Today's pollution of the parish pump."

1985 Sir Donald Acheson. Chief Medical Officer.
"Contributions to public health of past Chief Medical Officers."

1986 Professor Anthony Clare. Professor of Psychological Medicine, St Bartholomew's Hospital, London.
"Alcohol and the Medical Profession-a case of dependence."

1987 The Right Honourable Lord Dainton of Hallam Moore, FRS. Chancellor of the University of Sheffield.
"The University Medical Research and the NHS."

1988 David Owen, CH, PC, MP. Leader of the Social Democrat Party 1983-1987.
"Science and Medicine."

Appendix D: Eponymous Lecturers of the AAGBI

1989   Baroness Warnock of Weeke, DBE. Mistress of Girton College, Cambridge, Philosopher.
"The good of the child."

1990   Sir Bernard Lovell, OBE, FRS. Director of the Nuffield Radio Astronomy Laboratories, Jodrell Bank 1951-1981.
"The origin of the universe and of life on earth."

1991   Lord Asa Briggs of Lewes. Provost of Worcester College, Oxford. Historian.
"The health of the family."

1992   Professor P D Wall, MD. Professor of Anatomy, University College, London.
"Could we prevent pain as Snow prevented cholera?"

1993   *Professor Sir Donald Campbell, CBE. Professor of Anaesthesia, Glasgow.
"The leaven of science."

1994   Sir Robert Kilpatrick, CBE. President of the General Medical Council.
"To depart in peace."

1995   Dr R Whittington. HM Coroner for the Districts of Birmingham and Solihull.
"The coroner from one millenium to the next."

1996   *Dr Margaret Branthwaite. Consultant Anaesthetist, Physician and Barrister.
"Therapeutic options: who should decide."

1997   Professor D Bellamy.
"Mandrake and the herbal tradition."

1998   Sir John Carter. Chief Medical Officer, Scotland.
"The NHS: fifty years old and still going strong."

The Junior Anaesthetists' Group (Group of Anaesthetists in Training) Annual Guest and Pinkerton Memorial Lectures.

The first Guest Lecture was delivered by J Alfred Lee (President of the Association of Anaesthetists 1971-1973) at the Annual Meeting of the Junior Anaesthetists' Group at Sheffield in 1973. The series became the eponymous Pinkerton Memorial Lecture in 1982 in honour of H H (Tony) Pinkerton the

President of the Association (1965-1967) at the time the Junior Anaesthetists' Group was founded. A bronze medal, similar to that awarded to the John Snow Memorial Lecturers is presented to the Pinkerton Lecturer (Chapter 8).

Guest Lecturers

1973   J Alfred Lee. President of the Association of Anaesthetists 1971-1973. Consultant Anaesthetist, Southend-on-Sea.
"The history of anaesthesia in Britain during the last 50 years."

1974   A number of eminent anaesthetists addressed the Junior

1975   Anaesthetists' Group during these years but there were no
& 1976   specifically designated "guest lecturers".

1977   J Needham. Director, East Asian History of Science Library, Cambridge.
"Acupuncture and Anaesthesia."

1978   Mary Whittaker. University of Exeter.
"A new look at the importance of plasma cholinesterases to the anaesthetist."

1979   R de G Hanson. Surgeon Commander, RN.
"Physiological problems of saturation diving."

1980   A A Spence. Editor of the *British Journal of Anaesthesia* and later Professor of Anaesthesia Edinburgh and Glasgow.
"Writing for Medical Journals."

1981   C Armstrong-Esther. Professor of Nursing Studies, Guildford.
"Diurnal variations and confusions in hospital patients."

Pinkerton Memorial Lecturers

1982   C J Hull. Professor of Anaesthesia, Newcastle upon Tyne.
"Dangerous ground."

1983   D J Gee. Professor of Forensic Medicine, Leeds.
"Criminal view of life and death."

1984   D C Flenley. Professor of Respiratory Diseases, Edinburgh.
"Sleep, breathing and oxygen."

Appendix D: Eponymous Lecturers of the AAGBI 751

1985   A Maynard. Professor of Health Economics, York
"Rationing care and efficiency."

1986   K Rawnsley. Emeritus Professor of Psychological Medicine, Univesity of Wales.
"The sick doctor."

1987   J W Dundee. Professor of Anaesthesia, Queens University, Belfast.
"A travelling professor."

1988   M J Halsey. Reader, Medical Research Centre, Northwich Park.
"Basic science and anaesthesia."

1989   R Dyson. Professor of Clinical Management, University of Keele.
"Clinical and resource management. What are the options for anaesthetists?"

1990   W C Bowman. Professor of Pharmacology, University of Strathclyde.
"What's new at the neuromuscular junction?"

1991   T B Boulton. Consultant Anaesthetist, Oxford and Reading. President of the Association of Anaesthetists 1984-1986.
"From black gas to propofol."

1992   J S M Zorab. Consultant Anaesthetist, Bristol. President of the World Federation of Societies of Anaesthesiologists 1988-1992.
"Twenty five years of development in European and World Anaesthesia."

1993   Brian Edwards. Chief Executive of Trent Regional Health Authority.
"Have we seen the high point of the development of the health service."

1994   A Taylor, CBE. Solicitor. Past Chairman of the National Association of Health Authorities.
"A professional agenda for anaesthetists."

1995 S Brandon. Professor of Psychiatry and Postgraduate Dean, Leicester.
"The cost of caring."

1996 J S Milledge. Consultant Physician.
"High altitude medicine."

1997 I Calder. Consultant Anaesthetist, London.
"Follow the light."

1998 G Hume. Journalist.
"Medicine in the media."

The Critikon and Intavent lectures at Annual Scientific Meetings

The principal lecture on the first day of the Annual Scientific Meeting was sponsored by Critikon Ltd from 1988 to 1993 and thereafter it has been supported by Intavent Ltd. This funding has brought a succession of eminent physician anaesthetists and intensivists from abroad to speak to the delegates.

1988 R Kitz. Harvard Medical School, USA.
"Lessons from North America."

1989 J Viby-Morgensen. Copenhagen, Denmark.
"The abnormal phenotypes for cholinesterase and drug interaction."

1990 P F White. St Louis, USA.
"Come and go surgery."

1991 S Reiz. Umea, Sweden.
"Is postoperative cardiac risk affected by agent, technique or anaesthetist?"

1992 J L Vincent. Brussels, Belgium.
"The prevention of multiorgan failure."

1993 D Bevan. Vancouver, Canada.
"Half a century of relaxants."

1994 M F Roizen. Chicago, USA.
"Pre-operative care: a North American model."

1995 Elizabeth Frost. New York, USA.
"Postoperative pain organisation and complications."

1996 A D Rocke. Durban, Republic of South Africa.
"Obstetric anaesthesia: challenges for the future."

1997 J L Benum. San Diego, USA.
"The American Society of Anesthesiologists' difficult airway algorithm."

1998 P J F Baskett. Bristol, UK.
"It's alright so long as you take pleasure from it."

The OHMEDA Health Care Lecture

A guest lecture was sponsored by Radiometer Ltd at the second Winter Meeting in 1989 when Professor John Severinghaus (Seattle, USA) spoke on "The history and current status of oximetry"; subsequently, however OHMEDA has taken over the sponsorship of the guest lecture at the Winter Meeting (Council Minutes 2.6.1989).

1990 J F Nunn. Director of the Clinical Research Centre, Northwich Park, UK.
"The air we breath."

1991 W B Runciman. Adelaide, Australia.
"Balancing cost, benefit and risk - the major challenge for the future."

1992 Sir Keith Sykes. Oxford, UK.
"Clinic Measurement and Clinical Practice."

1993 Clayton Petty. National Institute of Health, Bethesda, USA.
"Risk management in anaesthesia."

1994 M F M James. Cape Town, South Africa.
"Magnesium - the once and future ion."

1995 J G Bovill. Leiden, Holland.
"The role of simulators in anaesthesia education."

1996 E O H Teik. Hong Kong.
"Intensive care - art or science?"

1997 R D Miller. San Francisco, USA
"Impact of health care reforms on USA Health Service."

1998 C Prys-Roberts. Bristol, England.
"A quality framework for anaesthesia."

APPENDIX E

Members of the Council of the Association of Anaesthetists of Great Britain and Ireland

1. **Officers and Elected Members of Council 1932-1995**

The Executive Officers are listed chronologically at the beginning of chapters 4-10. Elected Members who held office at some time during their period on Council are denoted by the following superscripts:-

President[1]: Vice President[2]: Honorary Treasurer[3]: Honorary Secretary[4]: Editor[5]: Chairman of the Junior Anaesthetists' Group (JAG) or the group of Anaesthetists in Training (GAT)[6]: Honorary Secretary of JAG or GAT[7].

An asterisk* indicates individuals who also served as "District Representatives" both before and after serving on council between 1933 and 1945. W T D Mart (Sheffield), W Daigan (Oxford) and A Mills (Dundee) were also "District Representatives" at various times but never served on Council.

Notes:

(i) This list includes those elected as the result of the elections in September 1998.

(ii) All Chairmen or Honorary Secretaries of JAG or GAT are listed as Elected Members of Council: originally, from 1967 to 1969, though elected by their peers, they were in fact, co-opted members of council and from 1970 to 1980 were uniquely, coopted members with a vote (Council Minutes 3.7.1970), but after 1981 they were included in the list of elected members of Council.

(iii) The dates in the column (a) are those of first election to Council, including services as JAG or GAT officer.

The dates in column (b) indicate re-election dates as a Council Member or Officer after an interval.

Appendix E: Members of the Council of the AAGBI 755

		(a)	(b)
Featherstone HW[1,4]	Birmingham	1932-42	
Blomfield J[1,2,4]	St George's, London	1932-41	
Mennell Z[1,3]	St Thomas', London	1932-47	
Jones Howard W[4]	Charing Cross, London	1932-35	
Chaldecott JH	St Thomas', London	1932-34	
Boyle HEG	St Bartholomew's, London	1932-34	
Phillips G Ramsey	St Mary's, London	1932-35	
Hadfield CF[2]	St Bartholomew's London	1932-43	
Hill E Faulkner	Manchester	1932-34	
Shipway Sir Francis	Guy's, London	1932-33	1935-37
Daly Ashley S	The London Hospital	1932-35	1938-47
Apperly RE	Middlesex Hospital, London	1932-35	
Hughes C	King's College, London	1932-34	
Flemming AL	Bristol	1932-34	
*Fairlie HP	Glasgow	1932-33	
*Mackenzie J Ross	Aberdeen	1932-33	
*Thompson H Torrance	Edinburgh	1932-33	
Magill (Sir) Ivan W	Westminster, London	1933-36	1937-43 1944-48
Morris CW	University College, London	1933-36	
Smith G Rowdon	Liverpool	1933-36	
Rowling S Thompson	Leeds	1933-36	
*Greaves H Gordon	Cardiff	1934-37	
Ashworth HK	Manchester	1934-37	
Crampton HP	Middlesex, London	1934-37	
Richards HA	Kings' College, London	1934-37	
Clausen RJ	Charing Cross, London	1935-38	
Hewer C Langton[1,2,5]	St Bartholomew's London	1935-38	1942-66
Sington HS[3]	Hospital for Sick Children, London	1935-42	
Challis JHT	The London Hospital	1936-42	1944-45
Webber HN	University College Hospital, London	1936-42	
*Phillips WJ	Durham	1936-41	
*Beckett J	Dublin; Irish Republic	1936-44	

Macintosh (Sir) Robert	Oxford	1937-43	1944-48 1953-56
Nosworthy MD	St Thomas', London	1937-38	
Vessell VE	St Thomas', London	1937-42	
Evans Frankis T	St Bartholomew's, London	1938-42	1944-45
Holroyd JBH	Sheffield	1938-42	
Marston AD[1,2,4]	Guy's, London	1938-48	
Minnitt RJ	Liverpool	1941-44	
Sykes CE	Manchester	1942-45	1946-49
Mathew AW	St Mary's, London	1942-44	
Hall Vernon F[1,2,3]	King's College, London	1942-45	1948-65
Hasler JK	West London	1942-44	
Gould R Blair	Golden Square, London	1942-45	
Bannister Freda B	Oxford	1943-46	
Davies H Woodfield	Postgraduate, London	1943-46	
Gillies J[1,2]	Edinburgh	1943-56	
Jarman R	Cancer Hospital, London	1943-46	1953-65
Johnson Bernard RM[2,3]	Middlesex, London	1943-53	
Rowbotham ES	Royal Free, London	1943-44	1947-50
Waddy FF	Northampton	1943-46	
Low WDA[1,2,3]	St Thomas', London	1943-53	
Murtagh BLS	Birmingham	1944-47	
Durrans SF	Bournemouth	1944-47	
Edwards G	St George's, London	1945-49	
Musgrove A Hugh	Cardiff	1945-48	
Murphy TIP	Plymouth	1946-49	
Budd CH	Cambridge	1947-50	
Lloyd-Williams Katherine G	Royal Free, London	1947-50	
Organe (Sir) Geoffrey SW[1,2,4]	Westminster, London	1947-56	
Wilson HB	St Thomas', London	1947-48	1954-57
Chester Aileen M	Princess Louise, London	1948-51	
Davies HM Armstrong	Newcastle uponTyne	1948-55	
Gray T Cecil[3]	Liverpool	1948-59	1962-64
Pinkerton HH[1,2]	Glasgow	1949-52	1960-63

Appendix E: Members of the Council of the AAGBI 757

Shackleton RPW[1,2,4]	Southampton	1949-58	1960-63
			1965-67
Steel GC	Royal Free, London	1949-52	
Woolmer RF	Bristol	1949-52	
Cope RW	University College, London	1950-53	
Galley AH	King's College, London	1950-53	
Mushin WW[2]	Cardiff	1950-59	
Harbord RP	Leeds	1951-54	
Helliwell PJ[1,2,4]	Guy's, London	1951-76	
Hopper GR	Liverpool	1951-54	
Morton HJV[2,3]	Uxbridge, Middlesex	1951-54	1959-69
Brennan HJ	Manchester	1952-55	
Bromage PR	Portsmouth	1952-55	
Wilton TNP	Bristol	1952-55	
Beard AJW[1,3,4]	Royal Postgraduate, London,	1953-63	1966-73
Machray R	Westminster and Brompton, London	1953-56	
Carnegie DM	Guy's, London	1954-57	
Finnie WJ	Bradford	1954-57	
Seward EH	High Wycombe, Bucks	1954-57	
McCormick VO[2]	Dublin	1955-58	1960-63
Pooler HE	Chesterfield, Yorkshire	1955-58	
Pask EA[3]	Newcastle uponTyne	1955-66	
Scurr CF[1]	Westminster, London	1956-59	1962-65
			1973-78
Wylie WD[1]	St Thomas', London	1956-59	1980-82
Forrester AC	Glasgow	1957-60	
Hunter AR	Manchester	1957-60	
Kerr GM	Chelmsford	1957-60	
Wood-Smith FG	Royal Postgraduate, London	1957-60	
Fraser AC	Lincoln	1958-61	
Gilmartin TJ[2]	Dublin	1958-61	1964-67
			1973-75
Lee J Alfred[1]	Southend-on-Sea	1959-62	1971-73
Davies Russell M	East Grinstead, Sussex	1959-62	
Wyman JB	Westminster, London	1959-62	
Dundee JW[2]	Belfast	1959-62	1979-81
Evans E Elwyn	Swindon, Wiltshire	1960-61	1963-64
Dinnick OP[2,4]	Middlesex, London	1961-68	1973-75

Appendix E: Members of the Council of the AAGBI

Loder RE	Peterborough	1961-64	1973-76
Rollason WN	Aberdeen	1961-65	
Youngman HR	Cambridge	1961-64	
Bodman RI	St Peters and St Pauls, London	1962-65	
Love SHS	Belfast	1962-65	
Smith JA	Plymouth	1962-65	
Hawksley Margaret	Hospital for Sick Children, London	1963-66	
Adams Aileen K[2,4]	Cambridge	1964-66	1968-73 1976-78
Binning RA	Brighton	1964-67	
Howat DDC[2,3]	St George's, London	1964-67	1969-81
Masson AHB	Edinburgh	1964-67	
Brown WM	Belfast	1965-68	
Coplans MP[4]	St George's, London	1965-72	
Lewis CB	Westminster and Royal Marsden, London	1965-68	
Powell KJ	Exeter	1965-68	
Wright RB	St Thomas', London	1965-68	
Enderby GE Hale	East Grinstead, Sussex	1966-68	
Leaming HL	Middlesborough	1966-68	
Thornton JA	Sheffield	1966-68	
Bryce-Smith R[5]	Oxford	1966-73	
Spence AA[6]	Glasgow	1967-69	1977-80
Crawford J	Glasgow	1967-70	
Culbert TD	Manchester	1967-70	
Kenny Sheila	Dublin	1967-70	
Pearce DJ	Southampton	1967-70	
Barron DW	Belfast	1969-70	
Hargrove RL	Westminster, London	1969-72	
Mason SA[1,3]	King's College, London	1969-72	1974-82
Riding JE	Liverpool	1969-72	
Simpson JC[6,7]	Hospital for Sick Children London	1969-70	
Thompson PW	Cardiff	1969-72	
Vickers MDA[1,2,4]	Royal Postgraduate, London, Birmingham, Cardiff	1968-70	1972-77 1981-84
Zorab JSM[2,4]	Bristol	1968-75	1979-81
Ellis G[2]	St Bartholomew's, London	1969-71	
Bland Eileen[7]	Birmingham	1969-71	
Ellis FR[6]	Leeds	1970-71	

Appendix E: Members of the Council of the AAGBI 759

Horsey PJ	Southampton	1971-74	
Inkster JS	Newcastle upon Tyne	1971-74	
Mair IMJ	Middlesborough	1971-73	
Macintosh FG	Leeds	1971-73	
Robertson JD	Edinburgh	1971-73	
Tomlin PJ	Birmingham	1971-75	
Wren WS[2]	Dublin	1971-74	1976-78
Vaughan RS[2,4,7]	Cardiff	1971	1992 et seq
Bryson THL	Liverpool	1972-75	
Williams PAD[6]	Brighton	1972-73	
Rosen M[1,2,3,4]	Cardiff	1972-88	
Thomas K Bryn	Reading, Berkshire	1972-75	
Healy TEJ	Nottingham	1973-76	
Boulton TB[1,2,5]	Reading, Berkshire and Oxford	1973-86	
Lewis EB[2]	Ashford, Kent	1973-76	1987-88
McDowall DG	Leeds	1973-76	
Nunn JF	Medical Research Council, Clinical Research Centre, Harrow	1973-76	1988-90
Smith G[6,7]	Glasgow and Leicester	1973-75	1983-87
Westwood DM[7]	Cambridge	1973-74	
Campbell Sir Donald[2]	Glasgow	1974-80	
Heath Margaret L[2]	Lewisham, London	1974-77	1988-93
Howells TH	Royal Free, London	1974-77	
Rimmer M[6,7]	Southampton	1974-77	
Black GW[2]	Belfast	1975-78	1981-82
Sugden JC[6]	Leeds	1975-76	
Ellis RH	St Bartholomew's, London	1975-78	
Robinson JS	Birmingham	1975-78	
Baskett PJF[1,2,4]	Bristol	1976-80	1986-92
Burn JMB	Southampton	1976-80	
Horton Jean[2,4]	Cambridge	1976-82	1985-87
Rimmer ME[6]	Reading, Berkshire	1976	
Nightingale DA	Liverpool	1976-79	
Scott DB	Edinburgh	1976-79	
Smith WDA	Leeds	1976-79	
Hughes RL[6,7]	Glasgow	1976-78	
Burrows MM[1,2,3]	Liverpool	1977-90	
Padfield A	Sheffield	1977-80	
Barham CJ[6,7]	King's College, London	1977-80	
Coultas RJ	Nottingham	1978-81	

Appendix E: Members of the Council of the AAGBI

Coleman D[2]	Cork	1978-80	
Rees G Jackson	Liverpool	1978-81	
Tunstall ME	Aberdeen	1978-81	
Atkinson RS[2]	Southend-on-Sea, Essex	1979-82	1987-89
Churchill-Davidson H	St Thomas', London	1979-82	
MacRae W R[1,2,3,4]	Edinburgh	1979-94	
Norman J	Southampton	1979-81	
Inman MT[2,4]	Plymouth	1980-89	
Lumley Jean	Royal Postgraduate, London	1980-82	
MacDonald AG	Glasgow	1980-82	
White WD[6,7]	Southampton	1980-82	
Chambers A[6,7]	Edinburgh	1980-83	
Bickford Smith PJ[6,7]	Leeds: Bradford	1981-82	1991-95
Cooper EA	Newcastle upon Tyne	1981-82	
Goodwin Julienne	York	1981-82	
Crawford J Selwyn	Birmingham	1981-82	
Leigh J	Guildford, Surrey	1981-82	
Lawson J Murray	Dundee	1981-82	
Lunn JN[2,5]	Cardiff	1982-93	
Eltringham RJ	Cheltenham, Glos	1982-86	
Haslett WHK	Ulster Hospital, Dundonald, Belfast	1982-86	
Morris P[2,4]	Manchester	1982-91	
Hatch DJ[7]	Hospital for Sick Children, London	1983-86	
Ogg TW	Cambridge	1983-87	
Wren WS	Dublin	1983-87	
Scott Wendy[6,7]	Stevenage, Milton Keynes	1983-86	1997 et seq
Whitaker D[7]	Manchester	1984-85	1997 et seq
Payne JP[2]	Royal College of Surgeons, London	1984-86	
Adams AP	Guy's, London	1984-88	
Bradshaw Elizabeth	Salford, Manchester	1984-88	
Searle JF[2]	Exeter	1984-88	1992-94
Hamlin W[6,7]	Leeds	1984-88	
Budd K	Bradford	1985-89	
Baird WLM[3,4]	Glasgow	1985 et seq	
Nimmo WS	Sheffield	1985-89	
Allan Lauren G[7]	Edinburgh	1985-87	1989-91
Edmonds-Seal J	Oxford	1986-90	
Nicholl ADJ	Cambridge	1987-88	

Appendix E: Members of the Council of the AAGBI 761

Wildsmith JAW	Edinburgh	1986-90	
Arthur DS	Glasgow	1987-90	
Charlton JE[4]	Newcastle uponTyne	1987-93	
Lyons SM[1,2]	Belfast	1987 et seq	
Paul DL[6]	Glasgow	1987-88	
Chestnut Rachel J[7]	Manchester	1988-89	
Hutton P	Birmingham	1988-92	
Marks RL	York	1988-91	
Weller RM[2]	Bristol	1988-92	1993 et seq
Heath PJ[6,7]	Southampton	1988-90	
McLaren CAB[2]	Royal Air Force	1989-91	
McLellan I	Leicester	1989-91	
Sykes Sir Keith[2]	Oxford	1990-92	
Aitkenhead AR[2]	Nottingham	1990-94	1995-97
Rollin Anna-Maria[2]	Epsom	1990-1996	
Sutcliffe Anne J	Birmingham	1990-94	
Spencer Elizabeth M[6,7]	Bristol	1990-93	
Geddes Susan M[6,7]	Glasgow	1990-95	
Morgan M[1,5]	Royal Postgraduate, London	1990 et seq	
Edwards A Eleri	Wrexham	1991-95	
Saunders DA[4]	Southampton	1991-1998	
Atkinson RE	Sheffield	1992 et seq	
Cahill JF	Cork	1992-1997	
Wilkinson DJ[3,4]	St Bartholomew's, London	1992 et seq	
Naylor Ann F[2]	Basildon	1993 et seq	
Wallace PGM[4]	Glasgow	1993 et seq	
Strunin L[2]	Royal London Hospital	1993-96	
Holder Kathryn[7]	Bristol	1993-96	
Cartwright DP	Derby	1994-98	
Mirakhur RK	Belfast	1994-98	
Sear JW	Oxford	1994-98	
Luntley JB[6,7]	Sheffield	1995-97	
Mackenzie PA[7]	Glasgow	1995-96	
Ballance JHW	Hereford	1995 et seq	
Buckland RW	Winchester	1995 et seq	
Stockwell Margaret C	Glasgow	1995 et seq	
McDowell G Carlos M	Drogheda	1996 et seq	
Ward ME	Oxford	1996 et seq	
Pollard BJ	Manchester	1996 et seq	

Maddock H[7]	Swansea	1996 et seq
Birks RJS	Sheffield	1997 et seq
Mallinson Claire[6]	London	1997 et seq
Shinde Samantha[7]	London	1997 et seq
Bogod DG	Nottingham	1998 et seq
Greenwell Stephanie K	North Shields	1998 et seq
McNicoll R	Glasgow	1998 et seq

2. Coopted Members of Council 1959-1995

Notes:

(i) Cooption to Council on a regular basis was rare prior to 1949. A resolution of Council (27.10.1948) established the power of council to coopt representatives of any organisation whose advice would assist the deliberations of Council. The immediate cooption was proposed of the Dean of the Faculty of Anaesthetists, the Adviser to the Ministry of Health, and the President of the Anaesthetic Section of the Royal Society of Medicine, but the only holder of the latter Office to have attended in that capacity seems to have been Ronald Jarman who was also coopted as Chairman of the Association Entertainments Committee for several years. It must be remembered, however, that in the forties and fifties prominent anaesthetists, who were officers or elected members of Council of the Association, quite often held office simultaneously in the Board of Faculty and/or the Royal Society of Medicine.

(ii) A representative of the Armed Forces has been coopted since 1961. This cooption was started at a time when the medical branches of the services were having particular manpower difficulties due to the end of the National Service, but the continuation of the practice has benefited Council; not least because of the value of having an independent view from outside the civilian NHS.

(iii) Cooption was regularised in the early sixties. It is a general rule that any anaesthetist who holds the Presidency or Chairmanship of a prestigious medical body, or is Chairman of a major Association Committee is coopted if he or she is not already an Officer or an Elected Member of Council.

Appendix E: Members of the Council of the AAGBI

(iv) Coopted members who also served on the Council of the Association at some time as Officers or Elected Members of council are distinguished by an asterisk*. See section 1 of this Appendix.

(v) See also Note (i) in Section 1 of this Appendix on Officers of the Junior Anaesthetists' Group(JAG).

(vi) This list is consecutive; some individuals appear more than once as holders of different offices.

*Jarman R	Chairman of the Association Entertainments Committee and later President of the Royal Society of Medicine Section of Anaesthetics	1946-50
*Marston AD	Dean of the Faculty Royal College of Surgeons of England and later Adviser to the Ministry of Health	1949-58
*Johnson BRM	Dean of the Faculty, Royal College of Surgeons of England	1952-55
*Evans Frankis T	Dean of the Faculty, Royal College of Surgeons of England	1955-59
*Organe GSW	Adviser to the Ministry of Health	1958-73
*Mushin WW	Member of the Health Services Council, Dean of the Faculty, Royal College of Surgeons of England	1959-70
Stephens KF	Armed Forces Representative	1961-63
Soper RL	Armed Forces Representative	1963-65
Galley AH	Chairman of the British Medical Association Anaesthetists' Group	1963-64
*Gilmartin TJ	Dean, Faculty of Anaesthetists, Ireland	1960-63
*Masson AHB	Royal Infirmary, Edinburgh, Scotland	1963-64
Woodcock J	Dean, Faculty of Anaesthetists, Ireland	1963-64
*Bryce-Smith R	Editor Elect of Anaesthesia	1963-65
O'Connor A	Armed Forces Representative	1965-66
*Ellis G	Chairman, 4th World Congress, London	1965-68
*Gray TC	Dean, Faculty of Anaesthetists, Royal College of Surgeons of England	1965-67
*Lee JA	Chairman, Editorial Board	1966-72

*Shackleton RPW	President, 4th World Congress, London	1966-67
Voller JJ	Armed Forces Representative	1966-69
Woodcock J	Dean, Faculty of Anaesthetists, Ireland	1966-77
*Wylie WD	Dean, Faculty of Anaesthetists, Royal College of Surgeons of England	1967-70
Davys GR	Dean, Faculty of Anaesthetists, Ireland	1967-69
*Howat DDC	Honorary Secretary, 4th World Congress, London	1967-68
*Boulton TB	Senior Assistant Editor of *Anaesthesia*	1967-72
Soper RL	Armed Forces Representative	1969-72
*Scurr CF	Dean, Faculty of Anaesthetists, Royal College of Surgeons of England	1970-73
*Dundee JW	Dean, Faculty of Anaesthetists, Ireland	1971-72
*Binning R	Chairman, British Medical Association Anaesthetists' Group	1971-72
*Bryce-Smith R	Chairman, Editorial Board	1973-75
Nicol APM	Armed Forces Representative	1972-75
*Lewis EB	British Medical Association Representative	1972-73
Robson JG	Dean, Faculty of Anaesthetists, Royal College of Surgeons of England	1973-76
*Wren WS	Dean, Faculty of Anaesthetists, Ireland	1973-76
*Coplans MP	Anaesthetists' Sub-Committee CCHMS	1973-76
Sanders CD	Armed Forces Representative	1975-78
*Riding JE	Dean, Faculty of Anaesthetists, Royal College of Surgeons of England	1976-79
*Love SHS	Dean, Faculty of Anaesthetists, Ireland	1976-79
*Burrows MM	Chairman, Anaesthetists Sub-Committee of the CCHMS (BMA)	1976-77
*Zorab JSM	Vice President, European Section of the WFSA	1976-78
Robson JG	Adviser in Anaesthesia to the Ministry of Health	1977-84
*Vickers MDA	Chairman, Anaesthetists Sub-Committee of the CCHMSN (BMA)	1977-78
*Helliwell PJ	Chairman, Editorial Board	1978-87

Appendix E: Members of the Council of the AAGBI

*Heath Margaret L	Chairman, Anaesthetic Sub-Committee CCHMS and DHSS Maintenance of Equipment Panel	1978-84
*Black GW	Northern Ireland Representative	1978-79
Merrifield AJ	Armed Forces Representative	1978
*Nunn JF	Dean, Faculty of Anaesthetists, Royal College of Surgeons of England	1979-81
*Lewis EB	Chairman, Representative Body BMA	1979-81
McCarthy JR	Dean, Faculty of Anaesthetists, Ireland	1979-81
*Thompson PW	Chairman, Safety Committee	1980-87
*Spence AA	Chairman, Education and Research Committee	1980-82
*Payne JP	Chairman, Manpower Advisory Standing Committee DHSS	1980-83
*Zorab JSM	Chairman, European Union of Medical Specialists and later Secretary General and President of the World Federation of Societies of Anaesthesiologists	1981-91
*Baskett PJF	British Representative and later Chairman of the European Union of Medical Specialists	1981-88
*Campbell D	Dean, Faculty of Anaesthetists, Royal College of Surgeons of England	1982-85
Hersey NGB	Armed Forces Representative	1980-81
Radford R	Armed Forces Representative	1981-84
*Burrows MM	Honorary Treasurer elect, Association of Anaesthetists	1982-83
*Black GW	Dean, Faculty of Anaesthetists, Ireland	1983-85
McEwen J	Armed Forces Representative	1983-85
Conway CM	Adviser in Anaesthesia to the DHSS	1984-86
*Adams Aileen K	Dean, Faculty of Anaesthetists, Royal College of Surgeons of England	1985-88
Keane P	Dean, Faculty of Anaesthetists, Ireland	1985-88
*McLaren CAB	Armed Forces Representative	1985-88
*Sykes MK	Adviser in Anaesthesia to the DHSS	1986-91
*Wylie WD	President, Medical Defence Union	1986-88
*Vickers MDA	President, European Academy of Anaesthesiology	1987-91

Moriarty DA	Dean, Faculty of Anaesthetists, Ireland	1988-91
Riordan D	Convenor, Irish Standing Committee	1988-91
*Adams AP	Chairman, Safety Committee	1988-89
Merrill SB	Armed Forces Representative	1989-94
*Rosen M	President, College of Anaesthetists	1988-91
Horton JN	Editor, *Anaesthesia News*	1990-92
Restall JR	Armed Forces Representative	1990-94
Blunnie WP	Convenor, Irish Standing Committee	1991-96
*Clarke RSJ	Dean, Faculty of Anaesthetists, Ireland	1991-94
*Spence AA	President, Royal College of Anaesthetists	1991-94
Willatts Sheila M	Adviser to the Department of Health	1991 et seq
*Vickers MDA	Secretary General and President from 1996, World Federation of Societies of Anaesthesiology	1992 et seq
*Charlton JE	Editor, *Anaesthesia News*	1993 et seq
Cooper JC	Dean, Faculty of Anaesthetists, Ireland	1994 et seq
Spencer I	Armed Forces Representative	1994-95
Prys-Roberts C	President, Royal College of Anaesthetists	1994-97
Swain D	Armed Forces Representative	1995 et seq
*Bickford-Smith PJ	Chairman, Safety Committee	1995-96
Breen PJ	Convenor Irish Standing Committee	1996 et seq
*Strunin L	President, Royal College of Anaesthetists	1997 et seq
Blunnie WP	Dean, Faculty of Anaesthetists Ireland	1997 et seq

Name Index

Honorific titles ("Lord", "Sir", etc.) are not included in this index; surnames are used except for those few instances where a territorial title differing from the surname is commonly employed (e.g., "Nuffield" and not "Morris W R"), and in the case of Royalty (e.g., "George VI"). The names of charitable foundations and commercial companies are included in this index, but those of medical societies and institutions will be found in the Subject Index.

A

ABBOT LABORATORIES plc. 164, 497, 620.
ABRAMS M E. 321.
ACHESON E D. 748.
ADAMS Aileen K. xv, 54, 177, 214, 231, 234, 236, 274, 279, 309, 328, 366, 498, 573, 580, 581, 725, 758, 765, *Fig 26.*
ADAMS A P. 343, 405, 436, 517, 537, 548, 591, 760, 766.
ADAMS Bodkin. 136.
AFRICAN MANGANESE COMPANY. 164.
AITKEN Hilary. 576.
AITKENHEAD A R. 506, 518, 537, 541, 572, 744, 761.
ALAN S N. 334/5, 592.
ALEXANDRA (Princess). 573.
ALLAN Lauren G. 760.
ALLISON A. 744.
ALLISON Celia. 543.
ALLMAN K. 539.
ANDERSON J. 738.
ANNAN N G. 748.
ANNE (Princess Royal). 584.
APPERLY R E. 23, 57, 755.
ARMSTRONG P. 539
ARMSTRONG W. 747.
ARMSTRONG-ESTHER C. 750.
ARNOTT M. 747.
ARTHUR GUINESS Ltd. 266.
ARTHUR D S. 761.
ASBURY J. 743.
ASHWORTH H K. 69, 755, *Fig 11.*
ATKINS Dorothy. 343.
ATKINSON R E. 562, 761.
ATKINSON R S. 343, 397, 405, 407, 727, 760.

AYIM E N. 409
AYRE T P. 337, 720.

B

BAILEY C P. 120.
BAIRD W L M. 413, 579, 601, 615, 625, 760, *Fig 31.*
BAKER D J. 738.
BAKER F. 143.
BALL G. 43.
BALLANCE J. 566, 761.
BANERJEE A K. 738.
BANNISTER Freda B. 756.
BARHAM C J. 279, 759.
BARKER J. 153.
BARLOW Angela. 543.
BARNARD C. 181.
BARRON D W. 758.
BASKETT P J F. xvi, 279, 328, 362, 394, 404, 405, 413, 425, 427, 428, 429, 432, 498, 513, 546, 574, 576, 577, 578, 729, 734, 753, 759, 765, *Figs 29 and 30.*
BATEMAN D V. 343, 402, 738.
BAXTER Joyce. 209, 210, 306, 308, 513.
BAXTER (TRAVENOL) plc. 540.
BEARD A J W. 114, 150, 177, 242, 244, 261, 265, 279, 318, 357, 597, 720.
BECK C S. 119.
BECKETT J. 755.
BEDFORD J R. 492.
BEECHER H K. 144, 148
BEINART Jennifer. vii.
BELLAMY D. 749.
BENAD G. 546.
BENAZON D. 147, 189.

BENNETT J A. 366, 543.
BENUM J L. 753.
BERGMAN Ingrid. 546.
BERRY C. 527.
BERRY Margaret. 744.
BESSER G M. 227.
BETCHER A M. 152.
BEVAN A. 63, 87, 160, 289, 441, 454, 464, 467.
BEVAN D. 752.
BEVAN P G. 565, 567.
BEVERIDGE W. 63, 86, 194.
BINNING R. 185, 214, 215, 425, 758, 764.
BIRKS R J S. 762.
BLACK A. 543.
BLACK G W. 759, 765.
BLAIR A L. 608.
BLAKE Doreen. 344.
BLAND Eileen. 758.
BLOGG C E. 343, 405, 518.
BLOMFIELD J. 6, 20, 22, 26, 28, 34, 36, 44, 49, 53, 57, 58/9, 62, 65, 73, 81, 96, 100, 101, 104, 105, 110, 755.
BLUNNIE W P. 766.
BODMAN R. 269, 276, 758.
BOEVE L A. 143.
BOGOD D G. 518, 762.
BONE J W. 34.
BONICA J J. 409, 722.
BONNEY V. 50, 52.
BOOTT F. 493.
BOTTOMLEY Virginia. 467, 473, 591.
BOULTON T B. iii, v, vi, vii, 212, 232, 266, 279, 324, 340, 369, 405, 413, 498, 515, 574, 618, 726, 734, 751, 759, 764, *Figs 17, 25 and 31.*
BOUREAU J. 157.
BOURNE J G. 239, 240, 241, 242, 244.
BOURNE W. 32, 38, 111, 137, 717.
BOVET D. 125.
BOVILL J G. 753.
BOWER A G. 186.
BOWKER K. 341.
BOWLES B J M. 744.
BOWMAN W C. 751.
BOYLE E G. 6, 18, 20, 22, 31, 38, 51, 52, 126, 716, 755.
BRADSHAW Elizabeth. 546, 760.

BRAIN A I J. 436, 437, 515, 731, 741.
BRANDON SA. 752.
BRANSTON P. 380.
BRANTHWAITE Margaret. 729, 749.
BRAUN H F W. 127.
BREEN P J. 530, 766.
BRENNAN H J. 33, 51, 757.
BRIGGS A. 483, 749.
BRITISH OXYGEN (MEDISHIELD) Ltd, later OHMEDA plc. 163, 164, 259, 260, 266, 275, 347, 348, 379, 502, 506, 507, 521, 538, 569, 577, 753.
BRITISH UNITED PROVIDENT ASSOCIATION. 540.
BROCK R C. 120.
BRODRICK W S F. 271, 272, 306.
BROMAGE P R. 757.
BROWN A C D. 338.
BROWN G. 88.
BROWN W M. 738, 758.
BRUCE J. 430.
BRYCE-SMITH R. 126, 177, 212, 236, 336, 340, 341, 618, 736, 758, 763, 764.
BRYSON T H L. 759.
BUCKLAND R W. 446, 761.
BUDD C H. 756.
BUDD K. 760.
BUGGY D. 745.
BULL P T. 738.
BURGESS A H. 45.
BURGESS Jane. 593.
BURN J M B. 759.
BURN N. 742.
BURNELL Mary. 153.
BURROWS M M. 357, 394, 413, 440, 443, 460, 461, 490, 498, 532, 564, 575, 583, 615, 726, 759, 764, 765, *Figs 25 and 31.*
BURY R. 476.
BUSHMAN J A. 226.
BUTLER P J. 740.
BUTTERFIELD J. 495. 748.
BUXTON D W. 5, 6.

C

CAHILL J. 529, 530, 531, 532, 533, 742, 761.
CALDER I. 752.

Name Index

CALMAN K. 338, 361, 466, 547, 608, 609, 610.
CAMPBELL D. 334, 580, 727, 749, 759, 765.
CAMPBELL E M M. 189.
CAMBPELL Susan. 344.
CAMPION M. 308.
CARNEGIE D M. 759.
CARTER J. 546, 749.
CARTER M. 542.
CARTWRIGHT D P. 522, 761.
CASALE F F. 227.
CASEY W. 544.
CASTLE Barbara. 290, 294, 394.
CHAIN E B. 30.
CHALDECOTT J H. 20, 22, 755.
CHALLIS J. 77, 755.
CHAMBERLAIN D. 425, 516, 578, 726.
CHAMBERS A. 279, 744, 760.
CHANTLER C. 443.
CHAREONTHEITAWEE. P. 591.
CHARLTON J E. xi, 413, 513, 522, 523, 619, 761, 766.
CHAWNER J. 456.
CHESTER Aileen M. 756.
CHESTNUT Rachel J. 576, 761.
CHILDERS E. 746.
CHURCHILL-DAVIDSON H. 150, 266, 760.
CIBA Foundation. 107.
CLARE A. 748.
CLARKE K. 408, 441, 455, 457, 461, 462, 463, 464, 465, 477.
CLARKE R S J. 728, 766.
CLAUSEN R J. 20, 755.
CLAYTON S. 391.
CLOTHIER C M. 401, 403, 495, 516, 724, 748.
CLOVER J T. xiv, 31, 103, 146.
CLOVER M. xiv, *Fig 15.*
CLUTTON-BROCK J. 128, 147, 185, 200, 216.
COATES M. 543.
COCHRANE A L. 350.
COHEN H M. xiv, 6, *Fig 2.*
COHEN H. 746.
COLE P V. 227, 232.
COLEMAN D. 760.
COLLINS (nee Jenner) Sally. xi, 500, 513.

CONWAY C M. 405, 765.
COOK T. 745.
COOPER Angela. 539.
COOPER E A. 200, 378, 541, 760.
COOPER J C. 729, 766.
COPE R W. 757.
COPLANS M. ix, 241, 244, 249, 250, 279, 306, 368, 390, 513, 547, 725, 736, 758, 764.
CORALL I. 343, 517.
COULTASS R J. 759.
COWAN J. 740.
COYLE Patricia. 367, 543, 738.
CRAMPTON H P. 20, 755.
CRAWFORD J. 758.
CRAWFORD J S. 378, 544, 760.
CRESSWELL Diana. 209.
CRIDLAND P Robin. 264, 266, *Fig 17.*
CRILE G W. 14.
CRITIKON Ltd. 752.
CROSSMAN R. 289.
CULBERT T D. 758.
CULL P. 336, 344, 714, 735, 739.
CULLEN S. 721.
CUMBERLEDGE Julia F. 473.
CUNNINGHAM A. 537.
CURSON I. 241, 250, 547.

D

DAIGAN W. 754.
DAINTON F S. 748.
DALY A S. 20, 22, 62, 66, 68, 69, 72, 78, 79, 80, 84, 85, 137, 717. 755.
DANKWERT L J. 130.
DAVIES H M A. 756.
DAVIES H W. 756.
DAVIES R M. 150, 757.
DAVIS Karen. 308.
DAVISON M H A. 142, 146, 173.
DAVY H. 528, 543.
DAVYS G R. 764.
DAWKINS C J M. 167, 337, 720.
DAY P. 457.
DeCAUX F P. 172.
DeDENEY G. 593.
DELAFRESNAYE Jean. 157.
DELAMOTHE T. 451, 479, 480.
DINNICK Margaret. 266, *Fig 17.*

DINNICK O P. 168, 177, 209, 214, 244, 254, 256, 260, 263, 265, 266, 271, 275, 336, 396, 598, 724, 736, 757, *Fig 17.*
DOBSON F. 608.
DOBSON M. 541, 545, 546, 742.
DOGMAGH G. 29.
DOUGHTY A G. 397, 401, 727.
DOWNING J W. 537.
DRÄGER plc. 497, 521.
DRINKER P. 30.
DRUMMOND A. 199
DRUMMOND-JACKSON S. 238, 239, 240, 241, 242, 244, 251.
DUBOIS F. 422.
DUDLEY M. 543.
DUDGEON L S. 43.
DUNCAN Elizabeth. 209.
DUNCAN P. 740.
DUNCUM Barbara M. 110.
DUNDEE J W. 125, 127, 143, 144, 200, 260, 378, 597, 725, 751, 757, 764.
DUNLOP D. 259, 747.
DURRANS S F. 756.
DYSON R. 486, 751.

E

EASTON K. 427.
ECCLES Audrey. 504, 513.
EDMONDS-SEAL J. 760.
EDWARDS A E. 761.
EDWARDS B. 298, 450, 454, 751.
EDWARDS G. 11, 12, 36, 99, 133, 146, 165, 174, 402, 723, 746, 756.
EDWARDS J C. 743.
EDWARDS Phyllis. 151.
EGAN E. 740.
EGER. 433.
ELAM J E. 82.
ELDON (J Scott). 493.
ELI LILLY plc. 164.
ELIZABETH II (Queen). 265, 344, 581, 590.
ELLIOTSON J. 493.
ELLIS F R. 153, 279, 321, 347, 378, 758.
ELLIS G H. 264, 265, 266, 321, 736, 758, 763, *Fig 17.*
ELLIS H. 350.
ELLIS R H. 343, 405, 611, 759.

ELTRINGHAM R J. 366, 541, 542, 544, 546, 579, 742, 760.
EMBLEY E H. 39.
ENDERBY G E H. 265, 266, 269, 758.
ENGLISH T. 587.
ENTHOVEN A. 455, 459.
EPSTEIN H G. 144, 201.
EVANS E E. 757.
EVANS F T. 144, 207, 719, 756, 763.
EVANS J. 348.

F

FAIRFIELD J E. 740.
FAIRLIE H P. 23, 755.
FARMAN J V. 231, 232.
FEATHERSTONE H W. v, viii, xiii, xxv, 1, 2, 16, 17, 19, 20, 21, 22, 23, 24, 26, 27, 28, 34, 35, 39, 43, 47, 48, 49, 50, 53, 57, 58, 59, 60, 61, 66, 76, 78, 79, 80, 99, 101, 103, 110, 112, 137, 144, 145, 577, 582, 620, 625, 626, 704-709, 717, 732, 755, *Figs Frontispiece and 3.*
FEE J P H. 518.
FELDMAN S. 153, 236.
FENTON P. 543, 743.
FINCH P M. 336, 735.
FINNIE W J. 757.
FLEMING A. 30.
FLEMMING A L. 26, 755.
FLENLEY D C. 750.
FLOREY H. 30.
FOLDES F. 144, 409, 721.
FORRESTER A C. 127, 200, 357, 722, 757.
FOWLER N. 441.
FRANKLIN C. 367, 546.
FRASER A C. 757.
FRASER I. 747.
FREEMAN M F. 740.
FRERK C. 745.
FREY R. 722.
FRIMPONG Lyn. 513.
FROST Elizabeth. 752.
FUGE C A . 492, 493.

G

GADSDEN P. 588.
GALLEY A H. 123, 171, 243, 354, 757, 763.

Name Index

GALLOON S. 147.
GAMAGE L. 85, 711.
GANDY E W. 26.
GARDNER H B. 80, 716.
GASK G E. 50.
GEDDES Susan. 524, 533, 601, 761.
GEE D J. 750.
GEORGE V (King). 20.
GEORGE VI (King). 85, 116, 711.
GEORGE D L. 85.
GEORGE WESTON HOLDINGS. 107, 163.
GERAGHTY I F. 738.
GIBBON J H. 120.
GILBERTSON A H. 232.
GILCHRIST Edith. 107.
GILL R. 37, 715.
GILLIES J. 51, 62, 94, 99, 100, 102, 104, 111, 114, 127, 133, 137, 153, 156, 157, 158, 159, 163, 718, 732, 756.
GILMARTIN T J. 200, 337, 495, 515, 721, 733, 757, 763.
GILMOUR J. 57.
GILSTON A. 190.
GLOVER J 60.
GODBER G. 287.
GOFF Catherine. 506, 507, 512, 513, 569.
GOGLER E. 427.
GOLDBLAT A. 157.
GOLDMAN V A. 69, 70, 80, 134, 172, 244, 723.
GOMEZ Q. 402, 723.
GOODCHILD C S. 574.
GOODMAN A. 296.
GOODWIN A. 527.
GOODWIN Julienne. 760.
GORBACHEV M. 414.
GORDH T. 127, 157, 337, 409, 721.
GORDON-TAYLOR G. 111.
GOULD R B. 102, 210, 211, 756.
GRANT-WHYTE H. 738.
GRAY T C. v, vi, 72, 73, 105, 106, 114, 127, 143, 145, 147, 150, 153, 163, 170, 200, 221, 232, 256, 335, 337, 402, 403, 722, 733, 756, 763, *Fig 14 and 31*.
GREAVES H G. 755.
GREEN R. 243.
GREENBAUM R. 518, 741.
GREENBOUGH S G. 744.

GREENWELL Stephanie G. 762.
GREY-TURNER E. 220.
GRIFFIN A. 504.
GRIFFITH H R. 31, 72, 137, 156, 157, 158, 159, 717.
GRIFFITHS D. 497.
GRIFFITHS E R. 438, 439, 440, 441, 442, 445, 446, 448, 449, 450, 452, 453, 454, 455, 456, 457, 469, 478, 480.
GRIFFITHS P. 349, 743.
GUILLEBAUD C W. 196.
GWATHMEY J T. 38.

H

HADFIELD C F. 20, 23, 43, 49, 755.
HALFORD F J. 74.
HALL G M. 537.
HALL V F. ix, 69, 70, 114, 163, 177, 201, 214, 244, 331, 719, 756, *Fig 11*.
HALL-DAVIES G. 215.
HALSBURY J A H G. 293.
HALSEY M J. 751.
HALTON J. 72.
HAMLIN W. 413, 760.
HAMMOND E. 745.
HANSELL P. 405.
HANSON R de G. 750.
HARBORD R B. 127, 757.
HARE R. xv, Fig 23.
HARGROVE R L. 397, 758.
HARMER M. 518, 618.
HARRIS T A B. 69, *Fig 11*.
HARROP-GRIFFITHS W. 518.
HASLER J K. 756.
HASLETT W H K. 215, 760.
HATCH D J. 760.
HAWKSLEY Margaret. 274, 758.
HAXHOLDT B. 736.
HAYES B. 742.
HAYES R. 619.
HEALY T E J. 378, 759.
HEATH E. 292, 602.
HEATH Margaret L. 215, 398, 440, 566, 573, 738, 759, 765.
HEATH P J. 413, 761.
HELLIWELL P. xv, 70, 108, 161, 177, 214, 264, 265, 279, 305, 309, 312, 313, 318,

Name Index

324, 325, 326, 337, 339, 340, 357, 358, 364, 368, 391, 405, 406, 408, 488, 513, 515, 517, 598, 617, 627, 722, 734, 757, 764, *Fig 19.*
HEMPSON'S Solicitors. 269, 313.
HERSEY N G B. 765.
HEWER C L. 13, 20, 59, 60, 62, 74, 100, 101, 102, 104, 114, 146, 177, 206, 207, 210, 211, 212, 213, 276, 340,409, 595, 618, 719, 732, 746, 755.
HEWITT F. 31, 83, 142, 143, 144, 146, 251, 252.
HICKMAN H H. 38, 103, 213, 716, 717.
HIGGS R H. 254, 256.
HILL C. 111.
HILL D W. 201.
HILL E F. 20, 22, 105, 207, 718, 755.
HILLARD E K. 737.
HINGSON R A . 232, 233, 234.
HITLER A. 28.
HODGKIN Dorothy. 747.
HOLDER Kathryn 761.
HOECSHT (UK) Ltd. 379.
HOLLAND W. 321.
HOLMDAHL M H. 516, 725.
HOLROYD J B H. 756.
HOPPER G R. 757.
HORSEY P J. 305, 343, 405, 759.
HORTON J N. 405, 520, 619, 741, 766.
HORTON Jean. 279, 405, 728, 759.
HOSFORD J P. 421.
HOWAT D D C. 159, 177, 261, 265, 279, 324, 328, 362, 366, 367, 397, 404, 492, 498, 724, 758, 764. *Fig 17.*
HOWELLS T H. 759.
HOYLE J. 425.
HUE C. 493.
HUGHES C H M. 20, 26, 755.
HUGHES R L. 279, 759.
HUGUENARD P. 125, 157.
HULL C J. 348, 405, 750.
HUME B. 591.
HUME G. 752.
HUNTER A R. 168, 213, 273, 331, 343, 379, 386, 723, 757.
HUTCHINSON Ruth. 741.
HUTTON A M. 108, 161, 214.
HUTTON P. 537, 583, 761.

I

IBSEN B. 118, 187.
IMPERIAL CHEMICAL INDUSTRIES plc. 164, 266, 504.
INKSTER J S. 305, 309, 343, 737, 759.
INMAN M. 413, 494, 495, 541, 542, 741, 760, *Fig 25.*
INTAVENT Ltd. 620, 752.
ISAAC J. 745.

J

JACK R D. 544.
JACK T M. 542.
JACOBSEN E. 336, 736.
JAMES E J F. 746.
JAMES M F M. 753.
JANSSEN PHARMACEUTICALS plc. 497.
JARMAN R. 32, 51, 85, 101, 102, 107, 109, 114, 133, 143, 147, 154, 156, 162, 163, 164, 177, 206, 207, 224, 226, 227, 265, 266, 719, 733, 756, 762, 763, *Figs 13 and 17.*
JENKINS B. 590.
JENKINS M T. 723.
JEWELL W E. 745.
JOHNSON B R M. 62, 100, 114, 153, 162, 165, 234/5. 91, 763.
JOHNSON Enid. 72.
JOHNSON M. 144.
JONSON-GILBERT R. 326, 329, 334, 335.
JOHNSTONE M W. 126, 725, 737.
JONES C G. 739.
JONES J G. 537, 572.
JONES P L. 215.
JONES R M. 518, 537.
JONES W H. 10, 11, 16, 17, 18, 20, 22, 26, 28, 41, 55, 755, *Fig 4.*
JOSEPH K. 289.
JOWITT M. 738.
JUBY James. 173.
JUNKER F E. 56.

K

KAUFMAN L. 343, 392, 393, 740.
KAYE G. 39, 152.
KEANE P. 537, 765.

KEARTON C F. 748.
KELLAR R J. 259.
KEMBER T. 453, 485.
KERWICK A. 32.
KENNEDY J F. 178.
KENNY Sheila. 274, 758.
KERR G M. 757.
KETTLER D F. 739.
KILPATRICK R. 591, 749.
KINDERSLEY H K M. 198.
KING A C. 60, 110, 143, 172, 173, 174, 260, 498, 502.
KING EDWARD'S HOSPITAL FUND FOR LONDON. 352.
KING M L. 178.
KINNOCK N. 416.
KITZ R. 752.
KLEIN Lisl. 380, 381, 382.
KLEIN R. 457.
KLOPPER A K. 1.
KNIGHT R J. 738.
KOLFF W J. 119.
KORNER Edith. 445.
KOUWENHOVEN W B. 119, 120, 185.

L

LABORIT H. 125.
LAMMIMAN D A. 200.
LANGA H. 249.
LASSEN H C A. 118, 187.
LASSNER J. 364, 365, 407, 409, 722.
LAURIE. 32.
LAWRENCE Ghislaine. 504.
LAWSON J M. 760.
LAYMAN P R. 744.
LEAMING H L. 758.
LEE J A. 10, 65, 211, 212, 279, 307, 311, 321, 324, 337, 348, 357, 596, 614, 721, 749, 750, 757, 763.
LEECH B C. 80, 716.
LEHMANN H. 516, 517, 723.
LEIGH J. 760.
LETT H. 50.
LETT Z. xv, 736, *Fig 20.*
LEVENTHAL F. 153.
LEWIN W S. 257, 258, 272, 306, 383, 384, 385, 386, 387, 389, 563.

LEWIS C B. 265, 758, *Fig 17.*
LEWIS E B. 305, 390, 759, 764, 765.
LIGHT D W. 462.
LIPTON S. 739.
LISTON R. 493.
LLOYD J. 193.
LLOYD'S BROKERS. 164.
LLOYD-WILLIAMS Katherine. 100, 143, 155, 156, 157, 165, 207, 274, 719, 756.
LOADER Sarah. 514.
LOCK S. 342.
LODER R E. 259, 757.
LOVE S H S. 758, 764.
LOVELL B. 749.
LOW W A. 62, 90, 91, 100, 114, 139, 140, 157, 158, 165, 170, 171, 756.
LUCAS B G B. 108, 271.
LUMLEY Jean. 541, 760.
LUNDY J S. 32, 722.
LUNN J N. 189, 279, 340, 343, 345, 350, 351, 352, 353, 405, 413, 515, 516, 518, 518, 618, 619, 728, 734, 760, *Fig 25.*
LUNTLEY J B. 601, 761.
LYONS S M. 545, 601, 603, 615, 616, 617, 761.
LYTHE J. 544.

M

McCARDIE W J. 697.
McCARTHY J R. 409, 765.
McCONNELL W S. 51, 69, *Fig 11.*
McCORMICK V O. 757.
McCOY E. 745.
MacDONALD A G. 760.
MacDONALD Alison M. 744.
McDOWALL D G. 153, 759.
McDOWELL G C M. 761.
McEWEN J. 765.
MACINTOSH F G. 759.
MACINTOSH R R. 30, 38, 53, 54, 61, 69, 71, 72, 74, 75, 84, 105, 111, 127, 137, 150, 153, 174, 187, 200, 206, 213, 239, 357, 401, 499, 545, 574, 596, 597, 718, 731, 733, 756, *Figs 6 and 7.*
MACKENZIE J R. 15, 23, 755.
MACKENZIE P A. 761.
McKESSON E I. 172.

McKHANN C F. 30.
McKINNERY M S. 744.
McKINSEY and Company. 290.
McLAREN C A B. 405, 575, 761, 765.
McLELLAN I. 503, 576, 742, 761.
MacLENNAN Fiona. 539.
McMECHAN F H. 6, 37, 48, 154, 715.
McMILLAN H. 415.
McNEILLY R H. 397.
McNICHOLL R. 762.
MACPHERSON G. 485.
MacRAE W R. 279, 363, 366, 405, 413, 477, 498, 502, 522, 567, 579, 588, 601, 609, 610, 729, 734, 760, *Figs 25 and 31*.
MACHRAY R. 757.
MADDOCK H. 762.
MAGILL I W. xiv, xvi, 20, 48, 49, 53, 57, 79, 137, 145, 156, 172, 207, 256, 401, 402, 437, 495, 502, 507, 514, 515, 574, 595, 717, 730, 755, *Fig 5*.
MAIR I M J. 759.
MAJOR J. 415, 416, 464, 470.
MAJOR Valerie. 739.
MAKEPIECE A W. 405.
MALLINSON Claire. 601, 762.
MALONE G. 615.
MALTBY R. 542.
MANLEY R W. 182.
MANSFIELD Ruth E. 739.
MAPLESON W W. 144, 201, 336, 516, 726, 736.
MARGARET (Princess). xv, xvi, 407, 408, 498, 499, 576, 577, *Figs 21 and 30*.
MARKS R L. 761.
MARRETT H R. 54.
MARRIOTT H L. 32
MARSH Sally. 514.
MARSDEN A. 582.
MARSTON A D. 62, 78, 80,84, 89, 95, 96, 99, 100, 103, 110, 111, 137, 156, 171,718, 756, 763.
MART W T D. 754.
MARTIN A J. 745.
MARY (Princess). 103, 110.
MASON Rosemary A. 518.
MASON S A. 266, 279, 305, 314, 324, 332, 357, 358, 390, 397, 405, 488, 492, 497, 723, 758, *Figs 17 and 31*.

MASSON A H B. 758, 763.
MATHEW A W. 756.
MATHEWS E T . iii, v, viii, xi, 577, 704.
MATHIAS J. 405.
MAWHINEY B. 473.
MAXWELL R. 516, 726.
MAY & BAKER Ltd. 164, 266.
MAYNARD A. 751.
MAYRHOFER O. 233, 263, 516, 726.
MEDAWAR P B. 119.
MEDICAL DEFENCE UNION. 357.
MELZACK R. 192.
MENNELL Z. 18, 19, 20, 22, 28, 36, 39, 45, 46, 55, 56, 57, 58, 62, 65, 66, 67, 76, 77, 78, 79, 81, 82, 84, 93, 99, 101, 137, 151, 153, 731, 732, 755.
MERRIFIELD A J. 739, 765.
MERRILL S B. 738, 766.
MERRISON A. 299, 300, 301, 302, 306, 354, 747.
MILBURN A. 463.
MILLEDGE J S. 752.
MILLER H. 747.
MILLER R D. 753.
MILLS A. 754.
MINNITT R J. 56, 79, 137, 172, 207, 718, 756.
MIRAKHUR R K. 541, 761.
MITCHELL Dorothy. 341.
MOIR D. 544.
MOIR E. 12, 13.
MONSON J R T. 422.
MOODY R A. 738.
MOORE J. 453.
MORAN C M. 110.
MORGAN M. xi, 343, 413, 517, 618, 761.
MORIARTY D A. 537, 766.
MORRIS C W. 18, 19, 43, 44, 51, 52, 755.
MORRIS P. 413, 494, 507, 526, 588, 728, 760, *Fig 25*.
MORRISON L G. 111, 732.
MORTLAKE J. 502.
MORTON H J V. 165, 166, 171, 177, 225, 226, 228, 271, 720, 757.
MORTON J. 496.
MORTON W T G. 72, 78, 102, 103, 109, 141, 619, 620.
MOUNTBATTEN L F V A N. 70.

Name Index

MOURET P. 422.
MOWBRAY M. 542, 740.
MOYERS J. 401, 737.
MUIR Ann H. xi, 308, 494, 498, 500, 512, 513, 514, 516, 727.
MURIRA Karungari. 514.
MURLEY R S. 128, 129, 167, 331.
MURPHY P B. 498.
MURPHY T I P. 756.
MURRAY A B. 45.
MURRAY J E. 119.
MURTAGH B. 108, 756.
MUSGROVE A H. 756.
MUSHIN W W. 125, 127, 133, 144, 153, 170, 189, 200, 214, 228, 243, 275, 335, 350, 351, 352, 353, 357, 409, 597, 721, 733, 746, 757, 763.
MYCROFT A W. 212, 341.

N

NAYLOR Ann F. 116, 566, 761.
NEEDHAM J. 750.
NEWTON D E F. 518.
NICHOL D. 458, 461, 468, 469, 473.
NICHOLL A D J. 760.
NICHOLSON Wendy. 514.
NICOL A P M. 764.
NIGHTINGALE D A. 759.
NILSSON E. 365.
NIMMO W S. 541, 744, 760.
NORLANDER O. 409.
NORMAN J. 332, 379, 405, 541, 611, 760.
NOSWORTHY M D. 51, 59, 109, 144, 206, 207, 719, 733, 756.
NUFFIELD PROVINCIAL HOSPITAL TRUST. 350, 351, 352.
NUFFIELD (W Morris). 30, 38, 53, 74, 372, 716.
NUNN J F. xvi, 116, 144, 153, 201, 215, 286, 333, 334, 350, 406, 409, 507, 514, 574, 580, 593, 594, 726, 730, 753, 759, 765, *Fig 27.*

O

O'CONNOR A. 763.
O'DONNELL M. 748.
O'DONOHOE B. 543.
OGG Lesley. xi, 500, 513, 514, 569.
OGG T W. 760.
OHMEDA plc formerly British Oxygen (Medishield) Ltd. 753.
O'KELLY T L. 432.
ORE SALES & SERVICES. 164.
ORGANE G S W. xiv, 62, 83, 101, 109, 114, 132, 133, 139, 142, 143, 149, 150, 153, 156, 157, 158, 159, 162, 163, 165, 174, 200, 201, 211, 231, 233, 234, 253, 262, 263, 265, 273, 325, 335, 357, 362, 401, 495, 720, 733, 756, 763, *Fig 15.*
ORGANE Peggy. xiv, *Fig 15.*
OSBORNE D. 380.
O'SULLIVAN Geraldine. 379, 539.
O'SULLIVAN Katrina. 543.
OWEN D. 290, 295, 297, 301, 394, 456, 748.

P

PADFIELD A. 343, 535, 759.
PAGE R. 543.
PAIGE V. 448.
PANTRIDGE J F. 425, 426.
PAPANTONOPOULOS G W. 136.
PAPPER E M. 495, 722.
PAPWORTH P P. 737.
PARBHOO N. vii.
PARBROOK E O. 343.
PARKHOUSE J. 213.
PARKS A. 333, 334, 580.
PARSLOE C. 516, 725.
PARSONS F B. 82.
PASK E A. 75, 106, 110, 127, 133, 142, 145, 162, 165, 177, 205, 207, 211, 225, 226, 231, 234, 335, 336, 337, 343, 402, 432, 515, 520, 575, 576, 732, 735, 757.
PASK Muriel. 336, 735.
PATERNOSTER Joan. 209.
PATERSON G M. 545, 574.
PATON W. 211, 337, 766.
PAUL D L. 413, 761.
PAYNE J P. 128, 143, 144, 170, 200, 440, 537, 725, 760, 765.
PEACH L. 448.
PEARCE D. 214, 758.
PENLON plc. 501.
PETTY C. 562, 753.

Name Index

PEUTRELL Jane. 539.
PHILIPS R. 499.
PHILLIPS G R. 17, 18, 22, 23, 755.
PHILLIPS W J. 755.
PILKINGTON H. 195, 196.
PINKERTON H H. 138, 177, 214, 264, 348, 720, 749, 756.
PINSON K B. 737.
PLANT Pat (Jasmine). 512, 514.
PLATT R. 139, 196, 197, 218, 219, 220, 221, 222.
PLEASANCE R E. 69.
PLUMPTON F S. 227.
POLLARD B J. 761.
POOLER H E. 208, 757.
PORRITT A. 196, 221, 272, 289, 440, 495.
PORTEX Ltd. 497.
POSWILLO D. 373, 547, 548, 550, 551, 552, 553.
POULSEN H. 427.
POWELL E. 195, 287.
POWELL K J. 758.
PRATT Freda. 54.
PRINCE Ann. 212.
PRIOR F N. 737.
PROBYN-WILLIAMS R J. 37, 715.
PROFUMO J D. 185.
PRYS-ROBERTS C. 151, 153, 401, 405, 528, 543, 615, 753, 766.
PUGH W R. 276.
PUTTICK N. 543.

R

RADFORD R. 765.
RAVENTOS J. 126.
RAWNSLEY K. 355, 356, 358, 516, 725, 751.
RAYNER P R. 739.
REES G A D. 498.
REES G J. 151, 153, 402, 515, 724, 734, 760.
REEVE P. 382.
REILLY C. 616.
REIZ S. 752.
RESTALL J R. 766.
REVELL A L. 200, 267, 405.
REW H. 50.
RICHARD Ray. 513.

RICHARDS H A. 755.
RICHARDSON B W. 175.
RICKARDS J F. 83.
RIDING J E. 300, 327, 364, 758, 764.
RIDLEY S A. 745.
RIGBY A. 502.
RIMMER M. 279, 759.
RIORDAN D. 530, 766.
ROBENS A R. 747.
ROBERTS F. 194.
ROBERTS F. 575, 577.
ROBERTS F W. 109.
ROBERTSON J D. 143, 144, 200, 737, 759.
ROBINSON J. 493.
ROBINSON J S. 200, 226, 350, 378, 537, 759.
ROBINSON K. 235, 289.
ROBSON J G. 200, 216, 325, 326, 327, 332, 339, 349, 350, 515, 724, 733, 764.
ROCHE PRODUCTS. 164.
ROCKE A D. 753.
ROGERS Karen xi.
ROIZEN M F. 752.
ROLLASON W N. 758.
ROLLIN Anna-Maria. iii, viii, xi, xiii, 504, 521, 522, 562, 601, 761.
RONEY Caroline. 405.
ROSEN M. 153, 160, 279, 301, 312, 314, 324, 348, 355, 356, 358, 365, 405, 407, 413, 490, 496, 498, 502, 505, 507, 512, 515, 565, 574, 575, 579, 582, 583, 587, 727, 730, 759, 766, *Figs 25, 26, 27, 28, 29* and *31*.
ROWBOTHAM E S. 31, 79, 111, 207, 718, 756.
ROWLING S T. 755.
RUBEN H. 516, 726.
RUNCIMAN W B. 508, 753.
RYLE J A. 81.

S

SABIN A. 118.
SALK J E. 118, 187.
SALMON B. 129, 288, 384.
SALT R. 737.
SANDERS C D. 764.
SANDO M. 409.

Name Index

SAUGMAN P. 341.
SAUNDERS D A. 526, 601, 761.
SAVAGE S. 740.
SCOTT D B. 349, 350, 759.
SCOTT Joan C. 378.
SCOTT R. 57.
SCOTT Wendy. 413, 575, 576, 740, 760.
SCURR C F. 143, 144, 211, 265, 267, 268, 279, 307, 320, 321, 326, 336, 349, 355, 364, 375, 392, 401, 406, 488, 489, 515, 579, 614, 724, 733, 757, 764, *Figs 17, 20 and 31.*
SEAR J W. 506, 541, 761.
SEARLE G D & Co. 164.
SEARLE J F. 192, 505, 506, 760.
SEBEL P S. 744.
SELLICK B A. 147, 166.
SELLORS T H. 220.
SEVERINGHAUS J. 507, 753.
SEWARD E H. 757.
SEWARD G. 369, 370, 371.
SHACKLETON R P W. 114, 133, 140, 150, 158, 159, 163, 177, 211, 214, 242, 256, 257, 261, 262, 264, 265, 268, 720, 733, 757, 764, *Fig 17.*
SHAW L A. 30.
SHEPHERD D. vii.
SHIELDS H J. 207, 718.
SHINDE Samantha. 762.
SHIPWAY F. 20, 22, 26, 80, 716, 755.
SHOCK M. 461, 463.
SHORT D H. 405.
SILK J F W. 5, 37, 80, 715, *Fig 1.*
SIMPSON B R J. 200.
SIMPSON J C. 177, 215, 279, 758.
SIMPSON J Y. 103, 111, 112, 259.
SIMPSON K. 747.
SIMPSON T B. 112.
SINCLAIR J R. 542.
SINGH Prittam. 722.
SINGTON H. 28, 62, 65, 78, 755.
SLANEY G. 580.
SMALL L. 739.
SMITH A C. 187, 200, 569.
SMITH G. 279, 405, 506, 507, 537, 541, 759.
SMITH G R. 755.
SMITH J A. 758.
SMITH P J B. 348, 398, 413, 760, 766.

SMITH R (B M J). 475.
SMITH R (R C S). 316, 325, 326, 516, 725.
SMITH W D A. 331, 379, 380, 381, 574, 708, 738, 759.
SNOW J. 75, 103, 109, 110, 137, 146, 175, 206, 213, 259, 335, 336, 348, 402, 495, 514, 515, 713, 723, 724, 729, 731, 732, 746, 747, 750.
SOMERS C L. 308.
SOPER R L. 763, 764.
SPALDING J M K. 187.
SPANNER Una J. xi, 344.
SPENCE A A. 177, 214, 216, 226, 286, 332, 372, 378, 405, 406, 408, 434, 537, 539, 541, 553, 578, 583, 586, 593, 750, 758, 765, 766.
SPENCER Elizabeth M. 217, 346, 413, 528, 533, 601, 761.
SPENCER G T. 189, 383.
SPENCER H. 114.
SPENCER I. 766.
SPENS W. 90, 196.
SQUIRES S J. 738.
STARZL T E. 181.
STEEL D. 180.
STEEL G. 77, 757.
STEINBEREITHNER K. 409.
STEINBERG J. 226.
STEPHENS K F. 199, 337, 713, 763.
STEVENSON R. 746.
STOCKING Barbara. 467.
STOCKWELL Margaret C. 761.
STOECKEL H O. 739.
STOOT G J. 738.
STRACHAN G I. 219.
STRANG T. 745.
STRATTON R. 741.
STRUNIN L. 537, 761, 766.
SUCKLING C W. 126, 144.
SUGDEN J C. 279, 759.
SUGG B R. 271, 741.
SUMNER E. 343.
SURGICON plc. 379
SUTCLIFFE Anne J. 761.
SUTHERLAND F M. 220.
SWAIN D. 766.
SWERDLOW M. 192.
SWISS R. 243.

SYKES C E. 756.
SYKES M K. 212, 343, 365, 508, 515, 545, 577, 727, 734, 753, 761, 765.
SYKES W S. 29, 31, 38, 77, 173.

T

TAYLOR A. 751.
TEIK E O H. 753.
THATCHER Margaret. 293, 296, 406, 414, 415, 416, 450, 453, 455, 457, 461, 463, 478.
THOMAS K B. 173, 174, 494, 503, 576, 759.
THOMAS STEVENS & SONS Ltd. 164.
THOMAS T. 544, 579.
THOMPSON H T. 23, 755.
THOMPSON P W. 396, 741, 758, 765, *Fig 29.*
THORNBURY E A. 744.
THORNTON J A. 201, 366, 758.
TIGHE S Q M. 738.
TINDAL A. 737.
TITE G. 492.
TODD A. 218, 272, 274, 337, 338.
TODD D D. 148.
TODD I. xvi, 580, 608, *Fig 28.*
TOMLIN P J. 320, 759.
TOMLINSON A. 542.
TOMLINSON B E. 474.
TOVELL R M. 80, 716.
TRICOMED plc. 501.
TROTTER W. 50.
TRUNKEY D D. 428.
TUNSTALL M E. 728, 760.
TYLER Betty. 512, 513.

U

UTTING J. 572.

V

VANDERVELL G A. 164, 207, 224, 227, 719.
Van ECK R. 144, 150.
VAUGHAN G. 377.
VAUGHAN R S. 405, 413, 507, 526, 575, 601, 741, 759.
VEIL Simone. 365.
VERMEULEN-CRANCH Doreen. 516, 724.
VERNER I R. 265, 405, 741, *Fig 17.*
VESSELL V E. 101, 102, 756.
VIBY-MORGENSEN J. 752.
VICKERS plc. 266.
VICKERS M D A. 159, 279, 301, 308, 309, 313, 320, 321, 322, 324, 331, 335, 339, 343, 365, 369, 378, 380, 402, 403, 404, 405, 410, 413, 489, 490, 491, 509, 515, 520, 521, 522, 525, 526, 535, 579, 614, 728, 734, 748, 758, 764, 765, 766, *Figs 29 and 31.*
VINCENT J L. 752.
VOLLER J J. 764.

W

WADDY F F. 13, 24, 45, 402, 738, 756.
WAGON R. 738.
WAKELEY T. 493.
WALDEGRAVE W. 463, 465, 466, 468, 473.
WALKER-SMITH D. 145.
WALKSMAN S A. 118.
WALL P D. 192, 286, 729, 749.
WALLACE Jacqui. 513.
WALLACE P G M. 761.
WALSH R G. 742.
WALTER C M. 59.
WALTER W G. 746.
WALTON J. 748.
WARBURTON E. 313, 315, 337, 344, 378, 405, 407, 412, 723.
WARD M E. 761.
WARING H. 48, 50.
WARNE S. 340.
WARNOCK H Mary. 749.
WATERS R M. 31, 32, 38, 148, 173, 716.
WATERSON A P. 420.
WATTS Louise. 514, 569.
WEAVER Barbara. 136, 147, 516, 727.
WEBBER H N. 755.
WEBB-JOHNSON A. 80, 81, 94, 95, 96, 98, 102, 104, 717.
WEESE H. 32.
WEIS K H. 736.
WELCH D B. 405.
WELLCOME FOUNDATION Ltd. 164, 497, 501.
WELLER R M. 562, 761.
WESTABY S. 432.

WESTWOOD D M. 759.
WHITAKER D. 760.
WHITAKER T K. 748.
WHITBY L. 140, 141.
WHITE D. 279.
WHITE I. 743.
WHITE P F. 752.
WHITE W D. 760.
WHITEHEAD A J. 110.
WHITEHOUSE Barbara. 501.
WHITTAKER Mary. 750.
WHITTINGTON R. 749.
WILDSMITH J A W. 506, 537, 541, 577, 761.
WILKINSON D. 503, 504, 601, 742.
WILKINSON R T. 379.
WILLATTS Shelia M. 766.
WILLIAMS L. xii.
WILLIAMS P A D. 279, 759.
WILLINK H. 86, 197.
WILSON Gwen. vii, 151.
WILSON H. 295, 300.
WILSON H B. 170, 756.
WILSON I H. 541, 542, 546.
WILTON N C T. 744.
WILTON T N P. 757.
WINDEYER B. 249, 250.
WINTERTON N. 468, 469.
WIRGMAN F. 315.
WOLFENDEN J. 747.
WOLFSON L J. 147, 431.
WOODCOCK J. 763, 764.
WOODHOUSE P G. 706.
WOOD-SMITH F G. 265, 266, 723, 757, *Fig 17*.
WOOLLAM C H M. 54.
WOOLMER R F. 71, 72, 127, 128, 143, 150, 171, 227, 757.
WOTHERSPOON G. 743.
WREN W S. 365, 531, 728, 759, 760, 764.
WRIGHT R A. 57.
WRIGHT R B. 265, 268, 758.
WRIGHT S. 50.
WYLIE W D. ix, xv, 109, 133, 153, 165, 166, 231, 234, 249, 250, 279, 307, 308, 313, 320, 321, 334, 335, 358, 368, 369, 370, 371, 372, 373, 402, 407, 409, 489, 491, 498, 515, 724, 734, 757, 764, 765, *Figs 21, 23, 25 and 31*.

WYMAN J B. 147, 757.

Y

YARNOLD Shirley. 209.
YATES A. 738.
YELTSIN B. 414.
YOUNG R B. 744.
YOUNGMAN H R. 758.

Z

ZENACA plc. 620.
ZORAB J S M. xv, 150, 159, 279, 313, 324, 326, 361, 362, 366, 390, 401, 404, 405, 515, 528, 541, 544, 546, 578, 729, 734, 751, 758, 764, 765, *Figs 22 and 29*.
ZORAB Shirley. xv, *Fig 22*.
ZUCK D. 743.
ZUCKERMAN. 257, 306.

Subject Index

Subject Index

References to medical societies and institutions are included in this index. The names of the Charitable foundations and commercial companies will be found in the Name Index.

A

Abortion Act *200, 326, 359, 415*
Academic Anaesthesia *43, 127, 200, 537*
Acknowledgements *12*
Acquired immune deficiency syndrome (AIDS) *417 - 420*
Acronyms and Abbreviations *xvii-xx*
Acupuncture *305*
Age Anaesthesia Society *554*
Anaesthesia (Clinical) *13-15, 30-33, 69-75, 121-127, 182-186, 283-286, 433-437, 602*
Anaesthesia Educational Research Foundation *232-234*
Anaesthesia (Journal) *100-107, 210-213, 340-345, 516-519, 618*
Anaesthesia News *519*
Anaesthetic Records *275*
Anaesthetic Research Society *201, 534, 653*
Anaesthetists
    Assistance for 383-389, 562-569
    Status and Representation 30, 39-47, 88-94
    Suicide 398
Anaesthetists Academic Foundation *327-329*
Antibiotics *29, 117*
Apparatus *30-33, 74, 182, 269-271, 503*
Armed Forces *66-71*
    New Deal 198-200
Armed Services *16, 66-71, 198-200, 255, 738*
Army *69-71*
Association of Anaesthetists of Great Britain and Ireland
    Advisory Committee 311, 617
    Annual Meetings and Dinners 110, 141-147, 258-261, 398-401
Art Competition 743
British Journal of Anaesthesia Library 503
Business of Council 33-47, 58-61, 89 - 94, 109, 131-136, 201-210, 272-277, 304-335, 354-358, 396-398, 410, 418, 487, 614-618
Coat of Arms 85, 710-714
Committees and Working Parties 133, 234, 242, 305, 308, 366, 377, 379-383, 504, 541-547, 562, 617
Cooperation with the Royal College of Anaesthetists and the Department of Health 614
Diamond Jubilee 576-578
Elections 26, 308-311
Eponymous Lecturers 746-753
Education and Research 108, 161-164, 224-228, 274, 377-379, 410, 505-508, 538-541, 569-575
Finance 313-315, 344
Foundation 16-26, 34-36
Historical Resources 502-504
Honours 137, 206, 335-337, 514-516, 715-745
Golden Jubilee 402
Headquarters 84, 306-308, 488-502
Historical Resources 502-504
Honours 137, 206, 335-337, 514-516, 715-745
Inaugural Meeting 23-26
International Relations 147-153, 305, 541-547
Irish Standing Committee 530
Joint Committee on the Higher training of Anaesthetists 338

780

Subject Index

John Snow Memorial Lecture **146, 746-749**
Junior Anaesthetists' Group (Group of Anaesthetists in Training) **213-217, 346-349, 523**
Legal Status **313, 492**
Linkman Organisation **339, 347, 520-523**
Members of Council **754-766**
Membership **24, 36, 38, 78-80, 133-136, 203-206, 304, 488**
Museum (Charles King) **172-174, 502**
Neck Ties **276**
Objects **23, 208**
Officers **28, 62, 114, 177, 279, 413, 601**
Prizes **228, 743-745**
Publications **see also**
  Anaesthesia (journal) and Anaesthesia News) **389-391, 508-512, 527**
Republic of Ireland **528-533**
Research Fellowships **107-109, 226, 379, 539**
Secretariat **208-210, 308, 512-514**
Seminar Programme **505**
Shop **575**
Silver Jubilee **143-145**
Specialist Societies **533-536**
Technical (Trade) Exhibition **260, 575**
Web Site **619**
Winter Scientific Meeting **506**
World War 2 **65-71**
Association of Cardiothoracic Anaesthetists **554, 556**
Association of Dental Anaesthetists **554, 556, 568**
Association of Paediatric Anaesthetists **534**
Association of Veterinary Anaesthetists **554, 727**
Australian and New Zealand College of Anaesthetist **16, 594**
Awareness during Surgery **185**

B

Bedford Square
  Number Nine **488-502**
  History **492-494**
  Official Opening **498-502**
  The move to 9 Bedford Square **494-498**
British Anaesthetic and Respiratory Equipment Manufacturers' Association **270**
British Association of Immediate Care **427, 534, 675**
British Dental Association (BDA) **139, 247, 374**
British Journal Of Anaesthesia **6, 58, 100-106, 503**
British Malignant Hyperthermia Association **554**
British Medical Association (BMA) **25, 200**
British Standards Institution **16, 194, 416**

C

Calman Report **608-614**
Chemotherapy **29, 117**
Chloroform centenary **111**
Coat of Arms
  Association of Anaesthetists **85, 710-714**
  (Royal) College of Anaesthetists **584**
  Committee on Safety of Medicine **194, 306, 398**
Cogwheel Report (NHS adminstrative organisation) **287**
College of Anaesthetists **see also**
  Faculty and Royal College of Anaesthetists **278, 579-590**
    Debate concerning foundation **315-335**
Complications of Anaesthesia **184**
Conclusion **625**
Confidential Enquiry into Perioperative Deaths (CEPOD) **169, 352, 354, 428**

Consultant Posts
    Contract and work load **389-391**
    Shortage **138**
    Unfilled **397**
Contents *xiii*
Controlled hypotension **124, 284, 640**
Copenhagen Anaesthesiology Centre **150**
Coroners **54- 57, 271, 278, 306, 428, 632, 658**
Curare **see also**
Anaesthesia (Clinical) and Muscle Relaxants **72**
Cyclopropane **13, 31, 60, 630**

D

Day-care surgery **282**
Death(s)
    Association with Anaesthesia **164-169, 349-354**
    Diagnosis **191**
    In Dental Surgery **240**
Dental Outpatient Anaesthesia **139, 204, 236-253, 367-368, 374, 547-556**
Developing Countries **230-236, 366, 541-547**
Diazepam **183, 648, 657**
Diploma in Anaesthetics (DA) **47-54, 96-98, 219, 612** see also
Fellowship of the Faculty of Anaesthetists
Distinction Awards
272, 306, 391, 398, 658, 670
Doctors with Domestic Commitments **273, 397**
Draw-over apparatus **74**

E

Emergency Medical Service (World War 2) **64**
Equipment Manufacturers **269-271, 740-741**
Ether **13, 31,**
    Centenary **109-111**
    Sesquicentennial **619**

Europe and the European Economic Community (European Union) **149, 261, 359-363, 602**
European Academy of Anaesthesiology **364**
European Congress of Anaesthesiology (1982) **405-410**
European Congresses **403-404**
European Diploma of Anaesthesiology **365**
European Journal of Anaesthesiology **365, 698**
European Society of Regional Anaesthesia **534, 545**
Explosions **170**-172, **646**
Extradural caudal and lumbar techniques
    Local anaesthesia **123**
    Narcotics **284**
    Obstetrics **123**

F

Faculty of Anaesthetists **98-100, 162**
Family Planning **394-396, 670**
Fatigue Working Party **379-383, 669**
Fees **see** Remuneration of Anaesthetists
Fellowship of the Faculty of Anaesthetists of the Royal College of Surgeons (FFARCS)**96-98**
Foreword *v-vi*

G

Gas Cylinders **59, 182**
General Dental Council (GDC) **237**
General Medical Council (GMC) **58, 237, 299-300**
Griffiths Report (NHS Management Inquiry) **437-450**
Group of Anaesthetists in Training (GAT) (**see** Junior Anaesthetists' Group)

H

Halothane **126, 184, 649**
Hepatitis B **420, 674**
Heroin **163, 169, 284**

History of Anaesthesia Society *534, 536, 619, 703*
Hospital Practitioner Grade *223*
Hospitals **See also** World War 2: National Health Service
    Organisation and staffing **8-13**
    Plan for England and Wales **195**

I

Illustrations *xiv-xvi*
Independent (private) practice **see** Remuneration
Industrial Unrest in the NHS
    Ancillary workers **292, 303**
    Nurses **293**
    Senior hospital doctors **293-296**
    Junior hospital doctors **296-299**
Inhalation Agents *13, 31, 109, 111, 183, 283, 433*
Intensive Care *186-191*
    Lectureship **583**
Intensive Care Society *190, 501, 534, 535*
International Congresses (1951) *154, 262*
International Congresses (1960-1969) *262, 366*
International Relations *38, 147-153, 230-236, 305, 366, 541-547*
Intravenous anaesthetic agents **see** Anaesthesia (Clinical)
Intravenous fluids *14, 73, 119*
Ireland (Republic of Ireland) *528-533*
    Private Practice **531**
Irish Senior Registrar Group *533*

J

Junior Anaesthetists' Group (Group of Anaesthesia in Training) *213-218, 346-349, 523-528*
    Junior Linkmen **347, 749-752**
    Pinkerton Lectures **348, 749-752**
Joint Subcommittee (Dental Anaesthesia) *243-248*

K

Ketamine *283, 660*
Kidney **see** Renal Disease

L

Laryngeal Mask *436, 679*
Lewin Report on Operating Theatre Staffing *383-386*
Lignocaine *127*
Linkman Organisation *339, 347, 520-523*
Liverpool Society of Anaesthetists *160*
Local Authorities *40-42, 91-93*
Local Anaesthetics *127, 183*

M

Manchester and District Society of Anaesthetists *160, 645*
Manchester Medical Society *160, 645*
Manufacturers of Medical Equipment *269-271*
Medical Assistant Grade *218-214*
Medical Students *274*
Medicine (Clinical) *7, 29, 117-121, 181, 193, 281-283, 417-424*
Medicines Act *193-194*
Methohexitone *127*
Midwives. Administration of Analgesia *55, 109*
Monitoring in Anaesthesia and Intensive Care *121, 191, 284, 435*
Monopoly and Mergers Commission Report *556-562*
Mortality **see** Deaths
Muscle Relaxants *72, 125, 433*

N

National Confidential Enquiry into Perioperative Deaths (NCEPOD) *353*
National Health Service (NHS) *63-65, 85-96, 128-131, 180, 194-198, 218-224, 236, 277, 286-306, 437-487, 603-607*
Neuroanaesthesia Society of Great Britain and Ireland *534*

Subject Index

Neuroleptanalgesia *182*
Neuromuscular blocking agents *see* Muscle Relaxants
NHS Reorganisation *289-292, 302, 440-450, 461-470*
Nine Bedford Square *see* Bedford Square
Nitroprusside *284*
Nurses and Midwives
    Anaesthesia *54-56, 70, 81-84, 109, 615-617*
    Professional organisation 288, 478-487, 606

O

Obstetrics
    Caudal and extradural anaesthesia 123
    Obstetric Anaesthetics Association 534
    Analgesia 55, 74, 109
    In vitro fertilisations (IVF) 282
Operating Department Assistants (Technicians) *254, 383-389, 562-569*

P

Paediatric Intensive Care Society *534*
Pain
    Chronic 192
    Obstetric 54, 74, 109, 123, 534
    Postoperative 284, 434
    Pain Society 534
Pethidine *124*
Phenothiazines *125*
Pilkington Report (Remuneration) *195*
Pinkerton Lecture *368, 470, 770*
Plastic Surgery and Burns Society *534*
Platt Report (staffing) *218-224*
Poliomyelitis *30, 118, 186*
Political Developments *28, 62, 114-117, 177-181, 280, 414, 470, 601, 607*
Pollution in Operating Theatres *285*
Porritt Report (BMA Medical Services Review) *440*
Postgraduate Specialist Training and Education *359-363, 410*
    Todd Report 337-339
    Calman Report 608-614
Postoperative Recovery *122, 188*
Poswillo Report (dental anaesthesia) *547-554*
Preface *viii-x*
Prehospital emergency Care *424-433*
Private Practice **see** Independent Practice under Remuneration
Prizes *228, 229, 743-745*

Q

no entries

R

References *626-703*
Regional Societies *160-161*
Recovery Wards **see** Postoperative recovery
Remuneration of Anaesthetists
    Academic *10-11, 42-46*
    Nineteen thirties *9-10, 39-42, 82*
    National Health Service *88-89, 138, 195-198*
    Outpatient Dental Anaesthesia *42, 236, 252, 374-377, 554-556*
    Independent (private) practice *40, 140, 253, 392-394, 556-562*
    Family Planning *394-396*
Renal Disease
    Dialysis *119*
    Transplantation *119, 181*
Research *75, 161-164, 224-228*
    Fellowships *107, 161, 226, 379, 539*
Resident Medical Anaesthetists *82*
Resuscitation
    Cardiopulmonary *14, 119, 185*
    Council of the United Kingdom *534*
Royal Air Force *69-71, 200, 608, 711, 718, 735*
Royal College of Anaesthetists **see also** College of Anaesthetists *590-594*
Royal College of Anaesthetists of Thailand *591*

Subject Index

Royal College of Obstetricians and Gynaecologists *109, 350, 727*
Royal College of Surgeons of England *84, 227, 428*
Royal Commission on Doctors' and Dentists' Remuneration (Pilkington Report) *195*
Royal Commission on Medical Education (Todd Report) *337*
Royal Commission on the National Health Service *288, 300-302, 340, 661-662*
Royal Navy *71*
Royal Society of Medicine *5*

S

Salmon Report (Nursing) *288*
Scottish Intensive Care Society *534*
Scottish Society of Anaesthetists *1, 160, 145*
Secrecy in the NHS *471-473, 683*
Seward Report (Dental anaesthesia) *369*
Sick Doctor Scheme *355, 356, 358, 411*
Society for Computing Technology *534*
Society for the Advancement of Anaesthesia in Dentistry (SAAD) *204, 238-240*
Society of Anaesthetic Laboratory Technicians *401, 737*
Society of Anaesthetists (1893) *5*
Society of Naval Anaesthetists *534*
Specialist Societies *535-536, 544, 617*
Spinal subarachnoid anaesthesia *123, 284*
Sterilisation
    Instruments *120*
    Syringes *120, 123*
Succinyl Choline *126*
Summary *620-625*
Surgery (Clinical) *7, 117-121, 181, 281-3, 417-424*
    Cardiac *120, 181, 281-3, 417-424*
    Minimal invasive (fibreoptic) *281, 421-424*

T

Teaching *35, 58, 89, 139, 201, 212, 255, 290, 392, 667*
Thalidomide *193*
Todd Report (Medical education)*337*
Tri-service Anaesthetic Society *534*
Trichloroethylene *74-75, 398, 635*
Tuberculosis *7, 117.*

U

no entries

V

no entries

W

Windeyer Report (Outpatient dental anaesthesia) *249*
World Congress of Anaesthesiology (1968) *263-269*
World Federation of Societies of Anaesthesiologist *154-160, 262, 403, 544, 578*
World War 2
    Armed Services *66-71*
    Civilian services *65-66*
    Clinical anaesthesia *72-75*
    Council Meetings *76-78*
    Research at Oxford *75*
Wylie Report (Outpatient dental anaesthesia) *368*

X

no entries

Y

no entries

Z

Zuckerman Committee on Scientific Services in the NHS *306*